Mesenteric Vascular Disease

Gustavo S. Oderich
Editor

Mesenteric Vascular Disease

Current Therapy

Springer

Editor
Gustavo S. Oderich
Division of Vascular and Endovascular Therapy
Mayo Clinic Gonda Vascular Center
Rochester, MN, USA

ISBN 978-1-4939-1846-1 ISBN 978-1-4939-1847-8 (eBook)
DOI 10.1007/978-1-4939-1847-8
Springer New York Heidelberg Dordrecht London

Library of Congress Control Number: 2014953223

Printed on acid-free paper

Springer is part of Springer Science+Business Media (www.springer.com)

To Gabriel and Victoria

Preface

Since the first successful mesenteric endarterectomy by Shaw and Maynard in 1958, significant progress has been made in the diagnosis and treatment of mesenteric vascular diseases. Improvements in imaging modalities, medical therapy, and open and endovascular reconstruction have allowed treatment of acute and chronic mesenteric artery diseases with satisfactory results. Yet, delay in diagnosis remains a major problem given that mesenteric diseases are uncommon and often present with unspecific symptoms.

Mesenteric Vascular Disease: Current Therapy has one purpose, which is to fill the gap between clinical knowledge and the technical expertise needed to master novel open and endovascular approaches to treat a variety of mesenteric arterial and venous diseases. In that, the book is organized in a logical fashion to address basic concepts, imaging methods, and novel techniques of revascularization for acute and chronic arterial and venous disorders.

Special attention has been devoted to technical aspects of mesenteric reconstructions, open and endovascular. Because these diseases are uncommon and most surgeons have limited experience, we felt it was important to summarize the evolution of surgical approaches over the last decades using as much illustration as possible in a didactic manner. Endovascular therapy, which has become an essential skill for the vascular clinician, has been emphasized in several chapters given that most patients with mesenteric ischemia are currently treated in this manner. Whereas in the 1990s angioplasty was reserved for the elderly or higher-risk patient, today this modality is used whenever possible in suitable lesions independent of the patient's clinical risk. Because this field rapidly evolves as new devices and the technology that drives them changes in fast pace, it is critical that physicians are familiar with novel approaches. It is also equally important that the vascular specialist recognizes its limitations and when open treatment is indicated or advantageous.

It is the editor's hope that this collection of 34 chapters provided by a multispecialty international panel of faculty experts will help enhance the diagnosis and treatment of mesenteric vascular diseases – and, most importantly, patients in need with these disorders.

Rochester, MN, USA Gustavo S. Oderich, MD, FACS

Acknowledgments

The editor would like to express great and humble thanks to all the individuals who made this book possible: first, my inspiring mentors who taught me the Mayo Clinic legacy and passed me their passion for mesenteric diseases and the skills needed to treat these patients by open or endovascular approaches; the authors, their secretaries, and members of the Mayo Clinic division of Scientific Publications, the staff from Springer, and especially our families, who supported us during this effort. I am especially appreciative of our publisher, Springer Science + Business Media, and grateful to my Development Editor, Ms. Margaret Burns, for her wonderful and tireless job putting this book together.

Contents

Part V Non-Occlusive Mesenteric Ischemia

Part VI Median Arcuate Ligament Syndrome

Part VII Isolated Mesenteric Artery Dissection

Part VIII Mesenteric Aneurysms

Contributors

Sadaf Sadie Ahanchi, MD Division of Vascular Surgery, Department of Surgery, Eastern Virginia Medical School, Norfolk, VA, USA

Sentara Heart Hospital, Norfolk, VA, USA

A.S. Bode, MD, PhD Department of Surgery, Catharina Hospital Eindhoven, Eindhoven, The Netherlands

Thomas C. Bower, MD Division of Vascular and Endovascular Surgery, Department of Surgery, Mayo Clinic, Rochester, MN, USA

Kenneth J. Cherry Jr., MD Division of Vascular and Endovascular Surgery, University of Virginia, Charlottesville, VA, USA

Mateus P. Correa, MD Division of Vascular and Endovascular Surgery, Department of Surgery, Mayo Clinic, Rochester, MN, USA

Thomas Curran, MD Department of Surgery, Beth Israel Deaconess Medical Center, Boston, MA, USA

Ramoncito A. David, MD Division of Vascular and Endovascular Surgery, Department of Surgery, Mayo Clinic, Rochester, MN, USA

Randall R. De Martino, MD, MS Division of Vascular and Endovascular Surgery, Department of Surgery, Mayo Clinic, Rochester, MN, USA

Leonardo Reis de Souza, MD Division of Vascular and Endovascular Surgery, Mayo Clinic, Rochester, MN, USA

Masters Degree Program from the Department of Surgery, Universidade Federal do Rio Grande do Sul, Porto Alegre, Brazil

M. Dekkers, MSc Department of Surgery, Catharina Hospital Eindhoven, Eindhoven, The Netherlands

Audra A. Duncan, MD Division of Vascular and Endovascular Surgery, Department of Surgery, Mayo Clinic, Rochester, MN, USA

Erik P. Dutson, MD, FACS Department of Surgery, Ronald Reagan UCLA Medical Center, Los Angeles, CA, USA

Jithinraj Edakkanambeth Varayil, MD Department of Internal Medicine, Mayo Clinic, Rochester, MN, USA

Young Erben, MD Division of Vascular and Endovascular Surgery, Department of Surgery, Mayo Clinic, Rochester, MN, USA

Kirk J. Giesbrandt, MD Department of Radiology, Mayo Clinic, Jacksonville, FL, USA

Shaun M. Gifford, MD Division of Vascular Surgery, Department of Surgery, Mayo Clinic, Rochester, MN, USA

Peter Gloviczki, MD Division of Vascular and Endovascular Surgery, Mayo Clinic, Rochester, MN, USA

Jihan Harki, MD Department of Gastroenterology and Hepatology, Erasmus University Medical Center Rotterdam, Rotterdam, The Netherlands

Ying Huang, MD, PhD Division of Vascular and Endovascular Surgery, Mayo Clinic, Rochester, MN, USA

Ryan T. Hurt, MD, PhD Division of General Internal Medicine, Mayo Clinic, Rochester, MN, USA

Juan Carlos Jimenez, MD, FACS Department of Surgery, Division of Vascular Surgery, Gonda (Goldschmied) Vascular Center, Ronald Reagan-UCLA Medical Center, David Geffen School of Medicine at UCLA, Los Angeles, CA, USA

Manju Kalra, MBBS Division of Vascular and Endovascular Surgery, Department of Surgery, Mayo Clinic, Rochester, MN, USA

Patrick S. Kamath, MD Division of Gastroenterology and Hepatology, Department of Medicine, Mayo Clinic, Rochester, MN, USA

Usah Khrucharoen, MD Department of Surgery, David Geffen School of Medicine at UCLA, Los Angeles, CA, USA

Rishi Kundi, MD Division of Vascular Surgery, Department of Surgery, University of Maryland School of Medicine, Baltimore, MD, USA

John H. Landau, MD Department of Vascular Surgery, London Health Sciences Centre, Victoria Hospital, Western University, London, ON, Canada

M.D. Luyer, MD, PhD Department of Surgery, Catharina Hospital Eindhoven, Eindhoven, The Netherlands

Thanila A. Macedo, MD Department of Radiology, Mayo Clinic, Rochester, MN, USA

Robert D. McBane II, MD Department of Medicine, Division of Cardiovascular Diseases, Gonda Vascular Center, Mayo Clinic, Rochester, MN, USA

Jason R. Moore, MD Division of Vascular Surgery, Department of Surgery, Eastern Virginia Medical School, Norfolk, VA, USA

Sentara Heart Hospital, Norfolk, VA, USA

Gustavo S. Oderich, MD, FACS Division of Vascular and Endovascular Surgery, Mayo Clinic, Rochester, MN, USA

Gonda Vascular Center, Mayo Clinic, Rochester, MN, USA

Jean M. Panneton, MD, FACS, FRCSC Division of Vascular Surgery, Department of Surgery, Eastern Virginia Medical School, Norfolk, VA, USA

Sentara Heart Hospital, Norfolk, VA, USA

Adam H. Power, MD, MPhil Department of Vascular Surgery, London Health Sciences Centre, Victoria Hospital, Western University, London, ON, Canada

Todd E. Rasmussen, MD US Combat Casualty Care Research Program, Fort Detrick, MD, USA

Uniformed Services University, Bethesda, MD, USA

Timur P. Sarac, MD Section of Vascular Surgery, Heart and Vascular Institute, Yale University School of Medicine, New Haven, CT, USA

Michael G. Sarr, MD Division of Subspecialty Surgery, Mayo Clinic, Rochester, MN, USA

Marc L. Schermerhorn, MD Chief, Division for Vascular and Endovascular Surgery, Department of Surgery, Beth Israel Deaconess Medical Center, Boston, MA, USA

Lars Stangenberg, MD, PhD Division of Vascular and Endovascular Surgery, Beth Israel Deaconess Medical Center, Boston, MA, USA

William M. Stone, MD Department of Surgery, Mayo Clinic, Scottsdale, AZ, USA

J.A. Teijink, MD, PhD Department of Surgery, Catharina Hospital Eindhoven, Eindhoven, The Netherlands

Eric T.T.L. Tjwa, MD, PhD Department of Gastroenterology and Hepatology, Erasmus University Medical Center Rotterdam, Rotterdam, The Netherlands

Désirée van Noord, MD, PhD Department of Gastroenterology and Hepatology, Erasmus University Medical Center Rotterdam, Rotterdam, The Netherlands

T.R. van Oudheusden, MD Department of Surgery, Catharina Hospital Eindhoven, Eindhoven, The Netherlands

Waldemar E. Wysokinski, MD, PhD Department of Medicine, Vascular Center, Mayo Clinic, Rochester, MN, USA

Phillip M. Young, MD Department of Radiology, Mayo Clinic, Rochester, MN, USA

Part I
Basic Concepts

Chapter 1
History of Mesenteric Vascular Disease

Kenneth J. Cherry Jr.

Although it is generally stated in any short historical introduction to an article concerning chronic mesenteric ischemia that Dunphy first correlated chronic abdominal pain to subsequent mesenteric artery occlusion and gut infarction in 1936, his paper did not arise suddenly from a barren field [1]. The problem with "mesenteric occlusion" and death from ischemic necrotic bowel had interested physicians for years previously. The problem was a complex one, but the impediments to understanding mesenteric ischemia and treating it were dishearteningly simple: neither diagnostic angiography nor vascular intervention was extant. Diagnosis was made during exploratory laparotomy for acute abdominal crises or at autopsy. Bowel resection was the sole surgical option.

Tiedemann had described mesenteric occlusion and bowel infarction in a patient in 1843 [2]. Seven years later, Virchow added two further such patients to the literature [3]. Welch, in 1887, had posited an 80 % stenosis of the SMA was necessary for ischemic bowel changes [4]. In 1904, Jackson, Parker, and Quinby described both arterial and venous occlusions of the mesenteric circulation [5]. Trotter, in 1913, reviewed 359 cases of infarcted bowel [5]. He proposed a relationship between heart disease and embolus to the superior mesenteric artery and a relationship between arteriosclerosis of the aorta and mesenteric vessels and local thrombosis of the visceral vessels. Klein pointed out in 1921 in his thesis on embolism and thrombosis of the superior mesenteric artery a relationship between superior mesenteric artery stenosis and episodic abdominal pain [6].

Cokkinis, a registrar at the London Lock Hospital, wrote a thesis in 1926, which is remarkable for several observations [7]. He reported 76 cases of "mesenteric occlusion" mostly from the London Hospital. He felt primary thrombosis of the mesenteric vessels rare, but reported one case with gangrene of the intestines and

K.J. Cherry Jr., MD (✉)
Division of Vascular and Endovascular Surgery, University of Virginia,
Charlottesville, VA, USA
e-mail: KJC5KH@hscmail.mcc.virginia.edu

G.S. Oderich (ed.), *Mesenteric Vascular Disease*,
DOI 10.1007/978-1-4939-1847-8_1

both lower extremities, and felt that atheromas of the aorta and mesenteric arteries themselves were causative, leading directly to thrombosis. He also described aortic-origin emboli.

Ten years before Dunphy's postmortem study could confirm a history of postprandial pain and subsequent gut infarction, Cokkinis wrote: "The patient complains of abdominal symptoms extending over a period of weeks or months. Among the commonest of these are: colicky abdominal pain, which may have some relation to food…The symptoms are colicky abdominal pain, 1½ to 2 h after meals, nausea and vomiting…they may last for years and then arterial thrombosis supervenes and leads to infarction…The pathological lesion is one of arteriosclerosis of the mesenteric arteries, interfering with the flow of blood to the intestines during digestion."

Given the lack of diagnostic modalities of the day, this is the most remarkable and accurate description of chronic mesenteric ischemia. All that is lacking for completeness sake is weight loss and fear of eating.

In 1936 in his famous report, Dunphy described 12 patients dying of mesenteric infarction studied at autopsy. Seven (58 %) had a history of recurrent abdominal pain proceeding the terminal event, a period of time ranging from weeks to years. The imperative for early treatment was thus identified, even if the means were not yet available.

Surgical Revascularization

In 1951, Klass performed direct embolectomy of the superior mesenteric artery in two patients [8]. One must remember at this point that the Fogarty catheter had not yet been invented. Both patients died, but the mesenteric circulation was free of thrombosis at the postmortem. Stewart, that same year, performed an SMA embolectomy [9]. Five years later Van Weel reported a successful thrombectomy, although the patient required subsequent resection of the distal ileum and cecum [10]. This would count as a success today. In 1957 Mikkelsen described the arteriographic findings of ostial mesenteric lesions [11].

The first embolectomy of the SMA to be successful and not to require subsequent bowel resection was performed in 1957 and reported by Shaw and Maynard [12]. Shaw with Rutledge in 1958 [13] reported endarterectomy of the SMA and paramesenteric aorta as treatment of chronic mesenteric ischemia. The remarkable Houston surgeons – Morris, Crawford, Cooley, and DeBakey – in 1962 reported retrograde reconstruction of the celiac and superior mesenteric arteries. It was associated with tortuosity and kinking of those grafts in some patients [14].

Wylie, Stoney, and Ehrenfield, in the 1970s, described both transaortic visceral endarterectomy and antegrade supraceliac bypass to the visceral vessels [15]. Initially, when performing endarterectomy, they employed a thoraco-retroperitoneal approach but modified this to medial visceral rotation in later years for appropriate patients.

Mayo Clinic Legacy

Hollier et al proposed in 1981 that complete revascularization of all three mesenteric vessels was the ideal [16]. He found that recurrence with one-vessel reconstruction was 26 % and that with 3-vessel reconstructions was less than 10 %. However, that Mayo Clinic cohort included no antegrade reconstructions. Further experience from the Mayo Clinic showed that obsession with three-vessel reconstruction increased mortality from the current 8–10 % in that day to 15–20 % [17]. The mortality in the 1980s was right around 8–10 %, second only to repair or thoracoabdominal aortic aneurysms in terms of risk to the patient. In the succeeding decades, with improved anesthetic techniques, refinement of operative approaches and appropriate patient selection, mortality has steadily decreased and is currently in the 2–5 % range.

Antegrade reconstruction was felt to be the gold standard of repair, but clamping of the paravisceral aorta was not without risk, especially in elderly patients with coronary artery disease, associated renal artery disease, and aortoiliac occlusive disease.

The group from Oregon modified infrarenal or retrograde bypass to bring the distal end of the graft in a curving manner such that the visceral artery anastomosis was constructed in an antegrade manner, to decrease turbulence of flow. Initially, they reconstructed both the celiac and superior mesenteric arteries [18, 19]. Later experience revealed that superior mesenteric artery reconstruction alone was satisfactory.

The Mayo group subsequently reported 91 cases [20]. That study was postulated on the premise that antegrade reconstruction would prove, albeit in a retrospective study, superior to infrarenal repair. That hypothesis was proved false. In properly selected patients, isolated retrograde reconstruction of the superior mesenteric artery was statistically no different than antegrade reconstruction. Further, reconstruction originating from a common or external iliac artery was felt to be superior to that originating from the infrarenal aorta, because the long axis of the graft is parallel to that of the aorta, as opposed to the perpendicular orientation seen with grafts originating from the infrarenal aorta, thereby eliminating the kinking seen in the latter group of grafts when the viscera are returned to their normal position. In addition, there is a subset of patients with densely calcific aortas whose iliac arteries are spared and thus provide superior donor sites.

Endovascular Therapy

Endovascular treatment of mesenteric disease was introduced in 1980. It is used in the majority of patients today, as its mortality is less in the hands of most practitioners than open repair. Further studies from the Mayo Clinic by Oderich et al detailing 229 patients, on the other hand, have shown that the mortality from open repair is less than 3 % and is in essence equal to that of endovascular repair. Nonetheless, these are retrospective studies from a high-volume institution with a long-standing interest in the problem, and the patients are carefully selected [21].

Those patients with flush occlusions of the celiac and superior mesenteric arteries and those with long calcific occlusions of the superior mesenteric artery are probably better treated by open repair. Multiple studies have shown less re-intervention after open repair (reflecting the same experience seen in most vascular beds when open and endovascular reconstructions are contrasted). Fortunately, open repair may be safely tailored to the patient's anatomy and physiology in this day and age, ranging from antegrade supraceliac reconstruction of the both the celiac and SMA, usually reserved for young relatively healthy patients whose life expectancy is long, to grafts originating from the iliac arteries and carried to the superior mesenteric artery in more elderly fragile patients. Whereas prosthetic grafts have historically outperformed saphenous vein for mesenteric reconstructions, retrograde saphenous mesenteric bypasses performed in the face of infection appear to have very acceptable patency rates.

The history of reconstructions for chronic mesenteric ischemia has been a progression. Currently, patients may be reconstructed via transaortic endarterectomy, antegrade graft reconstruction, or retrograde repair. The choice is usually made dependent on anatomy, physiology, and the applicability of endovascular techniques to these patients.

References

1. Dunphy JE. Abdominal pain of vascular origin. Am J Med Sci. 1936;192:109–13.
2. Tiedemann F. Von der Verengung and Schiessungder Pulsadern in Krankheiten, 3 pl. Heidelberg u Leipzig K Gross; 1843. xiv+316 pp.
3. Virchow RLK. Thrombose und Embolie, GBeassentzund sentische Infektion. In his Gesammelte zaur Wissenschaftlichen Medicin. Franmkfurr a. M.: Meidinger Sohn U. CO.; 1856. p. 219–732.
4. Welch WH. Thrombosis and embolism. In: Allbutt C, System of medicine. London: Macmillan; 1899, vol 4, p. 284–310; and in 2nd ed., 1909, vol 6, p. 691–821.
5. Jackson JM, Porter CA, Quinby WC. Mesenteric embolism and thrombosis: a study of 214 cases. JAMA. 1904; 42:1469:43:25; 43:110; 43:183.
6. Trotter LBC. Embolism and thrombosis of the mesenteric vessels. New York: Cambridge University Press; 1913.
7. Cokkinis AJ. Mesenteric vascular occlusion. London: Bailliere, Tindall and Cox; 1936.
8. Klass AA. Embolectomy in acute mesenteric occlusion. Ann Surg Gynec Obst. 1951;33:355–405.
9. Stewart GD, Sweetman WR, Westphal K, Wise RA. Superior mesenteric artery embolectomy. Ann Surg. 1960;151:274–73.
10. Van Weel MW. Acute mesenteric arterial occlusion, successful treatment of embolectomy and limited intestinal resection. Arch Chir Neerl. 1956;8:147–52.
11. Mikkelsen WSP. Intestinal angina; its surgical significance. Am J Surg. 1957;94:262–9.
12. Shaw RS, Rutledge RH. Superior-mesenteric artery embolectomy in the treatment of massive mesenteric infarction. N Engl J Med. 1957;257:595–8.
13. Shaw RS, Maynard III EP. Acute and chronic thrombosis of the superior mesenteric arteries associated with malabsorption: a report of two cases successfully treated by thromboarterectomy. N Engl J Med. 1958;258:874–8.

14. Morris GC, Crawford ES, Cooley DA, DeBakey ME. Revascularization of the celiac and superior mesenteric arteries. Arch Surg. 1962;84:95–107.
15. Stoney RJ, Ehrenfeld EK, Wylie EJ. Revascularization methods in chronic visceral ischemia. Ann Surg. 1977;186:468.
16. Hollier IH, Bernatz PE, Pairolerp PC, et al. Surgical management of chronic intestinal ischemia. A reappraisal. Surgery. 1991;90:940.
17. McAfee MK, Cherry KJ, Naessens JM, et al. Influence of complete revascularization for chronic mesenteric ischemia. Am J Surg. 1992;164:220.
18. Baur GM, Millay DJ, Taylor Jr LM, et al. Treatment of chronic visceral ischemia. Am J Surg. 1984;148:137.
19. Gentile AT, Moneta GI, Taylor Jr LM, et al. Isolated bypass to the superior mesenteric artery for intestinal ischemia. Arch Surg. 1994;129:926.
20. Park WM, Cherry KJ, Chua HK, et al. Current results of open revascularization for chronic mesenteric ischemia: A standard for comparison. J Vasc Surg. 2002;35:853.
21. Oderich GS, Bower TC, Sullivan TM, Bjarnason H, Cha S, Gloviczki P. Open versus endovascular revascularization for chronic mesenteric ischemia: risk-stratified outcomes. From the Society for Vascular Surgery. Presented at 2006 Vascular Annual Meeting, Society for Vascular Surgery, Philadelphia, PA, 1–4 June 2006.

Chapter 2
Normal and Variant Mesenteric Anatomy

Randall R. De Martino

The mesenteric vascular supply is a combination of rich collateral networks and commonly encountered variant anatomy. The effect of normal and variant anatomy has implications on pathology, treatment choices, and planning interventions. The goal of this chapter is to review the standard vascular anatomy with details of the potential collateral systems that may be present. Finally, a review of anatomic variants will assist in understanding the implications of abnormal anatomy on treatment for diseases associated with the mesentery.

Embryology

Understanding the vascular supply of the mesentery and the pathological implications of mesenteric vascular disease is best understood by a solid appreciation for the embryologic development of the mesenteric structures and their blood supply. This helps the clinician understand the pathological consequences of diseases of the mesenteric vasculature.

At three weeks, the early embryo consists of three flat germ layers (endoderm, mesoderm, and ectoderm) that will develop along separate paths to create each necessary organ system and tissue (endoderm will form the aerodigestive tract, and the mesoderm will form the mesenchymal tissue including the vasculature). The primitive gut is derived from the endodermal germ layer as it undergoes tubal formation. The cranial and caudal aspects fold to form the foregut and hindgut, while the intervening segment (midgut) remains open to the yolk sac, creating the yolk stalk

R.R. De Martino, MD, MS (✉)
Division of Vascular and Endovascular Surgery, Department of Surgery,
Mayo Clinic, Rochester, MN, USA
e-mail: demartino.randall@mayo.edu

G.S. Oderich (ed.), *Mesenteric Vascular Disease*,
DOI 10.1007/978-1-4939-1847-8_2

(the eventual omphalomesenteric or vitelline duct). These three distinct segments of the primitive gut have important implications for mesenteric vascular supply.

At about the same time, the embryo becomes too large to meet its metabolic needs by simple diffusion alone. The circulatory system begins its iterative development to support embryonic growth and formation. The paired dorsal aortae develop three sets of paired arterial branches: the dorsal intersegmental, the lateral segmental, and the ventral segmental vessels. The paired ventral segmental arteries course over the dorsal and lateral walls of the gut and yolk sac. Ultimately, as the dorsal aorta fuse, so do specific paired ventral vessels, namely, the 10th, 13th, and 21st. They fuse in the midline with gut closure and narrowing of the dorsal mesentery to form the celiac artery, superior mesenteric artery (SMA), and inferior mesenteric artery (IMA), respectively.

These three vessels go on to provide the blood supply for each segment of the developing gut. The foregut will form the lower esophagus to the duodenum and be supplied by the celiac artery. The midgut will form the lower duodenum to the cranial half of the transverse colon and be supplied by the SMA. Finally, the hindgut will form the caudal half of the transverse colon to the superior rectum and be supplied by the IMA [1].

Normal Anatomy

Normal mesenteric vascular anatomy is based on these three separate branches of the aorta [2]. Although not all patients will display normal mesenteric vascular anatomy, as this may have implications for disease treatment.

Celiac Artery

As the aorta passes below the crus of the diaphragm at the 12th thoracic vertebra, it immediately gives of the celiac artery (also referred to as the celiac trunk or celiac axis) a wide ventrally oriented branch that typically trifurcates during its 1.5 cm length. Of note, there may be a paired set of inferior phrenic vessels that come off the aorta more laterally to supply the inferior diaphragm at this location. Branches include [2]:

1. Left gastric artery
2. Splenic artery
    a. Dorsal and caudal pancreatic arteries
    b. Short gastric arteries
    c. Left gastroepiploic artery
    d. Posterior gastric artery

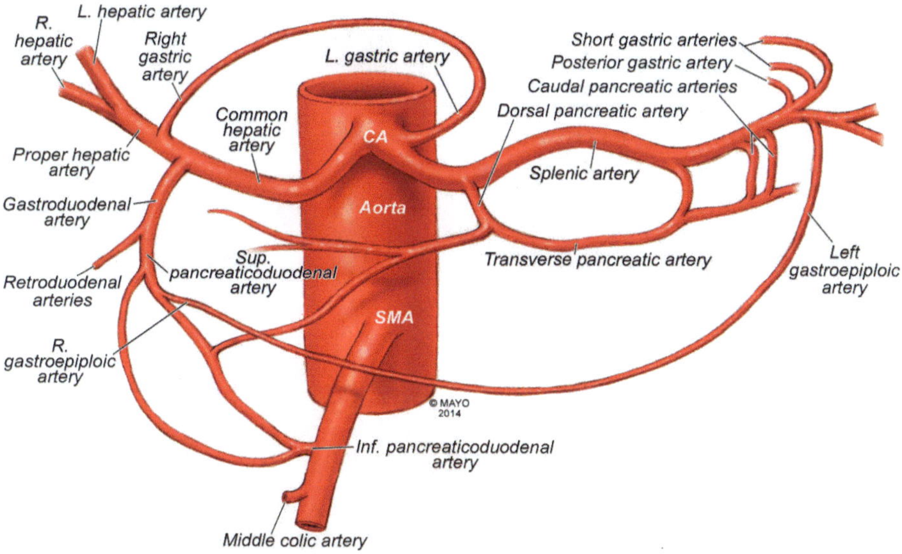

Fig. 2.1 Celiac artery anatomy and superior mesenteric artery collaterals. *CA* celiac artery, *SMA* superior mesenteric artery (By permission of Mayo Foundation for Medical Education and Research. All rights reserved)

3. Common hepatic artery
   a. Gastroduodenal artery
      i. Right gastroepiploic artery
      ii. Superior anterior and posterior pancreaticoduodenal arteries
   b. Right gastric artery
   c. Left hepatic artery
   d. Right hepatic artery

The typical configuration of the celiac artery is to give off a small left gastric artery and then divide into the splenic artery and the common hepatic artery (Fig. 2.1). This anatomy is present in approximately 50 % of the population. The left gastric and the splenic artery travel to the left, while the common hepatic artery turns towards the right and the porta hepatis.

The left gastric artery may originate from the aorta or anywhere along the celiac artery. It travels superiorly supplying the distal esophagus and then descends along the lesser curvature of the stomach to collateralize with the right gastric artery (Figs. 2.1 and 2.2a). Importantly, the left hepatic artery may be replaced, originating from the left gastric. When present, it is important to preserve this during access to the supraceliac aorta though the lesser sac. Conversely, the left hepatic artery may supply an accessory left gastric artery.

The splenic artery originates from the celiac artery 80 % of the time. As the splenic artery traverses to the left, it gives off segmental branches to the pancreas

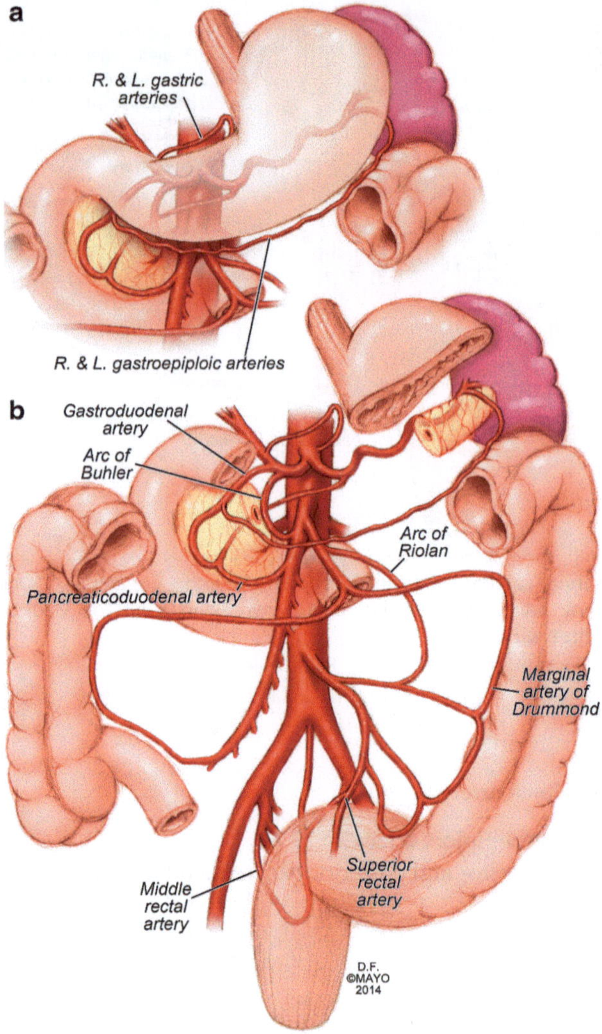

Fig. 2.2 Gastric and bowel collateral networks. (**a**) Gastric collaterals. Right and left gastric arteries collateralize along the lesser curvature, while the right and left gastroepiploic arteries collateralize along the greater curvature of the stomach. (**b**) Celiac to superior mesenteric artery (SMA) collaterals include the arch of Bühler and gastroduodenal arcade. SMA to inferior mesenteric artery (IMA) collaterals include the arc of Riolan and the marginal artery of Drummond. Perirectal collaterals form from the IMA, superior rectal artery, and internal iliac artery (By permission of Mayo Foundation for Medical Education and Research. All rights reserved)

(the dorsal pancreatic and caudal pancreatic arteries). These supply the body and the tail of the pancreas, respectively, collateralizing via the transverse pancreatic artery (Fig. 2.1). Distal branches of the splenic artery include the short gastric arteries, posterior gastric, left gastroepiploic, and the terminal splenic branches. The short gastric arteries number from 1 to 4 and collateralize to the greater curvature of the stomach and the aforementioned left gastric artery. The posterior gastric artery supplies the posterior fundus of the stomach. The left gastroepiploic artery often arises from the distal splenic artery in a common branch with the inferior splenic branch but may be a single branch. It travels along the greater curvature of the stomach giving off omental branches and collateralizing with the right gastroepiploic artery (Figs. 2.1 and 2.2a).

The common hepatic artery is the final branch of the celiac artery. It is of variable length and ends at the gastroduodenal artery branch, after which it continues as the proper hepatic artery to supply the liver and gallbladder. The proper hepatic artery bifurcates into the right and left hepatic arteries (Fig. 2.1). Alternatively, there may be a trifurcation of the common hepatic artery with no proper hepatic artery. The proper hepatic artery or only the right hepatic may arise from the SMA as variants. As mentioned, the left hepatic artery may arise from the left gastric artery. The right gastric artery may arise anywhere along the common or proper hepatic artery to collateralize along the lesser curvature with the left gastric artery (Figs. 2.1 and 2.2a).

The gastroduodenal artery passes inferiorly between the duodenum and the pancreas, giving rise to the right gastroepiploic artery and the superior pancreaticoduodenal artery. This has anterior and posterior divisions that are important collaterals to the superior mesenteric artery (Figs. 2.1 and 2.3).

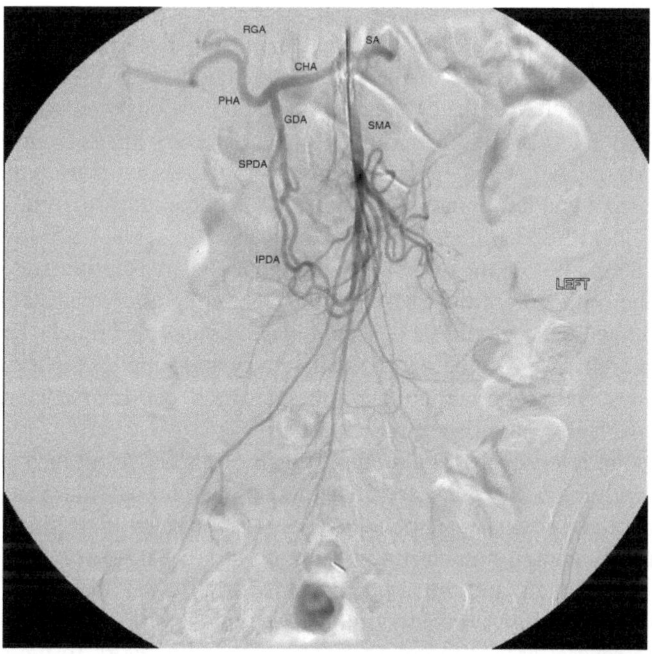

Fig. 2.3 Celiac artery and superior mesenteric artery collaterals. *CHA* common hepatic artery, *SA* splenic artery, *RGA* right gastric artery, *PHA* proper hepatic artery, *GDA* gastroduodenal artery, *SMA* superior mesenteric artery, *SPDA* superior pancreaticoduodenal artery, *IPDA* inferior pancreaticoduodenal artery

Superior Mesenteric Artery (SMA)

The SMA is the second ventral branch of the abdominal aorta. As mentioned above in the discussion of embryology, this artery will supply the distal duodenum, the small intestine, and the large intestine to the mid transverse colon. Given the vitally important structures its supplies and the important collaterals it provides to both the celiac and IMA, there is a very high morbidity associated with SMA occlusions. Anatomically, the SMA origin is about a centimeter distal to the celiac artery and accessible through the lesser sac near the superior border of the pancreas. The SMA comes off at an acute angle in comparison to the celiac artery. In this aortomesenteric angle, the left renal vein and the fourth portion of the duodenum pass. If this angle is too acute, it may lead to either nutcracker syndrome or SMA syndrome. Symptoms include flank pain and hematuria related to renal vein compression for the former and a gastric outlet obstruction syndrome related to the latter.

SMA branches include [2]:

1. Inferior anterior and posterior pancreaticoduodenal arteries
2. Middle colic artery
3. Right colic artery
4. Ileocolic artery
5. Jejunal and ileal branches

The first branches of the SMA include the inferior pancreaticoduodenal artery. This comes off the right side of the SMA and divides in to an anterior posterior branch that collateralize to the celiac artery via the previously mentioned collateral pathway (Figs. 2.1, 2.2, and 2.3). The middle colic artery arises from the proximal SMA after passing below the pancreas. This artery travels to the transverse mesocolon giving a right and left branch. During an infracolic exposure of the SMA, when this artery is identified within the transverse mesocolon, it can be followed down to identify the SMA. Within the mid SMA, the right colic artery originates. It is the last branch off the right side of the SMA. As the right colic artery traverses behind the parietal peritoneum, its supplies a descending and ascending branch. The ascending branch collateralizing with the middle colic artery and supplies the ascending right colon. The descending branch collateralizes to the ileocolic artery, supplying the more proximal right colon (Figs. 2.4 and 2.5).

The ileocolic artery is the final major branch of the SMA but may share a common origin with the right colic artery. The ileocolic artery vascularizes the terminal ileum, right colon, cecum, and appendix. There are four identifiable branches. These included the descending branch (to the right colon), cecal branch (an anterior and posterior), ileal branch, and the appendicular artery (to the appendix). Finally, on the left aspect of the SMA arise the multiple jejunal and ileal branches. These fan out, forming several arches to create a collateralized network to the small bowel (Figs. 2.4 and 2.5).

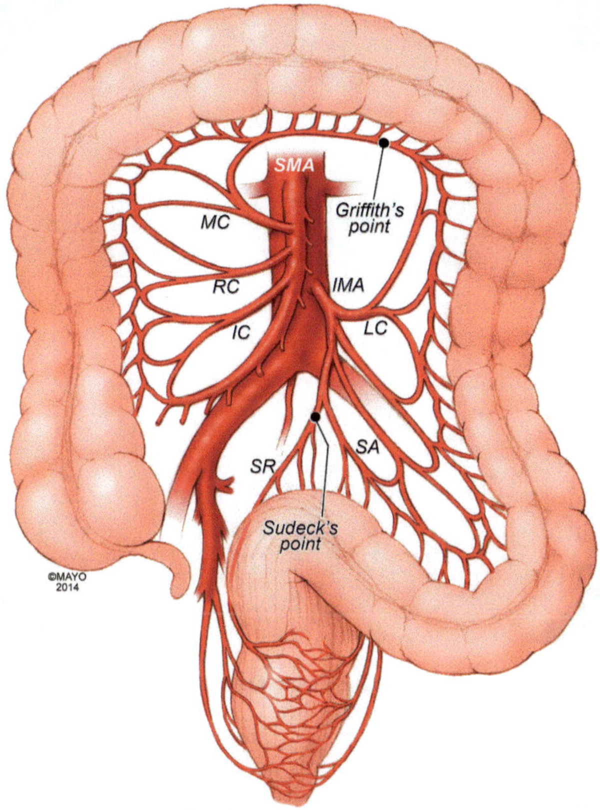

Fig. 2.4 Superior mesenteric artery and inferior mesenteric artery anatomy and collaterals. *SMA* superior mesenteric artery, *IMA* inferior mesenteric artery, *IC* ileocolic artery, *RC* right colic artery, *MC* middle colic artery, *LC* left colic artery, *SA* sigmoid arteries, *SR* superior rectal artery. The marginal artery of Drummond is formed by the arterial network from the ileocolic to the superior rectal. Critical regions of collateralization include Griffith's point (SMA to IMA) and Sudeck's point (IMA to internal iliac artery) (By permission of Mayo Foundation for Medical Education and Research. All rights reserved)

Inferior Mesenteric Artery

The inferior mesenteric artery is responsible for supplying blood flow to the distal third of the transverse colon, descending colon, sigmoid colon, as well as the upper rectum. It originates in an anterior lateral orientation to the left just above the aortic bifurcation, typically between the L2 and L4 vertebral bodies [3]. It travels in a retroperitoneal plane towards the sigmoid colon.

Branches include [2]:

1. Left colic artery
2. Sigmoid arteries
3. Superior rectal artery

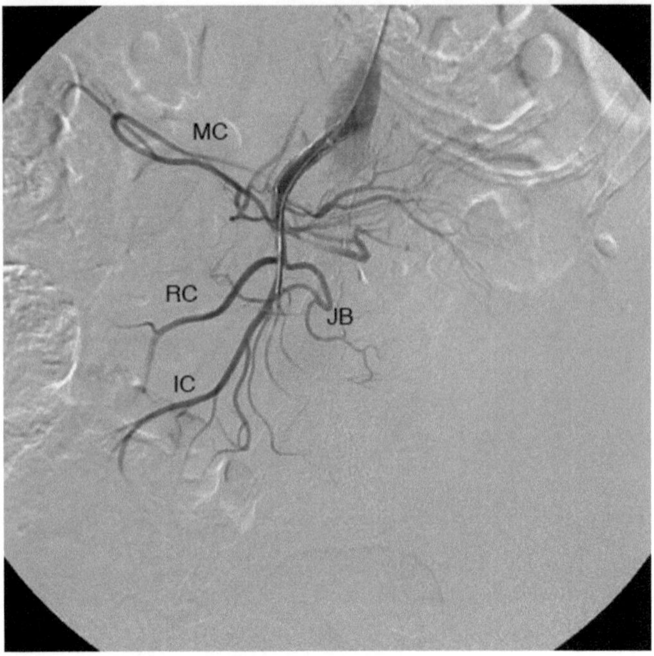

Fig. 2.5 Superior mesenteric artery angiographic anatomy. *IC* ileocolic artery, *RC* right colic artery, *MC* middle colic artery, *JB* jejunal branches

The left colic artery is comprised of an ascending and descending branch. The ascending collateralizes to the middle colic artery, distal transverse colon, and splenic flexure (Griffith's point [4], Fig. 2.4). This collateralization is important, as this area is at high risk for watershed ischemia in the setting of dehydration or mesenteric occlusive disease. The descending left colic artery branch collateralizes to the sigmoid arteries. These are comprised of two or three sigmoid artery branches within the mesocolon. The uppermost sigmoid artery collateralizes to the left colic artery, whereas the lowermost collateralizes to the superior rectal artery. The superior rectal artery descends into the pelvis dividing into right and left branches. The superior rectal artery collateralizes with both the middle rectal (branch of the internal iliac artery) and the inferior rectal artery (branch of the internal pudendal artery, Fig. 2.4).

Collateral Pathways

The mesenteric vasculature is rich with collateral blood supply. It is typically necessary to have disease in multiple vessels for clinical sequelae to develop due to the number of collateral networks. It is often ascribed that in chronic mesenteric ischemia, at least two of the three mesenteric arteries must be severely diseased, one of which being the SMA, for symptoms to be present due to this collateral network. The overall collateral blood supply can be thought of within three distinct patterns. These include collaterals within the same vessel distribution, between mesenteric vessels, and between the mesenteric and the parietal circulation [5].

Within Vessel Collaterals [5]

Celiac Axis

1. Collaterals between the left and right gastric and left and right gastroepiploic vessels to supply the stomach (Figs. 2.1 and 2.2a).
2. The fundus of the stomach possesses collaterals between the left gastric and short gastric arteries (from the splenic artery).
3. Pancreatic anastomotic collaterals between the pancreatic branches of the GDA and splenic origin (Fig. 2.1).

SMA

1. Collaterals between the inferior pancreaticoduodenal and jejunal vessels.
2. Collaterals between first and second jejunal vessels.
3. The collateral cascade between the right, middle, and ileocolic arteries as they formed the marginal artery of Drummond (Figs. 2.2b and 2.4).

IMA

1. Collaterals between the sigmoid, rectosigmoid, and superior rectal arteries and their formation of the latter part of the marginal artery of Drummond (Figs. 2.2b and 2.4).

Between Mesenteric Vessels

Celiac and SMA Collaterals

1. The arch of Bühler – an embryological remnant of an artery that linked the celiac and SMA (Fig. 2.2b) [6].
2. The pancreaticoduodenal arteries link the celiac and SMA via the superior and inferior pancreaticoduodenal arteries, respectively (Figs. 2.1, 2.2, and 2.3).
3. If present, an aberrant middle colic artery originating from the celiac would form collaterals to the SMA.

SMA and IMA Collaterals

The collateral circulation between the SMA and IMA is critically important, especially in the setting of chronic mesenteric ischemia. It is also a source of access for embolization of type II endoleaks after endovascular aneurysm repair. However, the terminology surrounding this collateral network is confusing. This is due to variations in nomenclature over time [7].

1. The marginal artery – the marginal artery (of Drummond) is a potential collateral pathway that connects the superior mesenteric and inferior mesenteric arterial systems. This anastomotic channel originates from the descending branch of the ileocolic artery. It involves the communication of this branch to the right colic artery via the right colic artery's descending and ascending branches, then the right and left branches of the middle colic artery, the ascending and descending branches of the left colic artery, and the sigmoid branches of the inferior mesenteric artery terminating in the superior rectal artery (Figs. 2.2b and 2.4). When well developed, this can be a rich source of collateral circulation to the colon, particularly in the event of colonic resection. The artery may run close to the bowel wall or in some instances more within the mesentery. Less than 50 % of the time, this collateral pathway may not be complete at the splenic flexure, a location named Griffith's point (Fig. 2.4). This void of collaterals from the left branch of the middle colic artery to the ascending left colic artery can result in colonic ischemia in the setting of bowel surgery or occlusive disease [4, 7].
2. Meandering mesenteric artery (also referred to as the arc of Riolan or meandering mesenteric artery of Moskowitz) [8] – this represents another collateral pathway between the SMA and IMA. It was named after anatomist Jean Riolan. When present, this connects the middle colic artery of the SMA with the left colic branch of the IMA (Fig. 2.2b). In the era of endovascular aneurysm repair, this is an important collateral pathway to permit coil embolization for type II endoleaks (Fig. 2.6).

Mesenteric and Parietal Arterial Collaterals

1. Collaterals flow may exist between the celiac artery and parietal circulation from the esophageal branches of the inferior phrenic artery to the left gastric and short gastric arteries.
2. Although typically obliterated, the falciform ligament, if recanalized, can be a source of collateral flow between the hepatic arteries and internal thoracic and superior epigastric arteries.
3. The IMA and the internal iliac artery form a perirectal plexus involving collaterals between the superior rectal, middle sacral, and middle and inferior rectal vessels (Sudeck's point – collateral communication between last sigmoidal branch and the superior rectal, Fig. 2.4) [3, 9].
4. The middle sacral artery can collateralize to the IMA circulation [3].

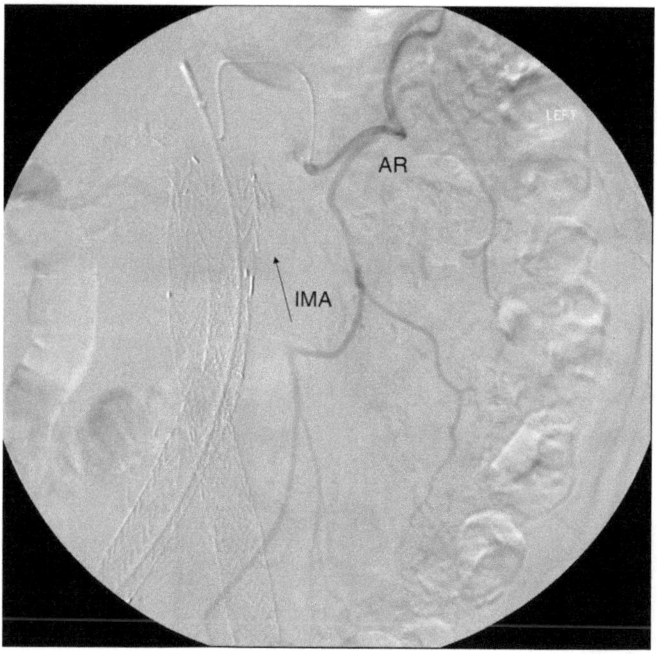

Fig. 2.6 Arc of Riolan. Catheter is placed in the middle colic artery through the SMA. The collateral connects to the IMA, in this case resulting in a type II endoleak after endovascular aneurysm repair. *AR* arc of Riolan, *IMA* inferior mesenteric artery

5. Less common collaterals can develop to permit collateral blood flow (1) to the liver via intercostal posterior abdominal wall arteries, (2) to the renal capsule via the marginal artery, and (3) from lumbar arteries on the posterior abdominal wall to the marginal artery [5].

Variant Anatomy

The anatomy of mesenteric vascular structures is highly variable. It is quite common to encounter patients with variations of either the celiac, SMA, or IMA, although the first two are much more common.

Celiac Artery Variants

The "normal" celiac artery consists of the left gastric, splenic, and common hepatic arteries as described above (Fig. 2.7a). This occurs in 55–89 % in series of anatomic dissections and arteriograms performed over the last 50 years [10–12]. In <10 % of

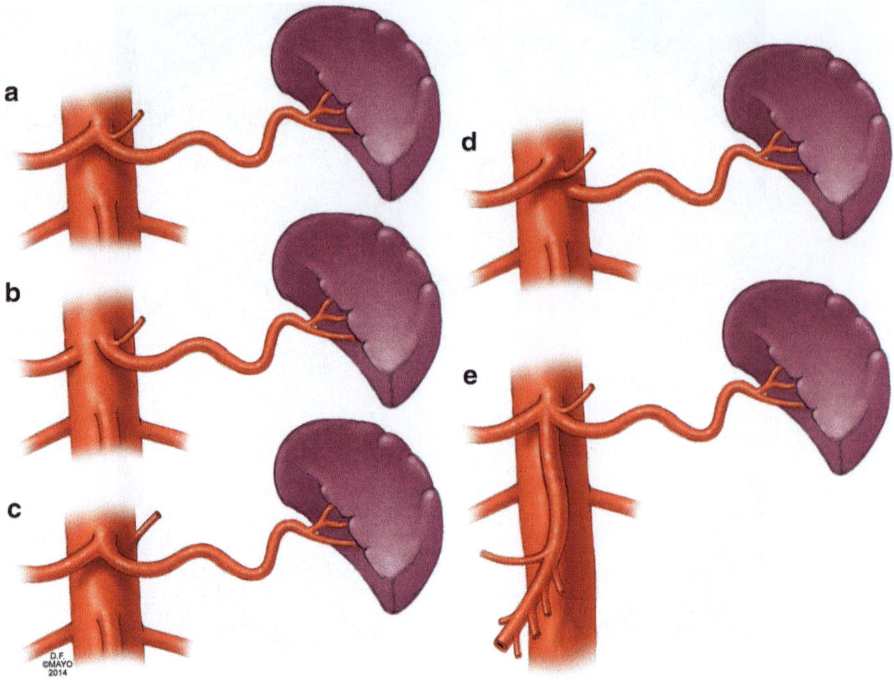

Fig. 2.7 Celiac artery anatomic variants. (**a**) Normal celiac artery anatomy with left gastric, common hepatic, and splenic artery, (**b**) gastrosplenic artery with separate common hepatic artery origin. (**c**) Hepatosplenic artery with separate left gastric origin. (**d**) Hepatogastric artery with separate splenic artery origin. (**e**) Celiacomesenteric axis – combined celiac and superior mesenteric artery origin (By permission of Mayo Foundation for Medical Education and Research. All rights reserved)

cases, the common hepatic artery originates separate from the aorta, while the left gastric and splenic arteries form a common origin (gastrosplenic trunk, Fig. 2.7b). Less commonly, a hepatosplenic (Fig. 2.7c) or hepatogastric trunk (Fig. 2.7d) is formed, with the remaining branch coming from the aorta. In rare circumstances, the SMA originates from the celiac artery as a common celiacomesenteric axis (Fig. 2.7e) [12]. The left gastric artery is a relatively constant structure. However, it may give rise to an accessory left hepatic artery (1–16 % of cases) or a replaced left hepatic artery 10 % of the time [10, 11, 13].

The common hepatic artery and the pancreaticoduodenal arcade anatomy can be highly variable. Variations can occur in all vessels and their branches. Detailed descriptions of all possible anatomic variants are beyond the scope of this chapter, and further descriptions are available in other texts [14]. The "typical" common hepatic artery arising from the celiac artery may occur in 80 % of cases. The most common variant is the absence of the common hepatic artery in 12 % of cases, while a common hepatic origin from the SMA occurs in <5 % of cases [12, 15]. If the common hepatic artery is absent, its branches may originate from the aorta, the SMA, or the celiac artery.

The left and right hepatic artery variants can occur with variations of the common hepatic artery or as isolated variants themselves. As mentioned previously, left hepatic arterial variations occur 20 % of the time in isolation and more often in combination with other variants. This is typically a replaced or accessory left hepatic artery from the left gastric artery. When the common hepatic artery is absent, the left hepatic artery may originate from the aorta or the celiac artery. Variations of the right hepatic artery occur in 6–18 % of cases as either a replaced right hepatic from the SMA (most common 6–11 % [10–15] or an accessory right hepatic artery (2–8 %) [10, 11, 13]). The replaced or accessory right hepatic artery may originate from the SMA (common) or the aorta when no common hepatic artery exists. The cystic artery commonly arises from the right hepatic artery in 70 % of cases; however, its relationship to the common hepatic duct is variable, and accessory cystic arteries may occur in 11 % of cases [15]. The "normal" gastroduodenal artery originating from the common hepatic artery occurs 75 % of the time [15]. Variations in its origin are commonly due to common hepatic artery variants. As such, it may arise from an aberrant common hepatic artery (off the SMA), a replaced right hepatic artery, or the left hepatic artery [12]. Finally, the right gastric artery is in its normal position in half of cases. Variations can include originating from the left or right hepatic artery or the GDA [15].

The splenic artery may be part of anomalous permutations of the celiac artery as discussed previously. The splenic artery can originate from the SMA as opposed to the celiac artery. It may also be duplicated with one or both branches originating from the aorta. Additionally, it may give rise to the left gastric, middle colic, or left hepatic artery [12].

SMA Variants

As noted above, the SMA can have a great number of variants related to arteries typically seen from the celiac axis. The SMA may originate from the celiac axis (Fig. 2.7e) or provide any combination of hepatic arteries, or accessory gastric, splenic, or pancreatic vessels. The "normal" SMA anatomy may be present in as many as 68 % of cases (Fig. 2.8a) [12]. The ileocolic artery appears to be the most consistent structure from the SMA. The other vessels have some degree of variability. Although normally a separate branch, the middle colic artery, can share a common trunk with the right colic artery (middle colic-right colic trunk, Fig. 2.8b) in up to 52 % of cases, representing the most common variant. If not involved in aberrant anatomy with the middle colic artery, the right colic artery may be an independent branch of the SMA (38 %) or a branch of the ileocolic artery in 8 % of cases (Fig. 2.8c). There may be an accessory right colic in 8–10 % of cases. Less commonly, the middle and right colic artery are absent (<10 % of the time), or the middle colic may send a large branch to the splenic flexure. In very rare cases, the middle colic artery may be a branch of the celiac artery [9, 12].

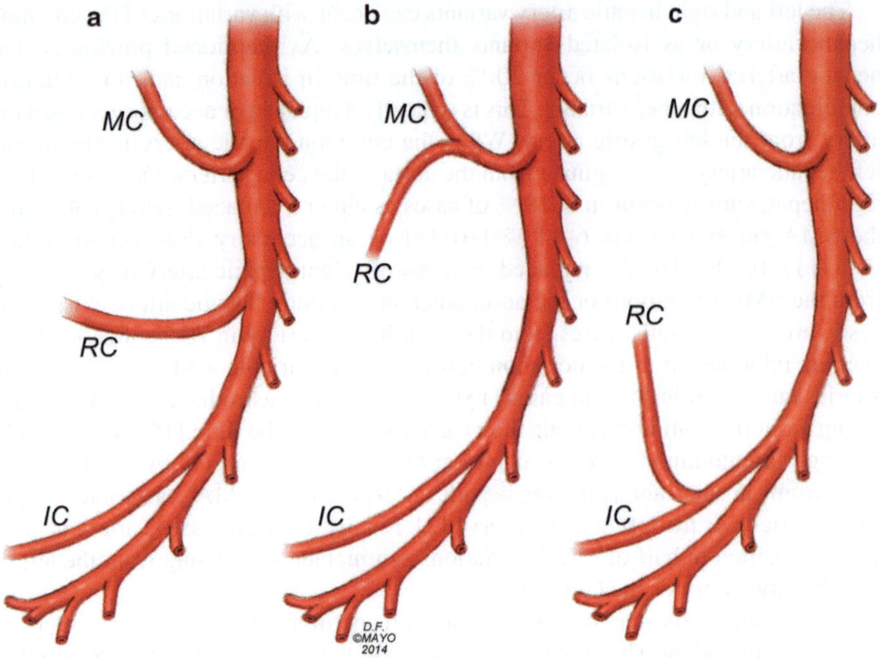

Fig. 2.8 Superior mesenteric artery anatomic variants. *IC* ileocolic artery, *RC* right colic artery, *MC* middle colic artery. (**a**) normal anatomy with separate IC, RC, and MC origins. (**b**) Combine MC and RC origin and separate IC origin. (**c**) Common RC and IC origin and separate MC origin (By permission of Mayo Foundation for Medical Education and Research. All rights reserved)

IMA Variants

The IMA has little variation in terms of position and origin. However, the left colic artery may be limited in its ascension to the splenic flexure in 86 % of cases, threatening the collateralization of the marginal artery in this region. In fact, adequate collateralization may only occur in 60 % of cases at the splenic flexure (Griffith's point) and in 50 % of cases in the upper rectum (Sudeck's point) (Fig. 2.4). The predominant variations of the IMA circulation involve the division of the sigmoidal arteries in forming the arterial arcades and collateralization to the internal iliac artery branches. Further details are available from Michels detailed description of these variations [9]. Rarely, there can sigmoidal artery origins from the internal iliac artery [12].

References

1. Carlson BM. Human embryology and developmental biology. 5th ed. Philadelphia: Elsevier/Saunders; 2013.
2. Uflacker R, Selby JB. Atlas of vascular anatomy : an angiographic approach. 2nd ed. Philadelphia: Lippincott Williams & Wilkins; 2007. xiv, 905 p.

3. Kahn P, Abrams HL. Inferior mesenteric arterial patterns; an angiographic study. Radiology. 1964;82:429–42.
4. Meyers MA. Griffiths' point: critical anastomosis at the splenic flexure. Significance in ischemia of the colon. Am J Roentgenol. 1976;126(1):77–94.
5. Geroulakos G, Cherry KJ. Diseases of the visceral circulation. London/New York: Arnold, Distributed in the USA by Oxford University Press; 2002. viii, 228 p., 12 p. of plates.
6. Rosenblum JD, Boyle CM, Schwartz LB. The mesenteric circulation. Anatomy and physiology. Surg Clin North Am. 1997;77(2):289–306.
7. Fisher Jr DF, Fry WJ. Collateral mesenteric circulation. Surg Gynecol Obstet. 1987;164(5):487–92.
8. Gourley EJ, Gering SA. The meandering mesenteric artery: a historic review and surgical implications. Dis Colon Rectum. 2005;48(5):996–1000.
9. Michels NA, Siddharth P, Kornblith PL, Parke WW. The variant blood supply to the descending colon, rectosigmoid and rectum based on 400 dissections. Its importance in regional resections: a review of medical literature. Dis Colon Rectum. 1965;8:251–78.
10. Covey AM, Brody LA, Maluccio MA, Getrajdman GI, Brown KT. Variant hepatic arterial anatomy revisited: digital subtraction angiography performed in 600 patients. Radiology. 2002;224(2):542–7.
11. Hiatt JR, Gabbay J, Busuttil RW. Surgical anatomy of the hepatic arteries in 1000 cases. Ann Surg. 1994;220(1):50–2.
12. Valentine RJ, Wind GG. Anatomic exposures in vascular surgery. 2nd ed. Philadelphia: Lippincott Williams & Wilkins; 2003. xiii, 577 p.
13. De Cecco CN, Ferrari R, Rengo M, Paolantonio P, Vecchietti F, Laghi A. Anatomic variations of the hepatic arteries in 250 patients studied with 64-row CT angiography. Eur Radiol. 2009;19(11):2765–70.
14. Michels NA. The anatomic variations of the arterial pancreaticoduodenal arcades: their import in regional resection involving the gall bladder, bile ducts, liver, pancreas and parts of the small and large intestines. J Int Coll Surg. 1962;37:13–40.
15. Daseler EH, Anson BJ, et al. The cystic artery and constituents of the hepatic pedicle; a study of 500 specimens. Surg Gynecol Obstet. 1947;85(1):47–63.

Chapter 3
Pathophysiology

Gustavo S. Oderich and Leonardo Reis de Souza

The first clinical and anatomical descriptions of intestinal ischemia were recognized by Chienne in 1869 and Councilman in 1884 [1, 2]. Goodman in 1918 associated the symptoms of postprandial abdominal pain to those of patients with angina pectoris [3]. Dunphy from the Peter Bent Brigham Hospital reported in 1936 the correlation between recurrent abdominal pain and fatal intestinal infarction from occlusive mesenteric arterial disease [4]. In that report, 60 % of patients who died of intestinal infarction had a history of recurrent abdominal pain, which preceded the fatal event by weeks, months, or years. Since then, the term *intestinal angina* has been coined to describe the classic symptom of chronic abdominal pain that occurs after meals, which is the cardinal symptom of *chronic mesenteric ischemia* (CMI).

Current estimates indicate that CMI accounts for <1 per 100,000 hospital admissions in the United States and <2 % of all admissions for gastrointestinal conditions [5]. Since the first successful mesenteric endarterectomy by Shaw and Maynard in 1958, techniques of revascularization have greatly evolved [6]. Advances in diagnostic imaging, medical therapy, surgical techniques, and endovascular technology resulted in improved outcomes. Balloon angioplasty was reported to treat mesenteric arterial stenoses by Uflacker, Furrer, and Gruentzig and colleagues in 1980 [7, 8]. During the last decade, mesenteric angioplasty and stenting gained

G.S. Oderich, MD, FACS (✉)
Division of Vascular and Endovascular Surgery, Mayo Clinic, Rochester, MN, USA

Gonda Vascular Center, Mayo Clinic, Rochester, MN, USA
e-mail: oderich.gustavo@mayo.edu

L.R. de Souza, MD
Division of Vascular and Endovascular Surgery, Mayo Clinic, Rochester, MN, USA

Masters Degree Program from the Department of Surgery,
Universidade Federal do Rio Grande do Sul, Porto Alegre, Brazil
e-mail: reissouza@gmail.com

G.S. Oderich (ed.), *Mesenteric Vascular Disease*,
DOI 10.1007/978-1-4939-1847-8_3

widespread acceptance and became the most frequently utilized treatment for CMI, relegating open surgery to patients who fail endovascular therapy or have complex lesions unsuitable to it [9]. This chapter provides a comprehensive review of the normal physiology of mesenteric circulation and pathophysiology of CMI.

Vascular Anatomy

The gastrointestinal tract is supplied by three direct aortic branches (Fig. 3.1), the celiac axis, superior mesenteric artery (SMA), and inferior mesenteric artery (IMA). The celiac axis supplies the upper gut including the stomach, liver, and spleen. The SMA is the largest single branch of the abdominal aorta and supplies the midgut, including the entire intestine, proximal portions of the colon, and the pancreas. The inferior mesenteric artery delivers blood to the distal colon. There is extensive collateral network between these three arteries, as well as other collateral pathways via phrenic, internal iliac, and parietal branches.

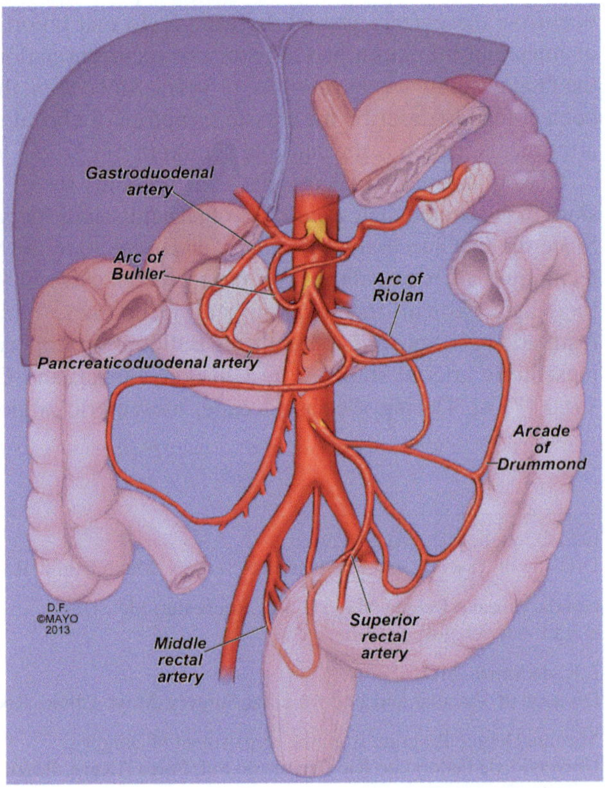

Fig. 3.1 Mesenteric circulation and its collateral networks between the celiac artery, superior mesenteric artery, and inferior mesenteric artery (By permission of Mayo Foundation for Medical Education and Research. All rights reserved)

Physiologic Response

Approximately 20 % of the cardiac output goes through the mesenteric arteries under normal conditions [10]. Blood flow to the gastrointestinal tract increases even before the ingestion of a meal, remaining elevated at levels approaching 100–150 % of normal (2,000 ml/min) over the next 3–6 h. There is still controversy if the blood flow is redirected selectively to the mesentery. In the 1930s, Herrick used a thermostromuhr to demonstrate that blood flow is increased 5 h after a meal in awaken dogs not only in superior mesenteric artery but also in carotid, coronary, and femoral arteries. Some speculated that these changes could be due to an increase in cardiac output [11]. Most of the early attempts to understand the physiologic response of mesenteric circulation after meal were based in extrapolation from animal data or from limited experiments using angiographic techniques or laparotomy with application of electromagnetic flowmeters [12].

The normal hyperemic postprandial response is mediated by cardiovascular changes that accompany the ingestion and digestion of food. It is well documented that these changes start even before food reaches the stomach. Anticipatory response usually represents a small increase in superior mesenteric artery blood flow. When meal doesn't reach the stomach, response tends to last only a few minutes. Studies in dogs and primates have shown that cardiac output, heart rate, and aortic pressure are increased in this phase but also that there is little change in mesenteric vascular resistance. After the anticipatory period, increase in cardiac output is not well documented [11].

Mesenteric vasodilatation starts 3–5 min after food enters the intestine, reaching its maximum 30–90 min later and lasting 4–6 h. The latency and duration of these responses depend upon the type and quantity of a meal, with high fat and protein-containing foods producing the most profound and sustained intestinal hyperemia [13]. Moneta and colleagues described variations in duplex scan measurements after ingestion of six different liquid meals by conscious humans: mixed, carbohydrates, fat, protein, mannitol, and water. Superior mesenteric artery blood flow measurements showed significant increases in peak systolic velocity, end-diastolic velocity, mean velocity, and volume flow after all meals, except water. Peak changes after carbohydrate meal tended to occur earlier and to be less intense than after mixed or fat meals. Although increases in duplex parameters in response to protein were less than those of carbohydrate, they appeared to be better sustained. Femoral and celiac arteries showed no significant changes. Minimal change in velocities in the celiac axis (CA) is presumably due to the relative low resistance on the splenic and hepatic circulations at baseline [12].

Postprandial mesenteric hyperemia is confined to organs in which digestion is occurring, but is not shared equally within the same mesenteric arterial territory or within the tissue layers of the intestine. The increased blood flow in the superior mesenteric artery (SMA) territory elicited by food in the intestine is associated with little to no change in blood flow to the stomach, pancreas, and colon.

Studies with introduction of food in specific parts of the intestine of dogs showed that even within the intestine, various regions are perfused in different degrees [11]. At the level of the intestinal wall, blood flow distribution favors the mucosa (70 to 80 % of total blood flow), rather than the submucosa and muscularis [14]. Mesenteric postprandial hyperemia is selective in its distribution to regions related to digestive and absorptive processes [11].

Several mechanisms have been proposed to explain postprandial hyperemia. Potential mediators are divided in five categories: direct effect of absorbed nutrients, enteric nervous system, gastrointestinal hormones and peptides, local nonmetabolic vasoactive mediators, and local metabolic vasoactive mediators [15]. Lipid micelles, some amino acids, carbon dioxide, and nitrogen ions are capable of diffuse across intestinal epithelial barrier to directly initiate autoregulation of blood flow in microvessels [16].

Effects of enteric nervous system are unclear. Postprandial hyperemia is not modified by pharmacological or surgical sympathetic blockade. Atropine infusion inhibits food-induced mesenteric vasodilatation, which is compatible with at least a partial influence of a hormonal mechanism, for cholinergic blockade reportedly prevents the release of cholecystokinin (CCK) [11]. Capsaicin-sensitive afferent fibers responsible for releasing CCK, substance P, and vasoactive intestinal polypeptide (VIP) are also potentially involved, since capsaicin and lidocaine can prevent hyperemia associated with micelle absorption. Therefore, a nonadrenergic, noncholinergic mechanism is possible [16].

Earlier studies with systemic infusion of secretin, gastrin, or CCK reported increases in superior mesenteric blood flow. CCK was also associated with increases in small intestinal and pancreatic blood flow [11]. Premen and colleagues questioned the importance of CCK as a physiological intestinal vasodilator, based on the finding that at physiological rates, it didn't alter intestinal blood flow. These authors performed intra-arterial infusion of secretin, neurotensin, CCK, and a combination of the three hormones in dogs. Results suggested that alone or in combination, none is of quantitative importance in regulating blood flow in postprandial state [17]. VIP, gastric inhibitory peptide, calcitonin gene-related peptide α, glucagon, enkephalins, somatostatin, and peptide YY also don't appear to have a role at physiological doses. It is acceptable, however, that specific sites in the digestive system may experience sufficient levels of these substances to produce a controlled local effect [16].

Serotonin, histamine, bradykinin, and prostaglandins are produced by small intestine in response to normal or pathological stimuli. Histamine release in the stomach has long been implicated in the control of blood flow. Its vasodilating effects are mainly mediated by H1 receptors. The proper role of local nonmetabolic vasoactive mediators probably depends on the balance of vasoconstrictors and vasodilators [11, 17].

Current knowledge suggests that metabolic products, mainly oxygen uptake and tissue PO_2, are the basic mediators of postprandial vascular response. Adenosine occupies fundamental positions in almost every metabolic process, and its levels are also elevated during hyperemia. Nitric oxide (NO) is a potent vasodilator product of endothelium, with important role as a regulator of intestinal motility, fluid balance, and electrolyte absorption. In rodents, NO appears to be essential for permucosal arteriolar dilation [16].

Collateral Pathways

The mesenteric circulation is rich in collateral network between the three main visceral artery territories (CA, SMA, and inferior mesenteric artery) and the internal iliac arteries (Fig. 3.1). Direction of blood flow is contingent on the location of the significant stenosis. The gastroduodenal and pancreaticoduodenal arteries provide collateralization between the CA and SMA. The marginal artery of Drummond and the arc of Riolan (Fig. 3.2) connect the left colic artery (inferior mesenteric artery) to the middle colic artery (SMA). The term meandering or central anastomotic artery describes marked enlargement that occurs in the arc of Riolan in patients

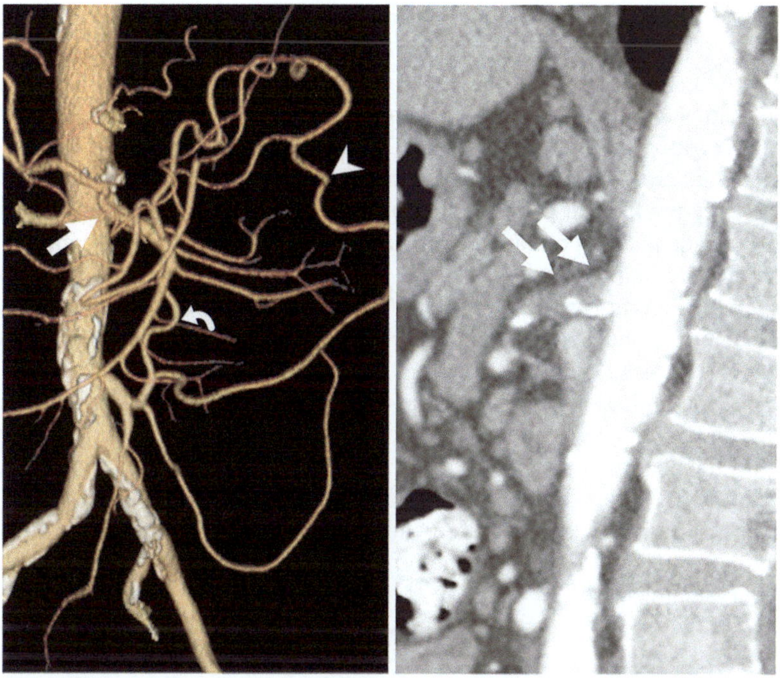

Fig. 3.2 Computed tomography angiography in a patient with severe symptoms of chronic mesenteric ischemia. Note the three-dimensional reconstruction with large meandering artery, which provides collateral flow into the superior mesenteric artery via arc of Riolan (*curved arrow*) and marginal artery of Drummond (*arrowhead*). The SMA connects to the celiac artery via gastroduodenal collaterals (*straight arrow*)

with high-grade stenosis or occlusion of the SMA and collateralization via a patent inferior mesenteric artery (IMA) [18]. The internal iliac arteries provide a collateral pathway via the hemorrhoidal branches.

Pathophysiology

Patients with chronic mesenteric ischemia fail to achieve the postprandial hyperemic response that is required to supply oxygen for the metabolic processes of secretion, absorption, and for increased peristaltic activity [19]. Just as in the patient with ischemic cardiomyopathy, where angina pectoris occurs as a result from inadequate supply of oxygen, intestinal angina results from the relative imbalance between tissue supply and demand for oxygen and other metabolites. At the tissue and cellular level, the lack of adenosine triphosphate metabolism affects intestinal mucosa, muscularis, and visceral nerves, causing failure of most intestinal mucosal transport pathways and contracture of the muscular layer with inadequate relaxation, resulting in malabsorption and abdominal pain [20, 21].

Because of the extensive collateral network, the majority of patients with symptoms of CMI have significant stenosis or occlusion of at least two of the three mesenteric arteries. In the last Mayo Clinic review of 229 mesenteric arteriographies, 98 % of patients with CMI had two- or three-vessel involvement, with occlusion or critical stenosis of the SMA in 92 % [22]. However, contrary to what has been propagated in many surgical textbooks, this is not an absolute requirement [23, 24]. The clinical significance of ischemia correlates not only to the extent of disease but also the adequacy of collateral pathways, acuteness of symptoms, and presence of arterial steal; approximately 2–10 % of patients with CMI have single-vessel disease, which affects primarily the SMA and patients with poorly developed collaterals or more acute presentation, as might be predicted from the postprandial hyperemic response [22].

Despite the limitations of using a non-complacent glass-model aorta with steady flow, Ku and colleagues demonstrated flow patterns that may explain the tendency of the infrarenal aorta in forming plaque. Flow separation and stagnation at the posterior wall of the aorta, mainly directly opposite the orifices of superior and inferior mesenteric arteries, were reported in resting and postprandial simulations. The shear stress could lead to plaque formation and eventually in both obstructive and aneurysmal disease.

Conclusion

The mesenteric arterial anatomy consists of a robust collateral network between the celiac, SMA, and IMA territories. The normal hyperemic response observed after a meal is triggered by humoral and metabolic factors, which result in a tenfold increase in blood flow. Patients with symptoms of chronic mesenteric ischemia are not able to mount this normal response; intestinal angina occurs as a result from inadequate supply of oxygen and from the relative imbalance between tissue supply and demand for oxygen and other metabolites.

References

1. Chienne J. Complete obliteration of celiac and mesenteric vessels. J Anat Physiol. 1869;3:363–72.
2. Councilman WT. Three cases of occlusion of mesenteric artery. Boston Med Surg J. 1894;130:410.
3. Goodman EH. Angina abdominis. Am J Med Sci. 1918;155(4):524–8.
4. Dunphy JE. Abdominal pain of vascular origin. Am J Med Sci. 1936;192(6):109–13.
5. Mitchell EL, Moneta GL. Mesenteric duplex scanning. Perspect Vasc Surg Endovasc Ther. 2006;18(2):175–83.
6. Shaw RS, Maynard 3rd EP. Acute and chronic thrombosis of the mesenteric arteries associated with malabsorption; a report of two cases successfully treated by thromboendarterectomy. N Engl J Med. 1958;258(18):874–8.
7. Furrer J, et al. Treatment of abdominal angina with percutaneous dilatation of an arteria mesenterica superior stenosis. Preliminary communication. Cardiovasc Intervent Radiol. 1980;3(1):43–4.
8. Uflacker R, Goldany MA, Constant S. Resolution of mesenteric angina with percutaneous transluminal angioplasty of a superior mesenteric artery stenosis using a balloon catheter. Gastrointest Radiol. 1980;5(4):367–9.
9. Schermerhorn ML, et al. Mesenteric revascularization: management and outcomes in the United States, 1988–2006. J Vasc Surg. 2009;50(2):341e1–8e1.
10. Kolkman JJ, et al. Diagnosis and management of splanchnic ischemia. World J Gastroenterol. 2008;14(48):7309–20.
11. Fara JW. Postprandial mesenteric ischemia. In: Shepherd AP, Granger DN, editors. Physiology of the Intestinal Circulation. New York: Raven; 1984.
12. Moneta GL, et al. Duplex ultrasound measurement of postprandial intestinal blood flow: effect of meal composition. Gastroenterology. 1988;95(5):1294–301.
13. Siregar H, Chou CC. Relative contribution of fat, protein, carbohydrate, and ethanol to intestinal hyperemia. Am J Physiol. 1982;242(1):G27–31.
14. Gallavan Jr RH, et al. Regional blood flow during digestion in the conscious dog. Am J Physiol. 1980;238(2):H220–5.
15. Chou CC, Coatney RW. Nutrient-induced changes in intestinal blood flow in the dog. Br Vet J. 1994;150(5):423–37.
16. Matheson PJ, Wilson MA, Garrison RN. Regulation of intestinal blood flow. J Surg Res. 2000;93(1):182–96.
17. Premen AJ, Kvietys PR, Granger DN. Postprandial regulation of intestinal blood flow: role of gastrointestinal hormones. Am J Physiol. 1985;249(2 Pt 1):G250–5.
18. Connolly JE. The meandering mesenteric artery or central anastomotic artery. J Vasc Surg. 2006;43(5):1059.
19. Poole JW, Sammartano RJ, Boley SJ. Hemodynamic basis of the pain of chronic mesenteric ischemia. Am J Surg. 1987;153(2):171–6.
20. Fu LW, Longhurst JC. Interleukin-1beta sensitizes abdominal visceral afferents of cats to ischaemia and histamine. J Physiol. 1999;521(Pt 1):249–60.
21. Kozar RA, et al. The type of sodium-coupled solute modulates small bowel mucosal injury, transport function, and ATP after ischemia/reperfusion injury in rats. Gastroenterology. 2002;123(3):810–6.

22. Oderich GS, et al. Open versus endovascular revascularization for chronic mesenteric ischemia: risk-stratified outcomes. J Vasc Surg. 2009;49(6):1472e3–9e3.
23. Mikkelsen WP. Intestinal angina: its surgical significance. Am J Surg. 1957;94(2):262–7; discussion, 267–9.
24. Carrick RP, et al. Chronic mesenteric ischemia resulting from isolated lesions of the superior mesenteric artery – a case report. Angiology. 2005;56(6):785–8.

Chapter 4
Epidemiology and Natural History

Thomas Curran and Marc L. Schermerhorn

Chronic Mesenteric Ischemia

Epidemiology

Chronic mesenteric ischemia (CMI) is characterized by recurrent postprandial abdominal pain and food fear secondary to small bowel hypoperfusion. Most frequently this condition is brought about by mesenteric atherosclerosis and subject to the same risk factors as coronary and cerebrovascular atherosclerosis. Unselected autopsy studies have shown incidence of mesenteric artery atherosclerotic stenosis to range from 30 to 80 % [1–4]. Roobottom et al prospectively assessed the prevalence of significant mesenteric stenosis (occlusion or stenosis > 70 %) using duplex ultrasonography in a population of 184 asymptomatic individuals undergoing ultrasound study for nonvascular indication [5]. As may be expected given the prevalence of atherosclerotic disease generally, they found that 18 % (N = 17/97) of individuals greater than 65 years met criteria for mesenteric stenosis, while only 3 % of patients (N = 3/87) less than 65 years met these criteria. Of those greater than 65 years, 11 % had single-vessel disease, while 7 % had multivessel disease. Aortograms, the gold standard for diagnosis of mesenteric stenosis, performed in elderly patients without abdominal symptoms have similarly demonstrated an 18 % (N = 97/553) prevalence of mesenteric artery stenosis [6]. However, only a small minority (1.3 %) was found to have multivessel disease. Accordingly while stenosis

T. Curran, MD
Department of Surgery, Beth Israel Deaconess Medical Center, Boston, MA, USA
e-mail: tcurran1@bidmc.harvard.edu

M.L. Schermerhorn, MD (✉)
Division for Vascular and Endovascular Surgery, Department of Surgery,
Beth Israel Deaconess Medical Center, Boston, MA, USA
e-mail: mscherme@bidmc.harvard.edu

G.S. Oderich (ed.), *Mesenteric Vascular Disease*,
DOI 10.1007/978-1-4939-1847-8_4

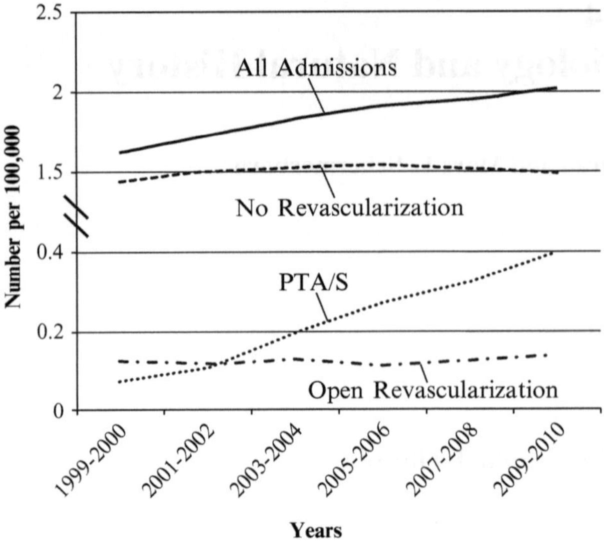

Fig. 4.1 Annual number of admissions per 100,000 persons for chronic mesenteric ischemia in the Nationwide Inpatient Sample

of at least one mesenteric vessel is common in the asymptomatic elderly population, those clinically diagnosed with CMI are far more frequently seen to have two or three-vessel disease. A report by Oderich and colleagues on 229 patients undergoing revascularization for CMI showed that 57 % (N=131/229) had three-vessel disease, 41 % (N=93/229) had two-vessel disease, while only 2 % (N=5/229) had single-vessel disease [7].

While multivessel mesenteric stenosis is found in 1 to 7 % of asymptomatic patients, it appears that the clinical manifestations of CMI are much more rare, though possibly increasing over time. Lo et al reviewed the Nationwide Inpatient Sample (NIS), a weighted 20 % sampling of nearly all United States (USA) hospital discharges, from 1998 to 2010 to show that the annual number of CMI-related admissions has risen 25 % over that time period from 1.6 to 2.0 admissions per 100,00 persons (Fig. 4.1) [8]. Similarly, the treatment of CMI has risen dramatically in recent years as evidenced by NIS data showing that overall treatment of CMI in the USA has increased from 200 repairs annually in 1994 to 1300 repairs in 2006, a trend largely driven by the increase in endovascular revascularization [9]. A follow-up study by Lo and colleagues using administrative data from Florida and California from 2006 to 2009 noted that while reintervention rates for endovascular treatment of CMI may range up to 10 % over 4 years, the vast majority of the observed increase in endovascular interventions for CMI stems from treatment of new cases [10]. However, it is unclear whether this increase in treatment is related to a true increase in the incidence of CMI or perhaps a lower treatment threshold following from the introduction of endovascular treatment options. Of CMI patients treated with mesenteric revascularization, a meta-analysis on all reported revascularizations from

1990 to 2008 showed a mean age of 59 years for those undergoing open revascularization and 64 years for those undergoing endovascular revascularization [11]. A strong majority of patients treated in both the open and endovascular groups were female [open: $N = 714/992$ (72 %); endovascular: $N = 306/409$ (75 %)]. Hence, while CMI remains a rare complication of mesenteric atherosclerotic disease, CMI related hospital admissions and treatment have increased in recent years.

Additionally, review studies estimate that approximately 10 % of CMI cases are attributable to etiologies other than atherosclerosis including primary vascular conditions such as dissection, fibromuscular dysplasia, or vasculitis; or other systemic conditions such as neurofibromatosis [12–16]. Dissection secondary to segmental arterial mediolysis (SAM), a non-atherosclerotic, non-inflammatory arteriopathy, with subsequent development of CMI, should also be recognized among these non-atherosclerotic causes though it is among the most rare with only 47 cases reported through 2011 [17]. The demographics of patients with non-atherosclerotic CMI vary widely according to the specific underlying pathology with most data restricted to single-center case series.

Natural History

The natural history of CMI has largely been elucidated by two prospective studies on the clinical course of patients found to have moderate to severe mesenteric atherosclerotic disease. From 1989 to 1995, Thomas and colleagues evaluated 980 aortograms of patients without CMI symptoms to identify 82 patients (8.3 %) with greater than 50 % stenosis of one or more mesenteric vessels [18]. These patients were then followed at six-month intervals with questionnaires on symptom status for a mean of 2.6 years (range: 1–6 years). Sixty patients meeting study criteria were available for follow-up during which time 4 patients (6 %) developed symptoms of mesenteric ischemia, 3 chronic and 1 acute. Notably, each of these 4 patients was among the 15 patients with three-vessel disease, while none of the remaining 45 patients developed symptoms. A subsequent study by Wilson et al studied 553 elderly patients undergoing visceral duplex ultrasonography to find 97 patients (18 %) with severe stenosis of either the celiac or superior mesenteric arteries [1]. Of the 20 patients with mesenteric artery stenosis who died during the mean 6.5 year follow-up period, no deaths were attributed to intestinal infarction. Further, of the 45 patients with mesenteric artery stenosis available for response at a mean follow-up of 6.8 years, no patient reported symptoms referable to chronic mesenteric ischemia. These two prospective studies have informed the recommendation for treatment of mesenteric artery stenosis only in symptomatic patients though the high incidence of symptoms in patients with three-vessel disease in the Thomas study may warrant further investigation of this subgroup.

Though results following treatment of CMI will be addressed separately in Chaps. 12 and 14, it is worthwhile to note that the number of in-hospital deaths associated with CMI are decreasing over time. Lo and colleagues, using the NIS, have shown a nationwide 25 % decrease in CMI-related in-hospital deaths from 1998 to 2010, from 0.16 deaths per 100,000 persons in 1998 to 0.12 deaths per 100,000 persons in 2010 [8]. Interestingly, the Centers for Disease Control Wide-ranging Online Data for Epidemiologic Research (CDC WONDER) database has demonstrated a relatively stable CMI attributable mortality ranging between 0.04 and 0.07 deaths per 100,000 persons over the same time period [8]. This discrepancy between in-hospital CMI-associated deaths as determined by the NIS and CMI attributable deaths as determined by the CDC WONDER database is likely due to the NIS inclusion of patients admitted to the hospital with CMI who go on to die of other causes (i.e., myocardial infarction or other catastrophic insult). Reconciling these two data sources, it appears that CMI-related deaths are either stable or falling in recent years. These compelling data are likely the result of multiple factors including improved medical prevention with statin agents, earlier diagnosis with the increased utilization of cross-sectional imaging, and, finally, earlier treatment with the increasing use of endovascular techniques.

Acute Mesenteric Ischemia

Epidemiology

Accounting for less than one in every 1,000 admissions [19], acute mesenteric ischemia (AMI) is a rare though highly morbid condition whereby acute onset of bowel hypoperfusion is brought on through a variety of mechanisms. In contrast to CMI, a condition for which hospitalizations have increased, hospital admissions for AMI have decreased from 9 per 100,000 US persons in 1999 to 7 per 100,000 US persons in 2010 (Fig. 4.2) [8]. Regarding the treatment of AMI, prior NIS data published by our group showed that from 1988 to 2006 the absolute number of procedures for the treatment of AMI in the United States remained largely stable at approximately 700 to 800 cases annually though the proportion of endovascular cases increased substantially [9]. Accordingly, population-adjusted data by Lo et al have shown that endovascular interventions for AMI have risen nearly threefold from 0.06 cases per 100,000 US persons in 1999 to 0.18 cases per 100,000 US persons in 2010 [8]. Yet, while AMI-related hospitalizations and AMI-related endovascular interventions appear to be trending in opposite directions, the reasons for this are likely multifactorial given the varied nature of AMI etiologies.

AMI is the final common pathway for several clinical entities, each of which has its own unique epidemiology: (1) mesenteric arterial thromboembolic disease, (2) mesenteric venous thrombosis (MVT), and (3) nonocclusive mesenteric ischemia (NOMI). Acosta and colleagues reviewed 270 AMI cases detected at either autopsy or operation at a regional hospital in Sweden to find the following distribution of etiology: 67 % thromboembolic, 16 % mesenteric venous thrombosis, 15 % nonocclusive mesenteric ischemia, and 2 % indeterminate [20]. Similarly, a clinical

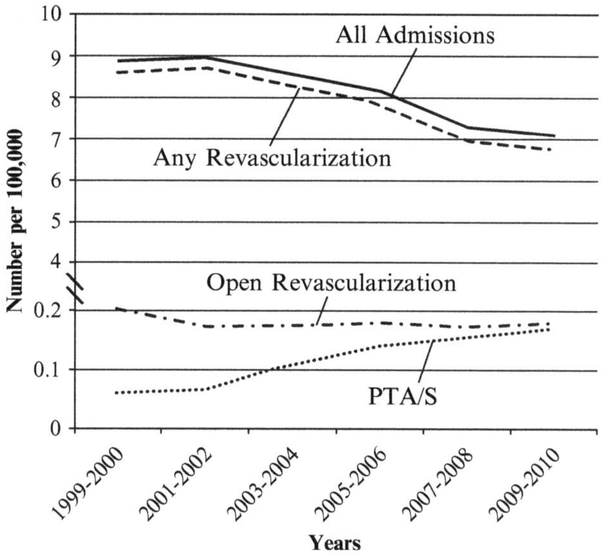

Fig. 4.2 Annual number of admissions per 100,000 persons for acute mesenteric ischemia in the Nationwide Inpatient Sample

series by Endean et al reported on 58 cases of thrombotic AMI, of which 38 % (N=22/58) were related to arterial embolism, 36 % (N=21/58) to arterial thrombosis, and 26 % (N=15/58) to venous thrombosis [21]. Other review data showed a similar etiologic pattern with superior mesenteric artery (SMA) embolism accounting for approximately half of all AMI cases, followed by SMA thrombosis in a quarter of cases and nonocclusive mesenteric ischemia and mesenteric venous thrombosis in 20 and 5 % of cases, respectively [19]. As each of these varies with respect to epidemiology, they will be addressed individually in this space.

Thromboembolic

Though data on the incidence of thromboembolic specific AMI have generally been limited to individual case series, a Swedish population-based autopsy study by Acosta et al has shed considerable light on this area. In Malmo, Sweden, a community in which 87 % of deaths are investigated by autopsy, 213 cases of thromboembolic AMI were identified from over 30,000 autopsies performed from 1970 to 1982; these were then added to the number of operations performed for AMI at the lone Malmo regional hospital over a 3-year sample period to produce a thromboembolic AMI incidence of 8.6 cases per 100,000 person-years [22]. Median age of those who died from thromboembolic AMI was 81 years with two thirds of cases being female. Incidence of AMI nearly doubles with each 5-year interval above age 70 with an incidence of 25 cases per 100,000 person-years for ages 70–74 that then rises to an incidence of 217 cases per 100,000 person-years for patients greater than 85 years. Interestingly, adjustment for the greater longevity of females in this population showed that female gender was not, in fact, an independent risk factor for AMI in this cohort.

The epidemiology of thromboembolic AMI may be influenced by the prevalence of conditions that place patients at increased risk. The pathophysiology of thrombotic AMI suggests that conditions such as prior cerebrovascular accident, aortic wall thrombosis, disseminated cancer, and CMI may increase risk of thrombotic events [20]. Not surprisingly, case series on AMI have documented rates of preexisting CMI in 0–43 % of cases [20, 23–25]. Risk for embolic AMI is increased by comorbid conditions suggestive of prior embolic events such as cerebrovascular accident or predisposing to embolic events including atrial fibrillation, congestive heart failure, and recent myocardial infarction among others [26]. A report by Batellier and colleagues on 82 consecutive patients treated for SMA embolism over a 22-year period (1966–1988) demonstrated a history of atrial fibrillation in 79 % ($N=65/82$) of cases and a history of prior embolic event in 35 % ($N=29/82$) [25]. Accordingly, autopsy study of 122 patients with AMI attributable death showed a cardiac source of thrombus in approximately half of cases ($N=58/122$) [27]. As the management of atrial fibrillation improves with better adherence to anticoagulation guidelines, it is hypothesized that the incidence of embolic AMI may also decrease though population level in this regard is lacking [26, 28]. Data from the National Health and Nutrition Examination Survey (NHANES) database supports this possibility as it demonstrates a sharp increase in the use of aspirin, clopidogrel, warfarin, and statin drugs over the period from 1999 to 2010 [8].

Mesenteric Venous Thrombosis – MVT is encountered in the acute form, which commonly presents as bowel infarction, or the chronic form, which may present more insidiously with nonspecific symptoms or esophageal varices in cases with portal vein involvement. Here we will focus on acute MVT. Again looking toward clinical and autopsy data from Malmo, Sweden, study periods from 1970 to 1982 and 2000 to 2006 showed a rising incidence of mesenteric venous thrombosis (MVT) with 2.0 cases per 100,000 person-years in the earlier period as compared to 2.7 cases per 100,000 person-years seen in the latter, this on the basis of 63 (56 % autopsy) and 51 (12 % autopsy) identified MVT cases, respectively [29, 30]. A rise in the use of abdominal imaging has certainly contributed to increased MVT detection as 69 % of patients in the period 2000–2006 were diagnosed with CT scan as compared to 0 % in the earlier period. Even within the period 2000 to 2006, a greater proportion of cases were diagnosed by CT scan in the latter half (2004–2006: $N=10/21$) than in the former (2000–2003: $N=25/30$); $p=0.026$. With an increasing proportion of cases diagnosed by cross-sectional imaging, it is likely that these data represent an increase in detection rather than an increase in true incidence. MVT involved secondary thrombus, or those cases in which an etiologic factor has been identified, in a majority of cases (80 %). As our understanding of congenital and acquired thrombotic states improves, the number of MVT cases attributed to primary thrombus, or those of unidentified etiology, has decreased [31]. Though men and women were equally likely to develop MVT, advancing age was correlated with increased incidence of MVT with septuagenarians having over twice the risk of those aged 60–69 years, 11.3 vs. 4.8 cases per 100,000 person-years, respectively.

Approximately two thirds of these patients ($N = 34/51$) were noted to have either a congenital or acquired thrombophilia with the remainder having either intra-abdominal infection or other pro-thrombotic conditions such as pancreatitis (18 %), post-surgical trauma (8 %), or inflammatory bowel disease (2 %). Rhee et al from the Mayo Clinic published on 72 cases of MVT (57 acute) from 1972 to 1993 with findings largely in agreement with the Swedish data [32]. Similar rates of secondary thrombus (75 %) were seen, and again thrombophilia or prior surgery were among the leading causes of MVT. CT scan was abnormal in all patients with acute MVT who were studied. Though rare, acute MVT diagnosis has increased over time owing to the improved quality and increased use of intra-abdominal vascular imaging.

Nonocclusive Mesenteric Ischemia

As the name would imply, NOMI refers to intestinal gangrene in the setting of patent mesenteric vessels [33]. First described in a 1949 case report from the Massachusetts General Hospital [34], NOMI describes a clinical syndrome comprising a number of entities which share the common pathophysiologic elements of mesenteric vasoconstriction, intestinal hypoxemia, ischemia–reperfusion injury, increased intestinal metabolic demand, and infection [35]. One in 5,000 hospital visits is attributed to NOMI [19] though given its nebulous description and frequent association with other pathologies, the true incidence may be difficult to define. Autopsy data from Sweden by Acosta and colleagues demonstrated an incidence of 2.0 cases per 100,000 person-years for fatal NOMI with incidence in octogenarians noted to increase to 40 cases per 100,000 person-years [36]. Nested case–control comparisons with non-NOMI autopsy patients identified fatal heart failure, history of atrial fibrillation, and recent surgery to be risk factors for fatal NOMI. Mesenteric stenosis also appears to have an association with NOMI as 25 of 62 patients in this series showed SMA stenosis at autopsy, with 14 of those also having celiac stenosis. Yet, importantly, the critical aspect in the development of NOMI is a low flow state, a state that may occur with or without concurrent mesenteric stenosis. Beyond these few epidemiologic studies, data on NOMI are primarily drawn from small case series and case reports relating it to varied conditions associated with either profound isolated vasoconstriction (e.g., cocaine use, digitalis toxicity) or low flow states with or without critical illness and vasopressor support [37–41].

Natural History

Though varying slightly according to etiology, the natural history of AMI, without intervention, follows an almost uniformly fatal progression from bowel infarction to sepsis and death. Even in the setting of operative intervention, outcomes remain poor. Case series prior to the endovascular era, with intervention rates ranging from

63 to 100 %, are confirmatory of this dismal prognosis with 30-day mortality rates for AMI ranging from 32 to 82 % [20, 21, 23–25, 42–45]. Contemporary series suggest that endovascular therapy may improve outcomes with a 30-day mortality rate of 24 % versus 42 % for endovascular versus open revascularization, respectively ($p=0.034$) [46]. However, it must be noted that these data were retrospective and most likely confounded by disease severity as 63 % of the open group underwent bowel resection as compared to 19 % in the endovascular group. A thorough treatment of open versus endovascular treatment for AMI will be presented in Chap. 20. Similarly, NOMI has an extremely poor prognosis though this is in part related to the nature of its association with critical illness in general [35]. In contrast, MVT has a slightly better prognosis than do AMI or NOMI with published reports showing operation for bowel resection in one to two thirds of patients and overall mortality rates of approximately 20 % [20, 30, 47, 48]. On a population level, Lo and colleagues, using the NIS, have shown that in-hospital mortality for AMI regardless of etiology or treatment approach has fallen from 1999 to 2010 [8]. Open repair has shown the most dramatic improvement for in-hospital mortality rate, from 43 % to 33 % over the study period. This was followed by the change seen in in-hospital mortality rate following endovascular revascularization, which has gone from 20 % to 15 %. CDC WONDER data, also reported by Lo et al, have similarly shown a decrease in AMI-related mortality going from 1.5 deaths per 100,000 US persons to 0.6 deaths per 100,000 US persons. Given these population-level figures, it appears that the overall management of AMI including diagnosis and treatment may be improving over time.

Median Arcuate Ligament Syndrome

Epidemiology

Alternately known as celiac artery compression syndrome or Dunbar syndrome, median arcuate ligament syndrome (MALS) refers to chronic, recurrent postprandial abdominal pain due to mesenteric ischemia in the setting of celiac artery compression by the median arcuate ligament (Fig. 4.3). From an anatomic perspective, Lipshutz and colleagues, in a 1917 cadaveric study reporting anatomic variants of the celiac axis in 83 patients, were the first to describe compression of the celiac origin by the diaphragm noting that such a configuration occurred "not infrequently"[49]. Further autopsy study by Derrick et al in 1959 reported that 44 % of unselected patients demonstrated stenosis of the celiac axis origin with half of these having stenosis >50 % [50]. Dunbar and colleagues then associated this anatomic finding with symptomatology when they noted that 15 of 27 patients with an abdominal bruit and unexplained postprandial abdominal pain showed compression of the celiac trunk on angiography [51]. This study as well as others prompted a dedicated autopsy study on the relationship of the celiac axis origin to the median arcuate ligament by Lindner et al who showed that in 75 unselected cadavers, 25

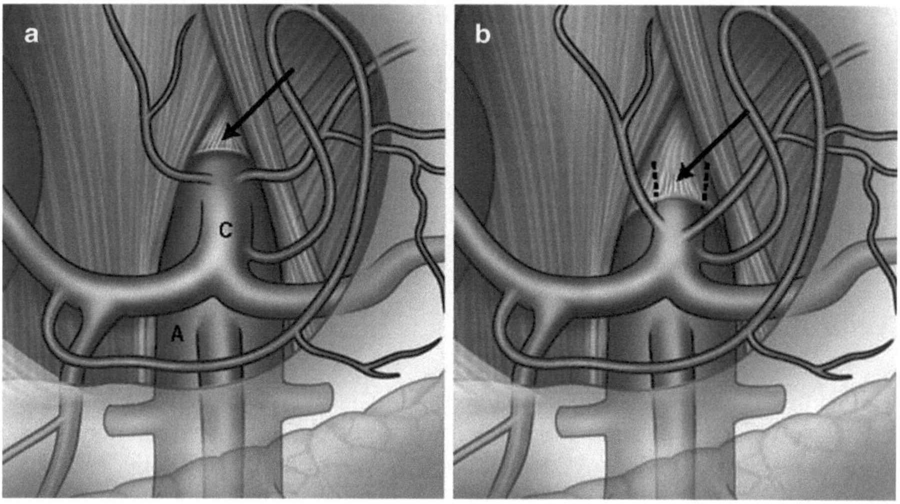

Fig. 4.3 (**a**) Normal relationship of celiac axis with respect to diaphragm. (**b**) Compression of the celiac axis by the median arcuate ligament

had a celiac artery origin cephalad to the median arcuate ligament with this configuration being more prevalent in females than males [52]. Thus, the anatomic conditions under which this pathology occurs have been shown in as many as one third of patients in general cadaveric studies with a preponderance of females showing celiac compression.

However, while cadaveric studies have demonstrated celiac artery compression in up to one third of patients, clinical manifestations of MALS occur much less frequently. Studies examining the correlation of clinical symptoms with anatomic findings have shown that celiac artery compression alone rarely, if ever, yields the symptoms of MALS as the gastroduodenal artery provides adequate collateral flow to the foregut. In fact, a 2001 study by Park and colleagues evaluated the celiac axis origin in 400 consecutive asymptomatic patients undergoing chemoembolization of hepatic tumors to find that 7.3 % ($N=29$) of patients had celiac axis stenosis, 3.5 % ($N=16$) due to median arcuate ligament compression and 2.5 % ($N=10$) of indeterminate etiology [53]. Thus, it is hypothesized that MALS may relate to a neuropathic mechanism secondary to compression of the celiac plexus by the median arcuate ligament. Given that anatomic configuration alone is insufficient to cause clinical symptoms, the association of celiac artery compression and clinical symptoms has been determined by analysis of symptom relief following celiac artery decompression. Reilly et al reported long-term outcomes on 51 highly selected patients undergoing celiac artery decompression with or without celiac artery revascularization [54]. Long-term symptom relief was achieved in 53 % ($N=8/15$) of patients receiving median arcuate ligament release alone and 76 % ($N=22/29$) of patients receiving ligament release with accompanying revascularization. This series, one of the largest published, reinforced a female predilection ($N=39/51$;

77 %) with a mean age of 47 years at time of treatment. MALS has also been reported in the pediatric population with one of the largest series showing a similar proportion of females ($N=42/46$; 91 %) and similar rates of symptom relief following surgery ($N=31/46$; 67 %) [55]. In summary, though population-level data on the incidence of MALS are lacking, case series suggest that MALS is a rare condition to be considered in patients, particularly females, with the appropriate symptoms and anatomy.

Natural History

The natural history of MALS is marked by diagnostic delay given that its mere existence is doubted by some and that it is a diagnosis of exclusion with nonspecific symptoms for the remainder. A contemporary series by Sultan and colleagues demonstrated a mean symptom duration of 34 months prior to diagnosis at a tertiary referral center [56]. Multiple reports have noted patients with MALS to have undergone other, unrelated abdominal procedures such as cholecystectomy, appendectomy, or others in attempts to characterize and/or alleviate abdominal pain [54, 57]. Definitive treatment is surgical, but reports of symptomatic relief have varied widely related to a heterogeneous case mix in many series with a wide variety of abdominal symptoms and often a high incidence of comorbid psychiatric illness [54, 58–64]. Results following surgical intervention will be discussed in greater detail in Chap. 32.

Isolated Mesenteric Artery Dissection

Epidemiology

Mesenteric artery dissection frequently occurs as a complication of abdominal aortic dissection; however, isolated mesenteric artery dissection (IMAD) is quite rare with only 106 total cases of isolated SMA dissection reported as of 2008 [65]. Though population-level data on the incidence of IMAD is unavailable, a flurry of case series in recent years suggests that IMAD diagnosis is increasing due to the widespread use and improving quality of abdominal imaging [66–72]. The vast majority of IMAD cases involve the SMA though reports have described the celiac or other visceral vessels in rare cases [65, 66, 72]. Demonstrating the growing need to better understand IMAD and facilitate its discussion in the literature, Sakamoto and colleagues have proposed a radiology-based, morphologic classification system on the basis of their institutional experience [73]. Pooled data on the 106 cases of isolated SMA dissection reported prior to 2008 show a mean age of 54 years and a 4:1 ratio of male-to-female patients [65]. Epidemiologic data for IMAD is lacking though certain risk factors have been suggested including hypertension, smoking, connective tissue disease, atherosclerosis, trauma, and inflammatory disorders [66]. Fourteen of 17 (82 %) of patients reported by Choi et al were smokers, while

Takayama and colleagues noted 2 of 19 patients to be have connective tissue disorders (systemic sclerosis and Sjogren's syndrome) [66, 72]. Rarer still are cases attributable to SAM as mentioned in the section on CMI. Further investigation will be required to better delineate the true incidence of IMAD and to better characterize the patients affected.

Natural History

The natural history of IMAD has been obscured by its relative rarity and the diverse clinical picture with which it presents. Patients with IMAD may be asymptomatic with dissection discovered incidentally on imaging obtained for another indication, but they may also present with abdominal pain; in either case IMAD has the potential to cause life-threatening mesenteric ischemia. The proportion of symptomatic patients with IMAD has varied significantly between case series ranging from 37 % in a report by Takayama et al to 88 % in a study by Choi and colleagues. However, while the literature clearly advocates for operative intervention in the event of current or impending bowel ischemia, many studies advocate for nonoperative management even in symptomatic patients. One of the largest published series on IMAD evaluates the natural history of 46 patients managed nonoperatively, with ($N=12$) or without ($N=36$) anticoagulation [71]. Only 18 % of the these patients were asymptomatic at presentation, and 79 % of those with pain rated their pain between 7 and 10 out of 10 in severity. At a median follow-up of 23 months, 90 % of patients had relief of abdominal pain with 75 % stating that the pain did not recur. On follow-up CT scan, no patient was found to have progression of disease. A number of other groups also champion a conservative approach when there are no signs of ischemia [66–68]. Jia et al defined SMA lumen compression > 80 %, SMA aneurysm > 2 cm, or bowel ischemia as reasons for endovascular intervention with others safely managed nonoperatively [68]. However, while all patients reported by Park et al demonstrated favorable outcomes with conservative management, Gobble and colleagues described 25 of 56 patients from prior literature in whom nonoperative management failed, and of these, 13 went on to die. IMAD then has been shown to most frequently manifest a benign course well managed with conservative therapy, though vigilance must be maintained given the catastrophic sequelae of unrecognized disease progression.

Mesenteric Aneurysms

Epidemiology

Though autopsy study has detected incidental splenic artery aneurysm in as many as 10 % of patients [74, 75], from a clinical perspective, mesenteric aneurysms are a rare entity whose scarcity has restricted our knowledge to small case series and meta-analyses. A pooled analysis by Shanley et al reviewed the literature from 1970 to 1995 to find only 29 celiac, 52 SMA, and 8 IMA-isolated aneurysms previously published [76, 77]. Further highlighting the particularly rare nature of IMA aneurysms, Edogawa and colleagues went so far as to review all English and Japanese language literature from 1861 to 2012 to still find only 54 cases of IMA aneurysm described [78]. Recognizing that biased conclusions may be drawn from a small sample size, the pooled data do reveal certain epidemiologic themes. Meta-analysis data by Shanley et al showed mean age of presentation for celiac, SMA, and IMA aneurysms to be in the early sixth decade of life with a majority of patients male for each aneurysm type. Early work by Busuttil et al noted visceral artery aneurysms to be multiple in up to a third of cases [79]. Celiac aneurysms were found in association with peripheral aneurysms in 18–67 % of cases [80].

Mesenteric venous aneurysms have also been described in the literature though these are encountered far less frequently than their arterial counterparts. A comprehensive review of the English and French literature by Sfyroeras and colleagues collected data on all mesenteric venous aneurysms reported through 2009 [81]. Approximately one quarter of these ($N=56/198$) involved the SMA or IMA, while the majority involved the intra- or extrahepatic portal veins. Diagnosis was incidental in approximately 40 % of cases with abdominal pain (45 %) or gastrointestinal bleed (7 %) the most common presenting complaints. A majority of patients had either portal hypertension (31 %) or cirrhosis (28 %).

Natural History

Mesenteric arterial aneurysms, according to pooled case report data, present with abdominal symptoms in over 85 % of cases regardless of location (celiac vs. SMA vs. IMA), yet the natural history of these aneurysms varies by location (Fig. 4.4) [76, 77]. The proportion of cases presenting with rupture varies with year of publication as increased utilization of high-resolution imaging has likely facilitated earlier diagnosis. While reports from the 1970s on celiac aneurysm noted a rupture rate greater than 80 % [82], collected reports from 1985 through 1995 observed a rupture rate of only 7 % [77]. In contrast, reports on SMA aneurysms have consistently described a rupture rate approaching 40 % [76, 83]. Eleven total cases of IMA rupture, all published after 2003, have been reported, though IMA aneurysm is so rare that this accounts for 20 % of all cases [78]. As expected, outcomes following aneurysm rupture are extremely poor in each of these series which places a high premium on early recognition and intervention.

Of the cases presented by Sfyroeras and colleagues, mesenteric venous aneurysms were seen to rupture in only 2 % of cases though thrombosis and compression of adjacent structures may also cause significant morbidity. Of the 87 patients for which treatment data were available, 53 were managed expectantly with active surveillance. Over a mean follow-up of 21 months, none of these 53 were taken for

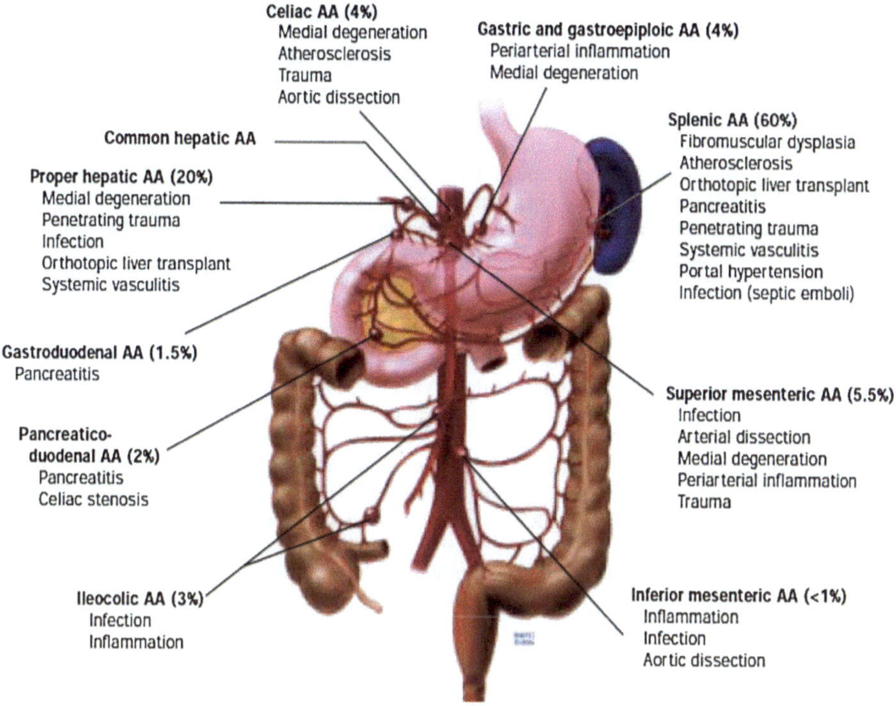

Fig. 4.4 Distribution of splanchnic artery aneurysms (From Pasha et al. [75], with permission)

operation. The remaining patients received a variety of surgical procedures to treat either thrombosis or rupture with specific procedure dictated by the local anatomy and clinical circumstance.

References

1. Wilson DB, et al. Clinical course of mesenteric artery stenosis in elderly Americans. Arch Intern Med. 2006;166(19):2095–100.
2. Reiner L, et al. Injection studies on mesenteric arterial circulation. III. Occlusions without intestinal infarction. Arch Pathol. 1962;73:461–72.
3. Glagov S, Ozoa AK. Significance of the relatively low incidence of atherosclerosis in the pulmonary, renal, and mesenteric arteries. Ann N Y Acad Sci. 1968;149(2):940–55.
4. Koikkalainen K, Laustela E, Tala P. Pathologic study of arteriosclerosis in the coeliac and mesenteric circulation. Ann Chir Gynaecol Fenn. 1968;57(2):234–8.
5. Roobottom CA, Dubbins PA. Significant disease of the celiac and superior mesenteric arteries in asymptomatic patients: predictive value of Doppler sonography. Am J Roentgenol. 1993;161(5):985–8.
6. Hansen KJ, et al. Mesenteric artery disease in the elderly. J Vasc Surg. 2004;40(1):45–52.
7. Oderich GS, et al. Open versus endovascular revascularization for chronic mesenteric ischemia: risk-stratified outcomes. J Vasc Surg. 2009;49(6):1472e3–9e3.

8. Lo RC, et al. The decline of mesenteric ischemia-related mortality in the last decade (in preparation).
9. Schermerhorn ML, et al. Mesenteric revascularization: management and outcomes in the United States, 1988–2006. J Vasc Surg. 2009;50(2):341e1–8e1.
10. Lo RC, et al. Readmissions and reinterventions after revascularization for mesenteric ischemia (in preparation).
11. Oderich GS, Malgor RD, Ricotta 2nd JJ. Open and endovascular revascularization for chronic mesenteric ischemia: tabular review of the literature. Ann Vasc Surg. 2009;23(5):700–12.
12. Oderich GS. Current concepts in the management of chronic mesenteric ischemia. Curr Treat Options Cardiovasc Med. 2010;12(2):117–30.
13. Rits Y, et al. Interventions for mesenteric vasculitis. J Vasc Surg. 2010;51(2):392e2–400e2.
14. Delis KT, Gloviczki P. Middle aortic syndrome: from presentation to contemporary open surgical and endovascular treatment. Perspect Vasc Surg Endovasc Ther. 2005;17(3):187–203.
15. Oderich GS, et al. Vascular abnormalities in patients with neurofibromatosis syndrome type I: clinical spectrum, management, and results. J Vasc Surg. 2007;46(3):475–84.
16. West CA, et al. Middle aortic syndrome: surgical treatment in a child with neurofibromatosis. J Vasc Surg. 2005;42(6):1236.
17. Tameo MN, Dougherty MJ, Calligaro KD. Spontaneous dissection with rupture of the superior mesenteric artery from segmental arterial mediolysis. J Vasc Surg. 2011;53(4):1107–12.
18. Thomas JH, et al. The clinical course of asymptomatic mesenteric arterial stenosis. J Vasc Surg. 1998;27(5):840–4.
19. Stoney RJ, Cunningham CG. Acute mesenteric ischemia. Surgery. 1993;114(3):489–90.
20. Acosta S. Epidemiology of mesenteric vascular disease: clinical implications. Semin Vasc Surg. 2010;23(1):4–8.
21. Endean ED, et al. Surgical management of thrombotic acute intestinal ischemia. Ann Surg. 2001;233(6):801–8.
22. Acosta S, et al. Incidence of acute thrombo-embolic occlusion of the superior mesenteric artery–a population-based study. Eur J Vasc Endovasc Surg. 2004;27(2):145–50.
23. Park WM, et al. Contemporary management of acute mesenteric ischemia: Factors associated with survival. J Vasc Surg. 2002;35(3):445–52.
24. Edwards MS, et al. Acute occlusive mesenteric ischemia: surgical management and outcomes. Ann Vasc Surg. 2003;17(1):72–9.
25. Batellier J, Kieny R. Superior mesenteric artery embolism: eighty-two cases. Ann Vasc Surg. 1990;4(2):112–6.
26. Wyers MC. Acute mesenteric ischemia: diagnostic approach and surgical treatment. Semin Vasc Surg. 2010;23(1):9–20.
27. Acosta S, et al. Clinical implications for the management of acute thromboembolic occlusion of the superior mesenteric artery: autopsy findings in 213 patients. Ann Surg. 2005;241(3):516–22.
28. Fuster V, et al. ACC/AHA/ESC guidelines for the management of patients with atrial fibrillation: executive summary a report of the American College of Cardiology/American Heart Association Task Force on Practice Guidelines and the European Society of Cardiology Committee for Practice Guidelines and Policy Conferences (Committee to Develop Guidelines for the Management of Patients with Atrial Fibrillation) Developed in Collaboration with the North American Society of Pacing and Electrophysiology. Circulation. 2001;104(17):2118–50.
29. Acosta S, et al. Mesenteric venous thrombosis with transmural intestinal infarction: a population-based study. J Vasc Surg. 2005;41(1):59–63.
30. Acosta S, et al. Epidemiology, risk and prognostic factors in mesenteric venous thrombosis. Br J Surg. 2008;95(10):1245–51.
31. Kumar S, Sarr MG, Kamath PS. Mesenteric venous thrombosis. N Engl J Med. 2001;345(23):1683–8.
32. Rhee RY, et al. Mesenteric venous thrombosis: still a lethal disease in the 1990s. J Vasc Surg. 1994;20(5):688–97.

33. Haglund U, Lundgren O. Non-occlusive acute intestinal vascular failure. Br J Surg. 1979;66(3):155–8.
34. Case 35082. New Engl J Med. 1949; 240(8):308–10.
35. Wilcox MG, et al. Current theories of pathogenesis and treatment of nonocclusive mesenteric ischemia. Dig Dis Sci. 1995;40(4):709–16.
36. Acosta S, et al. Fatal nonocclusive mesenteric ischaemia: population-based incidence and risk factors. J Intern Med. 2006;259(3):305–13.
37. Bjorck M, Wanhainen A. Nonocclusive mesenteric hypoperfusion syndromes: recognition and treatment. Semin Vasc Surg. 2010;23(1):54–64.
38. Sudhakar CB, et al. Mesenteric ischemia secondary to cocaine abuse: case reports and literature review. Am J Gastroenterol. 1997;92(6):1053–4.
39. Groesdonk HV, et al. Risk factors for nonocclusive mesenteric ischemia after elective cardiac surgery. J Thorac Cardiovasc Surg. 2013;145(6):1603–10.
40. Qureshi SS, et al. Fatal non-occlusive mesenteric ischemia after esophagectomy. J Cancer Res Ther. 2010;6(1):112–3.
41. Yu CC, et al. Factors associated with mortality from non-occlusive mesenteric ischemia in dialysis patients. Ren Fail. 2009;31(9):802–6.
42. Wadman M, Syk I, Elmstahl S. Survival after operations for ischaemic bowel disease. Eur J Surg. 2000;166(11):872–7.
43. Mamode N, Pickford I, Leiberman P. Failure to improve outcome in acute mesenteric ischaemia: seven-year review. Eur J Surg. 1999;165(3):203–8.
44. Jrvinen O, et al. Acute intestinal ischaemia. A review of 214 cases. Ann Chir Gynaecol. 1994;83(1):22–5.
45. Clavien PA, Muller C, Harder F. Treatment of mesenteric infarction. Br J Surg. 1987;74(6): 500–3.
46. Block TA, Acosta S, Bjorck M. Endovascular and open surgery for acute occlusion of the superior mesenteric artery. J Vasc Surg. 2010;52(4):959–66.
47. Morasch MD, et al. Mesenteric venous thrombosis: a changing clinical entity. J Vasc Surg. 2001;34(4):680–4.
48. Brunaud L, et al. Acute mesenteric venous thrombosis: case for nonoperative management. J Vasc Surg. 2001;34(4):673–9.
49. Lipshutz B. A composite study of the coeliac axis artery. Ann Surg. 1917;65(2):159–69.
50. Derrick JR, Pollard HS, Moore RM. The pattern of arteriosclerotic narrowing of the celiac and superior mesenteric arteries. Ann Surg. 1959;149(5):684–9.
51. Dunbar JD, et al. Compression of the celiac trunk and abdominal angina. Am J Roentgenol Radium Ther Nucl Med. 1965;95(3):731–44.
52. Lindner HH, Kemprud E. A clinicoanatomical study of the arcuate ligament of the diaphragm. Arch Surg. 1971;103(5):600–5.
53. Park CM, et al. Celiac axis stenosis: incidence and etiologies in asymptomatic individuals. Korean J Radiol. 2001;2(1):8–13.
54. Reilly LM, et al. Late results following operative repair for celiac artery compression syndrome. J Vasc Surg. 1985;2(1):79–91.
55. Mak GZ, et al. Median arcuate ligament syndrome in the pediatric population. J Pediatr Surg. 2013;48(11):2261–70.
56. Sultan S, et al. Eight years experience in the management of median arcuate ligament syndrome by decompression, celiac ganglion sympathectomy, and selective revascularization. Vasc Endovascular Surg. 2013;47(8):614–9.
57. Watson WC, Sadikali F. Celiac axis compression: experience with 20 patients and a critical appraisal of the syndrome. Ann Intern Med. 1977;86(3):278–84.
58. Kernohan RM, et al. Further evidence supporting the existence of the celiac artery compression syndrome. Arch Surg. 1985;120(9):1072–6.
59. Ghosn PB, et al. Celiac compression syndrome. Can J Surg. 1982;25(4):377–9.
60. Kokotsakis JN, et al. Celiac artery compression syndrome. Cardiovasc Surg. 2000;8(3): 219–22.

61. Daskalakis MK. Celiac axis compression syndrome. Int Surg. 1982;67(4 Suppl):442–4.
62. Lord RS, Tracy GD. Coeliac artery compression. Br J Surg. 1980;67(8):590–3.
63. Muqeetadnan M, et al. Celiac artery compression syndrome. Case Rep Gastrointest Med. 2013;2013:934052.
64. Williams S, Gillespie P, Little JM. Celiac axis compression syndrome: factors predicting a favorable outcome. Surgery. 1985;98(5):879–87.
65. Gobble RM, et al. Endovascular treatment of spontaneous dissections of the superior mesenteric artery. J Vasc Surg. 2009;50(6):1326–32.
66. Choi JY, Kwon OJ. Approaches to the management of spontaneous isolated visceral artery dissection. Ann Vasc Surg. 2013;27(6):750–7.
67. Cho BS, et al. Treatment guidelines for isolated dissection of the superior mesenteric artery based on follow-up CT findings. Eur J Vasc Endovasc Surg. 2011;41(6):780–5.
68. Jia ZZ, et al. Initial and middle-term results of treatment for symptomatic spontaneous isolated dissection of superior mesenteric artery. Eur J Vasc Endovasc Surg. 2013;45(5):502–8.
69. Jung SC, et al. Spontaneous dissection of the splanchnic arteries: CT findings, treatment, and outcome. Am J Roentgenol. 2013;200(1):219–25.
70. Min SI, et al. Current strategy for the treatment of symptomatic spontaneous isolated dissection of superior mesenteric artery. J Vasc Surg. 2011;54(2):461–6.
71. Park YJ, et al. Natural history of spontaneous isolated superior mesenteric artery dissection derived from follow-up after conservative treatment. J Vasc Surg. 2011;54(6):1727–33.
72. Takayama T, et al. Isolated spontaneous dissection of the splanchnic arteries. J Vasc Surg. 2008;48(2):329–33.
73. Sakamoto I, et al. Imaging appearances and management of isolated spontaneous dissection of the superior mesenteric artery. Eur J Radiol. 2007;64(1):103–10.
74. Bedford PD, Lodge B. Aneurysm of the splenic artery. Gut. 1960;1:312–20.
75. Pasha SF, et al. Splanchnic artery aneurysms. Mayo Clin Proc. 2007;82(4):472–9.
76. Shanley CJ, Shah NL, Messina LM. Uncommon splanchnic artery aneurysms: pancreaticoduodenal, gastroduodenal, superior mesenteric, inferior mesenteric, and colic. Ann Vasc Surg. 1996;10(5):506–15.
77. Shanley CJ, Shah NL, Messina LM. Common splanchnic artery aneurysms: splenic, hepatic, and celiac. Ann Vasc Surg. 1996;10(3):315–22.
78. Edogawa S, et al. Inferior mesenteric artery aneurysm: case report and literature review. Ann Vasc Dis. 2013;6(1):98–101.
79. Busuttil RW, Brin BJ. The diagnosis and management of visceral artery aneurysms. Surgery. 1980;88(5):619–24.
80. Stone WM, et al. Celiac arterial aneurysms: a critical reappraisal of a rare entity. Arch Surg. 2002;137(6):670–4.
81. Sfyroeras GS, et al. Visceral venous aneurysms: clinical presentation, natural history and their management: a systematic review. Eur J Vasc Endovasc Surg. 2009;38(4):498–505.
82. Stanley JC, et al. Clinical importance and management of splanchnic artery aneurysms. J Vasc Surg. 1986;3(5):836–40.
83. Stone WM, et al. Superior mesenteric artery aneurysms: is presence an indication for intervention? J Vasc Surg. 2002;36(2):234–7; discussion 237.

Chapter 5
Duplex Ultrasound of the Mesenteric Vessels

Thanila A. Macedo and Leonardo Reis de Souza

Angiography has been considered the gold standard technique for the diagnosis of chronic mesenteric ischemia. Due to its invasive nature and improvements in noninvasive diagnostic studies, angiography is currently reserved for patients with classic signs and symptoms of chronic mesenteric ischemia who have planned endovascular or open reconstruction. Among patients with atypical symptoms, it is not unusual to have significant delay in diagnosis [1]. Since the first published evaluation of the splanchnic human vasculature by duplex scanning in 1984 [2], the technique brought up intense interest in the medical community, mainly due to its noninvasive characteristic but also because it provides hemodynamic and anatomic information. In the last decades, duplex ultrasound has proved to be an accurate method to detect stenosis and is typically the first imaging study obtained in the evaluation of patients with suspected mesenteric artery occlusive disease.

Technique

Evaluation of the splanchnic circulation can be technically challenging. In experienced hands, the average time for exam completion is around 15–20 min. Besides experience and knowledge of vascular anatomy, some factors can potentially

T.A. Macedo, MD (✉)
Department of Radiology, Mayo Clinic, Rochester, MN, USA
e-mail: Macedo.Thanila@mayo.edu

L.R. de Souza, MD
Division of Vascular Surgery, Mayo Clinic, Rochester, MN, USA

Masters Degree Program from the Department of Surgery,
Universidade Federal do Rio Grande do Sul, Porto Alegre, Brazil
e-mail: reissouza@gmail.com

G.S. Oderich (ed.), *Mesenteric Vascular Disease*,
DOI 10.1007/978-1-4939-1847-8_5

contribute to increased difficulty. Obesity, previous abdominal surgery, dressings, anatomic variants, respiratory motion, and excessive bowel gas are the main factors contributing to a suboptimal examination. Modern and efficient equipment, an experienced sonographer, and appropriate patient selection are keys to a successful imaging.

The examination is performed in fasting state (at least 6 h) to minimize bowel gas and also because the established criteria used to diagnose mesenteric artery disease have been based on fasting velocities. Studies showed little or no improvement in accuracy when food challenges were used to detect stenosis. Furthermore, it is important to recognize that much of these patients are classically afraid of eating, due to intense pain [3, 4]. The postprandial state is induced by an 8-oz protein calorie supplement, and the exam is performed after 30 min [5].

The examination is typically performed with the patient in supine position. When bowel gas prevents adequate visualization of the vessels, patients may be turned to a lateral oblique decubitus position, which may provide a better window. Patient cooperation with breath hold is critical to record adequate Doppler spectral samples [6].

At the Mayo Clinic, we most commonly use the 1–5 MHz curved array or 9 MHz linear array transducers. Caution should be taken to keep the Doppler angle of insonation, ideally <60°. The variations of peak systolic velocity measurement as a function of angle of insonation is well documented [7]. This should be kept in mind especially in follow-up comparison examinations where similar technique should be used. Initially, the abdominal aorta is identified in transverse and sagittal planes, paying attention to diameter and atherosclerotic involvement. Spectral Doppler waveform is obtained with peak systolic velocity (PSV) and end-diastolic velocity (EDV) measurements in the area of mesenteric vessels origin. Color Doppler is used to identify the arteries and to guide sample volume placement for spectral Doppler analysis (Fig. 5.1). The superior mesenteric artery (SMA) and the celiac axis (CA) are best identified in the sagittal plane, arising from the anterior aspect of the aorta. The CA branches (hepatic and splenic) are best viewed in transverse orientation. Velocity measurements are obtained at the origin of the vessel and a few centimeters within the celiac artery during tidal breathing; specifically, measurements are obtained in deep inspiration and expiration for evaluation of median arcuate ligament compression syndrome (Fig. 5.2). Spectral Doppler sampling with PSV and EDV measurements are obtained at the origin and at the proximal, mid and distal SMA. Shortly after the origin, the SMA will curve inferiorly and course almost parallel to the aorta for several centimeters where it may be difficult to obtain a Doppler angle of <60°. Whenever possible, the inferior mesenteric artery (IMA) should be also evaluated. It is best identified using the transverse plane, arising from the anterolateral aspect of the aorta, generally a few centimeters above the aortic bifurcation. Measurements of PSV and EDV are obtained at the origin and distally as far as visible. Generally, only a short segment of the IMA near the origin is visualized, and because of its inferior trajectory nearly parallel to the aorta, optimal angle of insonation may not be obtained.

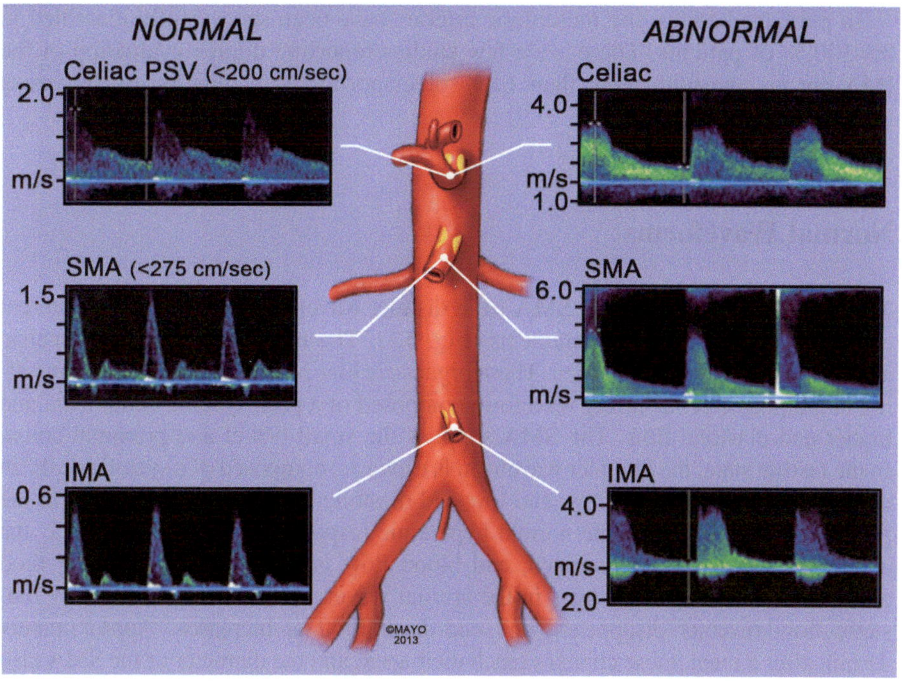

Fig. 5.1 Normal and abnormal mesenteric arteries' waveforms: The normal celiac artery has a low-resistance waveform. A peak systolic velocity of 2.5 m/s or greater is indicative of a significant stenosis. The normal superior mesenteric artery has a high-resistance waveform in the postprandial state and a peak systolic velocity of <2.75 m/s. The inferior mesenteric artery has a waveform similar to the superior mesenteric artery with high resistance. A peak systolic velocity of 2.75 m/s or greater is suggestive of a significant stenosis

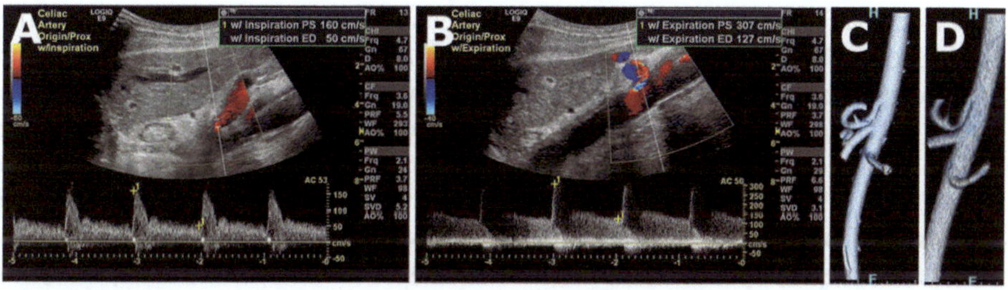

Fig. 5.2 Doppler ultrasound of the celiac artery in inspiration (**a**) reveals normal peak systolic velocity. During inspiration, the celiac artery moves caudally, and the median arcuate ligament moves anteriorly. With expiration, the opposite occurs, resulting in compression of the artery and elevated velocities (**b**). Volume rendered computed tomography images in inspiration (**c**) and expiration (**d**) are also elucidative.

In published series, the mesenteric arteries have been successfully identified in 85–100 % of patients. There are a few studies reporting duplex evaluation of the IMA but no one with more than 14 % of inappropriate evaluation of the vessel [7–10].

Normal Waveforms

The normal celiac artery and SMA have distinct waveforms reflecting the different end-organ blood supply requirements (Fig. 5.1). The major branches of the celiac artery supply the liver and spleen. These organs are low-resistance arterial beds, resulting in a biphasic celiac artery waveform composed of a peak systolic component and higher end-diastolic flow. The SMA supplies the small bowel and proximal colon. In the fasting state, the Doppler waveform is triphasic, composed of a systolic peak, an early diastolic reversal of flow, and low end-diastolic flow approaching zero. In the postprandial state, due to the normal hyperemic response described in Chap. 2, the end-organ resistance is decreased, and blood flow is increased for adequate food absorption, resulting in changes in the arterial waveform. PSV increases, early diastolic flow reversal disappears, and end-diastolic flow increases. Approximately 45 min after a meal, these changes reach their apex, and the diameter of the SMA also increases by a mean of 112 %. On the other hand, the CA waveform remains similar to the fasting state, basically because of the unchanged demands of the liver and spleen [11]. The Doppler arterial waveform is also affected by food composition, with mixed calorie meals resulting in the most pronounced change [12]. A low-resistance waveform can also be a normal finding if there is a replaced or accessory hepatic artery originating from the SMA. Although IMA examination can be difficult because of small size and posterior location, this vessel can be identified in up to 89 % of patients by skilled sonographers [8]. The IMA supplies the distal colon and upper rectum and therefore has a high-resistance waveform, similar to the triphasic SMA waveform.

Anatomic variations in the origin of the hepatic arteries, which occur in approximately 20 % of the population, can result in changes in the SMA waveform in the fasting state. The most common variation described above is a replaced right hepatic artery originating from the SMA, which occurs in up to 17 % of individuals. In these cases, the typical waveform has a lower-resistance pattern in the SMA, resembling the waveform of a CA. A normal PSV and the finding of a non-turbulent waveform with a clear systolic window favor the diagnosis of an anatomic anomaly as opposed to a stenotic lesion [1].

There is a paucity of data on duplex evaluation of the IMA; consequently its normal and pathological characteristics are not well described. Typically the IMA waveform shows a high-resistance pattern, similar to what is observed for the SMA during fasting state but with a higher resistance index [10]. The IMA is usually not affected by meals unless this vessel provides important compensatory collateral flow to the SMA [5].

Detection of Stenosis

In 1991, Moneta and colleagues reported the first retrospective study evaluating the role of duplex scanning of splanchnic arteries to identify SMA and CA stenosis (Fig. 5.3) in patients undergoing abdominal aortography [13]. In that study, a PSV of >275 cm/s for the SMA and >200 cm/s for the CA accurately detected stenosis >70 %. It also suggested that PSV was a better predictor than EDV and that an aorto-mesenteric ratio had no significant improvement in the ability to diagnose a significant stenosis. A few years later, the same group validated their findings in a prospective study of 100 patients who underwent duplex ultrasound and abdominal aortography, including 13 patients who had investigation for chronic mesenteric ischemia. Duplex ultrasound was able to adequately visualize the SMA in 92 % and the CA in 83 % of cases. Using the previously described PSV criteria, these authors found a sensitivity of 92 %, specificity of 96 %, positive predictive value (PPV) of 80 %, negative predictive value (NPV) of 99 %, and accuracy of 96 % to diagnose 70 % or greater stenosis. For the CA, the same parameters were 87, 80, 63, 94, and 82 %, respectively [14]. At the Mayo Clinic, we use the same criteria for the SMA but have adjusted the celiac artery criteria to 250 cm/s to improve diagnostic accuracy.

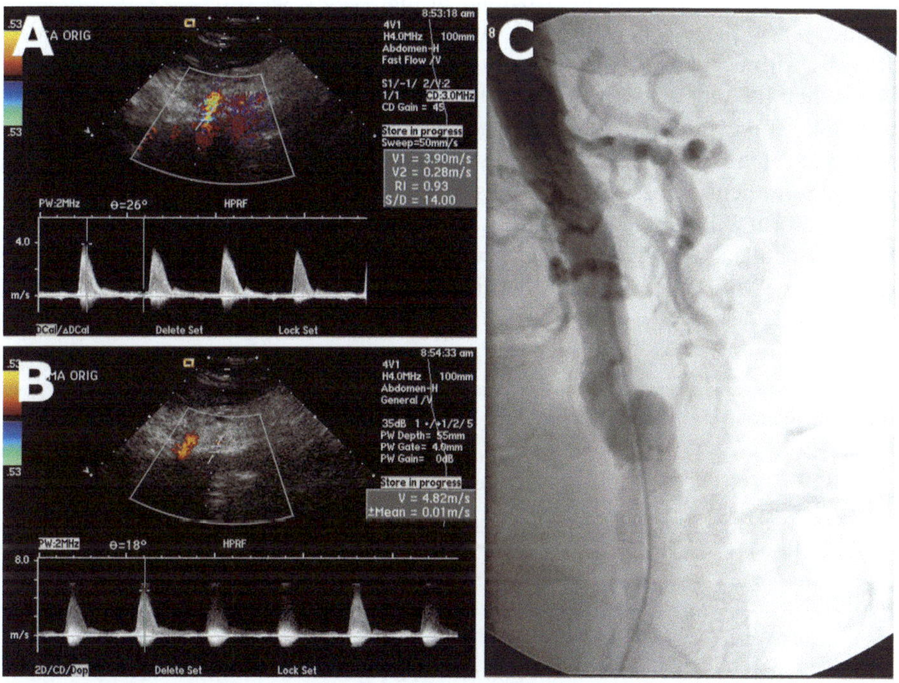

Fig. 5.3 Doppler ultrasound shows elevated peak systolic velocity at the origin of the celiac artery (**a**) and superior mesenteric artery (**b**) indicative of a significant stenosis. Angiogram correlation confirms significant stenosis of the celiac and superior mesenteric arteries (**c**)

Other velocity criterion has been proposed in the literature. In 1991, Bowersox and colleagues reported a retrospective study which identified EDV > 45 cm/s as the most accurate predictor of a >50 % SMA stenosis. [15]. Later, the same group published a prospective study validating these findings. An EDV of >45 cm/s had a sensitivity of 90 %, specificity of 91 %, PPV of 90 %, NPV of 91 %, and accuracy of 91 %. The same parameters for a >50 % stenosis in CA are, respectively, 93, 100, 100, 89, and 95 %.

More recently, AbuRahma and colleagues published results of a retrospective study of 153 patients who underwent angiography to evaluate for chronic mesenteric ischemia. In that study, the best PSV criteria to diagnose >50 and>70 % SMA stenosis were 295 cm/s (accuracy of 88 %) and 400 cm/s (accuracy of 85 %), respectively. The best PSV threshold to identify >50 and >70 % celiac stenosis were 240 cm/s (accuracy of 86 %) and 320 cm/s (accuracy of 85 %), respectively. Differences in velocity criteria in these studies need to be interpreted carefully given distinct methodology, equipment, and patient demographics [16].

Only a few studies have validated the criteria for IMA stenosis. The first one was published by Pellerito and colleagues in 2009, where he proposed the most accurate criteria was a PSV higher than 200 cm/s (specificity of 90 %, specificity of 97 %, PPV of 90 %, and NPV of 97 %) to diagnose >50 % stenosis [9].

AbuRahma and colleagues reported duplex evaluation of 85 patients with suspected chronic mesenteric ischemia. In that report, an IMA PSV of 250 cm/s predicted >50 % stenosis with 95 % of accuracy or 270 cm/s could predict a >70 % stenosis with accuracy of 92 %. In an ROC analysis, none of the criterion proved better than the others to diagnose >50 % stenosis [17]. Others have advocated the use of a test meal in cases where higher velocities are believed to occur for reasons other than stenosis, such as stented vessels. It is expected that, if a stenosis exists, a pressure gradient across the stenosis should develop, and consequent damping of the waveform will be detected. The CA and the IMA must be minimal or not affected by food challenge [5] The data concerning previous studies and the established criteria for SMA, CA, and IMA stenosis are summarized in Tables 5.1, 5.2, and 5.3.

Table 5.1 Most accurate cutoff points to diagnose stenosis of the superior mesenteric artery in different studies

Studies	Design	Stenosis grade	Cutoff (cm/s)	Sb (%)	St (%)	PPV (%)	NPV (%)	Ac (%)
Moneta (1993) [14]	Prospective	≥70 %	PSV ≥ 275	92	96	80	99	96
Zwolak (1998) [1]	Prospective	≥50 %	PSV ≥ 300	60	100	100	73	81
AbuRahma (2012) [16]	Retrospective	≥70 %	PSV ≥ 400	72	93	84	85	85
			PSV ≥ 410	68	95	88	84	85
			EDV ≥ 70	65	95	89	82	84
		≥50 %	PSV ≥ 295	87	89	91	84	88
			EDV ≥ 45	79	79	84	72	79

Sb sensitivity, *St* specificity, *PPV* positive predictive value, *NPV* negative predictive value, *Ac* accuracy, *PSV* peak systolic velocity, *EDV* end-diastolic velocity

Table 5.2 Most accurate cutoff points to diagnose stenosis of the celiac artery in different studies

Studies	Design	Stenosis grade	Cutoff (cm/s)	Sb (%)	St (%)	PPV (%)	NPV (%)	Ac (%)
Moneta (1993) [14]	Prospective	≥70 %	PSV ≥ 200	87	80	63	94	82
Zwolak (1998) [1]	Prospective	≥50 %	PSV ≥ 200	93	94	96	88	93
			EDV ≥ 55	93	100	100	89	95
AbuRahma (2012) [16]	Retrospective	≥70 %	PSV ≥ 320	80	89	84	86	85
			EDV ≥ 100	58	91	83	74	77
			EDV ≥ 110	56	92	85	74	77
			EDV ≥ 120	53	95	89	73	77
		≥50 %	PSV ≥ 240	87	83	93	72	86
			EDV ≥ 40	84	48	80	54	73
			EDV ≥ 45	80	58	82	53	73

Sb sensitivity, *St* specificity, *PPV* positive predictive value, *NPV* negative predictive value, *Ac* accuracy, *PSV* peak systolic velocity, *EDV* end-diastolic velocity

Table 5.3 Most accurate cutoff points to diagnose stenosis of the inferior mesenteric artery in different studies

Studies	Design	Stenosis grade	Cutoff[a]	Sb (%)	St (%)	PPV (%)	NPV (%)	Ac (%)
Pellerito (2009) [9]	Retrospective	≥ 50 %	PSV ≥ 200	90	97	90	97	95
			EDV ≥ 25	40	91	57	83	79
			MAR ≥ 2.5	80	88	67	93	86
AbuRahma (2012) [17]	Retrospective	≥ 50 %	PSV ≥ 250	90	96	90	96	95
			PSV ≥ 260	85	98	94	95	95
			EDV ≥ 80	60	100	100	83	96
			EDV ≥ 80	60	100	100	83	96
			MAR ≥ 4	75	100	100	92	93
			MAR ≥ 4.5	75	100	100	92	93

Sb sensitivity, *St* specificity, *PPV* positive predictive value, *NPV* negative predictive value, *Ac* accuracy, *PSV* peak systolic velocity, *EDV* end-diastolic velocity, *MAR* mesenteric/aortic velocity ratio
[a]PSV and EDV in cm/s; MAR is a ratio

Intraoperative Imaging

The main cause of early failure of arterial reconstructions is technical imperfection. Acute thrombosis of the mesenteric vessels is usually a life-threatening event, resulting in bowel infarction and its drastic consequences. Intraoperative duplex scanning emerges as a suitable option, providing anatomic and hemodynamic information with high accuracy. One of the first attempts to demonstrate the utility of the technique was published in 1987, by Okuhn and colleagues [18], and since then it has gained considerable interest.

In our institution, after the completion of the revascularization, a staff radiologist performs the intraoperative duplex ultrasound with assistance of an ultrasound technician. A 8–18 MHz linear probe is placed in a sterile plastic sheath previously filled with sterile acoustic gel. Sterile gel or saline solution is used for acoustic coupling between the probe and the vessel. Grayscale and color Doppler images are obtained in the native vessels proximal and distal to the revascularization, in the anastomosis, and in the conduct.

A normal exam is one where no technical defects are identified, waveforms have a normal expected appearance, and velocities are within normal range. Abnormal findings are divided into minor and major defects. Minor defects include residual plaque, small intimal flap, and graft kinks, which do not result in significant hemodynamic changes and are not necessarily repaired. Major defects (Fig. 5.4) require immediate revision and include residual stenosis, thrombus, larger intimal flap, dissection, and bypass graft kinks, which result in significant hemodynamic changes and are frequently corrected [19, 20].

Oderich and colleagues retrospectively reported their experience with this routine in 2003 [19]. The incidence of minor defects was 6.6 % and major defects 8.4 %. Major defects included severe residual stenosis [4], thrombus [2], kink [2], bidirectional flow [1], and intimal flap [1] and were promptly revised. One dissection was detected after revision and was treated again. Patients with persistent abnormal ultrasounds had increased risk of graft-related complications (45.5 % vs. 10.5 %; $p=0.01$), early graft thrombosis (11.7 % vs. 0.97 %; $p=0.04$), graft-related death (27.3 % vs. 3.5 %; $p=0.02$), and reintervention (17.6 % vs. 3.9 %).

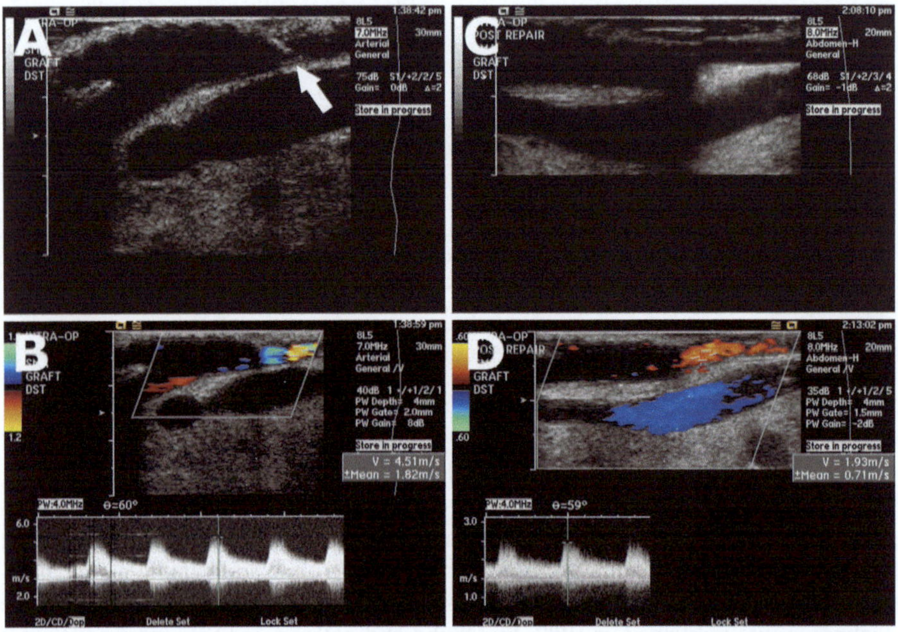

Fig. 5.4 Intraoperative ultrasound of a supraceliac bifurcated aorta to celiac and superior mesenteric artery bypass graft: Grayscale longitudinal image at the distal anastomosis reveals a linear filling defect (**a**, *arrow*). Spectral Doppler waveform confirms hemodynamic disturbance with elevated velocity >4 m/s (**b**). Post revision image reveals resolution of intimal flap and normalization of velocity (**c** and **d**)

Post-intervention Imaging

It is well known that clinical follow-up by itself has a sensitivity of as low as 33 % to predict graft occlusion [21]. This finding obviates the usefulness of a complementary imaging examination, which can detect a threat to the revascularization and prompt intervention to promote maintenance of primary-assisted patency. Unfortunately, there is no consensus on Duplex criteria to define significant recurrent stenosis that needs reintervention.

Prior to the examination, review of surgical notes or procedure report to clarify the type of intervention performed is critical for adequate imaging. Evaluation should include inflow and outflow arteries, anastomosis, and graft or stent.

There is no established criterion to diagnose recurrent stenosis in mesenteric bypass grafts. In our practice, we typically use the same threshold that is applied for native vessels (Fig. 5.5). Liem and colleagues showed their results in duplex scanning follow-up of visceral bypass procedures where ultrasound surveillance led to one reintervention due to stenosis at proximal anastomosis but failed to predict two graft occlusions [22]. An important observation was the finding that the mean PSV generally remains stable over time.

There is some evidence that the established duplex criterion that is used to diagnose stenosis in native arteries may overestimate stenosis rates in stented vessels [23, 24]. This has been more extensively studied in the carotid arteries. One of the possible explanations is that the stent may reduce vessel wall compliance, resulting in higher velocities, even when no narrowing is detected [5]. A retrospective study by Mitchell and colleagues compared mean PSV before and after stenting of the SMA and found post-stenting PSVs higher than 275 cm/s, despite reduction in

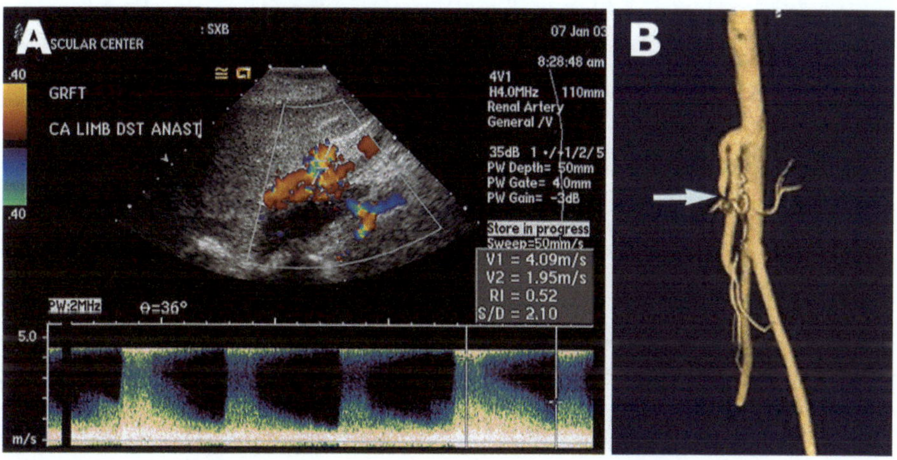

Fig. 5.5 Surveillance Doppler ultrasound of a supraceliac bifurcated aorta to celiac and superior mesenteric artery bypass graft: Longitudinal view of the distal celiac limb anastomosis reveals elevated peak systolic velocity with turbulent flow indicative of significant stenosis (**a**). Computed tomography angiography with volume-rendered 3D reconstructed image confirmed a severe stenosis at the distal anastomosis (**b**)

pressure gradients and satisfactory arteriographic image [25]. Similar findings were published by Baker et al. [23].

In our experience, we have found optimal criteria to identify 50 % or greater stenosis in stented superior mesenteric artery to be PSV of 350 cm/s (100 % sensitivity, 76 % specificity and 79 % accuracy) and in the celiac artery 270 cm/s (100 % sensitivity, 77 % specificity and 80 % accuracy). This is similar to the findings reported by AbuRahma and colleagues, who proposed a PSV over 325 cm/s to detect>50 % stenosis in stented SMA (89 % of sensitivity, 100 % of specificity, 91 % of accuracy) and 274 cm/s in the celiac artery (96 % of sensitivity, 86 % of specificity, 93 % of accuracy) [24]. Interestingly, in our experience, the majority of patients without significant (<50 %) in-stent stenosis had velocities in the normal range, with a mean stented superior mesenteric artery PSV of 260 cm/s.

An important aspect to consider when evaluating post-stent examinations is stability over time. An exam shortly after the procedure is helpful to establish a baseline, which serves for comparison with future follow-up studies. Although it has been suggested a potential role for meal tests to help differentiate elevated velocities related to stenosis or not in stented mesenteric arteries [5], to this date there is no convincing literature that it is helpful. Given the limitations of available studies and controversy regarding optimal criteria to identify in-stent restenosis, it is prudent to use caution interpreting elevated velocities on duplex ultrasound examinations (Fig. 5.6).

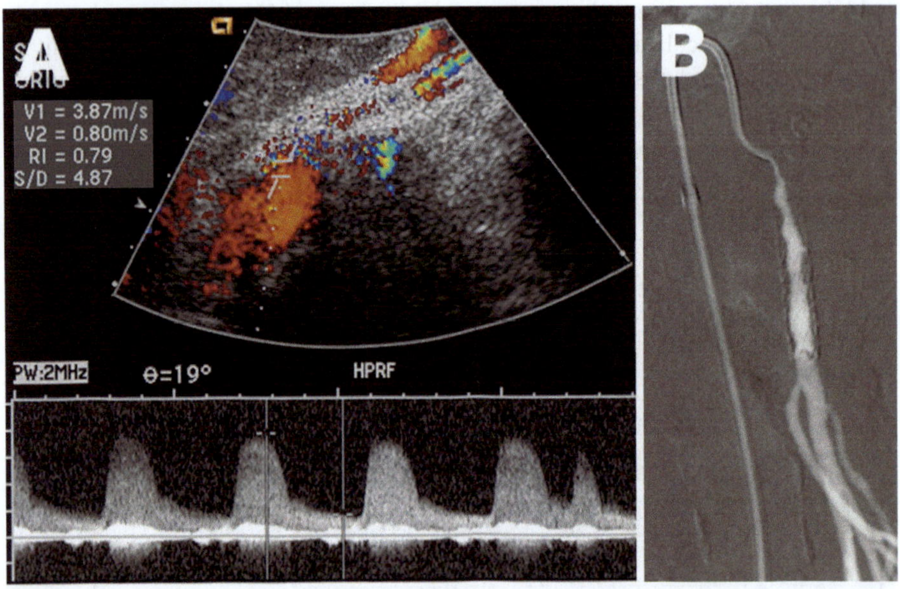

Fig. 5.6 Surveillance Doppler ultrasound of a stented superior mesenteric artery: Longitudinal view of the origin of the superior mesenteric artery reveals elevated peak systolic velocity with turbulent flow indicative of significant stenosis (**a**). Selective angiogram confirmed a severe in-stent stenosis (**b**)

Other Applications

Median Arcuate Ligament Syndrome

Median arcuate ligament compression syndrome (Fig. 5.2) remains a controversial entity. These patients often present with abdominal pain, which is believed to be related to compression of the celiac artery by the median arcuate ligament of the diaphragm. During inspiration, the celiac artery moves caudally, and the median arcuate ligament moves ventrally, which minimizes compression. During expiration, the opposite happens which results in maximal vessel compression. The questionable clinical significance of this entity is largely supported by the fact that a significant number of individuals in the general population have asymptomatic celiac axis compression [26]. Furthermore, although immediate relief has been widely reported with surgical decompression, the long-term success is poor with recurrence rates in the range of 50–83 %. There is a great deal of debate on the pathophysiology of this syndrome with respect to ischemia, steal phenomena, or ganglionic compression of the arterial adventitia causing pain.

Irrespective of these controversies, duplex ultrasound has been widely applied to screen patients with suspected median arcuate ligament syndrome. The variations in celiac artery compression related to respiration seen in celiac compression syndrome can be well documented with duplex ultrasound. Findings include a significant change in PSV between inspiration and expiration, associated with elevated PSV on expiration (Fig. 5.2). At times, the velocity during inspiration remains above the threshold for significant stenosis indicating a degree of fixed stenosis, which can develop over time. Commonly, another imaging modality such as computed tomography angiography (CTA) or magnetic resonance angiography (MRA) is used to anatomically delineate and confirm the diagnosis (see Chap. 7). Careful interpretation of the ultrasound findings seems prudent; it must be understood that respiratory changes in PSV are seen in patients with celiac compression syndrome but can also be seen in normal individuals. Clinical presentation and thorough evaluation are necessary to establish this diagnosis.

Acute Mesenteric Ischemia

Although duplex ultrasound has been obtained in patients with suspected acute intestinal ischemia, its applicability is limited, and it cannot be recommended as a test of choice in this setting [27, 28]. The last updated ACCF/AHA guideline for patients with peripheral arterial disease, published in 2013, considers duplex ultrasound as not an appropriate diagnostic tool for acute mesenteric ischemia, strongly not recommending its use [29].

Inflammatory Bowel Disease

Recent reports have raised interest in flow patterns at the splanchnic vessels to identify activity of Crohn's disease. These studies have shown that patients with active Crohn's often have hyperdynamic mesenteric circulation, which can be demonstrated by evaluating PSV, resistance index, and flow estimates in the SMA, as well as flow patterns at the aorta and distal small bowel vasculature. Even though it could be a useful tool in the future, the ability to detect disease activity still shows conflicting results [30].

Mesenteric Artery Dissection and Aneurysms

Ultrasound is frequently obtained in patients with abdominal pain. Isolated mesenteric artery dissections (Fig. 5.7) and aneurysms can be incidentally diagnosed or found to be a cause of the patient's symptoms. Among patients with aneurysms, ultrasound is often used for the assessment of size diameter during follow-up, prior or after an intervention.

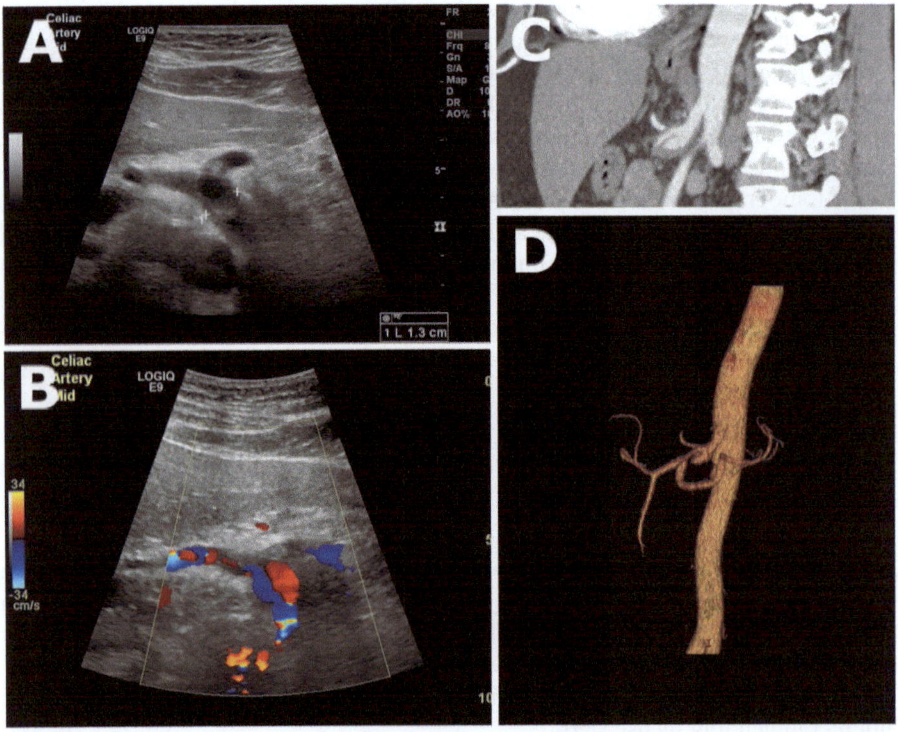

Fig. 5.7 Ultrasound performed during investigation of abdominal pain suggested celiac artery dissection (**a** and **b**). Computed tomography angiography confirms the diagnosis (**c** and **d**)

Conclusion

Duplex examination is widely used in the diagnosis and follow-up of mesenteric artery disease. It is well accepted as the first screening study in patients with symptoms of chronic mesenteric ischemia and suspected mesenteric artery occlusive disease. It is safe, noninvasive, low cost without ionizing radiation, and readily accessible. While well-established criteria are available for native vessel disease, caution should be used with elevated velocities in the stented arteries.

References

1. Zwolak RM, Fillinger MF, Walsh DB, LaBombard FE, Musson A, Darling CE, et al. Mesenteric and celiac duplex scanning: a validation study. J Vasc Surg. 1998;27(6):1078–87. [Comparative Study]; discussion 88.
2. Jager KA, Fortner GS, Thiele BL, Strandness DE. Noninvasive diagnosis of intestinal angina. J Clin Ultrasound. 1984;12(9):588–91 [Case Reports].
3. Gentile AT, Moneta GL, Lee RW, Masser PA, Taylor Jr LM, Porter JM. Usefulness of fasting and postprandial duplex ultrasound examinations for predicting high-grade superior mesenteric artery stenosis. Am J Surg. 1995;169(5):476–9 [Clinical Trial Comparative Study].
4. Zwolak RM. Can duplex ultrasound replace arteriography in screening for mesenteric ischemia? Semin Vasc Surg. 1999;12(4):252–60 [Review].
5. Hodjkiss-Harlow K. Interpretation of visceral duplex scanning: before and after intervention for chronic mesenteric ischemia. Semin Vasc Surg. 2013;26:127–32.
6. Revzin MV, Pellerito JS. Ultrasound assessment of the mesenteric arteries. Ultrasound Clinics. 2007;2(3):477–92.
7. Denys AL, Lafortune M, Aubin B, Burke M, Breton G. Doppler sonography of the inferior mesenteric artery: a preliminary study. J Ultrasound Med. 1995;14(6):435–9; quiz 41–2.
8. Mirk P, Palazzoni G, Cotroneo AR, di Stasi C, Fileni A. Sonographic and Doppler assessment of the inferior mesenteric artery: normal morphologic and hemodynamic features. Abdom Imaging. 1998;23(4):364–9 [Comparative Study].
9. Pellerito JS, Revzin MV, Tsang JC, Greben CR, Naidich JB. Doppler sonographic criteria for the diagnosis of inferior mesenteric artery stenosis. J Ultrasound Med. 2009;28(5):641–50.
10. Erden A, Yurdakul M, Cumhur T. Doppler waveforms of the normal and collateralized inferior mesenteric artery. Am J Roentgenol. 1998;171(3):619–27.
11. Jager K, Bollinger A, Valli C, Ammann R. Measurement of mesenteric blood flow by duplex scanning. J Vasc Surg. 1986;3(3):462–9 [Comparative Study].
12. Moneta GL, Taylor DC, Helton WS, Mulholland MW, Strandness Jr DE. Duplex ultrasound measurement of postprandial intestinal blood flow: effect of meal composition. Gastroenterology. 1988;95(5):1294–301.
13. Moneta GL, Yeager RA, Dalman R, Antonovic R, Hall LD, Porter JM. Duplex ultrasound criteria for diagnosis of splanchnic artery stenosis or occlusion. J Vasc Surg. 1991;14(4):511–8; discussion 8–20.
14. Moneta GL, Lee RW, Yeager RA, Taylor Jr LM, Porter JM. Mesenteric duplex scanning: a blinded prospective study. J Vasc Surg. 1993;17(1):79–84. [Comparative Study Research Support, U.S. Gov't, Non-P.H.S.]; discussion 5–6.
15. Bowersox JC, Zwolak RM, Walsh DB, Schneider JR, Musson A, LaBombard FE, et al. Duplex ultrasonography in the diagnosis of celiac and mesenteric artery occlusive disease. J Vasc Surg. 1991;14(6):780–6. [Comparative Study]; discussion 6–8.

16. AbuRahma AF, Stone PA, Srivastava M, Dean LS, Keiffer T, Hass SM, et al. Mesenteric/celiac duplex ultrasound interpretation criteria revisited. J Vasc Surg. 2012;55(2):428 e6–36 e6. [Comparative Study]; discussion 35–6.
17. AbuRahma AF, Scott DL. Duplex ultrasound interpretation criteria for inferior mesenteric arteries. Vascular. 2012;20(3):145–9.
18. Okuhn SP, Reilly LM, Bennett JB, Hughes 3rd L, Goldstone J, Ehrenfeld WK, et al. Intraoperative assessment of renal and visceral artery reconstruction: the role of duplex scanning and spectral analysis. J Vasc Surg. 1987;5(1):137–47 [Research Support, Non-U.S. Gov't].
19. Oderich GS, Panneton JM, Macedo TA, Noel AA, Bower TC, Lee RA, et al. Intraoperative duplex ultrasound of visceral revascularizations: optimizing technical success and outcome. J Vasc Surg. 2003;38(4):684–91.
20. Macedo TA, Oderich GS, Lee RA, Panneton JM. Intraoperative sonogram in mesenteric revascularization: spectrum of findings. Am J Roentgenol. 2005;184(5):1524–31 [Review].
21. McMillan WD, McCarthy WJ, Bresticker MR, Pearce WH, Schneider JR, Golan JF, et al. Mesenteric artery bypass: objective patency determination. J Vasc Surg. 1995;21(5):729–40. [Clinical Trial Comparative Study Research Support, U.S. Gov't, P.H.S. Review]; discussion 40–1.
22. Liem TK, Segall JA, Wei W, Landry GJ, Taylor LM, Moneta GL. Duplex scan characteristics of bypass grafts to mesenteric arteries. J Vasc Surg. 2007;45(5):922–7; discussion 7–8.
23. Baker AC, Chew V, Li CS, Lin TC, Dawson DL, Pevec WC, et al. Application of duplex ultrasound imaging in determining in-stent stenosis during surveillance after mesenteric artery revascularization. J Vasc Surg. 2012;56(5):1364–71; discussion 71.
24. AbuRahma AF, Mousa AY, Stone PA, Hass SM, Dean LS, Keiffer T. Duplex velocity criteria for native celiac/superior mesenteric artery stenosis vs in-stent stenosis. J Vasc Surg. 2012;55(3):730–8 [Comparative Study].
25. Mitchell EL, Chang EY, Landry GJ, Liem TK, Keller FS, Moneta GL. Duplex criteria for native superior mesenteric artery stenosis overestimate stenosis in stented superior mesenteric arteries. J Vasc Surg. 2009;50(2):335–40.
26. Szilagyi DE, Rian RL, Elliott JP, Smith RF. The celiac artery compression syndrome: does it exist? Surgery. 1972;72(6):849–63.
27. Baccoli A, Manni P, Sau M, Tuveri M, Tuveri A. Color Doppler ultrasound in acute mesenteric ischemia: 2 case reports. G Chir. 2003;24(4):148–51 [Case Reports].
28. Giannetti A, Biscontri M, Randisi P, Cortese B, Minacci C, Stumpo M. Contrast-enhanced sonography in the diagnosis of acute mesenteric ischemia: case report. J Clin Ultrasound. 2010;38(3):156–60 [Case Reports].
29. Anderson JL, Halperin JL, Albert NM, Bozkurt B, Brindis RG, Curtis LH, et al. Management of patients with peripheral artery disease (compilation of 2005 and 2011 ACCF/AHA guideline recommendations): a report of the American College of Cardiology Foundation/American Heart Association Task Force on Practice Guidelines. Circulation. 2013;127(13):1425–43.
30. Andrade TG, Fogaca HS, Elia CC, Pitrowsky MT, Souza HS. Crohn's disease activity assessed by Doppler sonography: the role of aortic flow parameters. Clinics (Sao Paulo). 2013;68(4):457–62 [Evaluation Studies Research Support, Non-U.S. Gov't].

Chapter 6
Functional Testing in the Diagnosis of Chronic Mesenteric Ischemia

Jihan Harki, Eric T.T.L. Tjwa, and Désirée van Noord

Chronic mesenteric ischemia (CMI) is a diagnostic challenge. Currently, there is no single test with high sensitivity and specificity to diagnose or exclude this condition. Chronic abdominal pain is a common symptom in the population, as are stenoses of the mesenteric arteries. Development of mucosal perfusion assessment techniques may be of additional diagnostic value in identifying and grading the severity of mesenteric ischemia. These functional tests may help to select patients who will benefit from treatment by revascularization. Until recently it was thought that CMI could only occur in the presence of minimal two occluded mesenteric arteries, but studies on diagnostic strategies including functional tests have shown that a significant stenosis of a single artery with insufficient collateral circulation can also lead to clinically relevant mesenteric ischemia [1, 2]. Functional testing also appeared to be of value in diagnosing nonocclusive causes of CMI [3–7].

A diagnostic approach combining assessment of clinical symptoms, radiological imaging of the mesenteric arteries, and functional testing is recommended in the work-up of CMI suspected patients [8]. Measurement of intragastric PCO_2 and mucosal oxygenation has been reported to be reliable in establishing mesenteric mucosal ischemia [3, 9–11]. In this chapter, we will highlight the two most relevant functional tests for such measurement, i.e., gastric tonometry and visible light spectroscopy.

J. Harki, MD (✉) • E.T.T.L. Tjwa, MD, PhD • D. van Noord, MD, PhD
Department of Gastroenterology and Hepatology, Erasmus University Medical Center Rotterdam, Rotterdam, The Netherlands
e-mail: j.harki@erasmusmc.nl; Eric.Tjwa@radboudumc.nl; d.vannoord@erasmusmc.nl

G.S. Oderich (ed.), *Mesenteric Vascular Disease*,
DOI 10.1007/978-1-4939-1847-8_6

Gastric Tonometry

Background

Mesenteric ischemia is one of the earliest events in circulatory stress and is being used as a monitoring technique for the intensive care. It is believed that hypoperfusion below a critical level of 50 % of the basal blood flow causes accumulation of carbon dioxide and acidosis in the mucosa of the intestine due to a switch to anaerobe glycolysis [9, 10]. The PCO_2 of the intestine may increase and the mucosal pH consequently decreases due to reduced washout of metabolically produced CO_2 and from buffering of anaerobically produced lactic acid and free H^+ protons by bicarbonate (Fig. 6.1) [11]. In parallel, a decrease in tissue PO_2 and oxygen consumption may be observed. This initiates tissue injury, increased permeability, bacterial translocation, and an aggressive inflammatory response which could result in acute ischemia of the mesenteric tract [12–15].

Studies dating back to the early 1970s have used measurement of PCO_2 in the mesenteric tract as an indicator of several pathophysiological processes and as a guide for treatment to improve the outcome of critically ill patients [16–19]. Measurement of PCO_2 can easily be performed using mesenteric tonometry. The tonometer is a balloon-tipped catheter, which can be placed in the stomach, jejunum, or colon and is attached to a modified capnograph.

Tonometry has the potential to detect ischemia defined as insufficient delivery and/or consumption of oxygen for metabolic demands irrespective of flow and mesenteric perfusion. Initially, tonometry calculated the mesenteric mucosal pH derived from the PCO_2 measured in the mesenteric lumen and the blood bicarbonate level using the

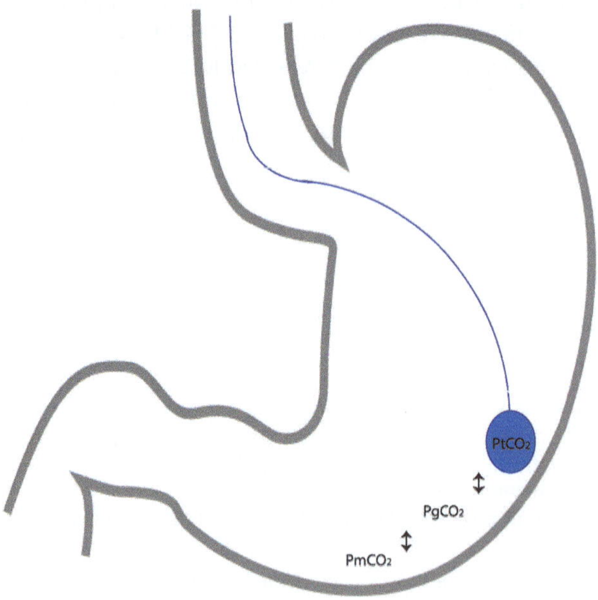

Fig. 6.1 Measurement of intraluminal PCO_2 by tonometry. The tonometer is placed in the stomach. The mucosal PCO_2 ($PmCO_2$) and the gastric PCO_2 ($PgCO_2$) are equal because of the rapid diffusion of CO_2 over the membrane layers. The balloon of the tonometer is also CO_2 permeable; therefore, the PCO_2 measured by the tonometer demonstrates the actual mucosal values (Adapted from Kolkman and Mensink [3], with permission)

Henderson-Hasselbalch equation [20]. However, this has major drawbacks as it is influenced by systemic variations in blood flow, which not necessarily reflects the true balance between oxygen supply and demand of the mesenteric tract [20, 21]. Therefore, it is replaced by the PCO_2 gradient, defined as the difference between luminal and arterial PCO_2. Since CO_2 diffuses rapidly over the membrane layers, the mesenteric PCO_2 in the lumen equals the PCO_2 in the mucosa. Mucosal ischemia will invariably be associated with increased mesenteric PCO_2 [3]. This is less influenced by systemic variation and is currently the preferred tonometric parameter for detection of ischemia.

Initially, the detection of mesenteric ischemia by tonometry was performed using meals as provocation [22]. However, this was not successful with an accuracy ranging from 0 to 100 % for ischemia as it was influenced by ongoing acid production of the stomach and direct influence of the meal on gastric PCO_2 [23–25].

It was not until the development of the gastric exercise tonometry (GET) and the 24-hour tonometry by Kolkman et al. that tonometry could be used as a practical, validated diagnostic test for the detection of ischemia [4, 26, 27]. GET requires submaximal exercise, i.e., cycling, to trigger mesenteric ischemia. The concept is very similar to the commonly used exercise testing for assessment of cardiac ischemia. The prolonged, 24-hour combined gastric and jejunal tonometry requires standardized test meals as a provocation of mesenteric ischemia [5, 8].

Procedure

Gastric Exercise Tonometry

Gastric exercise tonometry (GET) testing is performed according to a standard protocol [1, 27]. Patients are not allowed to drink or eat prior to the procedure and acid suppression will be administered. The tonometer, a balloon-tipped nasogastric tube, is placed 60 cm from the tip of the nose assuming intragastric position. Gastric and arterial PCO_2 measurements are performed before, during, and after the 10-min submaximal exercise. Gastric PCO_2 measurements are measured by inflation of a semi-permeable balloon with saline and repeated aspiration of the gas content of the balloon. The tonometer is attached to a modified capnograph. A radial catheter is inserted to allow for arterial PCO_2 measurements. To define a test result as pathologic, all three of the following criteria have to be met [4]:

1. Gastric-arterial gradient >0.8 kPa after peak exercise
2. Increase in gastric PCO_2 from baseline to peak exercise
3. Arterial lactate level <8 mmol/l

24-Hour Tonometry

This method consists of prolonged, 24-hour combined gastric and jejunal tonometry using standardized meals with a large metabolic demand as a provocation of mesenteric ischemia.

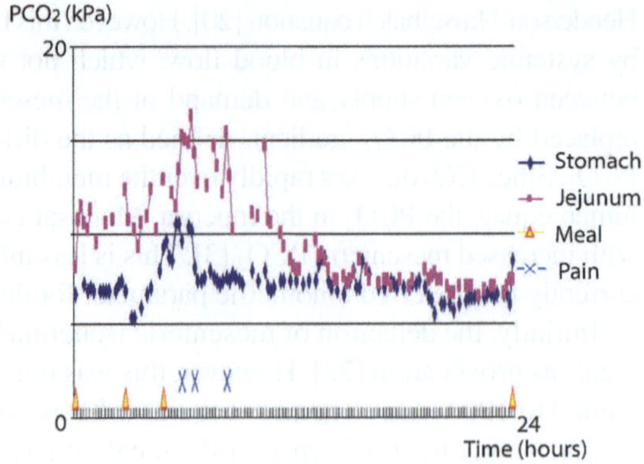

Fig. 6.2 Results of 24-hour tonometry in a patient with CMI. Abnormal postprandial increases in jejunal PCO_2 values are seen with a close association with the onset of abdominal pain symptoms

Tonometer catheters are inserted both in the stomach and jejunum by endoscopy and fluoroscopy. Gastric and jejunal PCO_2 levels are registered every 10 min using a computer assisted data-collection program. Continuous intravenous administration of proton pump inhibitors and gastric pH measurements are performed to maximally control acid suppression (Fig. 6.2).

Threshold values for elevated PCO_2 levels are gastric or jejunal $PCO_2 > 12.0$ kPa after breakfast or a bread meal, >13.6 kPa after dinner, or >10.6 kPa after ingestion of a compound solution. The criteria for a pathologic test result are [5, 28].

1. Elevated PCO_2 values after at least three meals or
2. Combination of elevated PCO_2 after at least one meal and a median $PCO_2 > 8.0$ kPa measured between meals

Test Meals

Patients are required to consume standardized meals during the test [5]. To minimize the disturbing effects of meals on the intragastric PCO_2 measurements explained by buffering and dilution, standardized meals are developed to optimally control the gastric and jejunal environment. The CO_2-producing and CO_2-absorbing capacities of these meals are minimal. Nevertheless, they maximally challenge the mesenteric arterial blood flow due to the large metabolic oxygen demand [29].

Meals consisting of a solution of carbohydrates, protein, and fat with a high caloric content and a low volume show the most significant increase in the blood flow of the mesenteric arteries [29, 30]. With this in mind, compound solution meals are the ideal meals showing maximum peak in PCO_2 after ingestion. Consumption of carbonated liquids is prohibited during the test.

Diagnostic Value of Tonometry

Sensitivity and Specificity

In two large cohort studies including patients suspected of CMI, the diagnostic efficacy of GET was evaluated. With a sensitivity of 78–85 % and a specificity of 82–92 % for the detection of CMI, GET appears to be a reliable diagnostic tool in the assessment of CMI [4, 31]. The sensitivity and specificity of 24-hour tonometry for the detection of CMI are similar to GET with a sensitivity and specificity of 77–91 % and 94–100 %, respectively [5, 28]. The combination of clinical features with 24-hour tonometry has a sensitivity of 88 %. Adding radiological imaging by means of CTA or MRA, this can raise up to 90–91 % [28, 32].

Tonometry After Intervention

Repeated GET showed normalization or improvement in 88–100 % of patients with sustained relief of symptoms after treatment [1]. In patients with persistent symptoms, repeated GET showed improved in only 29 % of the patients, whereas in 71 % unchanged or worsened results were observed [1]. This indicates an accurate correlation between gastric mucosal ischemia and tonometry results.

Visible Light Spectroscopy

Background

Functional tests such as gastric exercise tonometry (GET) and 24-hour tonometry both seem to be accurate for detection of mesenteric ischemia [1, 5, 31, 32]. Unfortunately, the wider use of mesenteric tonometry is hampered by its cumbersome and invasive nature; therefore, the need for a better, more patient-friendly test remained. This led to the development of visible light spectroscopy (VLS). VLS, also known as reflectance spectrophotometry, enables direct measurement of the adequacy of mucosal perfusion [7]. It is a relatively new technique that noninvasively measures capillary hemoglobin oxygen saturation using white light delivered by a fiberoptic probe during endoscopy. The marked difference in the absorption spectra of oxygenated and deoxygenated hemoglobin makes direct measurement of the percent saturation of the mucosal hemoglobin possible. Using real-time signaling, artifacts as those caused by scattering can also be eliminated [7]. Connected to a device, continuous display of the mucosal oxygen saturation on a screen is possible [6, 7].

VLS has been used for evaluation of intensive care patients and assessment of anastomotic strength in esophageal and colorectal anastomoses and to determine microvascular perfusion during reconstructive surgery [33–35]. It can also increase endoscopic detection of mesenteric tumors [36].

Furthermore, VLS appears to be of great value as a new and less invasive diagnostic tool in patients suspected of CMI [6]. Since the measured oxygen saturation measurements reflect the adequacy of mucosal perfusion, events that decrease the delivery of oxygen to the mesenteric mucosa (i.e., mesenteric artery stenosis) will result in lower mucosal hemoglobin oxygen saturations [6]. VLS can easily be incorporated in diagnostic strategies as endoscopy is often performed early in the diagnostic work-up of these patients with abdominal pain.

Procedure

VLS is performed during upper endoscopy under conscious sedation [6, 7]. Patients are not allowed to drink or eat before the procedure. Butylscopalamine is admitted intravenously before the start of VLS measurements in order to prevent luminal spasms and optimize the readings. Peripheral oxygen saturation and heart rate are continuously monitored and to minimize the effect of confounding factors of concomitant cardiopulmonary diseases, peripheral saturation should be above 94 %. If necessary, oxygen (FiO_2 21 %) can be administered.

The VLS measurements are performed using a fiberoptic catheter-based oximeter that can be passed through the endoscope. After irrigation of the target area to remove bile remnants, point measurements of the oxygen saturation are performed at three locations: antrum of the stomach, duodenal bulb, and descending duodenum. The probe is positioned approximately 1–5 mm above the mucosa (Fig. 6.3). Once a stable reading is obtained with less than 5 % variation in readout as seen on the display, the actual measurement can be performed. Three repeated readings will be taken of

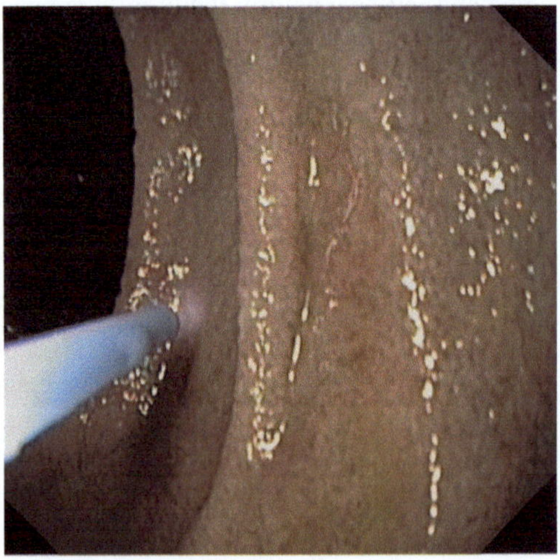

Fig. 6.3 Mucosal oxygen saturation using VLS. The probe is placed 1–5 mm directly above the mucosa of the stomach and duodenum

each location. The average of the three readings per location will be regarded as the most accurate reflection of mucosal oxygen saturation of that specific location.

Based on the cutoff values determined in a large cohort study in CMI suspected patients, measurements are positive for ischemia when the measured saturation is:

- <63 % in the antrum and/or
- <62 % in the duodenal bulb and/or
- <58 % in the descending duodenum [6]

Diagnostic Value of VLS

Sensitivity and Specificity

VLS is a validated diagnostic method to correctly detect CMI with a sensitivity and specificity of 90 % and 60 %, respectively [6]. The high sensitivity and low specificity are the consequence of the established cutoff values for each of the specific sites of the mesenteric tract as calculated by van Noord et al [6]. These cutoff values were based on a trainee data set of patients diagnosed with CMI using mesenteric tonometry and were additionally validated in a confirmation cohort.

With these cutoff values, the ability to distinguish patients with CMI from those without is the highest and no patients with CMI were missed, as earlier studies have shown that undiagnosed and untreated patients with ischemia have higher morbidity and mortality rates [10, 31]. However, the higher sensitivity results in a higher rate of false positives.

VLS After Intervention

After successful intervention, improved VLS measurements can be observed in patients with CMI [6]. Among the patients with relief of symptoms one year after intervention, 80 % showed improved or even normalization of the oxygen saturation measurements by VLS measurements. At the same time, in all patients with persistent symptoms after intervention, no improvement in the oxygen saturation measurements was observed [6]. Furthermore, selection for treatment based on standardized diagnostic work-up including radiological imaging and oxygen saturation measurements by VLS accommodates for a sustained response in 70 % of the patients with the clinical suspicion of CMI [37].

Clinical Considerations

Comparison Tonometry Versus VLS

Both VLS as tonometry have a high diagnostic accuracy for correctly diagnosing CMI [4, 5, 28, 31, 32]. In the assessment of CMI, tonometry allows the clinician to differentiate patients with asymptomatic single- or multivessel stenosis of the mesenteric arteries and patients in whom the abdominal symptoms are induced by mesenteric ischemia. The newly developed VLS has also shown its value and even appears to be slightly better in identifying patients with CMI [4–6, 28, 31].

Limitations of Tonometry

GET requires submaximal exercise to trigger mesenteric ischemia. However, many patients in this category are not able to perform suboptimal exercise for sufficient period of time to assess CMI due to age or concomitant disease [16]. Also, despite frequent monitoring of serum lactate as a measure for exercise intensity, the level of exercise in patients is still difficult to control.

As the name indicates, 24-hour tonometry requires 24-h hospitalization. This is inconvenient and expensive. Furthermore, suboptimal gastric acid suppression and meal-related CO_2 production may affect the tonometry results leading to false-positive outcomes therefore requiring the use of continuous gastric acid suppression and standardized meals [39].

Limitations of VLS

The measures of performance of VLS are based on data from only one large cohort study and has not yet been conducted or reproduced by other research groups [6]. This study compared mucosal oxygen saturation measurements in patients with CMI with a control group of non-CMI patients. However, the latter consisted of patients with a clinical suspicion of CMI, which is not the ideal. A control group consisting of healthy volunteers is needed to avoid selection bias and to obtain normal values for mucosal oxygen saturation measurements in order to optimize the cutoff values.

With the current cutoff values and the high sensitivity of 90 %, no patient with CMI should be missed. However, the mean of mucosal saturation measurements in patients with CMI shows great variation and the range of measurements is large. Due to small changes in the position of the probe during the measurements, small variations in the oxygen saturation can occur with the possibility of not acquiring the actual mucosal oxygen saturation. Especially if the obtained value is around the specified cutoff value, it can be difficult to classify the measurement as either positive or negative for mucosal ischemia. Therefore, the average of three repeated measurements of each location is regarded as the most accurate reflection of the mucosal oxygen saturation of that location [6].

Another limitation of mucosal oxygen measurements using VLS is that the current technique causes restrictions regarding the place and time of the measurements. Mucosal ischemia might be patchy and because VLS is limited to point measurements could therefore be missed with VLS [6, 7]. Furthermore, there is a possibility that mucosal ischemia only occurs postprandially, in response to an increased metabolic demand, or is exercise related indicating a time-dependent relation. VLS measurements are performed in a fasting state during endoscopy. In theory, patients with CMI with less impaired mesenteric blood flow could show low-normal or even normal mucosal saturation measurements in this fasting situation and can therefore be missed using VLS.

Conclusion

The choice for the functional test depends on the patient's condition, presence of comorbidity, and clinical symptoms. For instance, patients with exercise-induced symptoms are far better detected with GET rather than with 24-hour tonometry or VLS [38, 39]. For patients with postprandial complaints, 24-hour tonometry or VLS would be the most suiting technique. Furthermore, the experience of the treating physician with the technique and equipment is important.

VLS is minimally invasive and can be performed in almost all patients [6, 8]. Patients with a clinical suspicion of CMI have to undergo endoscopy early in the work-up, during which measurements with VLS can be easily performed. It only requires an additional two minutes during endoscopy which, in contrast to 24-hour tonometry, can be performed in the outpatient clinic. Therefore, it is also less expensive.

The diagnostic value of tonometry for the detection of CMI is more accurate than VLS. Reproducibility of tonometry has been shown in numerous studies, whereas these validations are lacking for VLS [4, 32, 37]. VLS is a promising diagnostic test for detection of CMI and shows excellent correlation with tonometry; however the established cutoff values need to be validated [37]. In conclusion, the strength of evidence for accurately detecting CMI is greater for tonometry than for VLS and is therefore the preferred method.

Best Practice

The current established approach for diagnosing CMI is based on three main components. The first includes assessment of medical history, clinical symptoms, and physical examination. The second component concerns radiological imaging of the mesenteric arteries and the third aims at detection of mucosal ischemia by means of a functional test [8, 10]. All patients and procedures are discussed in a dedicated multidisciplinary team consisting of a vascular surgeon, intervention radiologist, and gastroenterologist, all specialized in CMI, leading to a final expert-based consensus diagnosis [6, 8, 28].

The diagnosis CMI is made if patient fulfils two of the three following criteria [6]:

1. Distinctive clinical presentation including presence of postprandial pain and otherwise unexplained weight loss of >5 % of the normal body weight

2. Significant stenosis of >70 % of at least one of the mesenteric arteries demonstrated by radiological evaluation
3. Mucosal ischemia detected by tonometry or visible light spectroscopy

A definitive diagnosis of CMI is made after persistent relief of symptoms on follow-up after treatment. This is not the ideal gold standard; however, it is currently the most reliable way to establish CMI.

Future Aspects

Despite the success of tonometry and VLS, there still exist areas for continued development and improvement.

Optimizing Tonometry

The current method for measuring luminal PCO_2 is air tonometry using a balloon-tipped catheter, placed in the stomach (and jejunum), and the modified capnograph [19]. This allows for semi-automated PCO_2 measurements every ten minutes during which intraluminal CO_2 diffuses into the balloon. After a period of ten minutes, the air is then aspirated and measured ex vivo. As a result the maximum measurement frequency is once every 10 min, which is a great limitation. Second, during the measurement CO_2 is removed and O_2 is delivered which may influence the environment [40].

This led to the development of a new sensor, enabling continuous CO_2 measurement. However, in vivo tests show great temperature sensitivity, and therefore, it is too unstable for clinical use in current design [40].

Optimizing VLS

Sublingual VLS Measurements

Recently, the relationship between sublingual and intestinal microperfusion in critically ill patients has been investigated. This demonstrated a good correlation between sublingual microcirculatory perfusion and intestinal perfusion [41–43]. Against this background, a correlation with a decrease in sublingual oxygen saturation using VLS can theoretically be possible in patients with CMI with decreased mucosal oxygen measurements or elevated PCO_2 measurements, indicating impaired intestinal perfusion. Up until now, sublingual VLS measurements are performed in research setting [44]. However, they can be of great value in diagnosing patients with CMI. It is less invasive, more patient-friendly, and even less time-consuming than endoscopic VLS. However, further research is required to illustrate and to validate this hypothesis.

Postprandial VLS Measurements

The possibility remains that mucosal ischemia occurs only postprandially, in response to an increased metabolic demand. Currently VLS measurements are performed, while patients are in a fasting state. In theory, patients with CMI with less impaired mesenteric blood flow could show low-normal or even normal mucosal saturation measurements in this fasting situation and can therefore be missed. Postprandial mucosal saturation measurements using VLS may overcome the false negatives thus enhancing the specificity of the test.

Functional Tests of the Small Bowel Mucosa

Since the mucosa of the small bowel and colon is particularly sensitive to ischemia, potential markers for intestinal mucosal injury in patients with CMI were investigated like the sugar absorption test (SAT) consisting of an enzymatic measurement of mannitol, raffinose, sucrose, and lactose [45, 46].

The SAT has proven to be a sensitive measure of the small bowel function and thus the permeability of the mucosa as marked increases in the permeability are associated with intestinal diseases [47]. Assuming altered small bowel function in patients with CMI due to hypoperfusion by compromised blood flow, malabsorption of these sugars will occur causing unexplained diarrhea and weight loss [48]. However, it appears that the SAT can only be applied in acute cases of ischemia as it does not seem to be altered in patients with CMI. This can be explained by the reversible symptomatology of CMI and the fact that it is usually limited to certain provocating factors such as a meal or exercise [45]. Further research is needed to find a pathognomonic marker for CMI.

Biomarkers

Finding biomarkers pathognomonic for CMI could be an easy and patient-friendly way to recognize patients with CMI in an early stage. In the past, possible early markers like lactate dehydrogenase (LDH), leukocyte counts, C-reactive protein (CRP), and D-dimer testing for acute ischemia have been investigated in patients clinically suspected for CMI [45, 49–51]. However, in contrast to acute ischemia, the value of these markers in CMI is limited. Also, citrulline and intestinal fatty acid binding protein (I-FABP) have been thoroughly investigated [45, 52–55]. However, also these markers did not differ between patients with and without CMI [45].

Risk Stratification by Single-Nucleotide Polymorphisms

Due to the population's prolonged longevity, prevalence of cardiovascular diseases increases and is becoming a growing clinical problem. Several studies have been conducted to detect patients with genetic susceptibility for developing these diseases using single-nucleotide polymorphisms [56–58]. It seems that an inflammatory response is involved in the pathogenesis of ischemic diseases, with a prominent role for tumor necrosis factor-α (TNF-α) and tissue plasminogen activator (TPA) gene polymorphisms [57, 59]. Remarkably, given the high prevalence of cardiovascular disease among the population, only a relatively small number of patients develop abdominal symptoms due to stenosis of the mesenteric arteries [60, 61]. A promising future research topic would be to determine which patients are at risk for developing CMI by evaluating gene polymorphisms possibly associated with CMI.

References

1. Mensink PB, van Petersen AS, Kolkman JJ, Otte JA, Huisman AB, Geelkerken RH. Gastric exercise tonometry: the key investigation in patients with suspected celiac artery compression syndrome. J Vasc Surg. 2006;44(2):277–81.
2. van Noord D, Kuipers EJ, Mensink PB. Single vessel abdominal arterial disease. Best Pract Res Clin Gastroenterol. 2009;23(1):49–60.
3. Kolkman JJ, Mensink PB. Non-occlusive mesenteric ischaemia: a common disorder in gastroenterology and intensive care. Best Pract Res Clin Gastroenterol. 2003;17(3):457–73.
4. Otte JA, Geelkerken RH, Oostveen E, Mensink PB, Huisman AB, Kolkman JJ. Clinical impact of gastric exercise tonometry on diagnosis and management of chronic gastrointestinal ischemia. Clin Gastroenterol Hepatol. 2005;3(7):660–6.
5. Mensink PB, Geelkerken RH, Huisman AB, Kuipers EJ, Kolkman JJ. Twenty-four hour tonometry in patients suspected of chronic gastrointestinal ischemia. Dig Dis Sci. 2008;53(1):133–9.
6. Van Noord D, Sana A, Benaron DA, Pattynama PM, Verhagen HJ, Hansen BE, et al. Endoscopic visible light spectroscopy: a new, minimally invasive technique to diagnose chronic GI ischemia. Gastrointest Endosc. 2011;73(2):291–8.
7. Friedland S, Benaron D, Coogan S, Sze DY, Soetikno R. Diagnosis of chronic mesenteric ischemia by visible light spectroscopy during endoscopy. Gastrointest Endosc. 2007;65(2):294–300.
8. Mensink PB, Moons LM, Kuipers EJ. Chronic gastrointestinal ischaemia: shifting paradigms. Gut. 2011;60(5):722–37.
9. Kolkman JJ, Steverink PJ, Groeneveld AB, Meuwissen SG. Characteristics of time-dependent PCO2 tonometry in the normal human stomach. Br J Anaesth. 1998;81(5):669–75.
10. Kolkman JJ, Bargeman M, Huisman AB, Geelkerken RH. Diagnosis and management of splanchnic ischemia. World J Gastroenterol. 2008;14(48):7309–20.
11. Schlichtig R, Bowles SA. Distinguishing between aerobic and anaerobic appearance of dissolved CO2 in intestine during low flow. J Appl Physiol. 1994;76(6):2443–51.
12. Aneman A, Snygg J, Pettersson A, Johansson B, Holm M, Fandriks L. Detecting gastrointestinal hypoperfusion during cardiac tamponade in pigs: a role for nitric oxide tonometry? Crit Care Med. 1998;26(7):1251–7.
13. Sato Y, Weil MH, Tang W, Sun S, Xie J, Bisera J, et al. Esophageal PCO2 as a monitor of perfusion failure during hemorrhagic shock. J Appl Physiol. 1997;82(2):558–62.

14. Bjorck M, Hedberg B. Early detection of major complications after abdominal aortic surgery: predictive value of sigmoid colon and gastric intramucosal pH monitoring. Br J Surg. 1994;81(1):25–30.
15. Charpentier C, Audibert G, Dousset B, Weber M, Garric J, Welfringer P, et al. Is endotoxin and cytokine release related to a decrease in gastric intramucosal pH after hemorrhagic shock? Intensive Care Med. 1997;23(10):1040–8.
16. Rune SJ. The duodenal PCO2 in duodenal ulcer patients and normal subjects. Acta Hepatogastroenterol (Stuttg). 1972;19(5):386–7.
17. Gutierrez G, Brown SD. Gastric tonometry: a new monitoring modality in the intensive care unit. J Intensive Care Med. 1995;10(1):34–44.
18. Fiddian-Green RG. Gastric intramucosal pH, tissue oxygenation and acid–base balance. Br J Anaesth. 1995;74(5):591–606.
19. Groeneveld AB, Kolkman JJ. Splanchnic tonometry: a review of physiology, methodology, and clinical applications. J Crit Care. 1994;9(3):198–210.
20. Kolkman JJ, Otte JA, Groeneveld AB. Gastrointestinal luminal PCO2 tonometry: an update on physiology, methodology and clinical applications. Br J Anaesth. 2000;84(1):74–86.
21. Haisjackl M, Birnbaum J, Redlin M, Schmutzler M, Waldenberger F, Lochs H, et al. Splanchnic oxygen transport and lactate metabolism during normothermic cardiopulmonary bypass in humans. Anesth Analg. 1998;86(1):22–7.
22. Fiddian-Green RG, McGough E, Pittenger G, Rothman E. Predictive value of intramural pH and other risk factors for massive bleeding from stress ulceration. Gastroenterology. 1983;85(3):613–20.
23. Fiddian-Green RG, Stanley JC, Nostrant T, Phillips D. Chronic gastric ischemia. A cause of abdominal pain or bleeding identified from the presence of gastric mucosal acidosis. J Cardiovasc Surg (Torino). 1989;30(5):852–9.
24. Geelkerken RH, Schultze Kool LJ, Hermans J, Zarza MT, van Bockel JH. Chronic splanchnic ischaemia: is tonometry a useful test? Eur J Surg. 1997;163(2):115–21.
25. Kolkman JJ, Groeneveld AB, Meuwissen SG. Effect of gastric feeding on intragastric P(CO2) tonometry in healthy volunteers. J Crit Care. 1999;14(1):34–8.
26. Kolkman JJ, Groeneveld AB, van der Berg FG, Rauwerda JA, Meuwissen SG. Increased gastric PCO2 during exercise is indicative of gastric ischaemia: a tonometric study. Gut. 1999;44(2):163–7.
27. Otte JA, Oostveen E, Geelkerken RH, Groeneveld AB, Kolkman JJ. Exercise induces gastric ischemia in healthy volunteers: a tonometry study. J Appl Physiol. 2001;91(2):866–71.
28. van Noord D, Sana A, Moons LM, Pattynama PM, Verhagen HJ, Kuipers EJ, et al. Combining radiological imaging and gastrointestinal tonometry: a minimal invasive and useful approach for the workup of chronic gastrointestinal ischemia. Eur J Gastroenterol Hepatol. 2013;25(6):719–25.
29. Mensink PB, Geelkerken RH, Huisman AB, Kuipers EJ, Kolkman JJ. Effect of various test meals on gastric and jejunal carbon dioxide: A study in healthy subjects. Scand J Gastroenterol. 2006;41(11):1290–8.
30. Moneta GL, Taylor DC, Helton WS, Mulholland MW, Strandness Jr DE. Duplex ultrasound measurement of postprandial intestinal blood flow: effect of meal composition. Gastroenterology. 1988;95(5):1294–301.
31. Mensink PB, van Petersen AS, Geelkerken RH, Otte JA, Huisman AB, Kolkman JJ. Clinical significance of splanchnic artery stenosis. Br J Surg. 2006;93(11):1377–82.
32. Sana A, Vergouwe Y, van Noord D, Moons LM, Pattynama PM, Verhagen HJ, et al. Radiological imaging and gastrointestinal tonometry add value in diagnosis of chronic gastrointestinal ischemia. Clin Gastroenterol Hepatol. 2011;9(3):234–41.
33. Cornejo A, Rodriguez T, Steigelman M, Stephenson S, Sahar D, Cohn SM, et al. The use of visible light spectroscopy to measure tissue oxygenation in free flap reconstruction. J Reconstr Microsurg. 2011;27(7):397–402.
34. Karliczek A, Benaron DA, Baas PC, Zeebregts CJ, van der Stoel A, Wiggers T, et al. Intraoperative assessment of microperfusion with visible light spectroscopy in esophageal and colorectal anastomoses. Eur Surg Res. 2008;41(3):303–11.

35. Temmesfeld-Wollbruck B, Szalay A, Mayer K, Olschewski H, Seeger W, Grimminger F. Abnormalities of gastric mucosal oxygenation in septic shock: partial responsiveness to dopexamine. Am J Respir Crit Care Med. 1998;157(5 Pt 1):1586–92.
36. Maxim PG, Carson JJ, Benaron DA, Loo Jr BW, Xing L, Boyer AL, et al. Optical detection of tumors in vivo by visible light tissue oximetry. Technol Cancer Res Treat. 2005;4(3):227–34.
37. Sana A, Moons LM, Hansen BE, Dewint P, van Noord D, Mensink PBF, Kuipers EJ. Use of Visible Light Spectroscopy to Diagnose Chronic Gastrointestinal Ischemia and Predict Response to Treatment. Clin Gastroenterol Hepatol. 2014; doi:10.1016/j.cgh.2014.07.012. Epub ahead of print.
38. ter Steege RW, Kolkman JJ. Review article: the pathophysiology and management of gastrointestinal symptoms during physical exercise, and the role of splanchnic blood flow. Aliment Pharmacol Ther. 2012;35(5):516–28.
39. ter Steege RW, Kolkman JJ, Huisman AB, Geelkerken RH. [Gastrointestinal ischaemia during physical exertion as a cause of gastrointestinal symptoms] Maag-darmischemie tijdens lichamelijke inspanning als oorzaak van gastro-intestinale klachten. Ned Tijdschr Geneeskd. 2008;152(33):1805–8.
40. ter Steege RW, Herber S, Olthuis W, Bergveld P, van den Berg A, Kolkman JJ. Assessment of a new prototype hydrogel CO(2) sensor; comparison with air tonometry. J Clin Monit Comput. 2007;21(2):83–90.
41. Boerma EC, van der Voort PH, Spronk PE, Ince C. Relationship between sublingual and intestinal microcirculatory perfusion in patients with abdominal sepsis. Crit Care Med. 2007;35(4):1055–60.
42. Fries M, Weil MH, Sun S, Huang L, Fang X, Cammarata G, et al. Increases in tissue PCO_2 during circulatory shock reflect selective decreases in capillary blood flow. Crit Care Med. 2006;34(2):446–52.
43. Creteur J, De Backer D, Sakr Y, Koch M, Vincent JL. Sublingual capnometry tracks microcirculatory changes in septic patients. Intensive Care Med. 2006;32(4):516–23.
44. Singh DB, Stansby G, Harrison DK. Assessment of oxygenation and perfusion in the tongue and oral mucosa by visible spectrophotometry and laser Doppler flowmetry in healthy subjects. Adv Exp Med Biol. 2008;614:227–33.
45. van Noord D, Mensink PB, de Knegt RJ, Ouwendijk M, Francke J, van Vuuren AJ, et al. Serum markers and intestinal mucosal injury in chronic gastrointestinal ischemia. Dig Dis Sci. 2011;56(2):506–12.
46. Robinson JW, Mirkovitch V, Winistorfer B, Saegesser F. Response of the intestinal mucosa to ischaemia. Gut. 1981;22(6):512–27.
47. Hessels J, Snoeyink EJ, Platenkamp AJ, Voortman G, Steggink J, Eidhof HH. Assessment of intestinal permeability: enzymatic determination of urinary mannitol, raffinose, sucrose and lactose on Hitachi analyzer. Clin Chem Lab Med. 2003;41(1):33–8.
48. Meyers MA, Kaplowitz N, Bloom AA. Malabsorption secondary to mesenteric ischemia. Am J Roentgenol Radium Ther Nucl Med. 1973;119(2):352–8.
49. Block T, Nilsson TK, Bjorck M, Acosta S. Diagnostic accuracy of plasma biomarkers for intestinal ischaemia. Scand J Clin Lab Invest. 2008;68(3):242–8.
50. El-Awady SI, El-Nagar M, El-Dakar M, Ragab M, Elnady G. Bacterial translocation in an experimental intestinal obstruction model. C-reactive protein reliability? Acta Cir Bras. 2009;24(2):98–106.
51. Kurimoto Y, Kawaharada N, Ito T, Morikawa M, Higami T, Asai Y. An experimental evaluation of the lactate concentration following mesenteric ischemia. Surg Today. 2008;38(10):926–30.
52. Cronk DR, Houseworth TP, Cuadrado DG, Herbert GS, McNutt PM, Azarow KS. Intestinal fatty acid binding protein (I-FABP) for the detection of strangulated mechanical small bowel obstruction. Curr Surg. 2006;63(5):322–5.
53. Curis E, Crenn P, Cynober L. Citrulline and the gut. Curr Opin Clin Nutr Metab Care. 2007;10(5):620–6.

54. Mensink PB, Hol L, Borghuis-Koertshuis N, Geelkerken RH, Huisman AB, Doelman CJ, et al. Transient postprandial ischemia is associated with increased intestinal fatty acid binding protein in patients with chronic gastrointestinal ischemia. Eur J Gastroenterol Hepatol. 2009;21(3):278–82.
55. Peters JH, Wierdsma NJ, Teerlink T, van Leeuwen PA, Mulder CJ, van Bodegraven AA. Poor diagnostic accuracy of a single fasting plasma citrulline concentration to assess intestinal energy absorption capacity. Am J Gastroenterol. 2007;102(12):2814–9.
56. Ma Y, Wang SX, Liu Y, Peng GG, Wang XM, Zhang B, et al. Single nucleotide polymorphism of CD40 in the 5'-untranslated region is associated with ischemic stroke. Gene. 2013;529(2):257–61.
57. Sun X, Lai R, Li J, Luo M, Wang Y, Sheng W. The -7351C/T polymorphism in the TPA gene and ischemic stroke risk: a meta-analysis. PLoS One. 2013;8(1):e53558.
58. Gu L, Wu G, Long J, Su L, Yan Y, Chen Q, et al. The role of TNF-alpha 308G>A polymorphism in the risk for ischemic stroke. Am J Med Sci. 2013;345(3):227–33.
59. Cui G, Wang H, Li R, Zhang L, Li Z, Wang Y, et al. Polymorphism of tumor necrosis factor alpha (TNF-alpha) gene promoter, circulating TNF-alpha level, and cardiovascular risk factor for ischemic stroke. J Neuroinflammation. 2012;9:235.
60. Hansen KJ, Wilson DB, Craven TE, Pearce JD, English WP, Edwards MS, et al. Mesenteric artery disease in the elderly. J Vasc Surg. 2004;40(1):45–52.
61. Cardin F, Fratta S, Inelmen EM, Sergi G, Manzato E, Terranova C. Diagnosis of chronic mesenteric ischemia in older patients: a structured review. Aging Clin Exp Res. 2012;24(6):635–9.

Chapter 7
Noninvasive Arterial Imaging: Computed Tomography and Magnetic Resonance Angiography

Kirk J. Giesbrandt and Phillip M. Young

Mesenteric vascular disease can be challenging to diagnose as patients often present with relatively nonspecific clinical symptoms consistent with a number of intra-abdominal diseases including malignancy, inflammatory bowel disease, and motility disorders. Cross-sectional imaging has advanced at a rapid pace in recent years, allowing high-resolution imaging of both the mesenteric arteries and veins and also the abdominal viscera. These advances, in turn, have led to an increasing role for CT and MR in evaluated suspected cases of mesenteric vascular disease. Regardless of whether MR or CT is employed, cross-sectional vascular imaging has become a cornerstone in the evaluation of suspected acute and chronic mesenteric ischemia and can be used to help plan open surgical or percutaneous intervention.

Rationale for Computed Tomography and Magnetic Resonance Imaging

Multiple imaging options are available for patients with symptoms potentially attributable to mesenteric ischemia. Radiographs of the abdomen are generally of limited value; findings of early mesenteric ischemia are nonspecific and include either bowel dilatation or a paucity of bowel gas [1]. Radiographic findings more specifically associated with mesenteric ischemia (such as pneumatosis, portal venous gas, or pneumoperitoneum) are only present late in the course of the disease and are easily visible on CT and often MR as well.

K.J. Giesbrandt, MD (✉)
Department of Radiology, Mayo Clinic, Jacksonville, FL, USA
e-mail: Giesbrandt.Kirk@mayo.edu

P.M. Young, MD
Department of Radiology, Mayo Clinic, Rochester, MN, USA
e-mail: young.phillip@mayo.edu

G.S. Oderich (ed.), *Mesenteric Vascular Disease*,
DOI 10.1007/978-1-4939-1847-8_7

Duplex mesenteric ultrasound is an excellent screening study to evaluate patients with symptoms of chronic mesenteric ischemia, but its role is limited as an initial imaging study in the diagnosis of acute mesenteric ischemia [2]. Diagnostic angiography, covered in the following chapter, remains the gold standard for the diagnosis of acute and chronic mesenteric ischemia and allows for both diagnosis and treatment in the same procedure. However, given the invasive nature of catheter-based angiography, and often nonspecific clinical symptoms, an initial noninvasive test that can diagnose mesenteric ischemia and exclude other causes of acute or chronic abdominal pain is usually preferred.

Computed Tomography

Older CT scanners were limited by slow acquisition speed and low resolution. Spiral CT offered an improvement in the ability to image the mesenteric vasculature along with the bowel; however, the sensitivity for mesenteric ischemia remained too low to be used as a first-line diagnostic test [3]. In 2001, reports began to emerge in the literature about the use of multidetector CT (MDCT) scanners in the diagnosis of mesenteric ischemia [4, 5]. Shortly thereafter, the ability to use reformatted images permitted by MDCT was realized [6]. Current generation of MDCT scanners permit rapid acquisition times of high-resolution volumetric datasets during arterial phase contrast opacification (CT angiography) and delayed phase image allowing venous opacification and some assessment of bowel wall perfusion. These datasets are acquired quickly enough to overcome limitations of bowel peristalsis and can be reconstructed and viewed in three dimensions, improving confidence in diagnosis of mesenteric vascular disease [4]. These technological advances also aid in the diagnosis of other conditions which can mimic the clinical presentation of mesenteric ischemia, and the end result is increased sensitivity and specificity compared to earlier reports in the literature.

A meta-analysis of MDCT demonstrated a pooled sensitivity of 93 % and a specificity of 96 % [7], and CTA is the initial diagnostic test of choice for the diagnosis of both acute and chronic mesenteric ischemia. The American College of Radiology appropriateness criteria guide gives CTA a rating of 9, which is the highest possible rating for appropriateness in the imaging of acute and chronic mesenteric ischemia [2].

Clinical Role and Imaging Considerations for Computed Tomography Angiography (CTA)

Current generation CT scanners couple short acquisition times with the high resolution required to identify lesions in both main and branch mesenteric arteries and veins. Exact parameters vary between protocols and vendors, but with currently available technology sub-millimeter slices can be acquired and reconstructed at subcentimeter intervals providing volumetric data for multiplanar reformatting and three-dimensional (3D) reconstructions [8]. CT images are derived from X-rays, and CT angiography requires injection of intravascular contrast material timed to opacify vascular lumen. Contrast material used for CTA is iodine based, which attenuates X-rays more than the soft tissues and causes the opacified vasculature to appear bright and have higher Hounsfield units [9]. Ideal contrast agents are high in iodine concentration (350–370 mg I/mL), are nonionic, iso-osmolar compounds with low viscosity, and are injected at a high rate (4–6 mL/s for a total volume of 100–120 mL) [8, 9]. Because of the tight contrast bolus and small size of the vessels involved, the arterial and venous systems cannot be evaluated simultaneously, and dual-phase imaging is necessary. Usually, timing of the "arterial phase" involves either a test bolus or automated contrast tracking ("bolus triggering") system [9] to ensure peak arterial opacification during the scan acquisition. Following this, a "venous phase" is acquired, generally 70 s after the contrast injection. Typical CTA images are obtained from the diaphragm to the level of pubic symphysis in both the arterial and venous phases. A negative oral contrast agent may enhance visualization of the bowel wall and mucosa and permit easier 3D reconstructions without the need to subtract bowel contents or for positive contrast. One liter of water given to the patient 20 min prior to imaging serves as an adequate negative contrast source [8].

Because of the complex nature of the mesenteric vasculature and its variable anatomy, 3D reconstructions are valuable for assessment of mesenteric ischemia. Multiple reconstruction algorithms are used to more accurately assess the location and severity of stenosis, thrombus, emboli, or occlusion. For example, sagittal or sagittal oblique reconstructions are used to best visualize the origin of the celiac or superior mesenteric arteries, while the coronal oblique or axial oblique planes better demonstrate the distal branches of the mesenteric arteries [8, 10]. Advanced reconstructions such as volume rendering or maximum intensity projections further increase the sensitivity and specificity of CTA. Some authors suggest that maximum intensity projections are crucial for visualizing the most distal branches and the vasa recta. Other studies have shown that without multiplanar reconstructions and volume rendering, up to 66 % of lesions can be missed if the axial data is used alone [11].

Magnetic Resonance Angiography (MRA): Clinical Role and Imaging Considerations

MRA is not recommended as first-line imaging study for mesenteric vascular disease. The role of MRA in the diagnostic evaluation of these patients continues to evolve as new technologies emerge. MRA has a high sensitivity and specificity (comparable to CTA) in the detection of proximal occlusive disease and chronic mesenteric ischemia [12]. Some limitations occur in the diagnosis of stenotic or occlusive disease in the smaller, more distal mesenteric vessels, and visualization of the IMA has historically been difficult [13]. Logistical challenges also preclude the widespread use of MRA, as long scan times and the lack of MR availability can delay intervention in the acute setting. Much like CT, however, MR techniques continue to advance, and in addition to high-resolution MRA techniques which are increasingly available, complementary MRI techniques offer additional physiologic insights which can improve diagnostic confidence.

For contrast-enhanced MRA, gadolinium (Gd) chelates are used as T1 shortening agents to allow visualization of the abdominal vasculature when paired with gradient echo sequences. Similar to CTA, coordination of the imaging and injection of the contrast bolus is required to get optimal opacification of the mesenteric vasculature. Test bolus techniques and bolus tracking software exist, which work much in the same way as they do in CTA. The typical doses of most forms of Gd contrast is 10–20 mL (0.1–0.2 mmol/kg), which are injected over several seconds followed by a saline bolus of 20 mL [11, 14]. The sequences generate volumetric datasets, which can be reformatted into any plane or used to produce maximum intensity projections and volume rendered images, much like CT. Contrast-enhanced MRA can be performed in a single breath hold, optimally between 15 and 30 s in length. Each MRA examination involves a trade-off between spatial resolution, resistance to artifacts, and imaging time, so patients who are unable to hold their breath well are much more difficult to evaluate with MRA.

Unlike CT, there are additional MR techniques which can be used to perform angiographic type imaging without the use of IV contrast, avoiding potential complications in patients with renal insufficiency. Noncontrast MRA techniques are generally inferior to both CT and to contrast-enhanced MRA in terms of spatial resolution, acquisition time, and visualization of abdominal viscera, but can be useful given the frequency of concomitant vascular disease and renal insufficiency. Although these techniques can be used in select cases, intravenous gadolinium contrast for MR angiography is preferred as it increases the sensitivity and specificity of the examination [13].

A distinct advantage of MR imaging is the availability to discern physiologic as well as anatomic information in a noninvasive manner. The underlying principle is that when a normal person ingests calories, mesenteric blood flow is increased, and there is a compensatory increase in return of blood through the mesenteric veins to the liver. If a patient has limited mesenteric arterial flow reserve because of stenosis or occlusion, the decreased inflow will result in a less than expected increase in mesenteric venous return after a meal challenge and in increased oxygen extraction from the limited blood supply. By supplementing the anatomic exam with specialized MR pulse sequences to detect this altered physiologic state, the sensitivity, specificity, and diagnostic confidence of the overall exam are increased.

Chronic Mesenteric Ischemia

In the workup of chronic mesenteric ischemia, confident elimination of other abdominal pathologies that can lead to chronic abdominal pain is required. Chronic mesenteric ischemia is almost universally the result of atherosclerosis, and CTA and

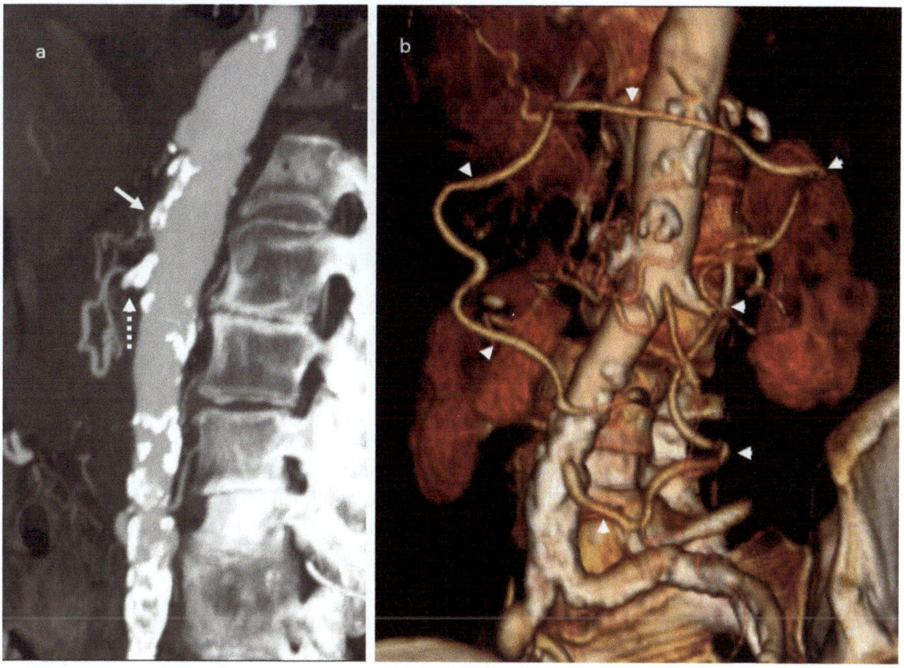

Fig. 7.1 CT angiographic images in a 78-year-old woman with chronic mesenteric ischemia. Sagittal oblique maximum intensity projection image (**a**) demonstrates occlusion of the celiac (*solid arrow*) and superior mesenteric (*dashed arrow*) artery origins. Volume-rendered image (**b**) demonstrates a markedly enlarged marginal artery of Drummond (*arrowheads*) from the inferior mesenteric artery supplying the celiac and superior mesenteric circulation

MRA typically demonstrate severe multivessel stenosis or occlusion of the proximal mesenteric arteries from calcified and noncalcified atherosclerotic plaques [8]. It is usually not until at least two of the three major mesenteric vessels (celiac artery, SMA, and IMA) are occluded that the patient becomes symptomatic, as collateral vascular supply of the intestines allows most patients to remain asymptomatic, even with severe stenosis of the mesenteric arteries. Due to the long time course over which chronic mesenteric ischemia develops, significant arterial collateral vessels are typically present (Fig. 7.1). Although it can happen, it is uncommon for chronic mesenteric ischemia to occur in the setting of single-vessel disease. Given the frequency of atherosclerotic disease in the general population (frequently incidentally visualized on CT), it is not uncommon to visualize greater than 50 % stenosis of a mesenteric artery in an asymptomatic patient [15–17], so pretest probability is an important consideration. Likewise, compression of the celiac axis by the median arcuate ligament is a frequent incidental anatomic finding, but frequently without associated clinical symptoms [8], so judicious use of the technology and clinical judgement are very important in interpreting exam results.

Although CTA is generally considered first-line imaging in cases of suspected chronic mesenteric ischemia, MRA is useful in equivocal cases or patients who

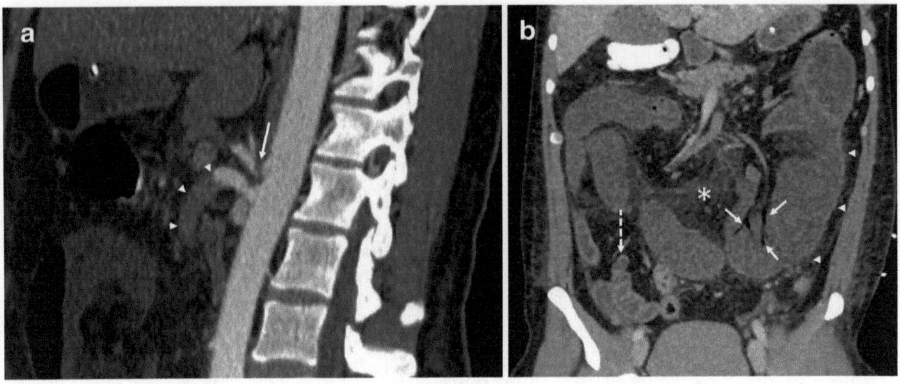

Fig. 7.2 A sagittal oblique MPR image (**a**) in a 40-year-old male with median arcuate ligament compression of the celiac axis (*arrow*) and an embolus lodged in the superior mesenteric artery (*arrowheads*). Coronal delayed phase CT image (**b**) demonstrates evidence of bowel ischemia with dilated, poorly enhancing loops of jejunum in the left mid-abdomen (*arrowheads*, contrasted with normal ileum in the right lower quadrant with a *dashed arrow*) and gas in portal venous tributaries (*arrows*). Also evident is mesenteric venous fat stranding indicating inflammation (*asterisk*)

have contraindications to CT contrast. MRA utilizing either specific gadolinium contrast agents or noncontrast techniques can also be advantageous to avoid potential complications of allergic reaction or contrast-induced nephropathy. MRA with contrast is well suited for the visualization of the proximal mesenteric arteries with an accuracy that is comparable to CTA [13]. Some authors have suggested that given the higher spatial and temporal resolution of CTA versus MRA, the IMA and distal mesenteric vessels are better assessed on CTA [13]. In our experience, with state-of-the-art MR techniques, non-visualization of a patent IMA or major SMA branches for technical reasons is very rare (Fig. 7.2), but with older scanners and less experienced operators, this certainly could still be a problem in routine clinical practice. Limited evaluation of the distal mesenteric vasculature is also less of a hindrance in the evaluation of chronic than acute mesenteric vascular disease.

In addition, MRA can be combined with functional physiologic data, which may additionally help to support or refute the diagnosis. Utilizing normal healthy volunteers, taking pre- and postprandial flow measurements, MR flow quantitation has demonstrated a postprandial increase in blood flow in the postprandial SMA and SMV due to the increased metabolic demands of the gut [14]. Studies have shown a correlation between the degree of SMA stenosis and the blunting of the normal postprandial blood flow increase in patients with varying degrees of SMA stenosis [16]. Other studies have shown a markedly decreased postprandial response in SMV flow in patients with chronic mesenteric ischemia versus healthy individuals [18]. Most commonly, flow in the SMV is measured prior to feeding and then at 15, 30, 45, and 60 min following a meal challenge. Increased flow in the SMV less than 50 % above baseline is considered abnormal and supportive of the diagnosis of chronic mesenteric ischemia [14, 16].

MR oximetry measures differences in T2 relaxation time of oxy- and deoxyhemoglobin. In normal healthy individuals, blood flow to the gut is increased following a meal to meet increased metabolic demands. In patients with stenosis or occlusions of the mesenteric arteries, blood flow cannot be increased, and therefore, oxygen extraction must be increased to attempt to meet the metabolic demand of the gut. Similar to flow quantitation, oximetry is performed in the SMV in the preprandial state and following a meal challenge. Studies have shown that in normal individuals the oxygen saturation in the SMV increases by about 5 % following feedings. In symptomatic patients with angiographically proven stenosis of two of the three mesenteric arteries, postprandial oxygen saturation decreases by about 9 % [14, 19].

Acute Mesenteric Ischemia

The major causes of acute mesenteric ischemia include embolus, mesenteric arterial thrombosis, mesenteric venous thrombosis, and nonocclusive mesenteric ischemia [8, 13, 14]. Acute embolus to the SMA is the most common cause of acute mesenteric ischemia, occurring in 40–50 % of the cases [13]. Most emboli to the SMA tend to lodge a few centimeters from the origin, just distal to the middle colic artery ostium. Smaller emboli can lodge further distally in the smaller splanchnic branches [13]. Nonocclusive emboli are visible on CTA as low-density filling defects within the vessel lumen, and occlusive emboli are visible as an abrupt termination of the vessel (Fig. 7.3). Given the acute nature of embolic phenomena, collateral vessels are frequently absent. Acute mesenteric artery thrombosis is the second most common cause of acute mesenteric ischemia, accounting for 20–30 % of all cases [13]. Thrombosis occurs following the rupture of an unstable atherosclerotic plaque leading to the accumulation of platelets and inflammatory mediators. Given that the thrombosis usually

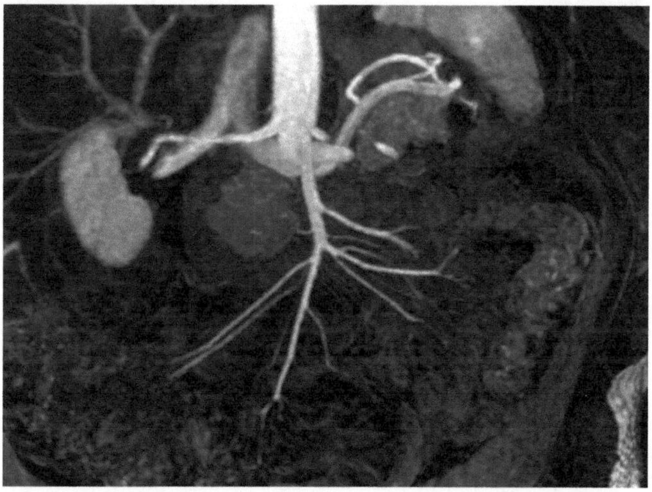

Fig. 7.3 Thin maximum intensity projection from a contrast-enhanced MR angiogram in a 55-year-old woman with a prior superior mesenteric artery (SMA) dissection demonstrates clear visualization of normal-appearing SMA and multiple jejunal and ileal branches

occurs in the setting of preexisting atherosclerotic disease, the site of thrombosis is typically at the origin of the SMA or within the proximal 2 cm [8]. Many patients presenting with acute SMA thrombosis have long-standing atherosclerotic disease, and their bowel is subjected to chronic ischemia. This leads to the development of small arterial collateral vessels, which can be readily seen on CTA. The typical imaging findings in SMA thrombosis are the complete occlusion of the origin or proximal SMA with poor visualization of the distal branches. This is in distinction to emboli, which tend to affect more distal branches. Intraluminal filling defects are uncommon in acute thrombosis [8]. Nonocclusive mesenteric ischemia and venous thrombosis together account for approximately 30–40 % of cases of acute mesenteric [8].

No matter the cause of the mesenteric ischemia, the sequela of bowel ischemia can be readily assessed with CTA. Hypoperfused bowel exhibits decreased peristalsis and retention of fluid and secretions. This leads to small bowel dilation (>3 cm), colonic dilatation (>9 cm), or bowel obstruction, with geographically dilated bowel. Edema and poor perfusion within the bowel wall commonly cause low attenuation and circumferential thickening up to 1.5 cm [8]. This severe degree of bowel thickening is more commonly seen in venous thrombosis than in arterial inflow causes, which tend to have bowel wall thickening of 8–9 mm [8] (Fig. 7.4). Occasionally, the bowel wall can be normal or even thinned. Although decreased contrast inflow and mural edema

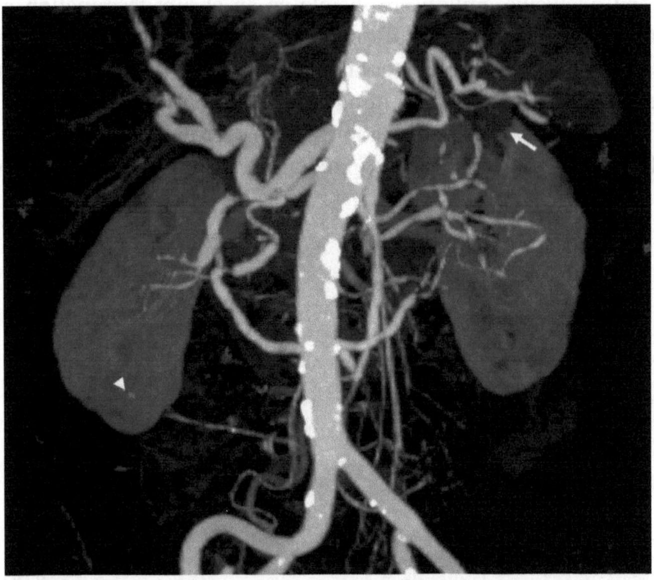

Fig. 7.4 Coronal oblique maximum intensity projection image from contrast-enhanced CT angiography in a 79-year-old female patient with a two-week history of abdominal pain, nausea, and anorexia. The exam was performed for suspicion of mesenteric ischemia. The image demonstrates diffuse segmental ectasia and stenotic "beading" of the mesenteric and renal circulation, as well as a small segmental infarct in the upper pole left kidney (*arrow*) and a tiny intrarenal aneurysm on the right (*arrowhead*). The findings are compatible with polyarteritis nodosa, and the patient's symptoms resolved on steroid therapy

can give the appearance of low density and hypoenhancement; hemorrhage within the bowel wall or compensatory hyperemia may paradoxically cause bowel wall hyperattenuation. Pneumatosis intestinalis is seen late in the course of ischemia, indicating transmural infarction with mucosal breakdown. This finding is commonly accompanied by gas within the portomesenteric system and carries a poor prognosis.

Cross-sectional imaging allows the evaluation of organs other than the bowel within the abdomen and pelvis, which aids in the differential diagnosis of conditions that can mimic acute mesenteric ischemia. Entities frequently seen on CTA in the absence of mesenteric ischemia include small bowel obstruction, cholecystitis, and diverticulitis [20, 21].

In the absence of definitive vascular findings, other findings can be seen due to decreased blood flow within the bowel. Mesenteric fat stranding or congestion, ascites or free abdominal fluid, and free abdominal air are generalized signs of a number of abdominal processes that can also be seen in mesenteric ischemia. Unfortunately, many of these secondary findings can be seen in a wide range of nonischemic conditions and lack specificity. The most common findings seen on CT in patients with acute mesenteric ischemia are mesenteric fat stranding, bowel wall thickening, bowel dilatation, and ascites [20–22]. These findings are suggestive of acute mesenteric ischemia, although their specificity ranges from 20 to 86 %. The most specific findings were those of late complications, including pneumatosis intestinalis, solid organ infarctions, and portal venous gas with specificities of 100 % reported in multiple studies [21, 22]. In an attempt to optimize the algorithm for diagnosis of acute mesenteric ischemia utilizing MDCT, one group diagnosed mesenteric ischemia with the single finding of pneumatosis intestinalis, portomesenteric venous gas, or visceral artery occlusion, or a combination of bowel wall thickening with portomesenteric venous thrombosis or solid organ infarction. This approach yielded a sensitivity of 93 %, specificity of 100 %, positive predictive value of 100 %, and negative predictive value of 96 % [21].

The use of MRA performed with intravenous contrast has a limited role in the diagnosis of acute mesenteric ischemia. MRA has a high accuracy in diagnosing arterial embolism or thrombosis of the proximal vasculature, but is usually more limited for evaluation of distal branches. Given the long acquisition times required for multiple sequences and the lack of widespread availability, the use of MRA may delay intervention in an acutely ill patient [14, 23]. In select cases, such as those patients with a severe iodine allergies or renal insufficiency, contrast-enhanced or noncontrast MRA may be a reasonable option.

Mesenteric Venous Thrombosis

Mesenteric venous thrombosis accounts for 5–15 % of cases of mesenteric ischemia [13]. The presentation can be variable and can occur as either an acute or a chronic disorder with patients clinically ranging from asymptomatic to critically ill, depending on the acuity and occlusiveness of the thrombosis [24]. The thrombus is seen as a filling defect at the site of venous obstruction, which can propagate peripherally. In cases attributable to a hypercoagulable state, venous thrombus is often first seen in the smaller branches as a low-density intraluminal filling defect and then spreads centrally towards the major venous trunks [24]. 3D reconstructions are especially useful for imaging the mesenteric venous system as these vessels can be easily identified and followed on the coronal and coronal oblique projections [10]. The confluence of the superior mesenteric vein and portal vein is a common site for venous thrombosis, and coronal reconstructions permit quick and accurate assessment of this area [8]. Several authors have found that other reconstructions, such as maximum intensity projections using thin slabs, are best used to display venous collaterals that occur in the presence of mesenteric venous thrombosis [8]. Due to the venous collateral system of the bowel, patients can be asymptomatic, even with a large degree of venous thrombosis, and evidence of bowel ischemia on CT or MR may not be present in isolated thrombosis. In acute or complete thrombosis, without robust venous collateral flow, severe venous hypertension results lead to engorgement of the veins with wall thickening and enhancement [13]. The bowel wall can be significantly thickened and congested due to venous obstruction. Intramural hemorrhage can be seen within the bowel wall as increased density on CT. With long-standing venous obstruction, transmural infarction can occur, which can cause complete lack of bowel wall enhancement [8]. This can lead to findings of pneumatosis intestinalis or portomesenteric gas, which portend a poor prognosis [8, 13] (Fig. 7.4). The generalized abdominal findings of bowel dilatation or ascites fluid are nonspecific and can be seen in venous thrombosis; however, hemorrhagic peritoneal fluid appearing hyperdense on CT suggests early bowel infarction [25].

Nonocclusive Mesenteric Ischemia

Nonocclusive mesenteric ischemia accounts for approximately a quarter of the cases of acute mesenteric ischemia, although it carries a high mortality rate that approaches 70 % [13, 26]. Nonocclusive ischemia is secondary to severe hypoperfusion of the bowel and is usually in association with cardiogenic shock or hypotension. Generalized findings of hypovolemic shock, including a slit-like appearance of the IVC, typically accompany this disorder. No focal vascular obstruction is identified, but rather global signs of hypoperfusion are present, including a “shock bowel” appearance. This term describes the segmentally dilated, commonly fluid-filled, small bowel with diffuse hyperenhancement of the wall seen in the setting of hypovolemic shock. This is thought to be the result of autoregulation and vasoconstriction of the mesenteric vasculature, which slows perfusion and shunts blood to the critical organs [27]. This hypoperfusion leads to vasoconstriction of the small mesenteric arteries, which can cause the vessels to appear very small on CTA and cause delayed filling of the mesenteric veins with no opacification during venous phase at 60–70 s after injection [13]. With prolonged vasoconstriction, intestinal mucosal permeability increases, allowing for entry of gas into the bowel wall and mesenteric vascular system, apparent as pneumatosis and portomesenteric gas on cross-sectional imaging.

Median Arcuate Ligament Syndrome

Median arcuate ligament syndrome is the result of the median arcuate ligament passing superior to the origin of the celiac trunk and compressing the vessel. This is best seen on the sagittal reconstructions as a smooth indentation along the superior margin of the proximal celiac artery. Both CTA and MRA images can be easily reconstructed in the sagittal format and can readily identify the median arcuate ligament and determine if there is any compression present. Compression of the proximal celiac artery is augmented on expiration with superior motion of the celiac trunk against the median arcuate ligament. It should be noted that isolated compression of the celiac trunk during expiration is not a specific finding and may not be clinically significant. Prior studies have shown that up to 50 % of asymptomatic patients exhibit some degree of compression of the celiac trunk during expiration [28]. More specific, but less commonly seen, findings of severe stenosis include prominent poststenotic dilatation and celiac artery compression which persists during inspiration [28]. Inspiratory and expiratory angiography may be helpful in equivocal cases.

Mesenteric Artery Dissection or Aneurysm

CTA is an ideal choice for first-line imaging in patients with isolated mesenteric artery aneurysms or dissections. Most commonly, celiac artery or superior mesenteric artery dissections are seen as an extension of an abdominal aortic dissection. The most common site of isolated mesenteric artery dissection is in the proximal few centimeters of the superior mesenteric artery [29]. As with dissections in other vessels, an intraluminal flap, thrombosis of the false lumen, and intramural hematoma are specific findings than can often be seen. Mild enlargement of the affected artery and fat stranding of the adjacent mesentery are less specific findings that may also be seen [30]. Isolated mesenteric artery aneurysms are a rare entity, which can be found incidentally or with the patient in extremis following rupture. Focal dilatation of a mesenteric artery clinches the diagnosis when seen on cross-sectional imaging. In one study of 21 patients with SMA aneurysms, the mean nonruptured size was 2.2 cm [31]. In that same study about 80 % of patients had an isolated superior mesenteric artery aneurysm, while about 20 % had multiple aneurysms. Both aneurysms and dissections may be also associated with either disorders of vascular connective tissue such as Ehlers-Danlos type IV or segmental arterial mediolysis or with a vasculitis such as polyarteritis nodosa (Fig. 7.5). Signs of aneurysm rupture on CTA include high-density peritoneal fluid corresponding to hemorrhage within the peritoneal cavity and active extravasation from the ruptured artery.

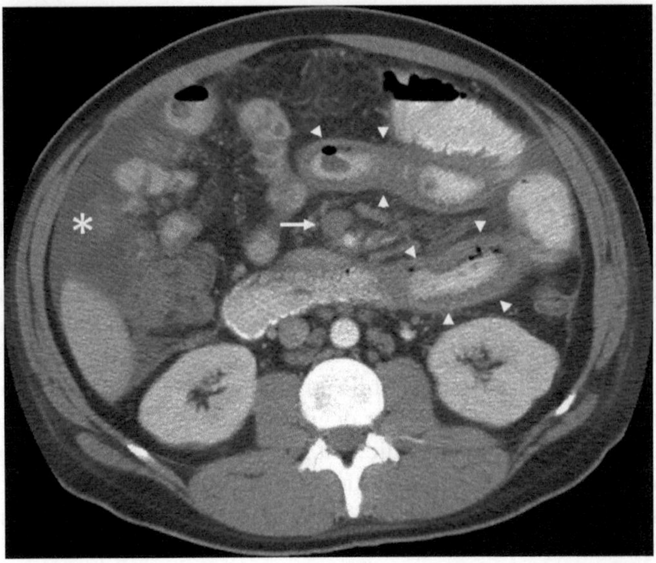

Fig. 7.5 Axial contrast-enhanced CT venogram in a 25-year-old male who developed severe and worsening abdominal pain after an episode of dehydration and vomiting from a gastroenteritis. CT demonstrates a thrombus in the superior mesenteric vein (*arrow*) and markedly thickened, poorly enhancing jejunal loops (*arrowheads*) and abdominal ascites (*asterisk*) secondary to mesenteric venous congestion

CTA Limitations

Although CTA is currently recommended as first-line imaging in the evaluation of mesenteric vascular disease, it does have limitations. CT uses ionizing radiation, with potential carcinogenic effects. The need for multiphase imaging in arterial and venous phases of enhancement increases the radiation exposure compared to a routine abdomen and pelvis CT for the evaluation of nonspecific abdominal pain. The American College of Radiology estimates the effective dose for an adult on the range of 1–10 mSv for CTA of the abdomen [2], and CTA for mesenteric ischemia can certainly double this. In most cases, the information obtained with CT is a benefit that outweighs the risk of radiation exposure. The potential adverse effects from radiation vary widely based on patient-based factors, particularly age, and the potential carcinogenesis is usually not a significant concern given the typical age of patients with suspected mesenteric ischemia. Pediatric patients are at higher risk for adverse effects from radiation exposure due to higher organ sensitivity to radiation and longer life expectancy, which increases the risk due to the long latent period that appears to accompany the adverse health effects of radiation [2]. In the evaluation of the pediatric patient with mesenteric vascular disease, forethought should be given to the possibility that they may need multiple serial follow-up examinations throughout the course of their lifetime. MRA may be a better choice in these cases due to the fact that no radiation exposure is incurred. Another limitation of CTA is the need for intravenous iodine-based contrast injection. In patients with allergies to iodinated contrast, premedication protocols exist to blunt the allergic response. In patients with anaphylaxis from prior contrast injection, clinicians may not feel comfortable administering contrast again, even with the use of premedication, so MRA would generally be a viable alternative.

There has been much discussion in the recent literature involving contrast-induced nephropathy, especially in those patients with mildly–moderately impaired renal function. The cause of contrast-induced nephropathy remains unclear, and it is common practice not to administer intravenous contrast material to patients with a GFR less than 45 mL/minute. Research published in 2013 suggests that *intravenous* contrast-induced nephropathy is not nearly as common as once thought – or may not exist at all. A study involving over 53,000 patients showed that the rate of contrast-induced nephropathy was no different from contrast material-independent acute kidney injury, suggesting that contrast material may cause renal insufficiency following contrast injection [32]. A large meta-analysis performed by the same group reviewed nearly 1,500 independent studies and found similar incidence of acute kidney injury, need for dialysis, and death in patients who received intravenous contrast and noncontrast control groups [33].

MRA Limitations

MRA has less widespread availability than CTA, so logistically the use of MRA in acute settings is discouraged because this may delay diagnosis and intervention. In general, MRI has lower spatial resolution than CT, and in cases that require evaluation of the small mesenteric branches, MRA may not be as useful. The acquisition of multiple sequences, some of which require breath holds for more than 20 s, create long imaging times compared to CTA, and the patient must remain still on the MRI table. This positioning and breath holding is challenging for some patients with multiple comorbidities. The nature of MR sequences make them more susceptible to motion artifact than CTA, and although glucagon can be given to inhibit peristalsis, bowel motion is a limiting factor when trying to evaluate the vasa recta or the intestines for early signs of ischemia. Additional susceptibility artifact from metal, namely, metallic stents, limits the use of MRA in evaluating patients status post-intervention with angioplasty and stent placement.

Nephrogenic systemic fibrosis is a scleroderma-like disease that has been seen after the administration of Gd-based contrast, primarily in patients on hemodialysis. The etiology of this disorder remains unclear; however, it is almost never seen in patients who do not have severe renal insufficiency and has not clearly been associated with all gadolinium formulations. Current guidelines recommend avoidance of administration of Gd-based contrast agents in patients on hemodialysis or with GFR rates less than 30 mL/min [2] or acute renal injury.

Lastly, many non-MR compatible implanted medical devices, such as pacemakers and spine or deep brain stimulators, preclude any MRI examination.

Future Directions

Cross-sectional imaging technology continues to advance rapidly, increasing the ability to provide accurate evaluation of the mesenteric vasculature and earlier diagnosis of mesenteric ischemia. Just as the development of MDCT revolutionized the diagnosis of mesenteric vascular disease with cross-sectional imaging, continued development of new technologies may change the way we diagnose and treat mesenteric vascular disease in the future. Dual-energy CT is an evolving technology that involves collecting helical CT data at two different energies, one low kVp and one high kVp. The differences of particular tissues at these various energies can then be exploited in many advantageous ways. For example, by utilizing post-processing software, calcium can be exclusively isolated and removed. This allows more accurate assessment of the true degree of stenosis occurring at the site of calcified atherosclerotic plaques [34]. Using the same calcium isolation and removal process, bone subtraction algorithms for volume rendering on dual energy systems can be optimized. Advances in CT perfusion technology may also permit evaluation of bowel viability and help us to better triage patients prior to laparotomy.

MR advances in rapid imaging and tissue characterization also have the potential to impact mesenteric ischemia diagnosis. Recent studies using 3 T magnets and animal models have shown that using diffusion-weighted imaging (DWI) can identify early ischemic changes. The ischemic bowel appears hyperintense on DWI and hypointense on the corresponding ADC map as early as 30 min after induction of ischemia, mimicking either occlusive or nonocclusive causes [35]. In the future, the more widespread availability of MRI and additional advances in functional imaging may be able to provide the earliest assessment of mesenteric ischemia and supersede CTA as first-line imaging.

Summary

Cross-sectional imaging, utilizing either CTA or MRA, is an ideal noninvasive method for the evaluation of patients with suspected mesenteric vascular disease. The high-resolution, widespread availability, and three-dimensional reconstructions afforded by the current generation of CTA yield a high sensitivity and specificity for diagnosing various causes of mesenteric ischemia and should be considered a first-line imaging study. CTA can also easily exclude other causes of acute or chronic abdominal pain and can provide detailed anatomic information, which can guide surgical or endovascular intervention. MRA has a lesser role than CTA for this indication, but given the lack of radiation, ability to image without intravenous contrast, and capacity to provide functional physiologic information, it can be useful as an alternative diagnostic tool. MRA is generally better suited for evaluating chronic mesenteric ischemia than acute mesenteric ischemia. Each imaging modality is with its own limitations, and the clinician should weigh the benefits and risks versus the limitations of each imaging modality in individual cases. Future directions with further advances in imaging technology will likely lead to increased functional data and early identification of patients at high risk for mesenteric vascular disease.

References

1. Wadman M, Syk I, Elmståhl B, Ekberg O, Elmståhl S. Abdominal plain film findings in acute ischemic bowel disease differ with age. Acta Radiol. 2006;47(3):238–43.
2. Oliva IB, Davarpanah AH, Rybicki FJ, Desjardins B, Flamm SD, Francois CJ, Dill KE. ACR appropriateness criteria® imaging of mesenteric ischemia. Abdom Imaging. 2013;38(4):714–9.
3. Taourel PG, Deneuville M, Pradel JA, Régent D, Bruel JM. Acute mesenteric ischemia: diagnosis with contrast-enhanced CT. Radiology. 1996;199(3):632–6.
4. Horton KM, Fishman EK. Multi-detector row CT of mesenteric ischemia: can it be done? Radiographics. 2001;21(6):1463–73.
5. Wiesner W, Mortelé KJ, Glickman JN, Ji H, Ros PR. Pneumatosis intestinalis and portomesenteric venous gas in intestinal ischemia: correlation of CT findings with severity of ischemia and clinical outcome. Am J Roentgenol. 2001;177(6):1319–23.
6. Yu CW, Lee WJ, Tsai YH, Liu KL, Chen SJ. Demonstration of extensive mesenteric venous thrombosis and intestinal infarction with multidetector row CT: value of curved planar reformations. Abdom Imaging. 2003;28(6):775–7.
7. Menke J. Diagnostic accuracy of multidetector CT in acute mesenteric ischemia: systematic review and meta-analysis. Radiology. 2010;256(1):93–101.
8. Horton KM, Fishman EK. CT angiography of the mesenteric circulation. Radiol Clin North Am. 2010;48(2):331–45.
9. Fleischmann D. CT angiography: injection and acquisition technique. Radiol Clin North Am. 2010;48(2):237–47.
10. Horton KM, Fishman EK. Mutidetector row and 3D CT of the mesenteric vasculature: normal anatomy and pathology. In: Seminars in ultrasound, CT, and MRI (Vol. 24, No. 5). Philadelphia: WB Saunders; 2003. p. 353–63.
11. Chen JK, Johnson PT, Horton KM, Fishman EK. Unsuspected mesenteric arterial abnormality: comparison of MDCT axial sections to interactive 3D rendering. Am J Roentgenol. 2007;189(4):807–13.
12. Laissy JP, Trillaud H, Douek P. MR angiography: noninvasive vascular imaging of the abdomen. Abdom Imaging. 2002;27(5):488–506.
13. Shih MCP, Hagspiel KD. CTA and MRA in mesenteric ischemia: part 1, role in diagnosis and differential diagnosis. Am J Roentgenol. 2007;188(2):452–61.
14. Chow LC, Chan FP, Li KCP. A comprehensive approach to MR imaging of mesenteric ischemia. Abdom Imaging. 2002;27(5):507–16.
15. Heiss SG, Li KC. Magnetic resonance angiography of mesenteric arteries. Invest Radiol. 1998;33(9):670–81.
16. Li KC, Whitney WS, McDonnell CH, Fredrickson JO, Pelc NJ, Dalman RL, Jeffrey RB. Chronic mesenteric ischemia: evaluation with phase-contrast cine MR imaging. Radiology. 1994;190(1):175–9.
17. Roobottom CA, Dubbins PA. Significant disease of the celiac and superior mesenteric arteries in asymptomatic patients: predictive value of Doppler sonography. Am J Roentgenol. 1993;161(5):985–8.
18. Burkart DJ, Johnson CD, Reading CC, Ehman RL. MR measurements of mesenteric venous flow: prospective evaluation in healthy volunteers and patients with suspected chronic mesenteric ischemia. Radiology. 1995;194(3):801–6.

19. Li KC, Dalman RL, Ch'en IY, Pelc LR, Song CK, Moon WK, Wright GA. Chronic mesenteric ischemia: use of in vivo MR imaging measurements of blood oxygen saturation in the superior mesenteric vein for diagnosis. Radiology. 1997;204(1):71–7.
20. Barmase M, Kang M, Wig J, Kochhar R, Gupta R, Khandelwal N. Role of multidetector CT angiography in the evaluation of suspected mesenteric ischemia. Eur J Radiol. 2011;80(3):e582–7.
21. Aschoff AJ, Stuber G, Becker BW, Hoffmann MHK, Schmitz BL, Schelzig H, Jaeckle T. Evaluation of acute mesenteric ischemia: accuracy of biphasic mesenteric multi-detector CT angiography. Abdom Imaging. 2009;34(3):345–57.
22. Kirkpatrick ID, Kroeker MA, Greenberg HM. Biphasic CT with mesenteric CT angiography in the evaluation of acute mesenteric ischemia: initial experience. Radiology. 2003;229(1):91–8.
23. Meaney JF, Prince MR, Nostrant TT, Stanley JC. Gadolinium-enhanced MR angiography of visceral arteries in patients with suspected chronic mesenteric ischemia. J Magn Reson Imaging. 1997;7(1):171–6.
24. Gore RM, Yaghmai V, Thakrar KH, Berlin JW, Mehta UK, Newmark GM, Miller FH. Imaging in intestinal ischemic disorders. Radiol Clin North Am. 2008;46(5):845–75.
25. Clavien PA, Dürig M, Harder F. Venous mesenteric infarction: a particular entity. Brit J Surg. 1988;75(3):252–5.
26. Bassiouny HS. Nonocclusive mesenteric ischemia. Surg Clin North Am. 1997;77(2):319–26.
27. Mirvis SE, Shanmuganathan K, Erb R. Diffuse small-bowel ischemia in hypotensive adults after blunt trauma (shock bowel): CT findings and clinical significance. Am J Roentgenol. 1994;163(6):1375–9.
28. Horton KM, Talamini MA, Fishman EK. Median arcuate ligament syndrome: evaluation with CT angiography. Radiographics. 2005;25(5):1177–82.
29. Okino Y, Kiyosue H, Mori H, Komatsu E, Matsumoto S, Yamada Y, Tomonari K. Root of the small-bowel mesentery: correlative anatomy and CT features of pathologic conditions. Radiographics. 2001;21(6):1475–90.
30. Suzuki S, Furui S, Kohtake H, Sakamoto T, Yamasaki M, Furukawa A, Takei R. Isolated dissection of the superior mesenteric artery. Abdom Imaging. 2004;29(2):153–7.
31. Stone WM, Abbas M, Cherry KJ, Fowl RJ, Gloviczki P. Superior mesenteric artery aneurysms: is presence an indication for intervention? J Vasc Surg. 2002;36(2):234–7.
32. McDonald RJ, McDonald JS, Bida JP, Carter RE, Fleming CJ, Misra S, Kallmes DF. Intravenous contrast material-induced nephropathy: causal or coincident phenomenon? Radiology. 2013;267(1):106–18.
33. McDonald JS, McDonald RJ, Comin J, Williamson EE, Katzberg RW, Murad MH, Kallmes DF. Frequency of acute kidney injury following intravenous contrast medium administration: a systematic review and meta-analysis. Radiology. 2013;267(1):119–28.
34. Kumamaru KK, Hoppel BE, Mather RT, Rybicki FJ. CT angiography: current technology and clinical use. Radiol Clin North Am. 2010;48(2):213.
35. Bruhn RS, Distelmaier MS, Hellmann-Sokolis M, Naami A, Kuhl CK, Hohl C. Early detection of acute mesenteric ischemia using diffusion-weighted 3.0-T magnetic resonance imaging in a porcine model. Invest Radiol. 2013;48(4):231–7.

Chapter 8
Diagnostic Angiography

Gustavo S. Oderich and Leonardo Reis de Souza

Diagnostic catheter-based arteriography is considered the "gold-standard" diagnostic study for evaluating mesenteric and visceral artery disease in patients with a variety of aneurysmal or occlusive mesenteric lesions [1]. During the last decade, its role as confirmatory test and for planning revascularization diminished, in favor of the less invasive modalities. Since 2002, the usage of contrast arteriography to plan mesenteric reconstructions for chronic mesenteric ischemia (CMI) has decreased from 97 to 57 % at the Mayo Clinic. This change occurred due to substantial increase in use of computed tomography angiography (55–88 %) and magnetic resonance angiography (12–33 %) [2]. Mesenteric arteriography is rarely needed to confirm the diagnosis, and it typically does not add anatomical detail to plan an intervention. More frequently, angiography is obtained in conjunction with a planned endovascular intervention. Exceptions are patients with suboptimal imaging studies and those with extensive calcification, small vessels, or multiple prior stents causing metallic artifact [3].

G.S. Oderich, MD, FACS (✉)
Division of Vascular and Endovascular Surgery, Mayo Clinic, Rochester, MN, USA

Gonda Vascular Center, Mayo Clinic, Rochester, MN, USA
e-mail: oderich.gustavo@mayo.edu

L.R. de Souza, MD
Division of Vascular and Endovascular Surgery, Mayo Clinic, Rochester, MN, USA

Masters Degree Program from the Department of Surgery,
Universidade Federal do Rio Grande do Sul, Porto Alegre, Brazil
e-mail: reissouza@gmail.com

G.S. Oderich (ed.), *Mesenteric Vascular Disease*,
DOI 10.1007/978-1-4939-1847-8_8

Technique

Diagnostic mesenteric angiography can be performed using either femoral or brachial approach. The later has higher risk of access-related complications and therefore should be avoided for purely diagnostic studies. Femoral approach is considered the first choice for diagnostic angiography. However, if diagnostic angiography is obtained in conjunction with a planned intervention, brachial or radial approach is used more liberally depending on the technical difficulty of the procedure and angle of origin from the aorta [4].

Percutaneous femoral access is established using a micropuncture set under ultrasound guidance. The 0.018-in. access guidewire is exchanged for a 0.035-in. floppy wire and a 5 Fr sheath is positioned in the external iliac artery. Systemic anticoagulation with 40 units/kg of heparin is recommended prior to selective catheterization; if intervention is anticipated, full heparinization (80 units/kg) is recommended. If brachial access is used in conjunction with anticipated intervention, the author's preference is to surgically expose the distal brachial artery at the elbow crease under local anesthesia, avoiding access-related complications. Other alternatives are total percutaneous access and radial access, which has been increasingly utilized. After access is established, mesenteric angiography consists of abdominal and selective views. A 5 Fr diagnostic flush catheter (pigtail, straight, or other) is positioned at T12 level over a 0.035-in. Glidewire for abdominal aortography. A complete study requires at least an anteroposterior (Fig. 8.1) and lateral views (Fig. 8.2). The later is ideal to demonstrate the origin of the celiac axis and superior mesenteric artery (SMA). The optimal projection to display the origin of the inferior mesenteric artery (IMA) it is a 15° right lateral-oblique view (Fig. 8.3).

Selective visceral artery angiography may be required to demonstrate anatomical detail and collateral patterns, to confirm severity of the disease, and to identify tandem lesions. Modest systemic anticoagulation (40 units/kg) is highly recommended prior to attempt selective catheterization. The choice of catheter shape is dependent upon access site, angle of origin, and individual preference (Table 8.1). For example, a multipurpose catheter (MPA, Fig. 8.4) is ideal for approaching the mesenteric arteries from brachial approach, whereas a secondary curve catheter (e.g., SOS or Simmons) is needed when these arteries are accessed via the femoral access. Other catheter shapes or guide catheters (Fig. 8.5) are useful for approaching the mesenteric arteries via either approach and may provide better support to assist with stent placement or other intervention.

Selective injection of the mesenteric arteries can be associated with abdominal discomfort, particularly in the patient with severe ischemia symptoms (Fig. 8.6). The use of a low-osmolar contrast agent (e.g., iodixanol) minimizes abdominal discomfort, frequently described as pain or warmth/cold sensation, during selective injections [5]. Pressure gradients can be useful in the case of a questionable lesion and be obtained by pressure wire and "pull-back" or simultaneous pressure measurement technique [6]. Intravascular ultrasound can also be useful in patients with lesions of questionable significance or to assess technical result after intervention

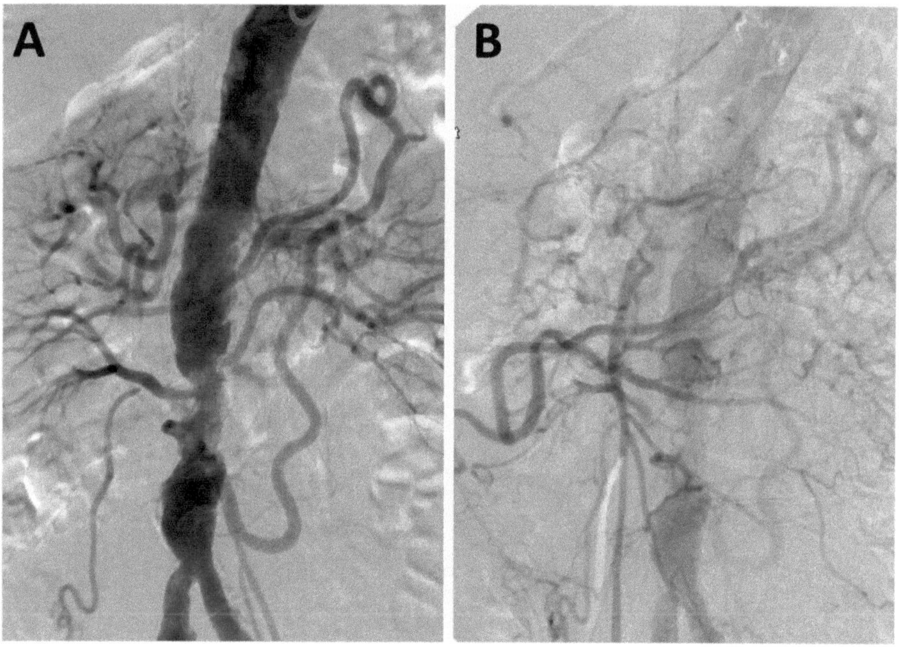

Fig. 8.1 Diagnostic aortography in a patient with chronic mesenteric ischemia. Note that both the celiac axis and superior mesenteric artery origin is not opacified in anterolateral projection (**a**). The inferior mesenteric artery is patent and provides collateral flow into the SMA and celiac via arc of Riolan. Lateral (**b**) views demonstrate occluded SMA and celiac axis with diseased inferior mesenteric artery

Fig. 8.2 Lateral aortography in a patient with moderate to severe celiac and superior mesenteric artery stenosis

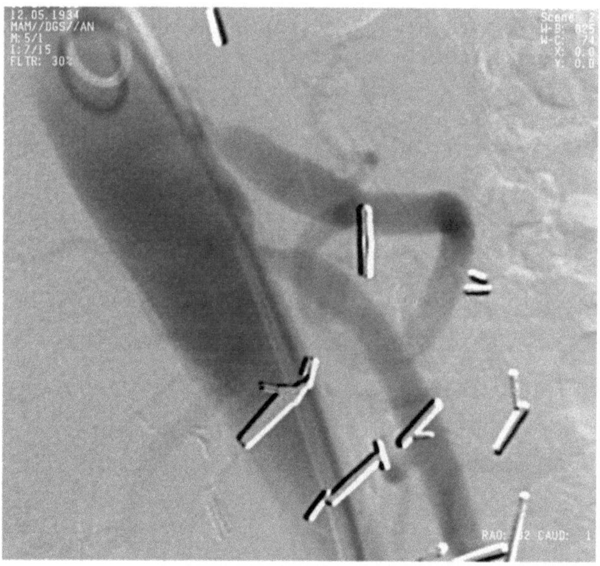

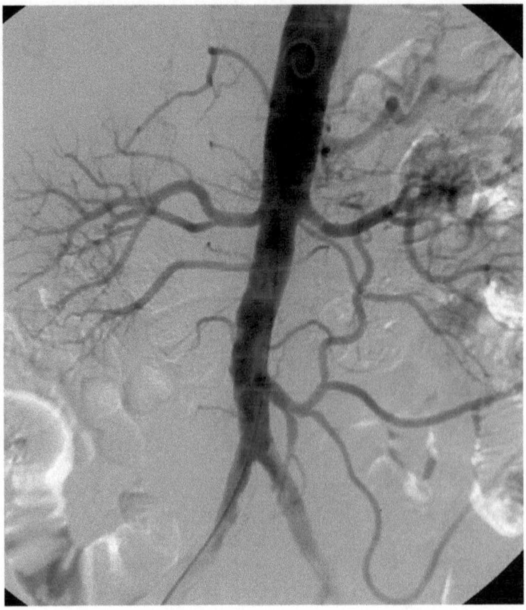

Fig. 8.3 Right anterior-oblique view and selective angiography of the inferior mesenteric artery demonstrate collateral networks to the superior mesenteric artery via arc of Riolan

Table 8.1 Catheters and injection rates used for selective mesenteric artery catheterizations

Artery	Catheter shape	Injection (mL/s)	Total volume	Filming (fr/s)
Celiac	Femoral: SOS Omni, Simmons, Cobra-2	5–7	15–20	2–4
	Brachial: MPA, MPB, Kumpe			
Splenic	Femoral: Simmons, Cobra 2	5–7	15–20	2–4
	Brachial: MPA, MPB, Kumpe			
Hepatic	Femoral: Simmons, Cobra 2	4–5	10–15	2–4
	Brachial: MPA, MPB, Kumpe			
Left gastric	Femoral: Simmons, Cobra 2	3–4	10–15	2–4
	Brachial: MPA, MPB, Kumpe			
Gastroduodenal	Femoral: Simmons, Cobra 2	3–4	10–15	2–4
	Brachial: MPA, MPB, Kumpe			
SMA	Femoral: SOS, Simmons, Cobra 2	5–7	15–20	2–4
	Brachial: MPA, MPB, Kumpe			
SMA branches	Femoral: Simmons, Cobra 2	3–4	10–15	2–4
	Brachial: MPA, MPB, Kumpe, micro-catheters			
IMA	Femoral: SOS, Simmons, Cobra 2	3–5	10–15	2–4
	Brachial: MPA, MPB, Kumpe			

SMA superior mesenteric artery, *IMA* inferior mesenteric artery

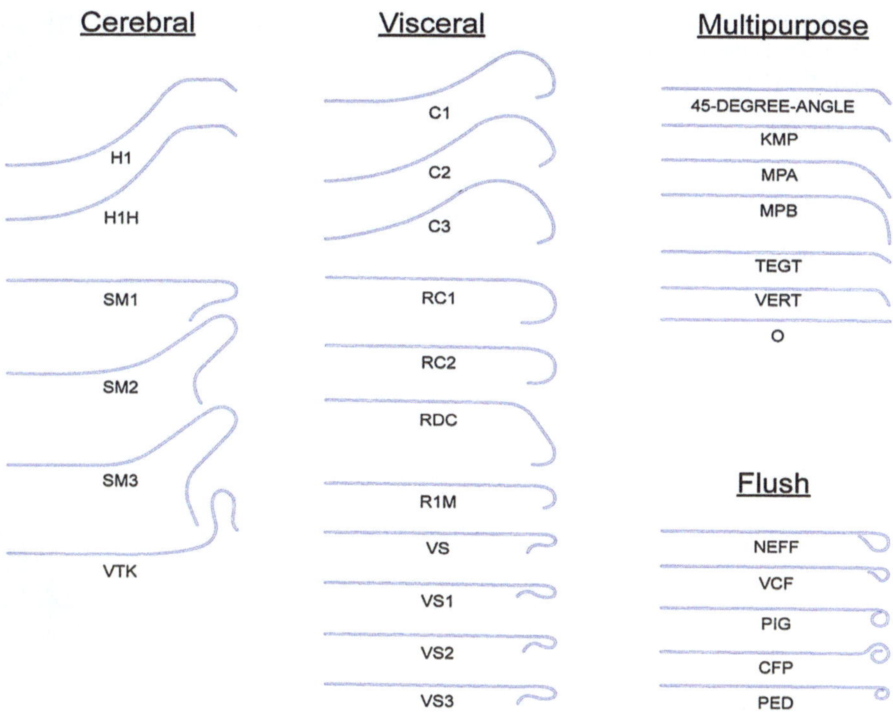

Fig. 8.4 Catheter shapes frequently utilized for diagnostic and selective visceral angiography

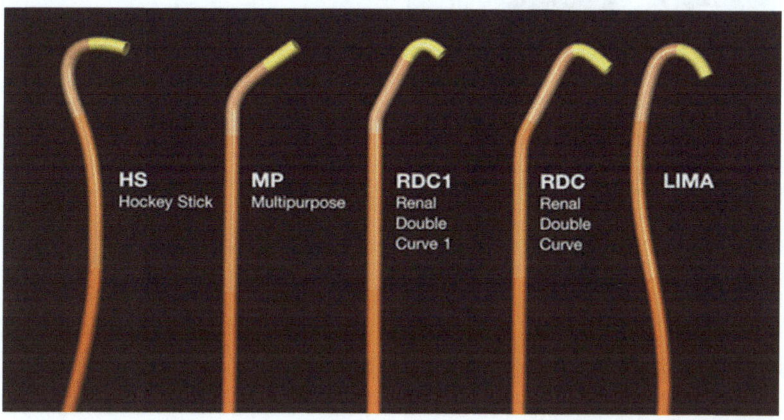

Fig. 8.5 Frequently utilized guide catheters for renal and mesenteric interventions

(Figs. 8.7, 8.8, and 8.9). Review of pre-procedure computed tomography or magnetic resonance imaging is helpful to guide access and choice of catheter shape. In patients with arteries that have angulated origin from the aorta or high-grade stenosis or occlusion, technical challenge can be anticipated from the femoral approach. In these cases, use of guide catheters (Fig. 8.5) may be necessary to provide adequate support and to facilitate exchanges if a stiffer system is needed for intervention.

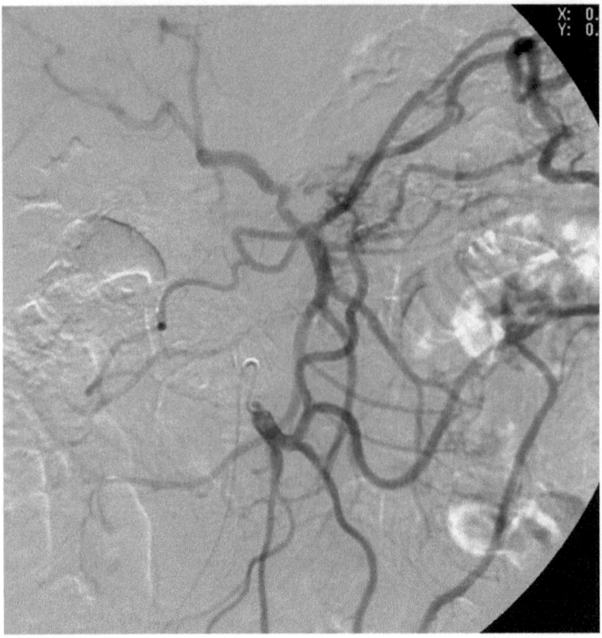

Fig. 8.6 Selective angiography of the inferior mesenteric artery demonstrates collaterals to the SMA and celiac axis

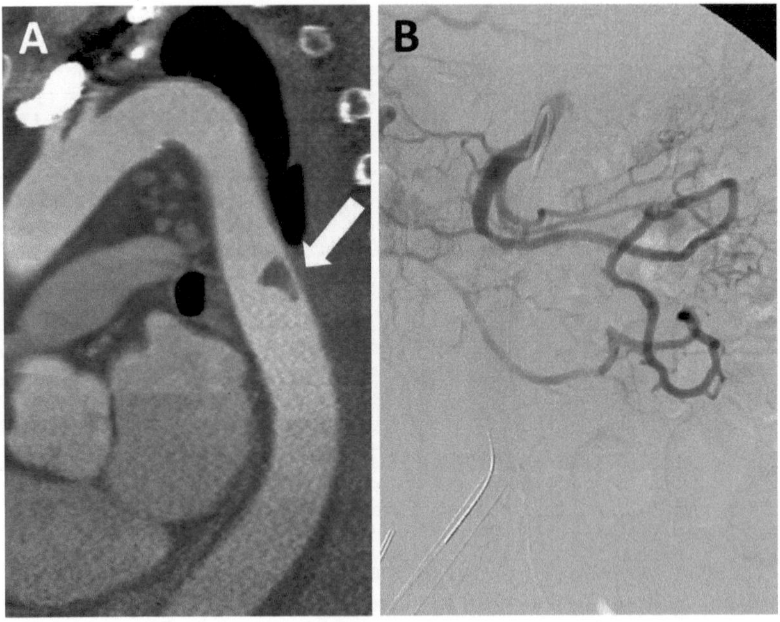

Fig. 8.7 Computed tomography angiography in a patient with large descending thoracic thrombus (**a**) which embolized to the SMA causing distal occlusion (**b**)

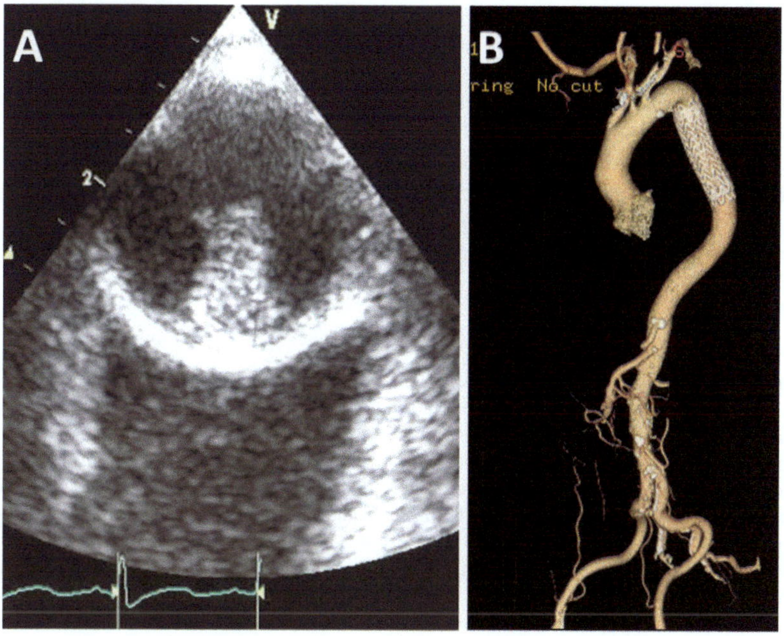

Fig. 8.8 Intravascular ultrasound was used to identify the location of the thrombus (**a**) to guide coverage by aortic stent graft (**b**)

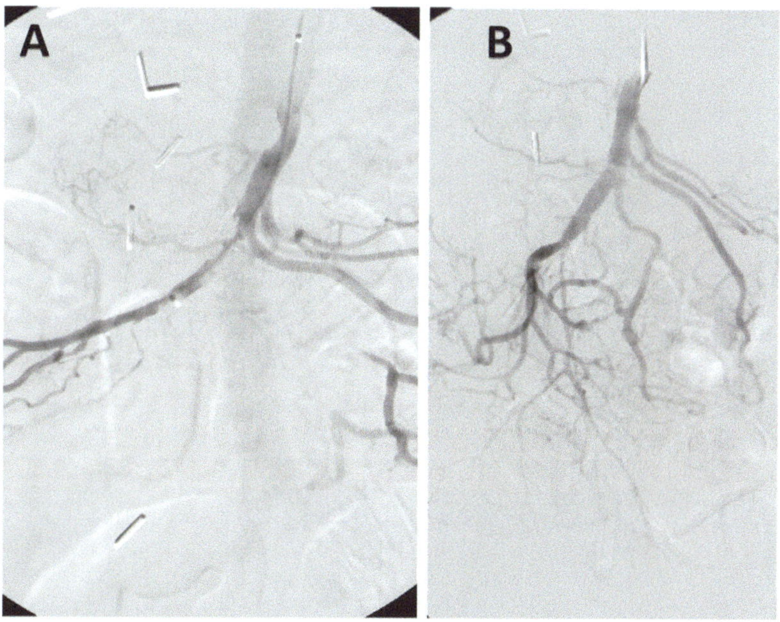

Fig. 8.9 Catheter-directed thrombolysis was used for treatment of the embolic lesion (**a**), with significant luminal improvement (**b**)

Conclusion

Diagnostic angiography is still considered the gold-standard study for most visceral artery pathology, but its role has decreased in the investigation of these disorders. Meticulous technique is recommended to avoid complications associated with diagnostic angiography and mesenteric interventions.

References

1. Bobadilla JL. Mesenteric ischemia. Surg Clin North Am. 2013;93(4):925–40. ix.
2. Ryer EJ, et al. Differences in anatomy and outcomes in patients treated with open mesenteric revascularization before and after the endovascular era. J Vasc Surg. 2011;53(6):1611e2–8e2.
3. Anderson JL, et al. Management of patients with peripheral artery disease (compilation of 2005 and 2011 ACCF/AHA guideline recommendations): a report of the American College of Cardiology Foundation/American Heart Association Task Force on Practice Guidelines. Circulation. 2013;127(13):1425–43.
4. Alvarez-Tostado JA, et al. The brachial artery: a critical access for endovascular procedures. J Vasc Surg. 2009;49(2):378–85. discussion 385.
5. McCullough PA, Capasso P. Patient discomfort associated with the use of intra-arterial iodinated contrast media: a meta-analysis of comparative randomized controlled trials. BMC Med Imaging. 2011;11:12.
6. Hannawi B, Lam WW, Younis GA. Pressure wire used to measure gradient in chronic mesenteric ischemia. Tex Heart Inst J. 2012;39(5):739–43.

Part II
Chronic Mesenteric Ischemia

Chapter 9
Clinical Presentation, Etiology, and Diagnostic Considerations

Lars Stangenberg and Marc L. Schermerhorn

Clinical Presentation

Chronic mesenteric ischemia (CMI) is a fairly uncommon disease that accounts for only 5 % of all cases of ischemic compromise of the gastrointestinal tract [1]. CMI poses thus a diagnostic challenge to the medical practitioner. There are numerous case reports of patients whose symptoms are vague and are treated for other causes than the actual underlying problem of CMI. Often they are diagnosed with colitis or other gastrointestinal diseases or even with depressive and eating disorders leading to poor oral intake and subsequently weight loss [2, 3]. This, however, reflects the nonspecific symptom complex and high prevalence of the other diagnoses such as colitis in the differential. This is further complicated by the fact that many people with stenoses of the mesenteric vessels do not show symptoms of CMI. The surgeon typically sees only a small proportion of patients with postprandial pain; patients that were oftentimes evaluated thoroughly by other specialists before presentation to a surgeon.

Part of the difficulty results from the rare occurrence of CMI. The prevalence is estimated at 1 in 100,000 individuals [4, 5]. This is in stark contrast to the prevalence of some degree of stenosis of the mesenteric vessels. In a cohort study of 553 participants aged 65 and older, Wilson et al found that 17.5 % of elderly patients had a critical stenosis of at least one vessel [6]. In another study researchers reviewed 205 consecutive angiograms of patients with aneurysmal or occlusive disease in the Veterans Affairs system. They found asymptomatic stenosis of mesenteric vessels in

L. Stangenberg
Division of Vascular and Endovascular Surgery,
Beth Israel Deaconess Medical Center, Boston, MA, USA
e-mail: lstangen@bidmc.harvard.edu

M.L. Schermerhorn (✉)
Chief, Division for Vascular and Endovascular Surgery, Beth Israel Deaconess
Medical Center, Boston, MA, USA
e-mail: mscherme@bidmc.harvard.edu

G.S. Oderich (ed.), *Mesenteric Vascular Disease*,
DOI 10.1007/978-1-4939-1847-8_9

40 % of patients with abdominal aortic aneurysms, 29 % in patients with aortoiliac occlusive disease, and 25 % in patients with peripheral occlusive disease [7]. Despite this rather common finding, it seems rare that the pathophysiologic process progresses to clinically detectable disease. In an observational study including 980 asymptomatic patients with at least 50 % stenosis of one of the visceral vessels, Thomas et al found only 4 patients that developed mesenteric ischemia. All patients had three-vessel involvement. The extensive collateralization between the three vessels that occurs over time in affected patients contributes to the slow progression of clinical symptoms and the low prevalence.

The classic patient is female and 75 years old. A female to male ratio of 2:1 has been reported [8]. She presents with postprandial abdominal pain, weight loss, and "food fear" (sitophobia). This triad of symptoms is present in about 50–60 % of patients [9]. The pain is often described as dull and cramping and located in the midepigastric area. The time course is important as it can distinguish CMI from other processes causing abdominal pain. The pain starts 15–45 min after a meal and lasts variably up to 4 h [1]. The intensity can be modulated by the size and the type of the ingested food with large fatty meals resulting in the most severe pain [10]. The pain eventually progresses to constant discomfort.

Two theories have been proposed to explain the timing of symptoms. One focuses on a mismatch between splanchnic blood flow and intestinal metabolic demand. Under resting conditions the intestinal circulation receives 10–20 % of the cardiac output. This increases to up to 35 % of the cardiac output after a meal in response to the increased activity of the gastrointestinal tract [11]. The stenotic mesenteric vessels cannot accommodate the doubling in flow and thus hypoperfusion ensues. The other theory suggests a shunting effect. Poole et al describe the use of tonometry to measure pH changes in stomach and small bowel of dogs [12]. They used ice cream to stimulate the tissues and cause hyperemia. They found that ice cream placed in the stomach causes a drop in pH in the small bowel indicative of a steel phenomenon. Due to the recurrent pattern of postprandial pain, patients develop an aversion to food and subsequently reduce the oral intake. This leads to an average weight loss of 20–30 lb at the time of diagnosis [13]. The weight loss is thus a result of decreased caloric intake rather than malabsorption (Fig. 9.1).

Other symptoms are vague and nonspecific. They include nausea and vomiting, fullness, and right upper quadrant discomfort. These symptoms are believed to be caused by hypoperfusion of the celiac artery (CA) territory rather than the superior mesenteric artery (SMA) territory leading to ischemic gastropathy. They occur in about 15 % of cases. Finally, changes in bowel habits can occur. Hematochezia and gastrointestinal bleeding due to CMI are rare.

Atherosclerosis is responsible for the majority of patients with CMI. Thus classical risk factors for atherosclerosis can often be elicited from the patients. In fact, half of the patients have known atherosclerosis in other vascular beds such as peripheral or coronary arteries [10]. Another study found the following comorbidities and risk factors at the time of presentation: hypertension 91 %, peripheral vascular disease 86 %, coronary artery disease 82 % with previous myocardial infarction 46 %, diabetes mellitus 66 %, hypercholesterolemia 48 %, and heavy smoking of >25 pack years 53 %.

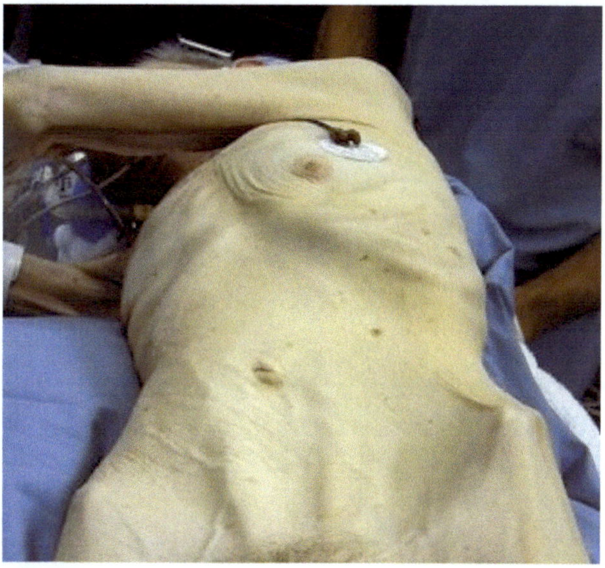

Fig. 9.1 Cachectic patient in right semilateral decubitus position in preparation to undergo retroperitoneal transaortic endarterectomy

The findings on physical examination are rather nonspecific. Often patients are underweight, sometimes to the point of cachexia due to poor oral intake related to food fear. Occasionally one can auscultate a bruit over the origin of the mesenteric vessels in the epigastrium. The bowel sounds, however, are frequently hyperactive. On palpation of the abdomen, there is rarely tenderness. Signs of peritonitis such as guarding or rebound tenderness are rarely found and suggest the possibility of acute or acute-on-chronic mesenteric ischemia. Similar to the physical examination, laboratory findings are nonspecific and often normal. Markers for the nutritional state of the patient such as albumin and prealbumin for long-term and short-term caloric intake are the exception and are low in many cases.

Etiology

Chronic mesenteric ischemia is usually caused by atherosclerotic changes of the three mesenteric vessels. However, as mentioned earlier, most patients have involvement of at least two vessels to cause clinically evident disease. According to some estimations, up to 95 % of cases of CMI are due to atherosclerosis [9]. The atherosclerotic changes occur at the ostium of the affected vessel. These changes are also found on the anterior aortic wall, and one might consider the ostial lesions of the mesenteric vessels as progressive aortic disease. This probably also explains the rare occurrence of isolated atherosclerosis-related disease of only one vessel.

Atherogenesis describes the multistep process of forming atheromatous plaques in arteries [14]. A brief synopsis of the involved steps is given below (Fig. 9.2). An early event in this process is the activation of endothelial cells (ECs). Usually resisting leukocyte attachment, ECs respond to irritants such as hypertension or

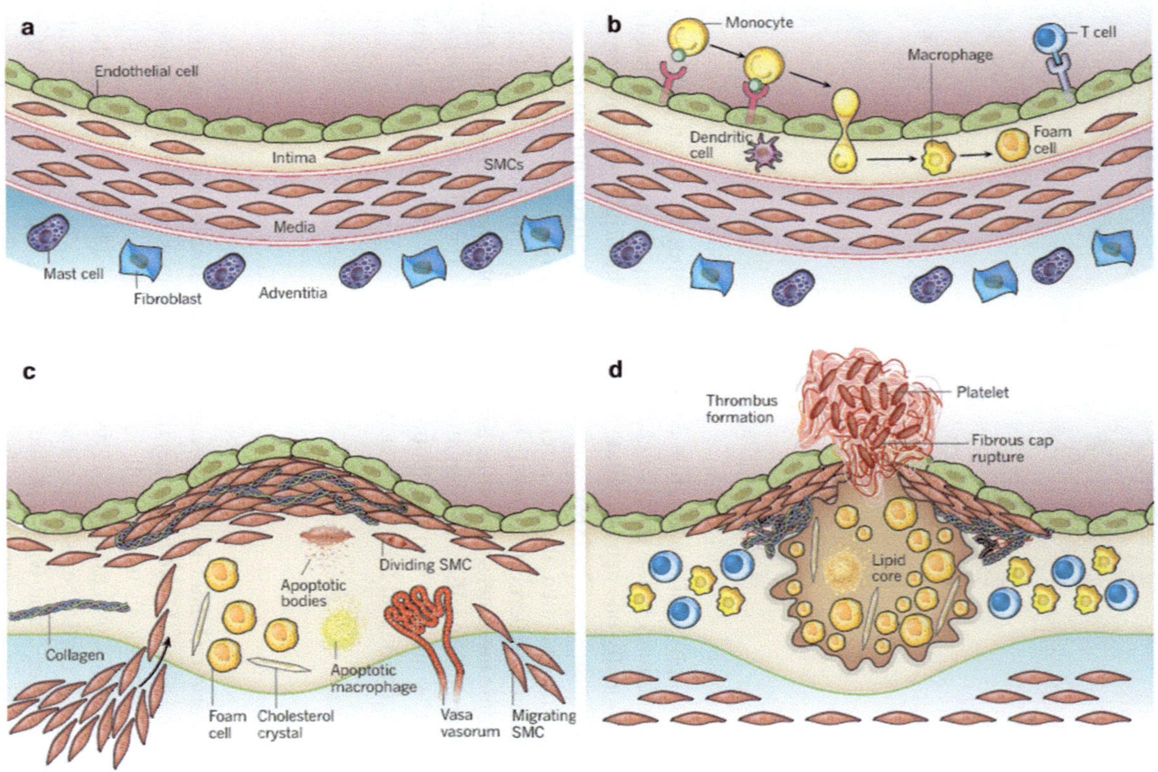

Fig. 9.2 Stages of development of atherosclerotic plaques and eventual rupture. (**a**) The normal muscular artery with its three layers. (**b**) Activation of ECs and subsequent attraction of monocytes, which eventually become foam cells. (**c**) Proliferation of smooth muscle cells and production of extracellular matrix proteins after cytokine stimulation by foam cells and other immune cells. (**d**) fracture of a fibrous cap (Adapted from Libby et al. [14], with permission of Macmillan Publishers, Ltd)

dyslipidemia by upregulation of cell adhesion molecules. Changes in endothelial permeability also lead to increased deposition of cholesterol-containing low-density lipoprotein (LDL) particles. Together with other chemoattractants, this leads to eventual leukocyte adhesion and migration to deep layers of the arterial wall. There, blood monocytes become tissue-resident macrophages and take up LDL. On pathological examination these macrophages have taken up such large amounts of lipid that they become foam cells. Foam cells and other cells of the immune system then further stimulate the process by releasing pro-inflammatory cytokines such as interleukin-1β (IL-1β) and tumor-necrosis factor (TNF). Smooth muscle cells from the intima as well as the media proliferate in response to these stimuli and produce extracellular matrix proteins including collagen and elastin, which form a fibrous cap over the plaques. This cap covers viable as well as apoptotic foam cells and extracellular debris and lipids. Over time the plaque grows and causes clinical manifestations by producing flow-limiting stenoses or by thrombus formation with distal embolization.

Beyond atherosclerotic changes causing mesenteric ischemia, there are a variety of systemic diseases that can affect the mesenteric vasculature. The prevalence of mesenteric compromise related to these diseases is difficult to estimate but certainly much lower than atherosclerosis as an etiology as mentioned above. Most available data are derived from case reports or small case series. A study from the Mayo Clinic seems to confirm this notion [15]. Over a period of 24 years, they treated only 15 patients (13 female and 2 male) for occlusive mesenteric vasculitis. Etiologies were Takayasu's arteritis in 7, polyarteritis nodosa in 4, indeterminate in 3, and giant cell arteritis in 1. The majority of patients underwent open revascularization. A few interesting points can be extrapolated from this paper. Patients with vasculitis as the underlying etiology are significantly younger than patients with mesenteric ischemia due to atherosclerosis. The mean age was 38 versus 65. These patients lack the classic cardiovascular risk factors of hypertension, hyperlipidemia, diabetes, and smoking. Finally, the Mayo experience confirms the low prevalence of mesenteric vasculitis (15 patients with vasculitis versus 163 patients with atherosclerosis).

Takayasu's arteritis was the most common form of vasculitis in this series. This finding is further supported by the majority of case reports on this subject [15]. Min et al, for example, report their experience with Takayasu's disease in 25 patients [16]. Two of them had involvement of the mesenteric vessels and were treated with stenting. Similarly, Kalangos et al report on 10 pediatric patients of whom 4 underwent endovascular or open repair of the SMA to treat ischemic symptoms [17].

Thrombangiitis obliterans, also known as Buerger's disease, is another inflammatory process that can lead to occlusion of the intestinal arteries over time. It is associated with smoking and usually affects the peripheral arterial beds [18]. It has long been known, though, that Buerger's disease can affect the visceral arteries on rare occasions [19]. Data are limited to case reports. Pfitzmann et al describe such a rare event. A patient with abdominal pain was found to have necrotic small bowel and hepatic hypoperfusion upon laparotomy [20]. Angiography eventually showed occlusion of celiac trunk and SMA. He was revascularized by SMA thrombectomy and vein bypass from SMA to hepatic artery.

Giant cell arteritis can also cause mesenteric ischemia [21]. Evans et al found smooth narrowing of the SMA and confirmed the diagnosis by temporal artery biopsy. The patient was started on steroids and improved slowly over a 6-month period. Other patients with giant cell arteritis can present more dramatically with intestinal infarction or perforation and subsequent mortality as high as 30 % [22, 23].

Other forms of vasculitis can cause mesenteric ischemia infrequently. Chubachi et al describe a patient with occlusive Behcet disease [24]. Churg-Strauss syndrome, Wegener's granulomatosis, microscopic polyangiitis, and other small-vessel arteriopathies can also on occasion affect the mesenteric circulation [25].

There are other unusual etiologies for mesenteric ischemia. Often there are only one or two patients described with a particular pathology. Krupski reviewed them in detail [26]. One patient suffered from an isolated spontaneous SMA dissection and presented with classic symptoms of CMI [27]. Resection of the intimal flap with vein patch angioplasty was performed with good result. Retroperitoneal fibrosis and neurofibromatosis can also cause mechanical obstruction by external compression [28, 29]. Median arcuate ligament syndrome is similarly recognized as an external lesion leading to external mechanical obstruction of the celiac trunk with ensuing ischemic symptoms. The syndrome is discussed in detail elsewhere in this book.

Diagnostic Considerations

The diagnosis of CMI remains a formidable challenge to the medical practitioner. It requires careful history taking to suspect mesenteric ischemia in a patient with vague abdominal symptoms. It has been shown, however, that the establishment of a multidisciplinary splanchnic diseases workgroup can lead to increased detection of CMI [30]. This Dutch group was able to increase the rate of diagnosis from 7 to 23 persons per million per year due to an increased degree of suspicion and an extensive investigation by several specialists.

Beyond a thorough history, the key to making a tentative diagnosis of CMI lies with various imaging modalities as well as physiologic testing. These imaging modalities include noninvasive techniques such as duplex ultrasonography (DUS), computed tomographic angiogram (CTA), and magnetic resonance angiography (MRA) and invasive techniques like conventional angiography, which served for a long time as the gold standard. Tonometry as a physiologic test has been employed to detect pH changes after stimulation. These tests can be used alone or in combination but even then a preoperative definitive diagnosis is impossible [9]. They can suggest a high confidence of the correctness of the diagnosis, but only the improvement of symptoms after a successful intervention, either open or endovascular, confirms the diagnosis definitively.

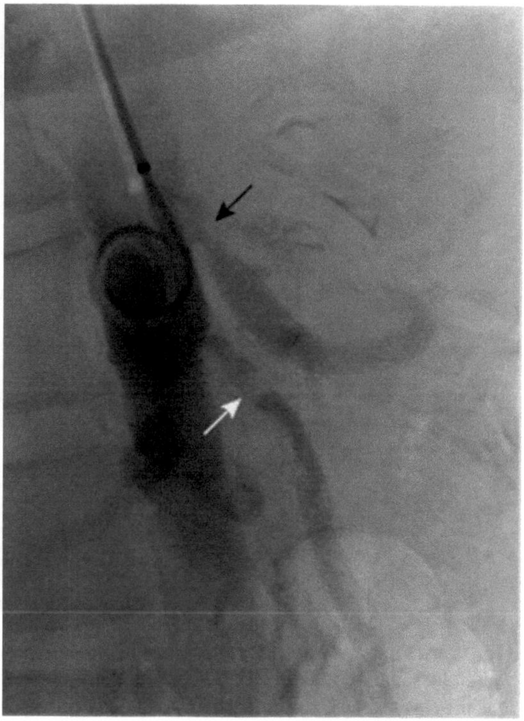

Fig. 9.3 Lateral projection aortogram with proximal mesenteric vessels (CA and SMA). Note the significant stenosis of the CA with post-stenotic dilation (*black arrow*) and the reduced intensity of contrast in SMA indicative of stenosis (*white arrow*). Further information can be obtained from selective cannulation of single vessels

Angiography

Biplanar selective angiography is the gold standard for detecting CMI against which all other modalities are tested (Fig. 9.3). It used to be the only test available to aid in diagnosis but has largely been replaced by newer technologies as outlined below. It is employed in therapeutic efforts, though, and in this capacity has gained importance due to the increase in endovascular treatment of CMI. If performed for diagnostic purposes, it is crucial to obtain several views of the ostia of mesenteric vessels. Plain anterior-posterior (AP) views do not allow for visualization of the vessel origins. Lateral views are better suited to assess this area of the vessel where most disease is located. Imaging should be performed early and late: early to visualize the CA and SMA origin and late to evaluate the retrograde flow, delayed proximal visualization, and collateral pathways between CA, SMA, and inferior mesenteric artery (IMA) [31].

Duplex Ultrasonography

Gene Strandness and colleagues at the University of Washington in Seattle demonstrated 30 years ago the utility of duplex ultrasonography (DUS) to detect stenoses and occlusions of mesenteric vessels [32]. This group found elevated velocities of

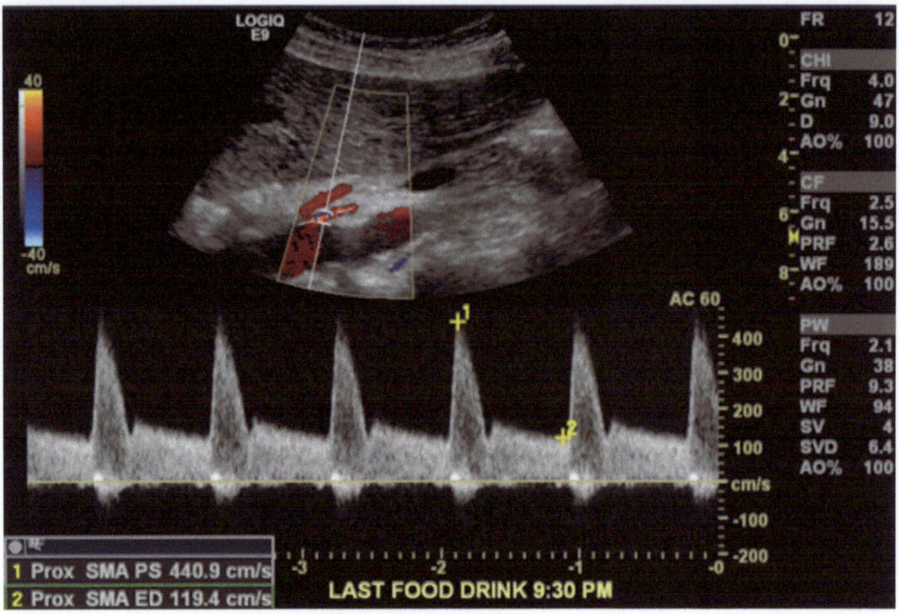

Fig. 9.4 Duplex ultrasonography examination of patient with symptoms of abdominal pain, weight loss, and food fear. DUS shows laminar flow in the aorta and CA. There is, however, turbulent flow at the SMA origin indicative of a stenosis, which was confirmed by pulse waveform analysis of this area. This showed PSV of 440.9 cm/s, a significantly elevated value

CA and SMA in a patient with postprandial abdominal pain and weight loss. Angiography confirmed the diagnosis. Since that time DUS has become the foremost screening tool to assess CMI due to its low cost, high speed, and general availability (Fig. 9.4). Starting in the early 1990s, several groups published retrospective reviews to establish velocity parameters and thresholds that would reliably predict critical stenoses of the mesenteric vessels. Moneta et al first published duplex criteria for diagnosis of SMA or CA stenosis in 1991 [33]. They used peak systolic velocities (PSV) and found that velocities >275 cm/s for the SMA and >200 cm/s for the CA predicted stenosis of at least 70 %. Sensitivity, specificity, and positive predictive values were 89, 92, and 80 % for the SMA and 75, 89, and 85 % for the CA, respectively. In their hands end-diastolic velocities (EDV) or calculated velocity ratios did not add additional accuracy to the test. This is in contrast to the data from Dartmouth where the authors found EDV more accurate than PSV in the diagnosis of SMA stenosis [34]. They reported an EDV>45 cm/s in the SMA to be the best indicator of severe stenosis (sensitivity 100 %; specificity 92 %). In their hands, PSV>300 cm/s was less sensitive (63 %) but highly specific (100 %) for severe SMA stenosis. They also reported issues with imaging the CA and correctly identifying threshold values. This was attributed to increased collateral flow through the gastroduodenal artery that would reduce the velocities across a CA lesion. In a later publication, the authors proved this to be the case and reported reversal of flow in the common hepatic artery to predict severe CA stenosis or occlusion [35].

Shortly after publishing the diagnostic threshold criteria using PSV, Moneta et al published a prospective study validating their initial results [36]. They studied 100 patients who underwent routine aortography and subsequently had DUS. Sensitivity, specificity, positive predictive value, negative predictive value, and overall accuracy for detection of a 70 % or greater SMA stenosis were 92, 96, 80, 99, and 96 % and for a 70 % or greater CA stenosis 87, 80, 63, 94, and 82 %, respectively. Similarly, Zwolak et al confirmed the Dartmouth criteria using EDV to diagnose stenoses [37]. An EDV threshold of 45 cm/s had a sensitivity of 90 %, specificity of 91 %, positive predictive value of 90 %, negative predictive value of 91 %, and overall accuracy of 91 % for detecting SMA lesions. For the CA, a threshold of 55 cm/s or no flow signal had best overall accuracy (95 %) with high sensitivity (93 %) and specificity (100 %). They also confirmed that a CA PSV > 200 cm/s or no signal has excellent accuracy (93 %), sensitivity (93 %), and specificity (94 %). The PSV data for the SMA were less convincing. It provided low overall accuracy (81 %), low sensitivity (60 %), but high specificity (100 %). The parameters that were established by both groups have been used for the last 2 decades to screen for and diagnose critical lesions of the mesenteric vessels. Recently though, a study by AbuRahma et al questioned these thresholds [38]. They found PSV > 295 cm/s to provide the highest accuracy for detecting SMA stenosis > 50 % and PSV > 400 cm/s for SMA stenosis > 70 %. The sensitivity for a 50 % stenosis was 87 %, specificity was 89 %, and overall accuracy 88 %, and for detecting a 70 % stenosis, it was 72, 93, and 85 %, respectively. Finally, DUS is a dynamic examination that relies on operator expertise as well as patient factors such as respirations, body habitus, timing of last meal, bowel gas, and anatomic variations [39].

The role for duplex extends beyond the initial diagnosis. Several studies show the utility of this powerful technology to follow patients after interventions. This allows for timely recognition of restenosis before it becomes clinically apparent and thus provides a window for a second intervention. There is, however, no clearly defined threshold for re-intervention. Baker et al document their experience of pre- and postprocedural duplex on 23 patients [40]. The mean PSV before intervention was 464 cm/s while it dropped to 335 cm/s afterwards. This number is still higher than the threshold of 275 cm/s used to diagnose the critical stenosis in the first place. From these rather preliminary data, they concluded that a threshold of PSV > 500 cm/s inside the stent or a change from baseline PSV obtained at 1-month follow-up should be used to trigger a re-intervention. Schoch et al come to a similar conclusion in their review of 107 patients having undergone endovascular therapy [41]. Eighty-three percent of patients had recurrent stenosis on surveillance duplex but 53 % remained asymptomatic. Thus clinical context and change from early baseline PSV values should trigger an intervention.

Computed Tomographic Angiography

Computed Tomographic Angiography (CTA) is a modern, fast, and accurate imaging modality to visualize the mesenteric vessels and their pathology. Especially since the introduction of multi-row detector technology in the late 1990s, the quality of temporal and spatial resolution is excellent [42].

Compared to conventional angiography, it allows for more complete assessment of the mesenteric vasculature [43]. It can be viewed in multiple planes and may include three-dimensional (3D) reconstructions (Fig. 9.5). CTA depicts vascular narrowing as well as the atherosclerotic plaque itself. A normal CTA virtually rules out CMI [44]. Finally, the CT part of the study enables evaluation of the bowel at the same time. Thickening of the bowel wall can indicate inflammatory changes associated with ischemia. A late finding of severe ischemic is the presence of pneumatosis intestinalis, air within the bowel wall. This might not be as critical for CMI as for AMI but is certainly beneficial and lends to a more thorough assessment. Similarly to conventional angiography, early and late phase images can be reacquired and thus provide more information. Late phase sequences examine the venous system including IMV, SMV, splenic vein, and portal vein.

Other findings include calcified and noncalcified atherosclerotic plaque, typically in the CA and SMA and less commonly in the IMA. The plaque is usually found in the proximal segment of the vessel within a few centimeters from its origin [45]. CTA is the superior modality to evaluate the plaque in detail as this has implications for treatment such as clamp placement and choice of inflow and target. Through adjustments of the window and level, and comparison to non-contrast images, calcified plaque can usually be distinguished from contrast. Changes in vessels in the proximity of a stenosis can increase the certainty of the diagnosis. One can detect the presence of collateral pathways, e.g., prominent vessels around the head of the pancreas that should raise immediate suspicion of a hemodynamically significant stenosis of the CA resulting in dilatation of the pancreaticoduodenal arteries [43]. This is somewhat similar to DUS, which can also assess the proximity of the stenotic vessel and detect ante- and retrograde flow in the hepatic artery. Detection of flow, however, is not possible with CTA, and only indirect findings such as the development of collaterals can hint at changes in flow.

Several studies evaluated the sensitivity and specificity of CTA compared with conventional angiography as gold standard. Cikrit et al performed a retrospective review of 32 patients, who had both angiography and CTA to evaluate stenoses of mesenteric arteries [46]. Spiral CTA had a sensitivity of 75 % and specificity of 100 % for detection of a 75 % celiac arterial stenosis. For detection of a similar stenosis in the SMA, sensitivity was 100 % and specificity was 91 %. By means of the Pearson correlation coefficient, significant correlation ($p<0.001$) was confirmed between spiral CT and arteriography for evaluation of stenosis of the SMA ($r=0.8991$) and celiac artery ($r=0.8260$).

Stueckle and colleagues confirmed this early experience and reported their results of 52 patients who underwent both CTA and angiography [47]. All aneurysms, occlusions, stenoses, and calcifications were diagnosed correctly by CTA in axial and multiplanar projections (sensitivity 100 %; specificity 100 %). The degree of stenosis was overestimated in three cases when using axial projections. Three-dimensional volume-rendered CTA showed a sensitivity of 91 % for aneurysms, 82 % for stenoses, 75 % for occlusions, and 77 % for calcifications. The specificity was 100 % in all cases.

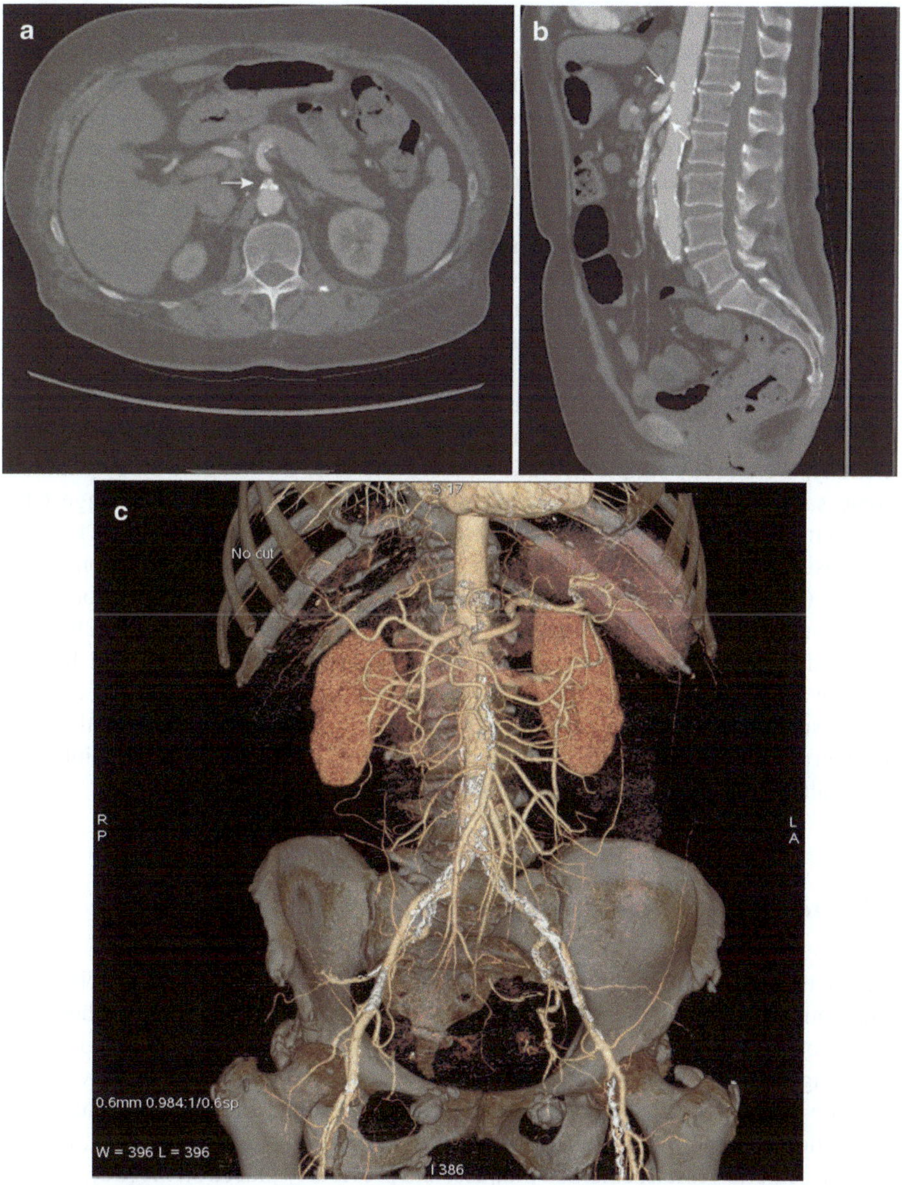

Fig. 9.5 (**a–c**) Axial and sagittal reconstructions of CTA. (**a**) The axial view is well suited to assess calcifications, stenoses, and occlusions at the origin of the mesenteric vessels as seen here (*white arrow*). (**b**) The sagittal reformat is particularly helpful in assessing the length of a stenosis as it allows for depicting the vessel in a longitudinal section. (**c**) Finally, 3D reconstructions are possible from CTA raw data that permits complete assessment of the mesenteric vasculature. These images can be viewed in all planes and help in preparation of endovascular interventions, e.g., choice of ideal projection angles to see the stenosis during angiography

The data generated from radiologic assessment of visceral vessels in setting of CMI is mirrored by data in the setting of AMI. A meta-analysis of six studies published between 1996 and 2009 on the diagnostic accuracy of MDCT in AMI showed a pooled sensitivity of 93 % and specificity of 96 % [48].

Given its widespread availability, low interobserver variability, noninvasiveness, moderate cost, and excellent diagnostic properties, CTA should be the anatomic imaging modality of choice for patients with clinical suspicion of CMI. In our practice, CTA is employed after initial screening with DUS but before any intervention for suspected CMI. Disadvantages of CTA include the use of ionizing radiation and the need for a contrast agent with its risk of allergic reactions and nephrotoxicity.

To overcome some of these issues, we have developed an institutional protocol to prevent allergic reactions (prednisone 50 mg at 13, 7, and 1 h before CTA; diphenhydramine 25 mg at 7 and 1 h before CTA) in those at risk. There is ongoing research and currently conflicting data on interventions to reduce the occurrence of nephrotoxicity. We employ simple hydration before and after the imaging study with isotonic saline [49]. We do not use bicarbonate or acetylcysteine. We suggest the following algorithm for the patient with elevated creatinine who is at risk for both contrast-induced nephropathy as well as nephrogenic systemic fibrosis from gadolinium (see MRA section below): hydrate and then perform CTA if the glomerular filtration rate is not prohibitively low (GFR < 30 cc/min). If this is the case, then we proceed straight to angiography based on a highly suggestive DUS and history. During angiography further techniques can be used to reduce the amount of contrast given such as only limited lateral views rather than both AP and lateral views. Furthermore, one can use carbon dioxide as a contrast agent and can add intravascular ultrasound or pressure gradient measurements if needed.

Magnetic Resonance Angiography

Magnetic resonance angiography (MRA) offers a second modality for obtaining anatomic imaging of the visceral vessels aside from CTA (Fig. 9.6). There are, however, important differences. Benefits of this technology are the avoidance of ionizing radiation and iodinated contrast agents. On the other hand, disadvantages include the long time to perform a study (~10 min) and the reduced degree of spatial resolution compared to CTA. It also has reduced visualization of the IMA, peripheral mesenteric vessels, calcified plaques, and previously placed stents [50]. Finally, MRA requires use of gadolinium-based contrast agents that are safer than iodinated agents used for CTA on a large scale. A rare but very severe adverse effect of gadolinium-based contrast agents is nephrogenic systemic fibrosis, a potentially lethal complication [51].

An early study by Wasser and colleagues proved the usefulness of this tool [52]. They performed conventional angiography on 24 patients and then performed cardiac-gated three-dimensional phase contrast MRA. They optimized the sequences and subsequently performed prospective studies on 10 patients with presumed CMI. Of six patients with stenoses on angiography, MRA identified four correctly

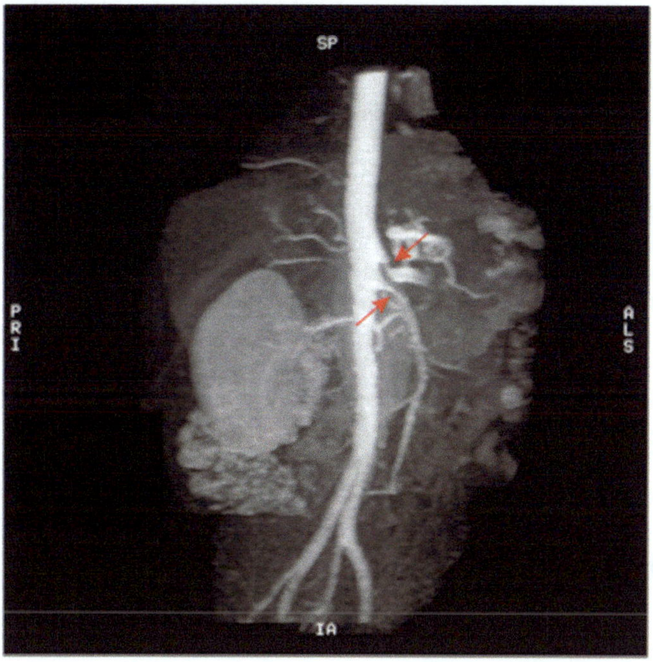

Fig. 9.6 3D reconstruction of aorta, mesenteric, and renal vessels from MRA raw data. Stenoses of the CA and SMA are clearly seen (*red arrows*)

which translates into a sensitivity of 66 %. Issues with their approach include the long acquisition time and susceptibility to motion artifact.

Another rather small study confirmed the general appropriateness of MRA to assess CMI. Meaney et al evaluated 14 patients with correlative angiograms and found stenosis in 7 CAs, 6 SMAs, and 4 IMAs. In two cases, IMA stenosis was overgraded. Overall sensitivity and specificity of MRA was 100 % and 95 %, respectively [53]. Similarly, Ernst et al assessed the degree agreement between angiographic and MR findings in a series of 24 patients by weighted kappa analysis [54]. Agreement was good or excellent for the hepatic artery (κ=0.78), the superior mesenteric artery (κ=0.65), the splenic artery (κ=0.70), the portal vein (κ=1.0), the superior mesenteric vein (κ=0.88), and the splenic vein (κ=0.75). Carlos et al showed a low degree of interobserver variability for mesenteric MRA [55]. Interobserver agreement for grading proximal splanchnic stenosis was 0.90 for CA, 0.92 for SMA, and 0.48 for IMA. The study also confirmed the rather poor imaging quality of MRA regarding the IMA.

MRA imaging can be combined with MRI and then yield functional information about splanchnic blood flow that is otherwise not attainable. Flow velocities and total flow volumes can be measured in the mesenteric vessels using two-dimensional cine phase contrast velocity mapping [9]. Flow volumes in both the SMA and the superior mesenteric vein (SMV) have been measured with MRI. Li and colleagues showed that postprandial flow augmentation in the SMA (exceeding 100 % in normal volunteers) was significantly reduced in a patient with high-grade stenosis

[56]. Burkhart et al performed a study of 10 volunteers and 10 patients to assess changes in SMV flow [57]. They showed that the difference between fasting and postprandial flows in the SMV was 245 ± 74 % in healthy volunteers. In four patients with angiographically proven stenosis of the mesenteric arteries, postprandial flow augmentation in the SMV was significantly reduced to 64 ± 28 %.

MRI can also be employed to measure the oxygen saturation of hemoglobin. The principle behind MR oximetry is that deoxyhemoglobin in erythrocytes is paramagnetic, but oxyhemoglobin (HbO2) is not. This allows for calculation of mesenteric oxygen extraction, which in turn is determined by the rate of mesenteric blood flow. As blood flow decreases, oxygen extraction will increase to maintain the level of oxygen uptake. Li et al measured the percentage of oxyhemoglobin (%HbO2) in the SMV before and after intake of a standard meal in a canine model [58]. Later they used this technology to assess patients with CMI. Normally, the %HbO2 in the SMV increases postprandially by 4.6±0.6 %, but in six patients with CMI, the %HbO2 in the SMV decreased by 8.8±0.7 % [59].

Tonometry

As described earlier, tonometry can be employed as a functional tool to assess mesenteric ischemia. The principle was initially reported in 1965 [60]. A tonometry catheter is inserted into the stomach or the intestine. This catheter includes a gas-permeable silicone balloon. Carbon dioxide freely equilibrates between the gastric mucosa, the lumen, and the content of the balloon. After equilibration the air is sampled from the balloon and analyzed. Theoretically, hypoperfusion below a critical level causes mucosal carbon dioxide accumulation. Since carbon dioxide diffuses easily across membranes, the PCO_2 in the lumen of the gut also increases, leading to an increase in the gap between tonometrically measured luminal PCO_2 and the conventionally measured PCO_2 in the peripheral blood. In the 1980s proof of principle studies were undertaken in dogs [61] as well as humans [62]. Since that time it has been advocated as a diagnostic tool without becoming a common modality [63]. The reason why it has not reached widespread routine use may lie with uncertainties regarding physiologic background and methodology [64]. For example, the diagnostic value of postprandial gastric PCO_2 levels is questionable [65], but gastric PCO_2 exercise tonometry seems more promising as a diagnostic test for gastrointestinal ischemia [66, 67]. Finally, the methodology is not simple as one has to avoid food in the stomach, acid buffering, and CO_2 generation.

Diagnostic Approach at Our Institution

As a summary of the presented data, we would like to offer the diagnostic approach we take at our institution. After a thorough interview focusing on cardiovascular risk factors, classic as well as subtle symptoms of mesenteric ischemia and a physical examination, we begin our diagnostic testing with duplex ultrasonography. It is cheap and readily available in our office. It sometimes can be performed at the same time if the referred patient is still NPO. Using DUS as an initial screening test, we usually order a CTA to confirm the putative diagnosis of CMI. It also serves other purposes such as evaluating the distal vessels that cannot be visualized during DUS, uncovering other potential vascular disease processes like aneurysms, and finally allowing for planning of an intervention. This can be an endovascular intervention – our preferred approach for most patients – or an open operation. In this situation a CTA delineates the entire aorta and iliac system and thus shows suitable clamp sites for bypasses. For an endovascular procedure, we like to use CTA to measure the vessels and size stents accordingly rather than to rely on intraprocedural angiographic measurements. Finally, we take patients to the angio-suite for definitive diagnosis and treatment in the same procedure.

References

1. Sreenarasimhaiah J. Chronic mesenteric ischemia. Best Pract Res Clin Gastroenterol. 2005;19(2):283–95.
2. Clifton WL, Kneitz A, Cohn WE, Delgado RM. Weight loss caused by visceral artery disease. Tex Heart Inst J. 2013;40(3):320–2.
3. Kilsby A, Pasha Y. Chronic mesenteric ischaemia: a battery of negative tests in a patient with episodic abdominal pain, weight loss and diarrhoea. BMJ Case Rep. 2013.
4. Marston A. Diagnosis and management of intestinal ischaemia. Ann R Coll Surg Engl Royal College of Surgeons of England. 1972;50(1):29.
5. Mitchell EL, Moneta GL. Mesenteric duplex scanning. Perspect Vasc Surg Endovasc Ther. 2006;18(2):175–83.
6. Wilson DB, Mostafavi K, Craven TE, Ayerdi J, Edwards MS, Hansen KJ. Clinical course of mesenteric artery stenosis in elderly Americans. Arch Intern Med Am Med Assoc. 2006;166(19):2095–100.
7. Valentine RJ, Martin JD, Myers SI, Rossi MB, Clagett GP. Asymptomatic celiac and superior mesenteric artery stenoses are more prevalent among patients with unsuspected renal artery stenoses. J Vasc Surg. 1991;14(2):195–9.
8. Cangemi JR, Picco MF. Intestinal ischemia in the elderly. Gastroenterol Clin North Am. 2009;38(3):527–40.
9. van Bockel JH, Geelkerken RH, Wasser MN. Chronic splanchnic ischaemia. Best Pract Res Clin Gastroenterol. 2001;15(1):99–119.
10. Moawad J, Gewertz BL. Chronic mesenteric ischemia. Clinical presentation and diagnosis. Surg Clin NA. 1997;77(2):357–69.
11. Zeller T, Macharzina R. Management of chronic atherosclerotic mesenteric ischemia. Vasa. 2011;40(2):99–107.
12. Poole JW, Sammartano RJ, Boley SJ. Hemodynamic basis of the pain of chronic mesenteric ischemia. Am J Surg. 1987;153(2):171–6.
13. Kazmers A. Operative management of chronic mesenteric ischemia. Ann Vasc Surg. 1998;12(3):299–308.
14. Libby P, Ridker PM, Hansson GK. Progress and challenges in translating the biology of atherosclerosis. Nature. 2011;473(7347):317–25.
15. Rits Y, Oderich GS, Bower TC, Miller DV, Cooper L, Ricotta JJ, et al. Interventions for mesenteric vasculitis. J Vasc Surg. 2010;51(2):392–2.

16. Min P-K, Park S, Jung J-H, Ko Y-G, Choi D, Jang Y, et al. Endovascular therapy combined with immunosuppressive treatment for occlusive arterial disease in patients with Takayasu's arteritis. J Endovasc Ther. 2005;12(1):28–34.
17. Kalangos A, Christenson JT, Cikirikcioglu M, Vala D, Buerge A, Simonet F, et al. Long-term outcome after surgical intervention and interventional procedures for the management of Takayasu's arteritis in children. J Thorac Cardiovasc Surg. 2006;132(3):656–64.
18. Cho YP, Kwon YM, Kwon TW, Kim GE. Mesenteric Buerger's disease. Ann Vasc Surg. 2003;17(2):221–3.
19. Wolf EA, Sumner DS, Strandness DE. Disease of the mesenteric circulation in patients with thromboangiitis obliterans. Vasc Surg. 1972;6(5):218–23.
20. Pfitzmann R, Nüssler NC, Heise M, Neuhaus P, Settmacher U. Mesenteric artery occlusion as a rare complication of thromboangiitis obliterans. Chirurg. 2002;73(1):86–9.
21. Evans DC, Murphy MP, Lawson JH. Giant cell arteritis manifesting as mesenteric ischemia. J Vasc Surg. 2005;42(5):1019–22.
22. Arguedas MR, Linder JD. Giant cell arteritis and intestinal angina. Dig Dis Sci. 2000;45(12): 2363–4.
23. Sujobert P, Fardet L, Marie I, Duhaut P, Cohen P, Grange C, et al. Mesenteric ischemia in giant cell arteritis: 6 cases and a systematic review. J Rheumatol. 2007;34(8):1727–32.
24. Chubachi A, Saitoh K, Imai H, Miura AB, Kotanagi H, Abe T, et al. Case report: intestinal infarction after an aneurysmal occlusion of superior mesenteric artery in a patient with Behçet's disease. Am J Med Sci. 1993;306(6):376–8.
25. Guillevin L, Dörner T. Vasculitis: mechanisms involved and clinical manifestations. Arthritis Res Ther. 2007;9 Suppl 2:S9.
26. Krupski WC, Selzman CH, Whitehill TA. Unusual causes of mesenteric ischemia. Surg Clin NA. 1997;77(2):471–502.
27. Krupski WC, Effeney DJ, Ehrenfeld WK. Spontaneous dissection of the superior mesenteric artery. J Vasc Surg. 1985;2(5):731–4.
28. Brunner H, Stacher G, Bankl H, Grabner G. Chronic mesenteric arterial insufficiency caused by vascular neurofibromatosis. A case report. Am J Gastroenterol. 1974;62(5):442–7.
29. Crummy AB, Whittaker WB, Morrissey JF, Cossman FP. Intestinal infarction secondary to retroperitoneal fibrosis. N Engl J Med. 1971;285(1):28–9.
30. Otte J, Geelkerken R, Huisman A, Kolkman J. Assessment of the incidence of chronic gastro-intestinal ischemia after institution of a multidisciplinary working group. Gastroenterology. 1999;116:A915.
31. Bakal CW, Sprayregen S, Wolf EL. Radiology in intestinal ischemia. Angiographic diagnosis and management. Surg Clin NA. 1992;72(1):125–41.
32. Jäger KA, Fortner GS, Thiele BL, Strandness DE. Noninvasive diagnosis of intestinal angina. J Clin Ultrasound. 1984;12(9):588–91.
33. Moneta GL, Yeager RA, Dalman R, Antonovic R, Hall LD, Porter JM. Duplex ultrasound criteria for diagnosis of splanchnic artery stenosis or occlusion. J Vasc Surg. 1991;14(4): 511–8; discussion 518–20.
34. Bowersox JC, Zwolak RM, Walsh DB, Schneider JR, Musson A, LaBombard FE, et al. Duplex ultrasonography in the diagnosis of celiac and mesenteric artery occlusive disease. J Vasc Surg. 1991;14(6):780–6; discussion 786–8.
35. LaBombard F, Musson A, Bowersox J, Zwolak R. Hepatic artery duplex as an adjunct in the evaluation of chronic mesenteric ischemia. J Vasc Technol. 1992;16:7–11.
36. Moneta GL, Lee RW, Yeager RA, Taylor LM, Porter JM. Mesenteric duplex scanning: a blinded prospective study. J Vasc Surg. 1993;17(1):79–84; discussion 85–6.
37. Zwolak RM, Fillinger MF, Walsh DB, LaBombard FE, Musson A, Darling CE, et al. Mesenteric and celiac duplex scanning: a validation study. J Vasc Surg. 1998;27(6):1078–87; discussion 1088.
38. AbuRahma AF, Stone PA, Srivastava M, Dean LS, Keiffer T, Hass SM, et al. Mesenteric/celiac duplex ultrasound interpretation criteria revisited. J Vasc Surg. 2012;55(2):428e6–36e6.

39. Geelkerken RH, Delahunt TA, Schultze Kool LJ, van Baalen JM, Hermans J, van Bockel JH. Pitfalls in the diagnosis of origin stenosis of the coeliac and superior mesenteric arteries with transabdominal color duplex examination. Ultrasound Med Biol. 1996;22(6):695–700.
40. Baker AC, Chew V, Li C-S, Lin T-C, Dawson DL, Pevec WC, et al. Application of duplex ultrasound imaging in determining in-stent stenosis during surveillance after mesenteric artery revascularization. J Vasc Surg. 2012;56(5):1364–71; discussion 1371.
41. Schoch DM, LeSar CJ, Joels CS, Erdoes LS, Sprouse LR, Fugate MW, et al. Management of chronic mesenteric vascular insufficiency: an endovascular approach. J Am Coll Surg. 2011;212(4):668–75; discussion 675–7.
42. Laghi A, Iannaccone R, Catalano C, Passariello R. Multislice spiral computed tomography angiography of mesenteric arteries. Lancet. 2001;358(9282):638–9.
43. Horton KM, Fishman EK. Multidetector CT angiography in the diagnosis of mesenteric ischemia. Radiol Clin North Am. 2007;45(2):275–88.
44. Fleischmann D. Multiple detector-row CT angiography of the renal and mesenteric vessels. Eur J Radiol. 2003;45 Suppl 1:S79–87.
45. Järvinen O, Laurikka J, Sisto T, Salenius JP, Tarkka MR. Atherosclerosis of the visceral arteries. Vasa. 1995;24(1):9–14.
46. Cikrit DF, Harris VJ, Hemmer CG, Kopecky KK, Dalsing MC, Hyre CE, et al. Comparison of spiral CT scan and arteriography for evaluation of renal and visceral arteries. Ann Vasc Surg. 1996;10(2):109–16.
47. Stueckle CA, Haegele KF, Jendreck M, Zipser MC, Kirchner J, Kickuth R, et al. Multislice computed tomography angiography of the abdominal arteries: Comparison between computed tomography angiography and digital subtraction angiography findings in 52 cases. Australas Radiol Blackwell Science Pty. 2004;48(2):142–7.
48. Menke J. Diagnostic accuracy of multidetector CT in acute mesenteric ischemia: systematic review and meta-analysis. Radiology. 2010;256(1):93–101.
49. Mueller C, Buerkle G, Buettner HJ, Petersen J, Perruchoud AP, Eriksson U, et al. Prevention of contrast media–associated nephropathy: randomized comparison of 2 hydration regimens in 1620 patients undergoing coronary angioplasty. Arch Intern Med Am Med Assoc. 2002; 162(3):329–36.
50. Shih M-CP, Hagspiel KD. CTA and MRA in mesenteric ischemia: part 1, role in diagnosis and differential diagnosis. Am J Roentgenol. 2007;188(2):452–61.
51. Cowper SE. Nephrogenic fibrosing dermopathy: the first 6 years. Curr Opin Rheumatol. 2003;15(6):785–90.
52. Wasser MN, Geelkerken RH, Kouwenhoven M, van Bockel JH, Hermans J, Schultze Kool LJ, et al. Systolically gated 3D phase contrast MRA of mesenteric arteries in suspected mesenteric ischemia. J Comput Assist Tomogr. 1996;20(2):262–8.
53. Meaney JF, Prince MR, Nostrant TT, Stanley JC. Gadolinium-enhanced MR angiography of visceral arteries in patients with suspected chronic mesenteric ischemia. J Magn Reson Imaging. 1997;7(1):171–6.
54. Ernst O, Asnar V, Sergent G, Lederman E, Nicol L, Paris JC, et al. Comparing contrast-enhanced breath-hold MR angiography and conventional angiography in the evaluation of mesenteric circulation. Am J Roentgenol. 2000;174(2):433–9.
55. Carlos RC, Stanley JC, Stafford-Johnson D, Prince MR. Interobserver variability in the evaluation of chronic mesenteric ischemia with gadolinium-enhanced MR angiography. Acad Radiol. 2001;8(9):879–87.
56. Li KC, Whitney WS, McDonnell CH, Fredrickson JO, Pelc NJ, Dalman RL, et al. Chronic mesenteric ischemia: evaluation with phase-contrast cine MR imaging. Radiology. 1994; 190(1):175–9.
57. Burkart DJ, Johnson CD, Reading CC, Ehman RL. MR measurements of mesenteric venous flow: prospective evaluation in healthy volunteers and patients with suspected chronic mesenteric ischemia. Radiology. 1995;194(3):801–6.
58. Li KC, Wright GA, Pelc LR, Dalman RL, Brittain JH, Wegmueller H, et al. Oxygen saturation of blood in the superior mesenteric vein: in vivo verification of MR imaging measurements in a canine model. Work in progress. Radiology. 1995;194(2):321–5.

59. Li KC, Dalman RL, Ch'en IY, Pelc LR, Song CK, Moon WK, et al. Chronic mesenteric ischemia: use of in vivo MR imaging measurements of blood oxygen saturation in the superior mesenteric vein for diagnosis. Radiology. 1997;204(1):71–7.
60. Dawson AM, Trenchard D, Guz A. Small bowel tonometry: assessment of small gut mucosal oxygen tension in dog and man. Nature. 1965;206(987):943–4.
61. Grum CM, Fiddian-Green RG, Pittenger GL, Grant BJ, Rothman ED, Dantzker DR. Adequacy of tissue oxygenation in intact dog intestine. J Appl Physiol Respir Environ Exerc Physiol. 1984;56(4):1065–9.
62. Fiddian-Green RG, McGough E, Pittenger G, Rothman E. Predictive value of intramural pH and other risk factors for massive bleeding from stress ulceration. Gastroenterology. 1983;85(3):613–20.
63. Boley SJ, Brandt LJ, Veith FJ, Kosches D, Sales C. A new provocative test for chronic mesenteric ischemia. Am J Gastroenterol. 1991;86(7):888–91.
64. Kolkman JJ, Otte JA, Groeneveld AB. Gastrointestinal luminal PCO2 tonometry: an update on physiology, methodology and clinical applications. Br J Anaesth. 2000;84(1):74–86.
65. Geelkerken RH, Schultze Kool LJ, Hermans J, Zarza MT, van Bockel JH. Chronic splanchnic ischaemia: is tonometry a useful test? Eur J Surg. 1997;163(2):115–21.
66. Kolkman JJ, Groeneveld AB, Meuwissen SG. Effect of gastric feeding on intragastric P(CO2) tonometry in healthy volunteers. J Crit Care. 1999;14(1):34–8.
67. Kolkman JJ, Groeneveld AB, van der Berg FG, Rauwerda JA, Meuwissen SG. Increased gastric PCO2 during exercise is indicative of gastric ischaemia: a tonometric study. Gut. 1999;44(2):163–7.

Chapter 10
Non-atherosclerotic Causes of Mesenteric Arterial Disease

Mateus P. Correa and Gustavo S. Oderich

The most common cause of occlusive mesenteric artery disease is ostial atherosclerosis. Non-atherosclerotic causes account for 5–10 % of all cases of chronic mesenteric ischemia (CMI). The vasculitides consist in a varied group of conditions characterized by an inflammatory response of vessel wall, with or without associated necrosis and granulomas, affecting 20 individuals per million a year. These diseases have different etiologies and pathogenic mechanisms, albeit most of them are not completely understood. Chronic inflammation can weaken the media and thin the arterial wall leading to aneurysm, or it can cause thickening of the arterial wall, resulting in stenosis and occlusions [1–4].

Although mesenteric manifestations of vasculitides are considered rare, accounting for less than five percent of all cases of mesenteric ischemia [1], reports have suggested that gastrointestinal (GI) manifestations of vasculitis are isolated and can be the first manifestation of this group of diseases in up to 13–16 % of cases. In addition, the clinical manifestations may be fatal and require early diagnosis and immediate management [3, 4].

This chapter presents the clinical features and approaches to diagnosis and treatment of non-atherosclerotic causes of mesenteric ischemia, including mesenteric vasculitis (MV), neurofibromatosis, and mid-aortic syndrome. Other causes such as median arcuate ligament compression syndrome are not discussed. Specific vasculitis disorder details such as American College of Rheumatology diagnostic criteria and treatment were not in our scope and will not be discussed.

M.P. Correa, MD
Division of Vascular and Endovascular Surgery,
Department of Surgery, Mayo Clinic, Rochester, MN, USA
e-mail: mateuspc@msn.com

G.S. Oderich, MD, FACS (✉)
Gonda Vascular Center, Mayo Clinic, Rochester, MN, USA

Division of Vascular and Endovascular Surgery, Mayo Clinic, Rochester, MN, USA
e-mail: oderich.gustavo@mayo.edu

G.S. Oderich (ed.), *Mesenteric Vascular Disease*,
DOI 10.1007/978-1-4939-1847-8_10

Anatomic Considerations

The bowel vasculature must be analyzed as a single functional unit. Whether ischemia develops depends mainly on the amount of blood that flows into the diseased segment from the other visceral arteritis.

The blood supply of the GI system has intramural and extramural components. The intramural vascular distribution is generally well developed with plexuses in the different layers of the bowel wall and with distinctive features in the liver, small intestine, and gastroesophageal junction that are adapted to their function. The extramural arterial supply for the esophagus is derived from thoracic aorta or its major braches. The blood supply to the abdominal organs is provided by three vessels, which arise from the anterior wall of the abdominal aorta, namely, the celiac axis (CA), superior mesenteric artery (SMA), and inferior mesenteric artery (IMA). CA supplies the distal esophagus to the second portion of the duodenum. The SMA provides blood supply to the third and forth segments of the duodenum, jejunum, ileum, and the large bowel to the splenic flexure. Anastomosis between these two vessels includes the gastroduodenal arteries and the nonconstant Bühler arch. The IMA supplies the colon from the splenic flexure to the rectum. Its anastomosis with the SMA includes the marginal artery of Drummond along the inner border of the splenic flexure. The collateral network of the IMA and distal aorta is formed by several connections to the lumbar arteries, the sacral artery, and internal iliac arteries.

The liver presents a double supply. The portal vein carries venous blood from the splenic and superior mesenteric veins, and the proper hepatic artery, which is a branch from the celiac axis, is the source of the arterial blood. The inferior mesenteric vein drains in the splenic vein. The superior and inferior mesenteric veins run parallel to their arteries draining the corresponding visceral territories.

Classification of Vasculitis

The different vasculitides are classified as primary or secondary (Table 10.1) [5]. Primary vasculitis was defined by the Chapel Hill International Consensus on the Nomenclature of Systemic Vasculitis [6]. Ten diseases were classified according to the size and type of involved vessels and the presence or absence of associated fibroid necrosis and/or granulomas. Large-sized vessel vasculitis affects the aorta and the largest arterial branches from the extremities, medium-sized vessel vasculitis affects the main visceral arteries and their branches, and small-sized vessel vasculitis affects arterioles, venules, and capillaries. They are also subclassified according to the particular features of the specific pathology, for example, age, type of inflammation, and serology.

Table 10.1 Classification of vasculitis

Primary vasculitis
Large-sized vessel vasculitis
Takayasu's arteritis
Giant cell (temporal) arteritis
Medium-sized vessel vasculitis
Polyarteritis nodosa
Kawasaki disease
Primary granulomatous central nervous system vasculitis
Small-sized vessel vasculitis
Antineutrophil cytoplasmic autoantibody
Wegener granulomatosis
Churg-Strauss syndrome
Microscopic polyangiitis
Immune complex small-sized vessel vasculitis
Henoch-Schönlein purpura
Cryoglobulinemic vasculitis
Secondary vasculitis
Connective tissue diseases
Systemic lupus erythematosus
Rheumatoid arthritis
Sjögren syndrome
Behçet syndrome
Infectious diseases
Bacteria
Virus
Drugs
Nonsteroidal anti-inflammatory drugs
Anticancer drugs
Antibiotics
Paraneoplastic vasculitis
Carcinoma
Lymphoproliferative neoplasm
Myeloproliferative neoplasm

Clinical Features

The diagnosis of the several GI vasculitides is often built on the correlation of clinical manifestations, image and laboratory findings, and histopathological features. As the clinical or image findings may not be distinct from diseases that can mimic systemic vasculitis (Table 10.2) and therefore may have limited value in making a specific diagnosis, a high suspicion rate is needed [7]. Nevertheless, the possibility of vasculitis must be considered whenever mesenteric ischemic changes develop in a young patient; are noted in atypical sites such as stomach, duodenum, or rectum; appear simultaneously in the large and small intestine; or are associated with

Table 10.2 Diseases that can mimic systemic vasculitis

Systemic multisystem disease	
Infection	Subacute bacterial endocarditis
	Neisseria
	Rickettsia
	Metastatic carcinoma
Malignancy	
Paraneoplastic	
Other	Sweet syndrome
	Scurvy
	Cocaine abuse
Occlusive vasculopathy	
Embolic	Cholesterol crystals
	Atrial myxoma
	Infection
Thrombotic	Antiphospholipid syndrome
	Procoagulant states
	Calciphylaxis
Others	Ergot
	Radiation
	Köhlmeier-Degos
Angiographic	
Aneurysmal	Fibromuscular dysplasia
	Neurofibromatosis
Occlusion	Coarctation
	Atherosclerosis

genitourinary involvement [1, 2]. As suggested by Ha and colleagues, knowledge of systemic clinical manifestations in affected patients may suggest a specific diagnosis [8] (Table 10.3).

The signs and symptoms of GI involvement in systemic vasculitis depend upon the size and location of the affected vessel. As a result, in the large-sized vessel diseases, abdominal manifestations may be indistinguishable from those of atherosclerotic or embolic mesenteric ischemia, except for evidences of systemic disease. In the medium-sized arteries, such as the CT and SMA, inflammation can lead to aneurysm formation (Fig. 10.1), as noticed in polyarteritis nodosa (PAN). Rupture of aneurysms may cause intra-abdominal or GI hemorrhage. In small-artery involvement, ulceration and stricture formation are common and can complicate with perforation.

The GI symptoms demonstrate a wide spectrum, ranging from mild transient abdominal pain to life-threatening complications requiring emergency surgery, such as bowel perforation, peritonitis, or hypovolemic shock (Table 10.4).

The GI tract may be involved in vasculitides in up to 50 % of the cases [9]. However, the majority of patients are asymptomatic. Rits and colleagues in a retrospective

Table 10.3 Systemic manifestations of vasculitis

	%
Fever	66
Peripheral nervous system involvement	61
Weight loss	60
Arthralgia	52
Cutaneous symptoms	44
Renal involvement	37
Myalgia	34
Hypertension	23
Lung involvement	19
Central nervous system involvement	13
Asthma	13
Ear, nose, and throat involvement	13
Cardiac involvement	10
Ophthalmologic involvement	10
Raynaud syndrome/digital ischemia	8

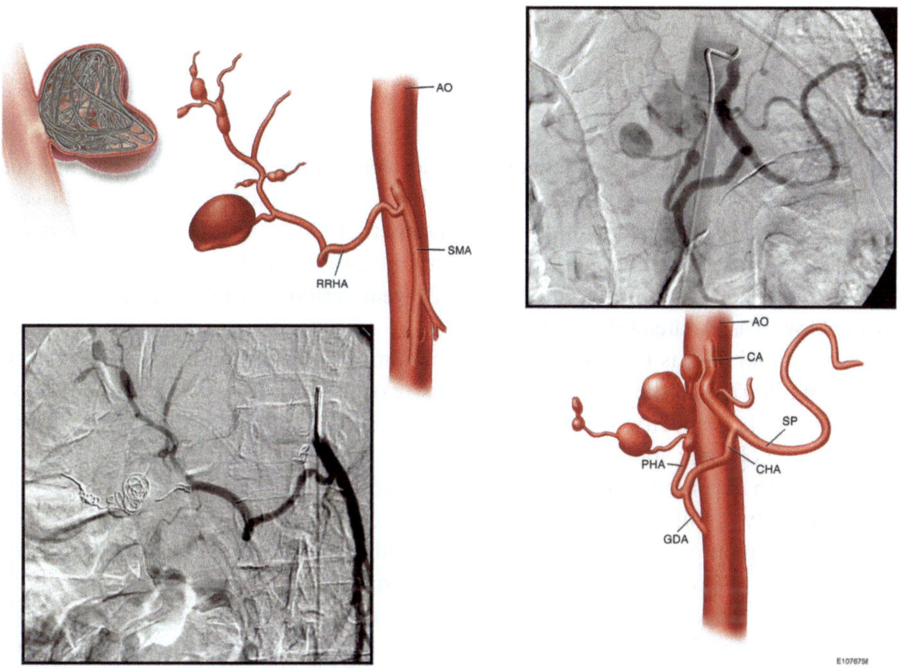

Fig. 10.1 Multiple intrahepatic aneurysms in a patient with polyarteritis nodosa who presented with ruptured intrahepatic artery aneurysm (By permission of Mayo Foundation for Medical Education and Research. All rights reserved)

Table 10.4 Gastrointestinal manifestations and radiologic findings

Abdominal findings in mesenteric vasculitis	
	%
Abdominal pain	97
Nausea or vomiting	34
Diarrhea	27
Hematochezia or melena	16
Hematemesis	6
Esophageal ulcerations	11
Gastroduodenal ulcers	27
Colorectal ulcerations	10
Gastritis	6
Peritonitis	18
Bowel perforations	15
Intestinal occlusion	6
GI ischemia/infarction	16
Appendicitis	10
Cholecystitis	8
Acute pancreatitis	5
Abnormal angiography	67
Abnormal abdominal CT	75
Surgical abdomen	34

review of the Mayo Clinic patients who underwent mesenteric revascularization due to mesenteric vasculitis evidenced 7,514 patients evaluated for vasculitis in a 24-year period, 102 (0.013 %) had symptoms of mesenteric ischemia, and only 15 underwent open or endovascular treatment for mesenteric vasculitis [1]. Pagnoux *et al.* reviewing 344 patients with systemic vasculitides in a 21-year period have evidenced 62 (0.18 %) patients with associated GI symptoms [3].

Abdominal pain is the most frequent and almost constant finding in these cases, occurring in 97 % of the patients. The intensity of the pain varies widely and usually does not lie in a specific location in the abdomen. Patients with GI vasculitis may also present chronic abdominal pain after eating, named intestinal angina, similar to patients with chronic atherosclerotic occlusion of the intestinal vessels. This symptom generally is followed by weight loss and cachexia and may be misdiagnosed as cancer. The pain can also be similar to the findings of acute mesenteric ischemia, which is out-of-proportion pain on the abdominal exam. However, a surgical abdomen was not systematically associated with intense abdominal pain or tenderness. Nausea and vomiting are present in one-third of the patients, and 27 % had diarrhea. Ischemic hepatitis, gastritis, esophagitis, pancreatitis, cholecystitis, and appendicitis were also reported in those patients [10–13]. Symptomatic patients may present with bleeding from gastrointestinal mucosal erosions or small aneurysms of the distal mesenteric or hepatic artery branches.

Image Findings

Duplex Ultrasound

Duplex ultrasound is an accurate screening test for ostial arterial lesions. A peak systolic velocity greater than 275 cm/s and an end-diastolic velocity greater than 45 cm/s seems to be highly specific for significant superior mesenteric artery (SMA) stenosis [14]. Moreover, patients with Behçet syndrome and GI involvement had increased flow in both the superior and inferior mesenteric arteries. These findings were not similar in patients with Behçet syndrome and no GI involvement. Altered pericolic fat may suggest presence of transmural necrosis [15, 16]. However, since the duplex scan has limitations, such as patients presenting with abdominal distention or intraperitoneal gas, and is operator-dependent, these findings may not be always reliable, and a second study with axial images of the abdomen is often necessary, in order to exclude other causes of pain and for analysis of the anatomy and planning of the procedure.

Endoscopy and Colonoscopy

Endoscopy and colonoscopy are useful exams in cases where symptoms of upper or lower GI involvement are suspected, proceeding with biopsy if ulceration is present. Despite the few reports on the subject, the combination of the tests and radiographic findings facilitates the precise diagnosis of the vasculitis [17]. Ischemic enteritis may suggest Kawasaki's disease, granulomatous enteritis can be present in Wegener granulomatosis, and mucosal edema and hemorrhage at the bowel may suggest systemic lupus erythematous or Churg-Strauss disease. During these procedures, the manipulation of the endoscopic device, the bowel insufflation, and biopsies must be performed with extreme caution and finesse, in order to prevent bowel perforation.

Computed Tomography

Contrast-enhanced computed tomography (CT) may provide useful information on inflammatory, neoplastic, and vascular diseases of the abdomen and have the advantage of assessment of emergent abdominal vascular conditions, ischemic bowel disease, and its complications. Bowel wall thickening, a "target sign," an increased attenuation of mesenteric fat, increased or delayed enhancement in the bowel wall due to hyperemia, or frank bowel infarction or perforation with *pneumatosis intestinalis*, portal venous air, or pneumoperitoneum are suggestive of acute ischemia.

Arterial-phase CT scans and particularly CT angiography (CTA) are of great value in the evaluation of mesenteric arteries. Arterial wall thickening is a characteristic

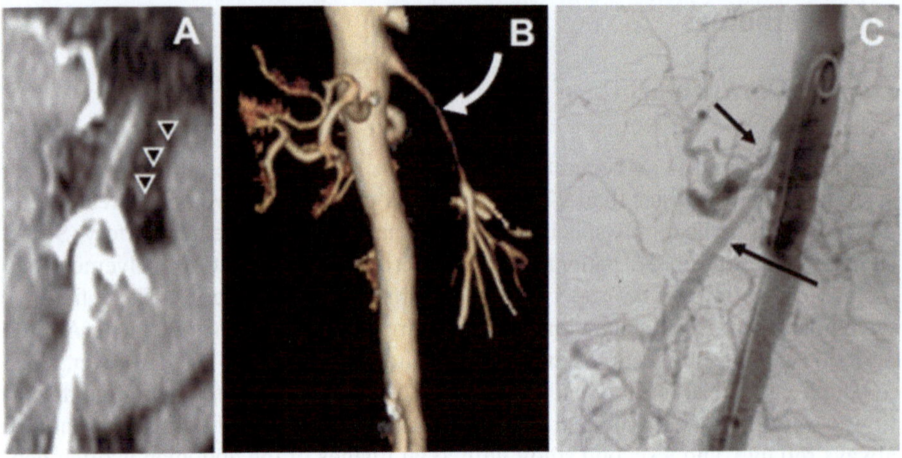

Fig. 10.2 Computed tomography angiography in a patient with mesenteric vasculitis. Coronal view demonstrates thickening of the arterial wall (**a**) also noticed in 3-D reconstruction (**b**). Angiography shows smooth lesion (**c**) sparing the origin of the mesenteric vessels

finding in patients with mesenteric vasculitis (Fig. 10.2). They help to identify site, level, and cause of bowel ischemia. In addition, venous phases may identify the mesenteric veins and the bowel wall itself, improving accuracy in the identification of bowel perforation and abscess [2, 8]. Limitations of the study are dye allergy and renal failure.

Angiography

Angiography remains the "gold standard" test for diagnosis of peripheral vessel splanchnic disease, particularly visceral aneurysms in polyarteritis nodosa and arterial narrowing in Takayasu's disease. Its role as confirmatory test and for planning revascularization diminished, in favor of the noninvasive modalities previously discussed. More frequently, angiography is obtained in conjunction with a planned endovascular intervention. Exceptions are patients with suboptimal imaging studies and those with extensive calcification, small vessels, or multiple prior stents causing metallic artifact.

Specific Disorders in Mesenteric Vasculitis

Although the ischemic symptoms and image findings may be similar regardless of the systemic vasculitis, distinct outcomes may result; hence specific syndromes deserve mention.

Takayasu's Arteritis

Takayasu's Arteritis (pulseless disease) is a large-sized vessel granulomatous vasculitis characterized by ocular disturbances and marked pulse weakening in the upper and lower extremities. It is related to fibrous thickening of the aortic arch with narrowing or obliteration of the ostia of the great vessels in the arch. TA involves the aortic arch, and in 32 % of the cases, it affects the rest of the aorta and its branches. Generalized symptoms and signs include malaise, fever, night sweats, arthralgia, and weight loss. GI symptoms are mainly nonspecific, such as anorexia, nausea, vomiting, and loss of weight, and start during the pulseless phase of the disease. GI morbidity is due to arterial stenosis; however, organ ischemia is rare. Chronic mesenteric ischemia has already been reported and is manifested similar to atherosclerotic presentation. Diagnosis is suspected by duplex scan and confirmed by arteriography or CTA. The findings consist in irregular thickening of the aortic wall with intimal wrinkling, stenosis, poststenotic dilatation, aneurysm formation, and occlusion with subsequent luxurious collateral circulation [2, 4, 8, 18].

Giant Cell Arteritis

Giant cell arteritis (GCA) is one of the most common vasculitides to present with occlusive mesenteric artery disease (Fig. 10.3). Giant cell arteritis is also known as temporal arteritis, cranial arteritis, or Horton disease. It most commonly involves large- and medium-sized arteries. Its original description affects branches of the external carotid artery and can lead to permanent blindness if not recognized and treated with corticosteroids. The name (giant cell arteritis) reflects the type of inflammatory cell involved and seen on a biopsy. The terms "giant cell arteritis" and "temporal arteritis" are sometimes used interchangeably, because of the frequent involvement of the temporal artery. However, it can involve other large vessels, such as the aorta ("giant cell aortitis") and its branches.

Polyarteritis Nodosa

Polyarteritis nodosa (PAN) is a fibrinoid necrotizing vasculitis that involves small- and medium-sized arteries. Multiple aneurysm formation (Fig. 10.1) is the characteristic finding of the disease and is present in 50–60 % of the patients [8]. The kidney is the most commonly involved organ (80–90 % of cases), followed by the gastrointestinal tract (50–70 %), liver (50–60 %), spleen (45 %), and pancreas (25–35 %). GI involvement increases mortality rates, due to the extensive destruction of the mesenteric arteries. The small intestine is the most commonly affected territory of the GI tract, followed by the mesentery and colon.

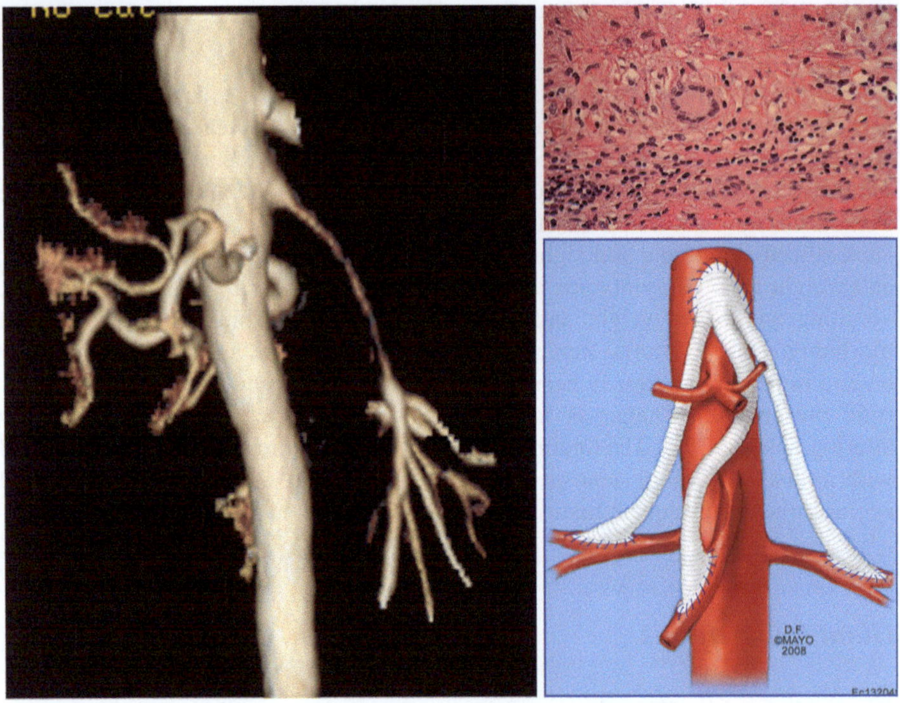

Fig. 10.3 Patient with long segment superior mesenteric narrowing and bilateral renal artery disease due to giant cell arteritis. Biopsy of arterial wall demonstrates giant cell (By permission of Mayo Foundation for Medical Education and Research. All rights reserved)

Approximately two-thirds of patients have abdominal pain, nausea, and vomiting. Other gastrointestinal signs and symptoms include peritonitis, mesenteric infarction, acute cholecystitis, appendicitis, and duodenal ulcers. In association with organ damage due to ischemia and infarction, GI hemorrhage occurs in 6 % of cases, bowel perforation in 5 %, and bowel infarction in 1.4 % of the cases [1, 3, 4, 7, 8, 19, 20].

The diagnostic is suggested by normochromic anemia and leukocytosis in CBC, an elevated ESR. A positive antineutrophil cytoplasmic antibody (ANCA) is found in 20 % of the patients. Angiography is the diagnostic modality to reach the diagnosis. The angiographic findings include multiple aneurysms up to 1 cm in diameter within the renal, mesenteric, and hepatic vasculature. Saccular aneurysms are found in 94 % of the patients. A "string-of-beads" appearance of the arteries is also frequently found. Colonoscopy with biopsy is useful for the diagnosis. If the bowel wall appears ischemic in a suspected patient, the biopsy must be performed and the exam must be immediately terminated. If left untreated, the disease is fatal in most instances, commonly related to renal failure, GI complications, or cardiovascular causes. Early detection of this pathology is the pillar of the treatment [2, 17].

Wegener Granulomatosis

Wegener granulomatosis (WG) is a characterized medium- and small-sized vessel granulomatous vasculitis of the upper and lower respiratory tract and kidneys, progressing with glomerulonephritis. WG may involve any part of the GI tract. Symptoms include odynophagia, abdominal pain, nausea and vomiting, and blood loss, occurring in 10–24 % of the WG patients. Typically, symptoms develop far from the disease onset. Clinical manifestations of severe intestinal disease are rare and may mimic inflammatory bowel disease, such as Crohn's disease and ulcerative colitis. Intestinal perforation, gangrenous gallbladder, and erosive esophagitis were also reported [2, 4, 8]. A positive ANCA is found in 90 % of patients with active WG. Granulomatous gastritis and colitis may be found [17].

Microscopic Polyangiitis

Microscopic polyangiitis (MP), also known as hypersensitivity vasculitis or leukocytoclastic angiitis, is a necrotizing small-sized vessel vasculitis, identical to PAN, except for the presentation in smaller vessels. Necrotizing glomerulonephritis occurs in 90 % of the patients, and GI manifestations include hemoptysis, hematuria, proteinuria, abdominal pain, or GI bleeding. When GI is involved, radiologic findings do not differ from those seen in other types of vasculitis, and bowel infarct and perforation rarely occurs. Unlike PAN, angiographic findings do not reveal microaneurysms and are usually normal [8].

Henoch-Schönlein Syndrome

Henoch-Schönlein syndrome (HSS) is a hypersensitivity-related acute small-sized vessel vasculitis. Many etiologies are demonstrated to start this vasculitis, but *Streptococcus* β-hemolytic from A group is the agent in 75 % of the cases. The GI manifestations are thought to be related to edema and intramural hemorrhage. When GI symptoms precede or predominate the appearance of skin lesions, the syndrome may mimic a number of acute abdominal diseases, resulting in unnecessary laparotomies. It may precede the typical rash in 36 % of the cases [2]. GI hemorrhage is mostly confined to the mucosa and submucosa, and full-thickness necrosis and bowel perforation is rare. Therefore, most GI manifestations are self-limited. Only 3–5 % of patients develop bowel infarct, perforation, or irreducible intussusception [21]. There is not a characteristic radiologic finding, although multifocal bowel wall thickening with unaffected areas along with clinical findings is important to establishing diagnosis [8]. The descending duodenum and terminal ileum are frequently involved with endoscopic findings of diffused mucosal redness, petechiae, hemorrhagic erosions, and ulcers [17].

Systemic Lupus Erythematous

Systemic lupus erythematous (SLE) is an autoimmune disorder that affects musculoskeletal system, kidneys, GI tract, or skin. Small blood vessel inflammation of the gut produces a variety of complications including intestinal ischemia, hemorrhage, ileus, ulceration, infarction, and perforation [12, 22, 23]. Lupus enteritis is a serious presentation of SLE. It may involve any part of GI tract from the esophagus to the colon. However, the superior mesenteric artery (SMA) territory is the most affected. Clinical signs and symptoms range from pain and hemorrhage from gastritis, perforation, gastritis, diarrhea, bowel perforation and infarct, ileus with ileitis, colitis, and intussusception [24]. The endoscopic features are ischemic enterocolitis and "punched-out" ulcers. Although histopathological diagnosis of lupus enteritis can be obtained, most endoscopic superficial biopsies might not yield a definitive result because the affected vessels are usually located in inaccessible areas [17]. Common CT findings include dilated bowel; focal or diffuse bowel wall thickening; most of the time multifocal, abnormal bowel wall enhancement; engorged mesenteric vessels in a comblike arrangement; ascites; and lymphadenopathy [13]. Angiography is not useful since the disease occurs in the small vessels. Unfortunately, there are no radiographic or histological pathognomonic findings suggestive of SLE [2].

Rheumatoid Vasculitis

Rheumatoid vasculitis (RV) is a classically leukocytoclastic lesion that predominantly involves the skin. Rarely, this disease can lead to life-threatening visceral infarction. RV occurs after long-standing rheumatoid arthritis (usually 15 years) in patients who exhibit advanced diseases with high titers of rheumatoid factor. Sometimes it may be difficult to determine whether the symptoms originate from the disease itself or from ongoing use of related medications [2, 4].

Behçet Syndrome

Behçet syndrome (BS) is a widely recognized necrotizing vasculitis involving multiple organ systems with well-known clinical manifestations. GI tract has been reported to be involved in 10–40 % of patients with BS. The usual stricked site is the terminal ileum and esophagus. BS manifests as large, deeply penetrating ulcerations of the submucosa, muscle layer, or entire intestinal wall. The ulcers can be localized in a specific territory or diffused throughout the visceral area. As a result, a considerable prevalence of complications such as hemorrhage, perforation, fistula, and peritonitis has been reported. Barium examination may show a large ovoid or irregular ulcer with marked thickening of the surrounding intestinal wall at the sites of involvement. At CT scan, the involved bowel demonstrates concentric wall thickening or polypoid mass. The presence of severe perienteric or pericolic infiltration raises the possibility of complications such as microperforation or localized peritonitis [2–4, 17, 25].

Thromboangiitis Obliterans

Thromboangiitis obliterans (TAO) or Buerger's disease is a distinct disease characterized by segmental, thrombosing, acute, or chronic inflammation of small- and intermediate-sized arteries and veins. Although it is not a classic vasculitis, the disease is considered as one due to the intense inflammatory response. GI tract manifestations are rare and preferentially involve the mesenteric vessels. The small intestine was more commonly affected than the colon [10, 11].

Differential Diagnosis

The diagnosis is based on a combination of clinical, laboratory, and histopathological features. Clinical manifestations should not be used alone for the diagnosis, as a variety of other diseases can mimic systemic vasculitides and mesenteric ischemia (Tables 10.5, 10.6, and 10.7). These other diseases can occur either with multiorgan features or similar findings of vascular imaging. Therefore, biopsy of the affected skin or involved organs is important to identify vessel changes.

Atherosclerosis is the most common cause of mesenteric ischemia due to occlusive disease or thrombus or cholesterol crystal embolism. Age >60 years, tobacco use, and diabetes mellitus are risk factors. Mesenteric vasculitis should be entertained in younger patients without other stigmata of arterial disease, such as calcifications. Fibromuscular dysplasia (FD) also occurs in young patients without calcifications, but less commonly affects mesenteric arteries, and a "string-of-beads" angiography appearance is typical. Although the disease can mimic Takayasu's arteritis and PAN, it does not present acute inflammatory response.

Calciphylaxis is a rare but potentially fatal disease. It occurs in patients with chronic renal failure and secondary hyperparathyroidism. Likewise in cardiac myxoma and infective endocarditis, it can be related to mesenteric and skin ischemia due to acute embolization. Chronic ergotism and cocaine abuse may develop mesenteric ischemia due to SMA vasoconstriction, and a careful history is required to establish their abuse.

Radiation vasculopathy depends on the territories included in the field, the type, and the radiation dose. It may present with endothelial thrombosis within 5 years of

Table 10.5 Differential diagnosis of mesenteric ischemia with arterial occlusion

Arterial occlusion
Thromboembolism
Left atrial origin
Aortic origin
Myxoma
Endocarditis
Cholesterol
Atherosclerosis
Arterial thrombosis
Arterial dissection
Aortic surgery
Stent placement
Therapeutic embolization
Antiphospholipid antibody syndrome
Systemic vasculitis
Takayasu's arteritis
Giant cell arteritis
Polyarteritis nodosa
Systemic lupus erythematous
Henoch-Schönlein purpura
Wegener granulomatosis
Churg-Strauss syndrome
Thromboangiitis obliterans
Rheumatoid vasculitis
Behcet syndrome
Thrombotic thrombocytopenic purpura
Hemolytic-uremic syndrome
Fibromuscular dysplasia
Miscellaneous
Diabetes mellitus
Amyloidosis
Oxalosis

therapy, progressive sclerosis and stenosis of arterioles and arteries within 10 years, or progressive atherosclerosis with 20 years of latency. It is distinguished from MV by the history of radiation therapy and lack of acute phase response.

Segmental arterial mediolysis (SAM) is a rare non-atherosclerotic noninflammatory arthropathy that affects small and medium-sized arteries and commonly affects visceral arteries. It involves most commonly the CA, SMA, and IMA branches and was also reported in hepatic and splenic branches. It is mislabeled as vasculitis

Table 10.6 Differential diagnosis of mesenteric ischemia with venous occlusion

Venous occlusion
Venous thrombosis
Infiltrative conditions
Neoplastic conditions
Inflammatory conditions
Abdominal infectious conditions
Hypercoagulable conditions
Polycythemia vera
Sickle cell disease
Thrombocytosis
Thrombophilia
Carcinoma
Pregnancy
Drugs
Systemic vasculitis
Wegener granulomatosis
Systemic lupus erythematous
Behcet syndrome
Complicated bowel obstruction
Strangulated hernia
Strangulated closed loop obstruction
Volvulus
Intussusception
Intestinal overdistension
Enterocolic lymphocytic phlebitis

given its clinical features. The disease may present with abdominal pain associated with intra-abdominal bleeding. SAM leads to microaneurysm formation and a "string-of-beads" appearance in angiography, which can mimic PAN. Both can be difficult to distinguish without histological examination [13].

Köhlmeier-Degos disease is also known as malignant atrophic papulosis. It is a rare and lethal condition, which involves skin, gut, and nervous system. The arterial lesion found in affected patients is luminal stenosis leading to bowel infarction, fever, and acute phase response. The diagnosis is based on skin biopsy and lesion appearance, which begins as erythematous, pink and red papules and which evolves into circular porcelain white scars with an atrophic depressed center. This disease can mimic vasculitis and there is no specific treatment. The usual cause of death is intestinal perforation [7].

Table 10.7 Differential diagnosis of mesenteric ischemia from nonocclusive diseases

Nonocclusive disease
Narcotics
Cocaine
Heroin
Shock bowel
Familial dysautonomia
Pheochromocytoma
High-endurance athletes
Chronic renal failure
Trauma
Radiation
Corrosive injury
Prostaglandins antagonist
Iatrogenic
Immunotherapy
Chemotherapy
Vasoconstriction
Digitals
Ergotamine
Vasopressin
Epinephrine
Hypotension
Antihypertensive drugs
Diuretics
Antidepressants

Treatment

Medical Treatment

Since vasculitides are primarily inflammatory processes, corticosteroids alone or combined with other immunosuppressants are the cornerstones of medical therapy [1]. Even in the presence of severe GI vasculitis, medical therapy must be initiated [3]. The medical regimen at Mayo Clinic is based on previous work published in our institution [26, 27]. The treatment includes a daily dose of 40–60 mg of prednisone, which is preferred over a lower dose or alternate day corticosteroid therapy, and aspirin. Prednisone is maintained at this dosage for approximately 4–6 weeks, after which is tapered by 10 % every 2–4 weeks, depending on absence of symptoms and level of inflammatory markers. The addition of an antimetabolic or steroid-sparing agent may allow reduction of the prednisone dose, although these medications are reserved for patients without initial response to prednisone. The medical treatment resolved mesenteric symptoms in >87 % of our patients [1].

Surgical Approach

Patients who present signs or symptoms of acute mesenteric ischemia, with bowel necrosis, bowel perforation, or peritonitis, should be treated with bowel resection. Other surgical abdomen presentations, such as appendicitis, acute pancreatitis, and GI bleeding, also should be treated at once. Levine and colleagues reported a lower (23 %) overall mortality for surgical patients presenting with less severe GI involvement. However, severe GI involvement has been associated with high mortality [20]. According to uni- and multivariate survival analysis of 62 patients that presented with GI vasculitides, the only high mortality predictors were peritonitis, bowel perforation, GI ischemia or infarction, and intestinal occlusion [3].

Mesenteric revascularization is reserved for failure of medical therapy in the acute or chronic setting or because of severe side effects from immunosuppressive medications. The most commonly disorders implicated in this setting are the large- and media-sized vessel vasculitides: Takayasu's arteritis due to aortic involvement proximal to or at the ostia of the mesenteric arteries, giant cell arteritis, and polyarteritis nodosa.

According to our experience in the management of occlusive lesions from Takayasu's arteritis [28], we prefer open arterial reconstruction in most patients with vasculitis, independent of vascular territory. The best results are achieved in patients who are operated on when arteritis is quiescent and preferably when are absent of steroids intake. Late outcomes are uncommon and the majority of patients remained asymptomatic after 41 months of follow-up. All patients remained alive. Freedom of mesenteric symptoms at 10 years was 83 % for patients with vasculitis, in comparison with 75 % in those where mesenteric reconstruction was due to atherosclerotic disease [1].

Mesenteric revascularization is performed just for symptomatic patients and selectively for those who effectively have three-vessel involvements, either with mesenteric trunk disease or aortic coarctation involving the origins of all the three arteries. We do not perform prophylactic reconstruction of visceral arteries, owing to difficulties in reoperation to revascularize a visceral artery.

There are no guidelines for how to approach open mesenteric reconstruction in MV. The general principle is for the inflow and outflow anastomoses to be done to noninflamed arteries. Similar to patients with atherosclerotic mesenteric disease, we favor an antegrade bypass from the supra-celiac aorta, whenever it is possible. If the patient is older or has cardiac disease or a calcified aorta, iliomesenteric retrograde bypass with straight or C-shaped configuration should be performed. Both celiac and SMA arteries are reconstructed, so late failure of one graft does not necessarily result in recurrent symptoms. Although concomitant renal or aortic reconstructions are avoided in atherosclerotic disease, these may not be the case in MV. Seven of 15 patients (47 %) with MV in our institution also had refractory renal hypertension and required associated renal bypass. None of our patients have died [1, 28, 29]. Late outcomes are not common, and 93 % patients remained asymptomatic.

Endovascular Treatment

Endovascular treatment should be reserved for embolization of aneurysms and for focal and isolated lesions. The durability of angioplasty and stenting of mesenteric lesions has not matched the results obtained with open surgery. This should be considered an as important argument that favors to open surgery in young patients affected by MV and with normal life expectancy. Furthermore, long lesions are prone to recoil, which may lead to poor technical result; and angioplasty and stent placement contradicts the basic principle of avoiding the inflammatory bed, especially in patients with active disease, acute inflammation, or those with chronic disease still on corticosteroids [18, 20, 29–31].

Neurofibromatosis and Other Causes of Mid-aortic Syndrome

Neurofibromatosis type I (NF-I), or von Recklinghausen disease, is an autosomal dominant disorder affecting one in 3,000 individuals. Cardinal features of NF-I include multiple café au lait macules, benign neurofibromas, and iris hamartomas (Fig. 10.4). Other common manifestations are learning disabilities, short stature, and skeletal abnormalities. Vascular lesions of medium- and large-sized arteries and veins are a well-recognized, albeit rare, feature. The term "*NF-I vasculopathy*" has been coined in the medical literature to describe aneurysms, stenoses, and arteriovenous malformations occurring in patients with NF-I. The pathogenesis, clinical spectrum, and natural history of these abnormalities are unknown.

The majority of patients with NF-I vascular abnormalities are asymptomatic but have involvement of multiple vessels. Symptoms usually occur in childhood or early adulthood. The renal artery is the most frequent site of involvement and renovascular hypertension is the most common presentation. Abdominal aortic coarctation, internal carotid artery aneurysms, and cervical vertebral arteriovenous malformations are other common manifestations.

Abdominal aortic coarctation or mid-aortic syndrome involving the visceral segment can be manifested by symptoms of mesenteric ischemia. The most common presentation is lower extremity claudication or difficult to control hypertension. Etiologies include Takayasu's arteritis, giant cell arteritis, and neurofibromatosis type I. Mesenteric artery stenosis is found in approximately one-third of the patients and can present with symptoms of CMI or require revascularization combined with aortic reconstruction in patients with critical lesions.

The aorta may be aneurysmal or stenotic. Aneurysms predominate in patients over age 50, whereas abdominal aortic coarctation occurs more often in younger patients. In our opinion, the indications for treatment in either circumstance should be the same as for patients without NF-I. In general, we offer repair of abdominal aortic aneurysms 5.5 cm in diameter or larger, and thoracoabdominal aneurysms of at least 6.0 cm, depending on the patient age and comorbidities. Although there are

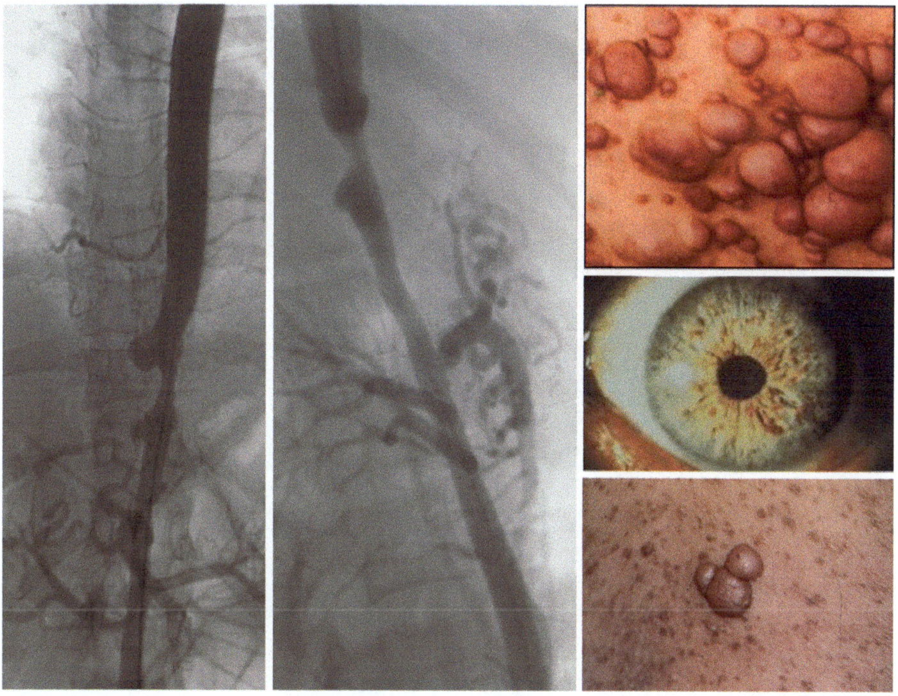

Fig. 10.4 Patient with neurofibromatosis type I and long segment narrowing of the visceral aortic segment with symptoms of chronic mesenteric ischemia

no reports of endovascular repair for aneurysms associated with NF-I, this approach could be applied to select older patients. We noted no fragility of the aorta or abdominal branch arteries during open repair but had two patients with aneurysms, one jugular vein and the other subclavian artery, who had friable vessels. Therefore, some precautionary measures are appropriate. We recommend gentle, atraumatic, and delicate handling of tissues, careful placement of retractors, and use of soft, protected arterial clamps. We are unaware of any reports showing increased risk of complications with diagnostic angiography and other catheter-based procedures in NF-I patients.

Open reconstruction is offered to patients with abdominal aortic coarctation who have renovascular hypertension unresponsive to medical therapy, chronic mesenteric ischemia, disabling claudication, or combinations thereof (Figs. 10.5 and 10.6). The aorta is frequently narrowed in the para-visceral segment though we and others have reported distal thoracic involvement. Supra-celiac to infrarenal aortic bypass or patch aortoplasty are the treatment options. We favor a midline, transperitoneal approach with medial visceral rotation in most patients or a low left thoracoabdominal approach if the distal thoracic aorta is involved. A supra-celiac to infrarenal aorta bypass with end-to-side anastomoses is preferred for patients with a long (>5–6 cm) narrowed aortic segment. This technique minimizes renal and

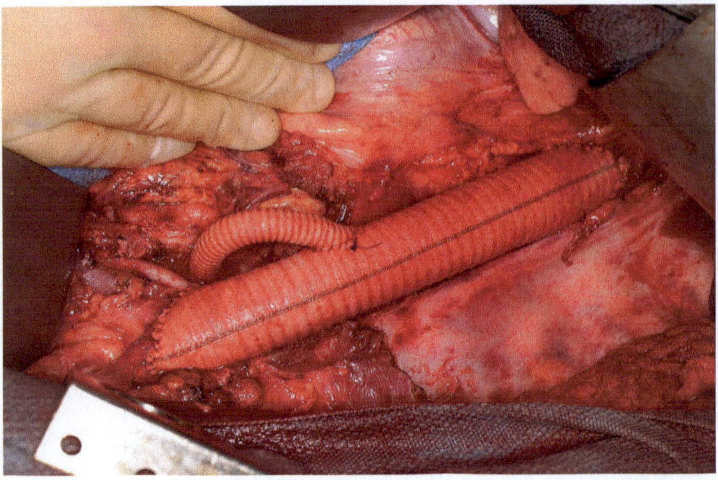

Fig. 10.5 Mid-aortic syndrome treated by aorto-aortic bypass and mesenteric bypass

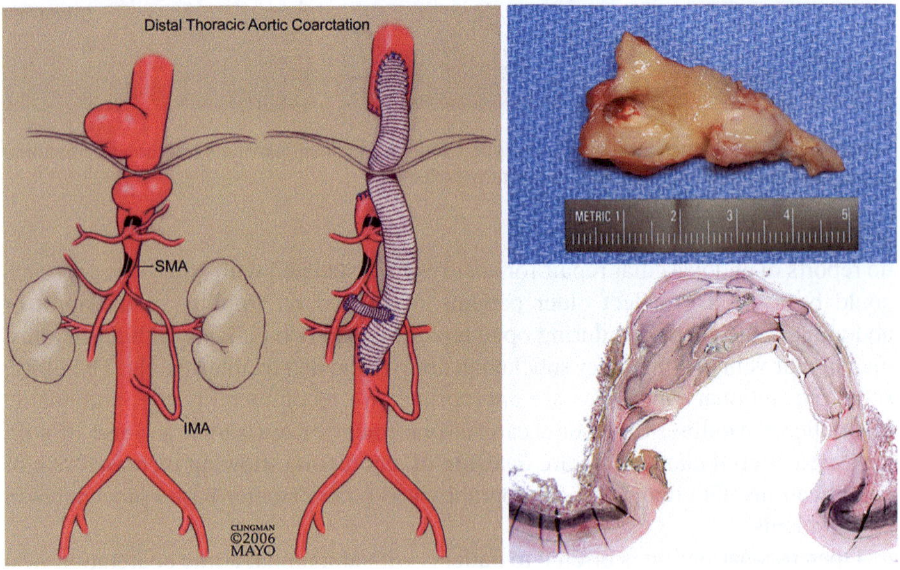

Fig. 10.6 Illustration of aorto-aortic bypass with mesenteric graft as depicted in Fig. 10.5 (By permission of Mayo Foundation for Medical Education and Research. All rights reserved)

mesenteric ischemia time and allows placement of a larger graft in children whose aorta will still "grow." Additional grafts to the renal and mesenteric arteries are done as needed. Abdominal aortoplasty is reserved for patients with a focal narrowing of the aorta but may be used in conjunction with aortic bypass in cases of long segment stenosis.

Although endovascular treatment has been used in select patients, open reconstruction remains the treatment of choice for most. Fibromuscular dysplasia can affect the mesenteric arteries and responds well to balloon angioplasty, similar to renal artery lesions.

Conclusion

Non-atherosclerotic causes account for 5–10 % of cases of chronic mesenteric ischemia. Mesenteric vasculitis is a rare manifestation of systemic vasculitis, and the involvement of other vascular territories is common. Clinical manifestations can range from mild discomfort, often mistaken as side effects from the underlying treatment, to potentially life-threatening bowel rupture. Hence it should be suspected when younger patients present with clinical features of mesenteric ischemia, and an early diagnose is paramount. Severe GI symptoms have major mortality rates and should be aggressively treated with corticosteroids and surgery. The choice of arterial reconstruction depends on the associated aortic inflammation, but surgical reconstructions are durable and effective when needed.

References

1. Rits Y, Oderich GS, Bower TC, Miller DV, Cooper L, Ricotta 2nd JJ, Kalra M, Gloviczki P. Interventions for mesenteric vasculitis. J Vasc Surg. 2010;51:392–400. e392.
2. Ragab G. Vasculitic manifestations in the gastrointestinal tract. In: Ball GV, Bridges Jr SL, editors. Vasculitis. New York: New York Oxford University Press; 2008. p. 181–98.
3. Pagnoux C, Mahr A, Cohen P, Guillevin L. Presentation and outcome of gastrointestinal involvement in systemic necrotizing vasculitides: analysis of 62 patients with polyarteritis nodosa, microscopic polyangiitis, wegener granulomatosis, churg-strauss syndrome, or rheumatoid arthritis-associated vasculitis. Medicine. 2005;84:13.
4. Ahn E, Luk A, Chetty R, Butany J. Vasculitides of the gastrointestinal tract. Semin Diagn Pathol. 2009;26:115–28.
5. Hunder C, Arend W, Bloch D. al. e. The american college of rheumatology 1990 criteria for the classification of vasculitis. Arthritis Rheum. 1990;33:1065–7.
6. Jennette J, Falk R, Andrassy K, Bacon P, Churg J, Gross W, Hagen E, Hoffman G, Hunder G, Kallenberg C. Nomenclature of systemic vasculitides. Proposal of an international consensus conference. Arthritis Rheum. 1994;37:187–92.
7. Watts R, Scott D. Vasculitis mimics. In: Watts RA, Scott DG, editors. Vasculitis in clinical practice. London: Springer; 2010. p. 143–54.
8. Ha H, Lee S, Rha S, Kim J, Byun J, Lim H, Chung J, Kim J, Kim P, Lee M, Auh Y. Radiologic features of vasculitis involving the gastrointestinal tract. Radiographics. 2000;20:15.
9. Casella G, Bonzino B, Cutrino L, et al. Vasculitis and gastrointestinal involvement. Minerva Gastroenterol Dietol. 2006;52:137–214.
10. Hassoun Z, Lacrosse M, Ronde T. Intestinal involvement in buerger's disease. J Clin Gastroenterol. 2001;31:85–9.
11. Sujobert P, Fardet L, Marie I, Duhaut P, Cohen P, Grange C, Gaultier JB, Arrive L, Cabane J. Mesenteric ischemia in giant cell arteritis: 6 cases and a systematic review. J Rheumatol. 2007;34:1727–32.

12. Tian XP, Zhang X. Gastrointestinal involvement in systemic lupus erythematosus: insight into pathogenesis, diagnosis and treatment. World J Gastroenterol. 2010;16:2971–7.
13. Krupski W, Selzman C, Whitehill T. Unusual causes of mesenteric ischemia. Surg Clin North Am. 1997;77:471–502.
14. Ryer E, Oderich G, Bower T, Macedo T, Vrtiska T, Duncan A, Kalra M, Gloviczki P. Differences in anatomy and outcomes in patients treated with open mesenteric revascularization before and after the endovascular era. J Vasc Surg. 2011;53:1611–8.
15. Siğirci A, Senol M, Aydin E, Kutlu R, Alkan A, Altinok M, Yoloğlu S, Baysal T, Saraç K. Doppler waveforms and blood flow parameters of the superior and inferior mesenteric arteries in patients having behçet disease with and without gastrointestinal symptoms: preliminary data. J Ultrasound Med. 2003;22:449–57.
16. Ripollés T, Simó L, Martínez-Pérez M, Pastor M, Igual A, López A. Sonographic findings in ischemic colitis in 58 patients. Am J Roentgenol. 2005;184:777–85.
17. Hokama A, Kishimoto K, Ihama Y, Kobashigawa C, Nakamoto M, Hirata T, Kinjo N, Higa F, Tateyama M, Kinjo F, Iseki K, Kato S, Fujita J. Endoscopic and radiographic features of gastrointestinal involvement in vasculitis. World J Gastrointest Endosc. 2012;4:50–6.
18. Ozdil E, Parikh D, Krajcer Z, Angelini P. Stent placement in a patient with takayasu's arteritis. Cathet Cardiovasc Diagn. 1996;38:373–6.
19. Kendirli T, Yuksel S, Oral M, Unal N, Tulunay M, Dilek US, Yalcnkaya F. Fatal polyarteritis nodosa with gastrointestinal involvement in a child. Pediatr Emerg Care. 2006;22:810–2.
20. Levine S, Hellmann D, Stone J. Gastrointestinal involvement in polyarteritis nodosa (1986–2000): presentation and outcomes in 24 patients. Am J Med. 2002;112:386–91.
21. Wang HL, Liu HT, Chen Q, Gao Y, Yu KJ. Henoch-schonlein purpura with intestinal perforation and cerebral hemorrhage: a case report. World J Gastroenterol. 2013;19:2574–7.
22. Janssens P, Arnaud L, Galicier L, Mathian A, Hie M, Sene D, Haroche J, Veyssier-Belot C, Huynh-Charlier I, Grenier PA, Piette JC, Amoura Z. Lupus enteritis: from clinical findings to therapeutic management. Orphanet J Rare Dis. 2013;8:67.
23. Lin YJ, Chen PC, Chen HA. Mesenteric vasculitis causing ileocecal intussusception as the initial presentation of systemic lupus erythematosus: a case report. Clin Rheumatol. 2013;32 Suppl 1:S37–40.
24. Yuan S, Ye Y, Chen D, Qiu Q, Zhan Z, Lian F, Li H, Liang L, Xu H, Yang X. Lupus mesenteric vasculitis: clinical features and associated factors for the recurrence and prognosis of disease. Semin Arthritis Rheum. 2014;43(6):759–66.
25. Yokota K, Akiyama Y, Sato K, Shindo Y, Yoshida Y, Miyoshi F, Akiba H, Nakajima K, Asanuma Y, Mimura T. Vasculo-behcet's disease with non-traumatic subcapsular hematoma of the kidney and aneurysmal dilatations of the celiac and superior mesenteric arteries. Mod Rheumatol/Japan Rheumatism Assoc. 2008;18:615–8.
26. Warrington K, Matteson E. Management guidelines and outcome measures in giant cell arteritis (gca). Clin Exp Rheumatol. 2007;25:137–41.
27. Hunder G, Sheps S, Allen G, Joyce J. Daily and alternate-day corticosteroid regimens in treatment of giant cell arteritis: comparison in a prospective study. Ann Intern Med. 1975;82:613–8.
28. Fields C, Bower T, Cooper L, Hoskin T, Noel A, Panneton J, Sullivan T, Gloviczki P, Cherry KJ. Takayasu's arteritis: operative results and influence of disease activity. J Vasc Surg. 2006;43:64–71.
29. Park W, Gloviczk IP, Cherry KJ, Hallett JJ, Bower T, Panneton J, Schleck C, Ilstrup D, Harmsen W, Noel A. Contemporary management of acute mesenteric ischemia: factors associated with survival. J Vasc Surg. 2002;35:445–52.
30. Tyagi S, Jolly N, Khalilullah M. Multivessel angioplasty in takayasu's arteritis. Indian Heart J. 1993;45:215–27.
31. Golden DA, Ring EJ, McLean GK, Freiman DB. Percutaneous transluminal angioplasty in the treatment of abdominal angina. Am J Roentgenol. 1982;139:247–9.

Chapter 11
Techniques of Open Mesenteric Reconstructions

Thomas C. Bower

Over the past decade, endovascular therapy has changed the role for open reconstructions to treat atherosclerotic mesenteric artery stenoses. While initially reserved for high-risk patients, endovascular therapy is now routinely used at most institutions to treat all patients with favorable lesions. However, there still is a role for open surgery. Patients with flush occlusions, thick calcified lesions, those with long stenoses, and individuals who have failed angioplasty and stenting are best served with an open operation. Herein, the surgical exposures and techniques of antegrade and retrograde reconstructions will be reviewed.

Surgical Treatment

A number of techniques are used to reconstruct either single or multiple mesenteric arteries. The reconstructions can be done in an antegrade or retrograde fashion, though each has advantages and disadvantages. There are differing opinions as to how many visceral arteries require reconstruction, which artery is most important to revascularize, and how the graft limb(s) ought to be configured.

Exposure

Mesenteric artery bypass is done through an upper midline or bilateral subcostal incision when the origin of the graft is from the supraceliac aorta. A midline incision is used to isolate the infrarenal aorta or iliac arteries as inflow for retrograde grafts.

T.C. Bower, MD (✉)
Division of Vascular and Endovascular Surgery, Department of Surgery,
Mayo Clinic, Rochester, MN, USA
e-mail: bower.thomas@mayo.edu

G.S. Oderich (ed.), *Mesenteric Vascular Disease*,
DOI 10.1007/978-1-4939-1847-8_11

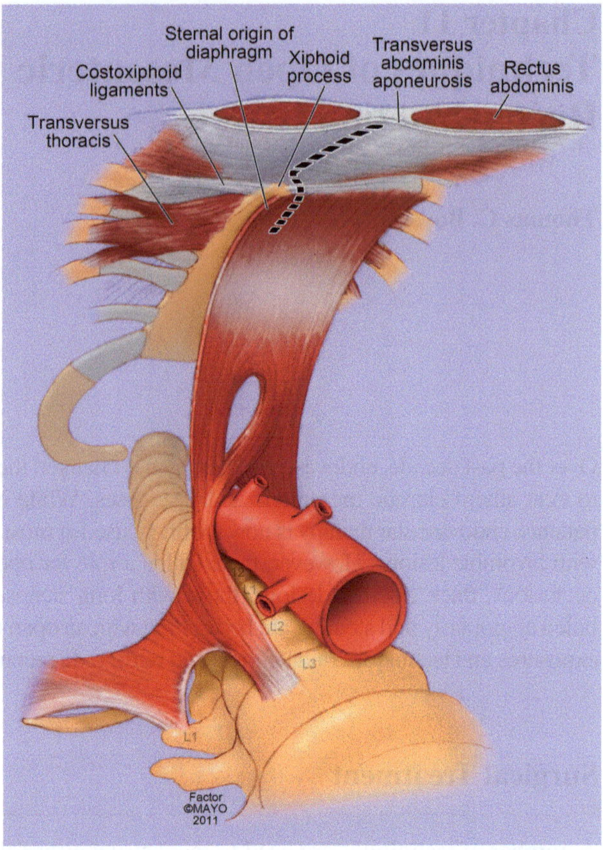

Fig. 11.1 Schematic drawing of additional upward and lateral retraction of the abdominal wall obtained incising the sic musculoaponeurotic attachments along the site of the xiphoid process (By permission of Mayo Foundation for Medical Education and Research. All rights reserved)

An upper midline incision provides excellent exposure of the supraceliac aorta in most patients, especially those with narrow costal margins. A bilateral subcostal incision is used in patients with wide costal flares and in the rare patient who requires a left medial visceral rotation to isolate the paravisceral aorta and mesenteric arteries for endarterectomy. Extension of the midline incision along the xiphoid process releases six muscular and aponeurotic attachments and is the lynchpin of the abdomen (Fig. 11.1). This maneuver allows better upward and lateral retraction of the abdominal wall and costal margin than what a standard incision provides and facilitates a near straight on view of the supraceliac area. A self-retaining retractor is helpful to maintain abdominal wall and visceral retraction. The aorta is isolated by taking down the left triangular ligament of the liver and gently retracting it to the right side of the patient. The lesser sac is entered and the crura of the diaphragm are divided. Care must be taken to avoid injury to the esophagus during the aortic exposure, and a nasogastric tube helps in this regard. Attachments with padded salts are used to gently retract the esophagus and stomach to the left side. Approximately 5–8 cm of the aorta is dissected free (Fig. 11.2). At times, the right or left pleura is inadvertently

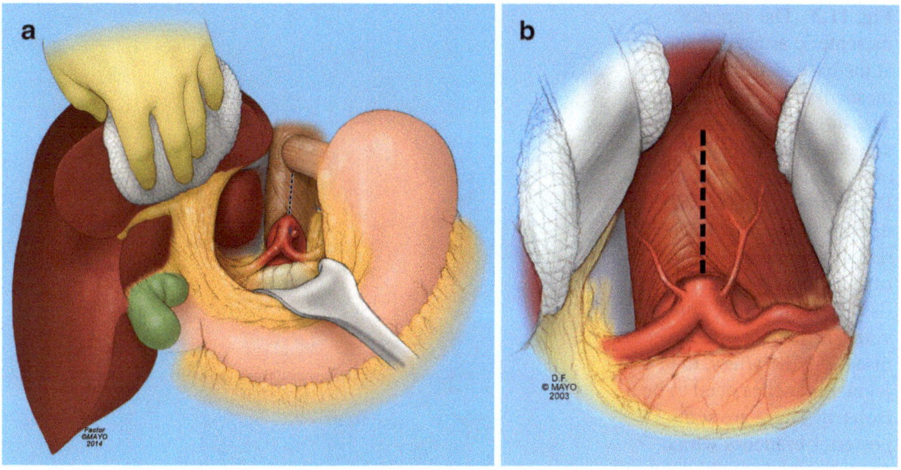

Fig. 11.2 Transperitoneal exposure of the supraceliac aorta and the celiac artery. First, the left triangular ligament of the liver is divided so that the liver can be retracted toward the patient's right side. With a nasogastric tube in place, the stomach and esophagus are gently retracted to the left side (**a**). The patient can be placed in a slight reverse Trendelenburg position and the pancreas and the viscera retracted caudally to achieve exposure of the celiac. The crural fibers are divided longitudinally over the top of the aorta (**b**). As much as 5–8 cm of the supraceliac or lower descending thoracic aorta can be exposed through this approach (By permission of Mayo Foundation for Medical Education and Research. All rights reserved)

opened and requires closure. Rarely, the supraceliac aorta is diseased and inflow is best obtained from the lower descending thoracic aorta. Several centimeters of the thoracic aorta can be isolated after complete division of the crura of the diaphragm and cephalad retraction of the central tendon of the diaphragm. However, as a general rule, it is always best to not work in a keyhole when sewing a graft to the aorta.

The celiac artery is isolated first when a two-vessel antegrade reconstruction is planned. The patient is placed in a gentle head up position (reverse Trendelenburg), and the viscera and pancreas are gently retracted caudally by retractor blades with pads beneath them. The artery can be isolated by first exposing the common hepatic artery above the pancreas, then tracing it to the celiac bifurcation. Occasionally, there are a couple of periarterial veins which cause nuisance bleeding when disrupted. The splenic artery then is isolated, which allows for circumferential dissection of the celiac to its origin. Periarterial ganglionic and fibrous tissue requires excision. One or more small branches may be present and are ligated and divided. The left gastric artery often is ligated and divided too, which helps facilitate a retropancreatic tunnel for a superior mesenteric artery (SMA) graft limb. Complete isolation of the celiac is needed when that trunk is the target for bypass, and it also allows placement of a hypogastric clamp across the lower supraceliac aorta from below (caudal) the celiac origin, if needed (see below under Technique). The celiac is not isolated if the target for bypass is the common hepatic artery.

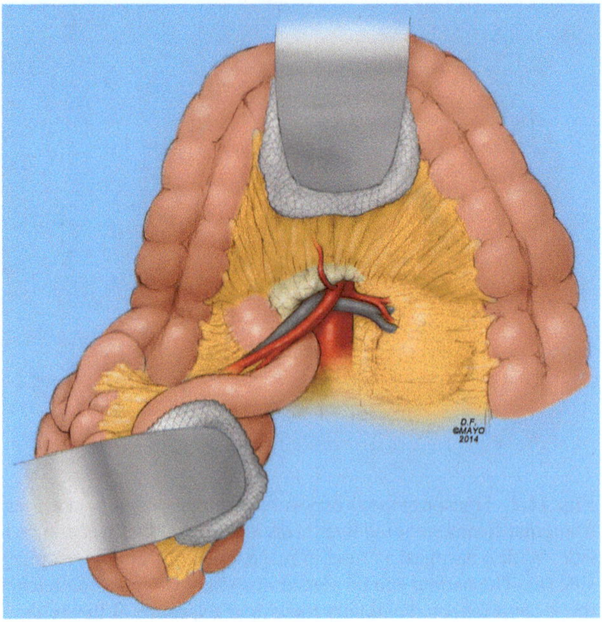

Fig. 11.3 The superior mesenteric artery is exposed at the base of the transverse mesocolon in most patients. The surgeon can palpate the artery running along the base of the small bowel mesentery. Dissection should be carried directly to the artery, which requires ligation and division of some overlying fibro-fatty tissues, lymphatics, and small veins. If there is extensive disease in the artery, the jejunal branches need to be isolated. There are some posterior branches which cause troublesome bleeding if injured (By permission of Mayo Foundation for Medical Education and Research. All rights reserved)

The superior mesenteric artery may be exposed above or below the pancreas, depending on patient anatomy and the extent of disease. If the artery is isolated above the pancreas, care must be taken not to disrupt the pancreatic capsule. This approach is reserved for rare patients whose disease is isolated to the origin of the artery. In most patients, it is safer to isolate the SMA near the base of the transverse mesocolon beyond the ligament of Treitz (Fig. 11.3). The transverse colon is retracted cephalad. The small bowel is retracted to the right side of the abdomen. The SMA can usually be palpated within the proximal mesentery. There are often lymphatic and fibro-fatty tissues along the proximal SMA which require meticulous ligation and division. Within several centimeters of the SMA origin, there are a number of jejunal branches which can be isolated with Silastic loops. Care must be taken not to injure a replaced right hepatic artery during this dissection should one be present. A patient with extensive atherosclerosis in the proximal SMA needs dissection to be carried further distally in the mesentery until a softer artery is palpated. Rare patients, who have had abdominal radiation years earlier, can have calcification of almost every branch artery. A retropancreatic tunnel is created between the supraceliac aorta and the infracolic SMA for patients having an antegrade two-vessel bypass. The tunnel is made by careful blunt dissection on top of the left renal vein and just along the left anterolateral aorta. The tunnel must be free of fibrous bands and of adequate size to accommodate the graft limb. Plasma tubing is placed through the tunnel.

A midline incision is used to isolate the infrarenal aorta or iliac arteries when retrograde bypass is planned. Retrograde bypass from the iliac artery or infrarenal

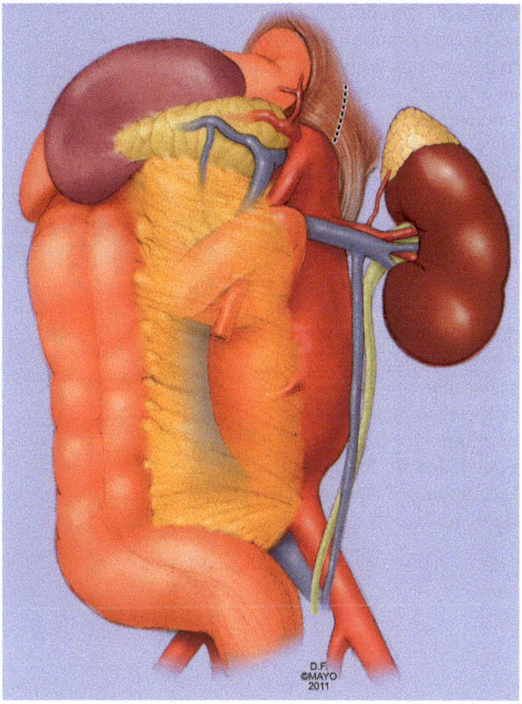

Fig. 11.4 A left medial visceral rotation is another approach to the celiac and superior mesenteric arteries, similar to the exposure used to treat patients with aneurysms which extend to the suprarenal level. This approach is useful for visceral artery endarterectomy and bypass in select patients. The left kidney is kept down. The crura of the diaphragm require division to gain access to the supraceliac aorta (By permission of Mayo Foundation for Medical Education and Research. All rights reserved)

aorta may be preferable in patients with diseased supraceliac aortas, those with compromised cardiac or pulmonary function, and in older patients. The retroperitoneal tissues are opened vertically to isolate the aorta and iliac arteries, similar to a transperitoneal infracolic exposure for open aortic aneurysm repair.

Transaortic visceral artery endarterectomy is an infrequent but a useful technique for good-risk patients with orificial disease, those who have concomitant symptomatic renal artery atherosclerotic stenoses, and in select patients with acute mesenteric ischemia who have peritoneal contamination. Midline, extended/bilateral subcostal, or thoraco-retroperitoneal incisions can be used to perform a medial visceral rotation for exposure of the paravisceral aorta and visceral arteries (Fig. 11.4). Choice of incision is based on body habitus, costal flare, and the location of the mesenteric artery origins relative to the inferior extent of the xiphoid process on sagittal CT imaging. The left kidney is kept down. Care is taken to avoid injury to the spleen and pancreas. The aorta is isolated from the supraceliac to the juxtarenal segment in most patients, as the aortotomy must be made from above the celiac artery origin to below (caudal) the SMA origin. In patients with a short distance between the SMA and renal origins, the upper infrarenal aorta requires isolation. The left crus is divided as part of the exposure. Phrenic or other side branches are ligated and divided. An occasional patient has small aortic branches near the celiac origin which cause pesky bleeding if injured. The celiac and SMA are circumferentially dissected free for 3 or 4 cm, a key step to allow for eversion endarterectomy.

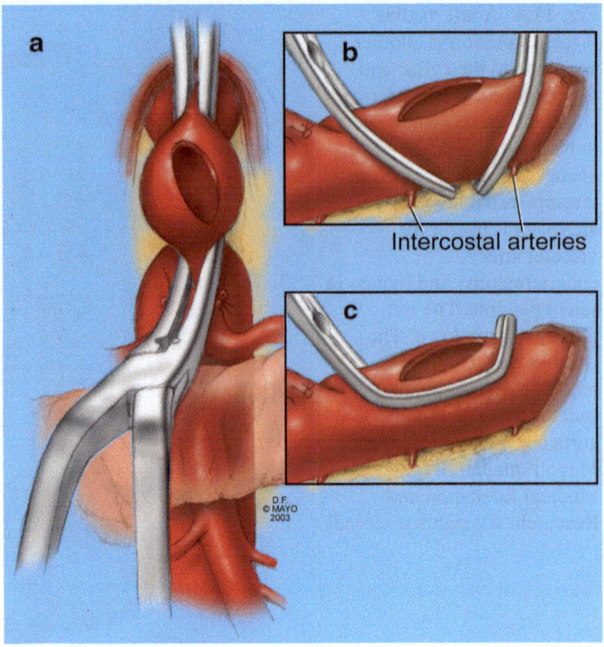

Fig. 11.5 A supraceliac-aortic based mesenteric bypass begins with making an elliptical aortotomy on the anterior wall of the aorta, often done obliquely (**a**). Some patients need double clamping of the aorta to perform the anastomosis as shown in **a** and **b**. Partial occlusion clamping is possible as shown in **c**, though the author prefers a deeper all-purpose clamp rather than the Satinsky clamp shown here (By permission of Mayo Foundation for Medical Education and Research. All rights reserved)

Technique

For antegrade reconstructions based on the supraceliac aorta, the patient is given intravenous heparin (50–100 units/kg) and 12.5 g of mannitol before aortic cross-clamping (Figs. 11.5 and 11.6). The aorta either can be fully or partially cross-clamped (Fig. 11.5). Complete aortic clamping may be needed in deep patients or those with plaque in the aorta. This is best facilitated with a straight or mildly angled aortic clamp for the proximal supraceliac aorta and a hypogastric clamp for the lower supraceliac aorta. In some patients, the latter clamp can be placed from behind the celiac artery origin. This is a useful maneuver for patients with a short length of supraceliac aorta below thc hiatus. This two-clamp technique allows a good view of the aortic lumen after aortotomy is made and occludes backbleeding from the lumbar arteries. Although partial aortic occlusion is preferred when possible, adequate visualization of the aortic lumen is necessary to perform the proximal anastomosis. Since this anastomosis can be done within 15 min or less in most patients, the risk of renal and lower extremity ischemia is lower than the risk of an imperfect anastomosis that requires revision. Moreover, the cardiac risk from increased afterload with complete aortic clamping should also be low with good anesthesia management. The latter requires close communication between surgeon and anesthesiologist. For these reasons, I do not hesitate to fully occlude the aorta. The author prefers an all-purpose aortic clamp to partially occlude the aorta. This clamp has deeper blades than other such clamps. Once the aorta is clamped and provided the hemodynamics remain stable, a slightly oblique aortotomy is made. A stay stitch can be

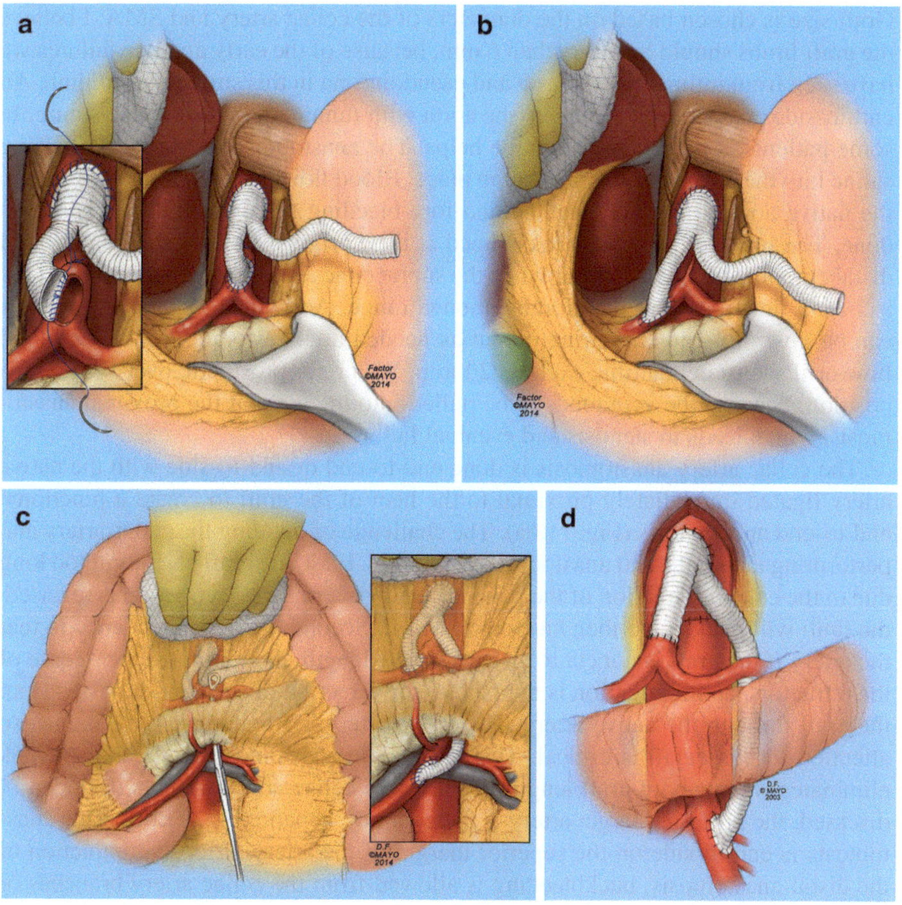

Fig. 11.6 The steps of performing a supraceliac-based reconstruction to the celiac and superior mesenteric arteries are illustrated. Once the aortic anastomosis is completed, a limb either is sewn to the celiac artery end-to-side with ligation of the artery immediately proximal to the anastomosis to create a functional end-to-end anastomosis (**a**) or can be carried to the common hepatic artery for patients who have diffused atherosclerotic disease or occlusion of the celiac artery (**b**). Once blood flow has been restored through the celiac system, the superior mesenteric artery graft limb is passed through a retropancreatic tunnel to where the SMS has been exposed. The graft is cut to length in an end-to-side anastomosis is completed (**c**). A schematic of the final position of the bifurcated graft is shown in (**d**) (By permission of Mayo Foundation for Medical Education and Research. All rights reserved)

placed in the aortic wall if it affords better exposure of the lumen and does not interfere with sewing. For patients with aortas of 16 mm or greater diameter, removing a sliver of aortic wall aids the view of the lumen and obviates the need for a stay stitch. If there is debris or loose plaque in the aorta, this needs to be removed to avoid distal embolization into the kidneys and/or extremities. Bypass in most patients is done with a 12×7 mm, 14×7 mm, or a 16×8 mm knitted polyester graft.

Graft size is chosen based on the diameters of the celiac artery and SMA. I believe the graft limbs should be larger than 6 mm, because of the early and late failures we have seen from intimal hyperplasia and pseudointima in this smaller-sized limb. An end-to-side anastomosis is done to the aorta with running polyproprolene suture. In some patients, a parachute technique helps. The anastomosis is tested by infusing saline into the graft with clamps still in place. Blood flow is restored slowly through the native aorta after backbleeding and fore-bleeding through the limbs has been done. The limbs of the graft are clamped at their origins. Acute kidney injury and distal embolization rarely occur when the supraceliac aorta is free of disease and the ischemia time is within the aforementioned range. Additional mannitol and Lasix can be given to stimulate urine output as needed after restoration of aortic blood flow or if the ischemia time exceeds 20 min. We prefer prosthetic over vein in this position, because the vein tends to be pulled into the aorta at the proximal anastomosis, which leads to stenosis and eventual failure.

The celiac artery anastomosis is done end-to-end or end-to-side with the native artery ligated immediately proximal to the heel of the graft to create a functional end-to-end anastomosis (Fig. 11.6a). The challenge of dividing the celiac artery and performing an end-to-end anastomosis is twofold. First, the graft can be cut too long due to the caudal retraction of the pancreas and viscera. Once retraction is released, the limb will buckle and then has to be revised. Second, there is a tendency to tear the artery if the graft is not cut to an appropriate length, there is not some release of the retractors, and if attention is not paid to the direction of suture as it passes from the graft through the native artery. The celiac artery is fragile in some patients, so attention to this detail is critical. The end-to-side anastomosis to the celiac trunk eliminates worry about graft length. If the entire celiac artery trunk is occluded or diseased, the preferred target artery is the common hepatic (Fig. 11.6b). This anastomosis is end-to-side on the superior margin of the artery. Prior to completion of the distal anastomosis, backbleeding is allowed from the celiac artery branches or hepatic artery with the distal graft limb clamped or compressed immediately proximal to the heel to keep the graft limb clean. Fore-bleeding is allowed through the SMA graft limb; it is flushed with saline and any blood and fibrin within it removed with suction. The SMA limb is clamped at its origin, and blood flow is established into the celiac artery branches.

A ringed forceps is clamped to the plasma tubing that had been placed through the tunnel during the exposure (Fig. 11.6c). With an assistant gently lifting up the transverse colon, the clamp is slowly guided to the supraceliac position by pulling on the plasma tubing with one hand and guiding the ringed forceps with the other hand. The SMA graft limb is placed into the forceps and passed through the tunnel to the infracolic position. The upper retractors on the liver and stomach are relaxed, and retraction is reset for exposure of the SMA anastomosis. This anastomosis is done in an end-to-side fashion with the arteriotomy often on the left lateral or anterolateral side of the artery. It is important to gently relax the small bowel to be certain the graft is cut to appropriate length. Patients with more extensive disease in the SMA trunk may require a focal endarterectomy and patch angioplasty before the distal anastomosis is done.

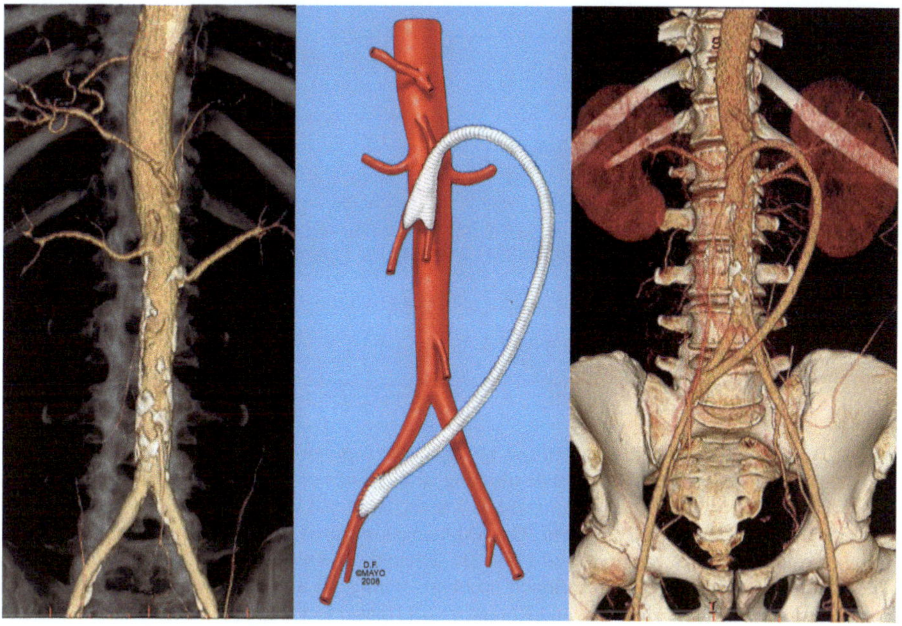

Fig. 11.7 High-risk patients who would not tolerate aortic clamping, and those with extensive calcification in a non-stenotic aorta, can be treated with a retrograde bypass from the iliac artery. Illustrated is a 3-D CT image of a high-risk patient with aortic calcification who was treated with a retrograde bypass in a C-shape configuration. The postoperative CT angiogram is shown on the right (By permission of Mayo Foundation for Medical Education and Research. All rights reserved)

Our group favors isolation of the common iliac arteries and less often the external iliacs for origin of retrograde bypasses (Fig. 11.7). Generally, a 7-mm or 8-mm polyester graft is used for the bypass, though PTFE and good-quality saphenous vein can also be chosen. Most patients have this graft taken to the SMA, either directly or in a C-shape as espoused by the Oregon Health Sciences University surgical group. Rarely, a two-vessel reconstruction is done to the SMA and common hepatic arteries. In this case, the graft is sewn side-to-side to the SMA, passed through either a retropancreatic tunnel or on top of the pancreas, gently curved, and then sewn end-to-side to the common hepatic artery. If the bypass is carried straight to the SMA, the iliac artery anastomosis is performed first, with both anastomoses done end-to-side. If a C-configuration is performed, either the proximal or distal anastomosis is done first based on surgeon preference. Origin of the graft from the right iliac artery is preferable, though the left iliac artery can be used as an inflow source if it is less diseased than the right one. The author's preference is to sew the distal anastomosis end-to-side of the SMA first, let the bowel relax, and then fill the graft with saline to properly position it in a C-shape. The graft is then cut to length, spatulated, and sewn end-to-side to the iliac artery. The advantage of the C-shape is that blood flow is antegrade vis-à-vis the SMA. If the infrarenal aorta is used for inflow, the challenge is to avoid buckling or kinking of the graft. Figure 11.8 shows

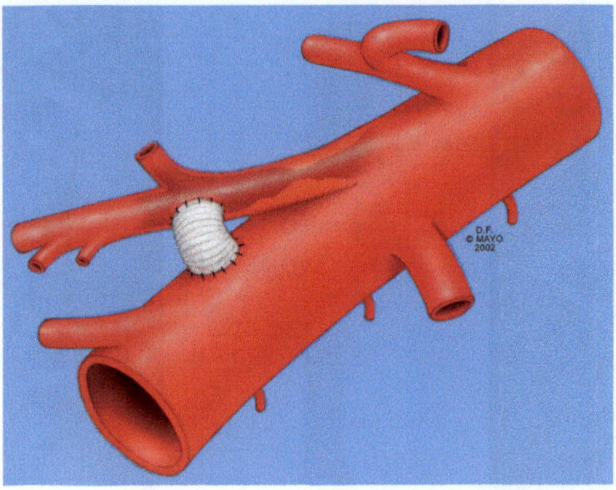

Fig. 11.8 The challenge with originating a bypass to the superior mesenteric artery from the infrarenal aorta is that the graft often is made too long, and it kinks or buckles when the small bowel is returned to its normal position. Illustrated is the technique of a short (stovepipe) bypass graft between the SMA and infrarenal aorta. The SMA anastomosis is done first. The bowel is relaxed, and the graft is cut short, no more than 1.5–2 cm in length, and sewn end-to-side to the aorta. This reconstruction avoids the aforementioned problems with graft kinking (By permission of Mayo Foundation for Medical Education and Research. All rights reserved)

a technique of placing a short infrarenal aorto-SMA bypass graft. This technique leaves a graft that is about 1.5–2-cm in length, like a short stovepipe hat. The advantage with this configuration is that it will not kink nor twist when the small bowel resumes its normal position.

Transaortic visceral artery endarterectomy requires full aortic clamping (Fig. 11.9). After intravenous heparin and mannitol are administered, the celiac and SMA are occluded with atraumatic clamps or Silastic loops, lumbar arteries are controlled with loops or bulldog clamps, and aortic clamps are placed distally below the SMA or renal arteries and on the supraceliac aorta. A trapdoor or curvilinear incision is made from the anterior wall of the supraceliac aorta, carried along the left lateral side of the aorta, and then turned anteriorly caudal to the SMA origin. A freer or spatula is used to develop a plane between the aortic wall and the occlusive plaque, similar to a carotid endarterectomy. The intra-aortic plaque is freed circumferentially around the orifices of the celiac and SMA. Eversion endarterectomy is done on each mesenteric artery. The aortotomy is closed with running 4–0 polypropylene suture. Backbleeding and fore-bleeding are allowed before restoration of blood flow. In the rare patient who needs concomitant endarterectomy of the renals and/or aortic reconstruction, the initial aortotomy is carried anteriorly below the SMA and renal arteries. Once the endarterectomy is completed and the aortotomy is closed below the renals, blood flow is reestablished. If aortic reconstruction is needed, a padded aortic clamp is placed across the aorta and suture line below the renals once the aortotomy is closed to that level. In any of these latter situations, diuresis is induced with a bolus of mannitol (12.5 g) and Lasix (20, 40, or 60 mg), with the Lasix dose based on ischemia time and the presence of chronic kidney disease. Some patients

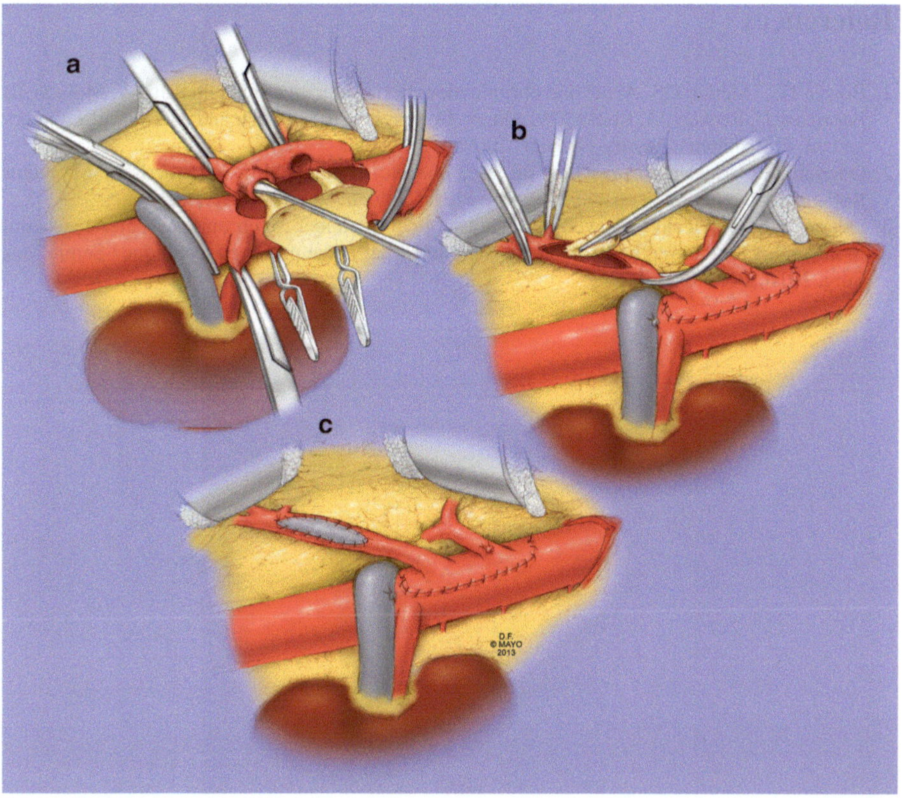

Fig. 11.9 Transaortic visceral artery endarterectomy and completion superior mesenteric endarterectomy. Exposure is done via a left medial visceral rotation leaving the kidney down. This can be done through a midline or bilateral subcostal incision. The aorta and visceral arteries are clamped as shown in **a**. In some patients, the renal arteries require temporary occlusion to perform the operation. A trapdoor incision is made, beginning above the celiac artery, carried along the anterolateral wall of the aorta to below the visceral artery origins, and then curved to the anterior aorta. Endarterectomy is done via an eversion technique. Patients with disease extending for 2–3 cm into the SMA require completion endarterectomy and patch angioplasty as shown in **b** and **c** (By permission of Mayo Foundation for Medical Education and Research. All rights reserved)

have a tongue of plaque that extends beyond the first 2 cm of the SMA and cannot be easily removed. A completion endarterectomy of the SMA is done after the aorta is closed. This is accomplished via a transverse or longitudinal arteriotomy. Once the plaque is removed, the artery is closed primarily or with a patch.

After completion of any mesenteric reconstruction, intraoperative duplex imaging is used to be certain the arteries, graft, and anastomoses are widely patent and there are normal blood flow velocities. Imaging should be done with the bowel relaxed to alleviate any stretch on the celiac or SMA trunk. Any technical abnormalities are corrected in the operating room. It is important to assure the graft is covered to avoid contact with the bowel, and omentum works well.

References

1. Bower TC, Oderich GS. Acute and chronic mesenteric ischemia. In: Hallett Jr JW, Mills Sr JL, Earnshaw JJ, Reekers JA, Rooke TW, editors. Comprehensive vascular and endovascular surgery. 2nd ed. Philadelphia: Mosby Elsevier; 2009. p. 339–50.
2. Oderich GS. Mesenteric vascular disease: chronic ischemia. In: Schermerhorn M, editor. Rutherford's textbook of vascular surgery. 8th ed. Philadelphia: Elsevier; 2013.
3. Oderich GS, Gloviczki P, Bower TC. Open surgical treatment for chronic mesenteric ischemia in the endovascular era: when it is necessary and what is the preferred technique? Semin Vasc Surg. 2010;23(1):36–46.

Chapter 12
Results of Open Mesenteric Reconstructions

Thomas C. Bower

Chronic mesenteric ischemia (CMI) is most often associated with atherosclerosis affecting at least two of the three mesenteric arteries. Rarer causes include vasculitis, fibromuscular dysplasia, neurofibromatosis, dissection, trauma, embolization, and distal thoracic or abdominal aortic coarctation. Treatment goals are to relieve symptoms, restore normal weight, and prevent bowel infarction. Mesenteric revascularization is indicated for symptomatic patients and is rarely undertaken prophylactically, because the risk of bowel ischemia is low in the absence of symptoms. Mesenteric revascularization sometimes is necessary during concomitant aortic-based procedures in patients with asymptomatic high-grade three-vessel mesenteric artery disease [1, 2]. Symptomatic patients are best treated without much delay, since 43 % of patients who develop acute mesenteric ischemia have preexisting symptoms of chronic ischemia [3].

Open revascularization has been the time-honored treatment and provides immediate relief of symptoms in most patients. Mesenteric angioplasty and stenting first emerged as an alternative to surgical bypass in the elderly or higher-risk patient. Now, endovascular therapy is the primary treatment modality in most patients with anatomically suitable lesions, independent of their surgical risk. Mesenteric bypass continues to have an important role in the treatment of CMI in the endovascular era. This chapter summarizes contemporary outcomes of open mesenteric revascularization in patients treated for CMI caused by atherosclerosis.

T.C. Bower, MD (✉)
Division of Vascular and Endovascular Surgery, Department of Surgery, Mayo Clinic, Rochester, MN, USA
e-mail: bower.thomas@mayo.edu

G.S. Oderich (ed.), *Mesenteric Vascular Disease*,
DOI 10.1007/978-1-4939-1847-8_12

Outcomes

Patient outcome after open mesenteric artery reconstruction depends on anatomic factors, patient-specific risk, surgeon experience, and perioperative management. Anatomically, the key issues are the extent of disease in the native arteries, size of the target arteries, associated aneurysmal or symptomatic aortic disease, and source of inflow. Age, cardiac, pulmonary, liver and renal function, and the physical and nutritional status of the patient affect the choice of operation and influence the ability of the patient to tolerate the stress of surgery. Since these operations are infrequently performed compared to other open surgical procedures, operator experience matters. Most patients do well if the operation is planned and executed well. Some patients experience an inflammatory response to revascularization and may have significant fluid shifts the first 48 postoperative hours because of the loss of mesenteric arteriolar autoregulation. Meticulous care early after operation is critical to outcome, and close monitoring of the intravascular volume, cardiac function, and acid–base status is imperative [4].

Important lessons have been learned over the last 20 years in the surgical management of these patients [1–20]. First, tailor the operation to what the anatomy and patient risk allow. Not every patient needs complete revascularization or a supraceliac aortic-based bypass. While low mortality rates are achieved at high-volume centers, mortality as high as 13–20 % is reported in the community [4, 5, 20]. Second, avoid concomitant aortic reconstruction unless absolutely needed for inflow. Operative mortality is reported as high as 8–10 % by experienced groups when the primary indication for operation is chronic mesenteric ischemia but when mesenteric revascularization is combined with aortic replacement [1, 2, 6]. In contrast to prior years, patients with diffuse aortoiliac disease precluding inflow can now be offered hybrid retrograde mesenteric revascularization [7, 8]. Isolated open surgical bypass can be performed with low mortality in good-risk patients operated at institutions with a wealth of experience in these types of reconstructions, even with redo open procedures [6, 9–17]. The Mayo Clinic group used the SVS comorbidity scoring system in 229 patients treated for CMI with open and endovascular procedures to risk stratify patients. Outcomes were assessed by whether a patient was deemed high or low risk. The overall mortality was similar for the open (2.7 %) and endovascular (2.4 %) revascularization groups. Mortality was 1 % for low-risk and 6.7 % for high-risk patients treated by open bypass, with the highest mortality encountered in patients who had concomitant aortic reconstruction (8.9 %) [6].

Even in experienced hands, the risk of perioperative complications can be high. Complication rates after open mesenteric revascularization average 20 % to 40 % [1, 2, 4–6, 9–17]. In the last report from the Mayo Clinic group, the incidence of any complication was 36 %. The most common problems were pulmonary (15 %), gastrointestinal (14 %), cardiac (10 %), and renal (4 %). Prolonged ileus occurs in 8 % of patients, and many are malnourished and/or have vitamin and trace element deficiencies. Perioperative nutritional support is often needed [6]. Meticulous wound closure is important because the risk of wound-related complications ranges between 4 % and 8 % [4]. Moreover, ascites is a risk early after operation because the bowel weeps fluid, which highlights the importance of meticulous abdominal wall closure. Rarely, compartment syndrome from severe ascites requires abdominal decompression, though this problem is more likely to occur in the patient with subacute on chronic mesenteric ischemia [4, 6]. High index of clinical suspicion is needed to detect early graft occlusion or intestinal ischemia. These latter two problems manifest with an increase in fluid volume requirements and a drop in urine output, thrombocytopenia and/or leukocytosis, a narrowing of the A–aO2 gradient and/or pulse pressure, and metabolic acidosis which may be subtle at first. Early graft thrombosis is uncommon (<2 %) and may lead to intestinal ischemia, infarction, or death of the patient. Early graft failure is usually due to a technical problem and can be minimized by completion intraoperative duplex imaging of the reconstruction. The routine use of ultrasound imaging of the completed reconstruction has reduced our early graft failure rate to less than 1 % [21]. Other causes of early graft thrombosis include poor runoff or a hypercoagulable state [4, 6]. Open operations carry higher morbidity and longer hospital stays and recovery times compared to endovascular therapy based on single-center reports and a systematic review (Table 12.1) [19]. Morbidity and length of stay average 11 % and 3 days with endovascular, compared to 33 % and 14 days with open surgery [19].

Postoperative medical therapy should include smoking cessation and antiplatelets and cholesterol-lowering agents. Patients may develop diarrhea after surgery because the absorptive capacity of the gut changes, and for some individuals, the diarrhea lasts weeks and can be problematic. Surveillance imaging with duplex ultrasound is done every six months during the first year and annually thereafter [4].

Symptom Relief, Recurrent Symptoms, and Re-intervention

Outcomes of mesenteric revascularization should include analysis of mortality, morbidity, symptom relief, and freedom from restenosis, recurrence, and re-intervention. There needs to be reporting standards, stratification of patient risk, and methods to compare anatomic severity of disease if comparisons of open and endovascular treatment are to have meaning. Currently, interpretation of data and comparison of outcomes between published reports is difficult for several reasons [6]. Studies often mix patients with acute and chronic presentations, including median arcuate ligament syndrome, and cover a long period of time; reports vary in the definition of technical success; analyses lack time-dependent outcomes such as patency rates, symptom recurrence, restenosis, and re-intervention; patient follow up is limited; and there is no consistent objective determination of patency.

Open revascularization provides excellent symptom relief and better durability than endovascular treatment. In a systematic review, symptom improvement averaged 93 % with open and 88 % with endovascular revascularization [18]. Most single-center reports and a systematic review suggest that bypass is associated with lower rates of restenosis, better patency, and higher freedom from recurrent symptoms or re-interventions compared to mesenteric angioplasty and stenting.

Table 12.1 Patient outcome after open mesenteric artery reconstruction

Author (year)	*n*	Vessels	Mortality	Morbidity	Recurrence	Re-intervention	Primary patency	Follow-up (months)
			%					
Leke (2002)	17	25	6	41	0	0	100 at 34 months	34
Cho (2002)	25	41	4	–	32	20	57 at 5 years	64
Brown (2005)	33	51	9	30	9	7	100 at 6 months	34
Sivamurthy (2006)	46	66	15	46	32	12	83 at 6 months	9
Biebl (2007)	26	48	8	42	11	8	–	25
Kruger (2007)	39	67	2.5	12	5	3	92 at 5 years	39
Atkins (2007)	49	88	2	4	22	22	90	42
Mell (2008)	80	120	3.8	26	11	11	90	46
Oderich (2009)	146	265	2.7	36	6	5	88 at 5 years	36
Low risk	101	–	0.9	37	6	6	94 at 5 years	–
High risk	45	–	6.7	38	11	11	90 at 5 years	–
Concomitant aortic reconstruction	23	–	8.4	–	–	–	–	–
Rawat (2010)	52	75	13	32	15	13	81	41
Ryer (2012)	116	203	2.5	50	14	16	86 at 5 years	43
Total	629	1049	6.3	32	14	11	–	38

Primary patency of open bypass averaged 89 % at 5 years in a recent review of the pooled literature (57 % to 92 %), with freedom from re-intervention in 93 % [20]. The systematic review by van Petersen et al. [19] showed open surgery to have better primary (86 % versus 51 %) and secondary patency rates (87 % versus 83 %), lower restenosis (15 % versus 37 %), less symptom recurrence (13 % versus 30 %), and fewer re-interventions (9 % versus 20 %) than endovascular intervention., respectively. Nonetheless, endovascular therapy is now the first option for treatment of atherosclerotic mesenteric artery stenoses at most centers, with stenting preferred because of its better patency. A contemporary report by Ryer and colleagues [15] indicated that open bypass is increasingly performed in patients with more comorbidities and worse anatomy than those treated with endovascular techniques. Despite this evolution toward more difficult reconstructions, open surgery had a respectable primary patency rate of 76 % at 5 years.

Reoperation for Failed Open Mesenteric Reconstructions

Redo open reconstruction may be needed in the patient who presents with chronic graft occlusions, recent graft occlusion with acute mesenteric ischemia, and in those who are not candidates for endovascular therapy to treat a failed or failing graft . In these patients, hybrid retrograde stenting or an iliac artery-based reconstruction should be considered [7, 8, 22, 23]. Reoperation is technically more challenging because of intra-abdominal and periarterial scar tissue and more extensive disease in the target artery which requires more distal isolation and because of the risk of damage to important collaterals during the operative dissection to isolate the artery. Giswold and associates [24] reported operative mortality of 6 % and primary patency at 4 years of 62 % among 22 patients who underwent redo mesenteric revascularization. In the rare patient with an inadequate source of inflow from the abdominal aorta or iliac arteries, mesenteric bypass can be originated from the thoracic or ascending aorta [22, 25, 26].

Patient Survival

Poor prognostic indicators for long-term patient survival after mesenteric revascularization include advanced age and severe cardiac, pulmonary, or renal disease [6]. The type of revascularization has not been shown to affect survival, but comparative analysis is limited by selection bias favoring open bypass for good-risk patients and endovascular revascularization for higher-risk ones. Tallarita and associates [27] reported long-term survival in a cohort of 343 patients treated for CMI, with nearly identical 5-year survival rates using propensity-matched scores for patients treated by open (57 %) or endovascular (60 %) techniques [27]. Five-year patient survival averaged 71 ± 4 % for low-risk, 49 ± 6 % for intermediate-risk, and 38 ± 7 % for high-risk patients. Freedom from mesenteric-related death was 91 ± 2 % after open and 93 ± 4 % after endovascular revascularization at 5 years. Independent predictors for any cause mortality were age >80 years (OR 3.3, CI 1.03–1.06, p=<0.001), chronic kidney disease stage IV or V (OR 5.5, CI 1.4–16.6, $p<0.01$), diabetes (OR 1.7, CI 1.2–2.6, $p<0.01$), and home oxygen therapy (OR 3.7, CI 1.2–9.1, $p<0.001$). Stage IV or V chronic kidney disease (OR 3.4, CI 3.3–345, $p=0.003$) and diabetes (OR 4.2, CI 1.7–10.5, $p=0.005$) were independently associated with mesenteric-related death. In this study, the most common causes of late death in decreasing order of frequency were cardiac events, cancer, respiratory complications, and mesenteric-related complications. The combined rate of early and late mesenteric-related death was 8 % for patients treated by open reconstruction and 6 % for those who had endovascular revascularization [27].

Summary

Our management of patients with CMI has evolved over the years. Currently over 70 % of the patients are treated with mesenteric angioplasty and stent placement. This option is preferred in the high-risk group and is also considered in low-risk patients with ideally suited lesions. Open mesenteric revascularization continues to have an important role in the endovascular era. Surgical bypass or, rarely, endarterectomy may be required because of unfavorable anatomy (flush or extensive occlusions, severe calcification, tandem lesions, small-sized vessels, or occluded stents) and younger patients with non-atherosclerotic lesions. Recent reports have shown that mesenteric bypass can be done safely in the hands of experienced surgeons with mortality rates that compare favorably to endovascular treatment. Open revascularization should focus on mesenteric artery revascularization as the primary goal and should avoid, if possible, extensive aortic or renal artery reconstruction. Anatomically, low-risk patients with flush or long-segment occlusions or stenosis, heavily calcified lesions, or atheromatous debris may be better suited for open repair. Young patients or women with small vessels may also be better candidates for open repair. Our preference in these patients has been a supra-celiac aorta to celiac and SMA bypass.

References

1. Hollier LH, Bernatz PE, Pairolero PC, Payne WS, Osmundson PJ. Surgical management of chronic intestinal ischemia: a reappraisal. Surgery. 1981;90(6):940–6.
2. McAfee MK, Cherry KJ, Naessens JM, et al. Influence of complete revascularization on chronic mesenteric ischemia. Am J Surg. 1992;164:220–4.
3. Ryer EJ, et al. Revascularization for acute for acute mesenteric ischemia. J Vasc Surg. 2012;55:1682–9.
4. Bower TC, Oderich GS. Acute and chronic mesenteric ischemia. In: Shermerhorn M, editor. Rutherford's textbook of vascular surgery. 8th ed. Philadelphia: Elsevier; 2013.

5. Schermerhorn ML, Giles KA, Hamdan AD, Wyers MC, Pomoselli FB. Mesenteric revascularization: management and outcomes in the United States, 1988–2006. J Vasc Surg. 2009;50:341–8.
6. Oderich GS, Bower TC, Sullivan TM, Bjarnason H, Cha S, Gloviczki P. Open versus endovascular revascularization for chronic mesenteric ischemia: risk-stratified outcomes. J Vasc Surg. 2009;49:1472–9.
7. Wyers MC, Powell RJ, Nolan BW, Cronenwett JL. Retrograde mesenteric stenting during laparotomy for acute occlusive mesenteric ischemia. J Vasc Surg. 2007;45:269–75.
8. Milner R, et al. Superior mesenteric artery angioplasty and stenting via a retrograde approach in a patient with bowel ischemia – a case report. Vasc Endovasc Surg. 2004;38:89–111.
9. Park WM, Cherry Jr KJ, Chua HK, Clark RC, Jenkins G, Harmsen WS, et al. Current results of open revascularization for chronic mesenteric ischemia: a standard for comparison. J Vasc Surg. 2002;35(5):853–9.
10. Kasirajan K, O'Hara PJ, Gray BH, Hertzer NR, Clair DG, Greenberg RK, et al. Chronic mesenteric ischemia: open surgery versus percutaneous angioplasty and stenting. J Vasc Surg. 2001;33(1):63–71.
11. Cho JS, Carr JA, Jacobsen G, Shepard AD, Nypaver TJ, Reddy DJ. Long-term outcome after mesenteric artery reconstruction: a 37-year experience. J Vasc Surg. 2002;35(3):453–60.
12. Illuminati G, Calio FG, D'Urso A, Papaspiropoulos V, Mancini P, Ceccanei G. The surgical treatment of chronic mesenteric ischemia: results of a recent series. Acta Chir Belg. 2004;104(2):175–83.
13. Kruger AJ, Walker PJ, Foster WJ, Jenkins JS, Boyne NS, Jenkins J. Open surgery for chronic atherosclerosis mesenteric ischemia. J Vasc Surg. 2007;46:941–5.
14. Atkins MD, Kwolek CJ, LaMuraglia GM, Brewster DC, Chung TK, Cambria RP. Surgical revascularization versus endovascular therapy for chronic mesenteric ischemia: a comparative experience. J Vasc Surg. 2007;45(6):1162–71.
15. Ryer EJ, et al. Differences in anatomy and outcomes in patients treated with open mesenteric revascularization before and after the endovascular era. J Vasc Surg. 2011;53:1611–8. e2.
16. Leke MA, Hood DB, Rowe VL, Katz SG, Kohl RD, Weaver FA. Technical consideration in the management of chronic mesenteric ischemia. Am Surg. 2002;68(12):1088–92.
17. Mell MW, Acher CW, Hoch JR, Tefera G, Turnipseed WD. Outcomes after endarterectomy for chronic mesenteric ischemia. J Vasc Surg. 2008;48:1132–8.
18. Gupta PK, et al. Chronic mesenteric ischemia: endovascular versus open revascularization. J Endovasc Ther. 2010;17:540–9.
19. van Petersen AS, et al. Open or percutaneous revascularization for chronic splanchnic syndrome. J Vasc Surg. 2010;51:1309–16.
20. Oderich GS, Malgor R, Ricotta II JJ. Open and endovascular revascularization for chronic mesenteric ischemia: a tabular review of the literature. Ann Vasc Surg. 2009;23(5):700–12.
21. Oderich GS, Panneton JM, Macedo TA, Noel AA, Bower TC, Lee RA, et al. Intraoperative duplex ultrasound of visceral revascularizations: optimizing technical success and outcomes. J Vasc Surg. 2003;38:684–91.
22. Foley JI, Moneta GL, Abou-Zamsam AM, et al. Revascularization of the superior mesenteric artery alone for treatment of intestinal ischemia. J Vasc Surg. 2000;32:37–47.
23. Taylor LM, Moneta GL, Porter JM. Treatment of chronic visceral ischemia. In: Rutherford RB, editor. Vascular Surgery. 5th ed. Philadelphia: WB Saunders; 2000. p. 1532–41.
24. Giswold ME, et al. Outcomes after redo procedures for failed mesenteric revascularization. Vasc Endovas Surg. 2004;38:315–9.
25. Farber MA, et al. Distal thoracic aorta as inflow for the treatment of chronic mesenteric ischemia. J Vasc Surg. 2001;33:281–7; discussion 287–8.
26. Chiche L, et al. Use of the ascending aorta as bypass inflow for treatment of chronic intestinal ischemia. J Vasc Surg. 2005;41:457–61.
27. Tallarita T, et al. Patient survival after open and endovascular mesenteric revascularization for chronic mesenteric ischemia. J Vasc Surg. 2013;57:747–55.

Chapter 13
Techniques of Endovascular Mesenteric Revascularization

Gustavo S. Oderich and Leonardo Reis de Souza

The most common cause of chronic mesenteric ischemia (CMI) is atherosclerotic disease, accounting for over 90 % of cases in most series. Atherosclerotic lesions usually affect the origin or the proximal 2–3 cm of the mesenteric arteries, frequently with associated plaque in the aorta and renal arteries. Because of the extensive collateral network, the majority of patients with symptoms of CMI have significant stenosis or occlusion of at least two of the three mesenteric arteries. However, contrary to what has been propagated in many surgical textbooks, this is not an absolute requirement [1, 2]. The clinical significance of ischemia correlates not only to the extent of disease but also the adequacy of collateral pathways, acuteness of symptoms, and presence of arterial steal; approximately 2–10 % of patients with CMI have single-vessel disease, which affects primarily the SMA and patients with poorly developed collaterals or more acute presentation, as might be predicted from the postprandial hyperemic response [3].

Despite the lack of prospective randomized comparisons between open surgery and endovascular treatment, mesenteric angioplasty and stenting has been widely adopted in most centers, resulting in a decline in the number of open surgical reconstructions. Currently, open surgery is relegated to patients who are not suitable candidates for endovascular therapy or who failed treatment. Based on systematic reviews, endovascular revascularization has been associated with decreased morbidity, length of stay, and convalescence time. Mortality rates are similar with an average 30-day mortality of 6 %

G.S. Oderich, MD, FACS (✉)
Division of Vascular and Endovascular Surgery, Mayo Clinic, Rochester, MN, USA

Gonda Vascular Center, Mayo Clinic, Rochester, MN, USA
e-mail: oderich.gustavo@mayo.edu

L.R. de Souza, MD
Division of Vascular and Endovascular Surgery, Mayo Clinic, Rochester, MN, USA

Masters Degree Program from the Department of Surgery,
Universidade Federal do Rio Grande do Sul, Porto Alegre, Brazil
e-mail: reissouza@gmail.com

G.S. Oderich (ed.), *Mesenteric Vascular Disease*,
DOI 10.1007/978-1-4939-1847-8_13

(0–15 %) for open and 5 % (0–21 %) for endovascular revascularization [4]. Because the selection of type of treatment is dependent on physician's preference and the patient's comorbidities, results of the two techniques may not be comparable unless outcomes are analyzed using clinical risk stratification. This chapter summarizes the indications and techniques of endovascular revascularization for chronic mesenteric disease.

Indications

There is no role for a conservative approach with chronic parenteral nutrition and non-interventional therapy in patients with symptomatic mesenteric artery disease. Excessive delays in proceeding with definitive revascularization or use of parenteral nutrition alone have been associated with clinical deterioration, bowel infarction, and risk of sepsis from catheter-related complications [5, 6].

Revascularization is indicated in all patients with symptoms of symptoms of mesenteric artery occlusive disease, acute or chronic. Treatment goals are to relieve symptoms, restore normal weight, and prevent bowel infarction. The indication of prophylactic revascularization in patients with asymptomatic disease remains controversial. Based on the report by Thomas and colleagues, there may be a role for prophylactic revascularization in patients with severe three-vessel disease, particularly for those with difficult access to medical care who live in remote or underserved areas [7]. Our approach in these patients has been close surveillance and counseling regarding symptoms of mesenteric ischemia, with a low threshold to proceed with revascularization if any gastrointestinal symptoms (e.g., bloating, diarrhea, atypical pain) arise. Revascularization has been advised in asymptomatic patients with severe three-vessel disease undergoing aortic reconstructions for other indication.

Choice of Open Versus Endovascular Revascularization

Treatment selection has evolved in most centers. The number of mesenteric revascularizations has increased tenfold in the United States in the last decade, largely because of improved diagnosis and decreased morbidity of endovascular therapy (Fig. 13.1). In most centers, angioplasty and stenting surpassed open bypass as the first option and is currently utilized in over 70–80 % of the patients treated for CMI [3, 8, 9]. These changes in treatment paradigm have occurred despite the lack of prospective randomized comparisons between the two techniques. Endovascular revascularization has been associated with decreased morbidity, length of stay, and convalescence time, but similar mortality compared to open repair [3, 4]. Mesenteric bypass offers improved patency, with lower rates of re-interventions and better freedom from recurrent symptoms [3, 4, 9–20].

In most centers, including ours, mesenteric angioplasty and stenting is currently the first choice of treatment in patients with CMI who have suitable lesions, independent

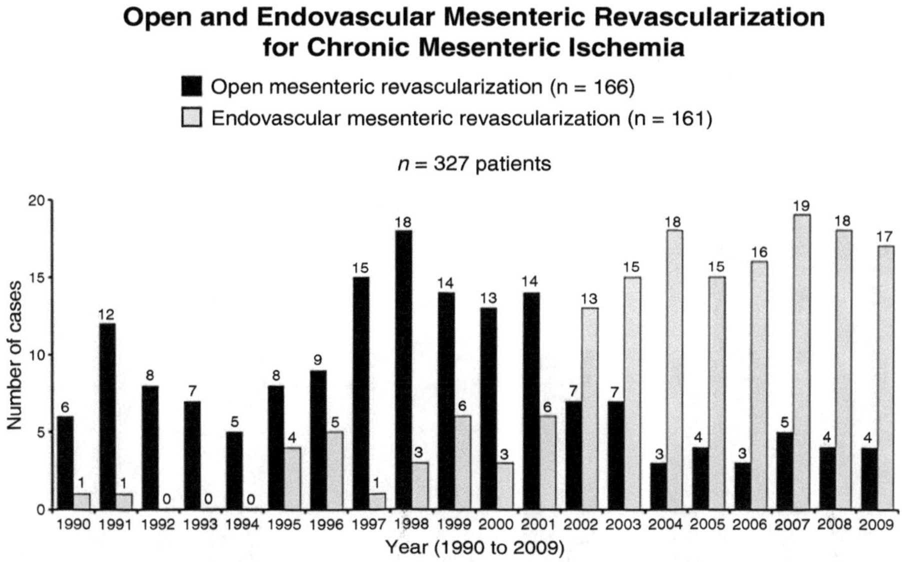

Fig. 13.1 Treatment trends in patients with chronic mesenteric ischemia treated by open or endovascular revascularization at the Mayo Clinic

of their clinical risk. A careful review of pre-procedure CTA with attention to anatomical factors determines selection of open or endovascular approach. The SMA is the primary target for revascularization, and as such the anatomy of the SMA is the most important determinant of choice of therapy. The ideal lesion for angioplasty and stenting is a short, focal stenosis or occlusion with minimal to moderate calcification or thrombus (Fig. 13.2). For celiac axis (CA) lesions, angioplasty and stenting carries higher rates of restenosis [21], and should not be performed if there is active compression by the median arcuate ligament, unless this has been surgically released. We found no benefit for two-vessel stenting [21]. The technical difficulty of endovascular procedures is increased by presence of severe eccentric calcification, flush occlusion, and in patients with longer lesions, small vessels, and tandem lesions affecting branches. Although these anatomical features do not contraindicate the use of stents, technical result is often not optimal with higher rates of arterial complications (e.g., distal embolization, dissection) and restenosis [22, 23]. Our preference in lower-risk group has been to offer open revascularization if the anatomy is unfavorable for angioplasty and stenting [24, 25]. Mesenteric bypass has also been increasingly performed in patients who have failed a percutaneous intervention or in those with multiple recurrences or other non-atherosclerotic lesions, such as vasculitides and neurofibromatosis. Finally, for patients who are not good candidates for open repair because of severe comorbidities or cachexia, stenting can be used as a "bridge" to open surgical bypass, or endovascular recanalization can be attempted to treat complex lesions.

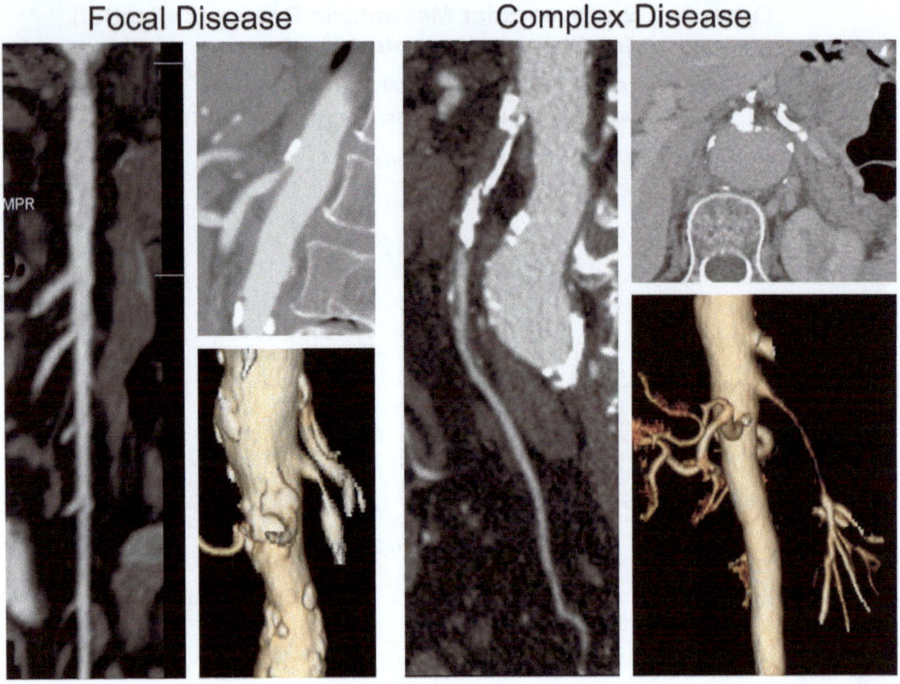

Fig. 13.2 Computed tomography angiography is the most useful imaging study to plan revascularization. Anatomical characteristics of the superior mesenteric artery (SMA) can be used to identify patients with focal disease where angioplasty and stenting is favored or patients with complex disease where endovascular therapy is technically more challenging. Lesions with unfavorable anatomy for stenting include heavily calcified occlusions, long-segment occlusions, and long-segment stenosis involving multiple branches

Pre-procedure Evaluation

Endovascular mesenteric revascularization carries definitive risk. The average 30-day mortality in a recent systematic review was 6 % (0–21 %), surpassing the mortality reported for other types of endovascular interventions, including aortic, renal, and carotid procedures. Even though most interventions are done using local anesthesia, these patients typically undergo a comprehensive medical evaluation to identify and optimize cardiovascular risk factors and their nutritional status. Many of the comorbidities may require medical therapy to be started prior or after the intervention, depending on its severity. Revascularization should not be excessively delayed. Patients who present with deterioration of symptoms should be admitted, started on intravenous heparin, and treated urgently within 24–48 h. Patients with iodinated contrast allergy should be premedicated with steroid preparation. Those with chronic kidney disease who have serum creatinine level >1.5–2.0 mg/dL (133–177 Mmol/L) undergo intravenous hydration with sodium bicarbonate and oral acetylcysteine, starting the day prior to intervention. Review of pre-procedure imaging (CTA, MRA, or conventional angiography) is key to select the ideal approach based on the angle of origin of the mesenteric vessels in relation to the aortic axis, the amount of calcium and thrombus load, and the presence of important collaterals or unusual anatomy (e.g., replaced hepatic) in proximity to the target lesion.

Selection of Access Site

The choice of ideal access is dependent on vessel anatomy, extent of occlusive disease, angle of origin from the aorta, and physician preference. The advantages of femoral approach include the frequent use and familiarity, ability to use shorter delivery system, and most importantly the exceedingly low rate of access site complications. However, because the CA and superior mesenteric artery (SMA) have acute angle of origin from the aorta, mesenteric interventions can be difficult to perform via the femoral approach. Excessive angulation often results in added time and radiation exposure, multiple guidewire exchanges, and in some cases, treatment failure.

Therefore, the ideal approach remains controversial. The author's preference is to use the left brachial artery access with a small 1–2 cm incision to surgically expose the artery. This is done under local anesthesia. Brachial access is particularly beneficial in the patient with difficult anatomy, such as those with flush occlusions, acute aortic angles, or long-segment lesions affected by very high-grade stenosis. Although the use of brachial access has been associated with higher rate of local complications when done totally percutaneously, it may reduce rate of severe mesenteric artery complications including dissections, vessel perforations, and embolization. Finally, we have increasingly utilized the radial artery access, but this is limited by need for longer delivery system and smaller profile sheath and devices.

Diagnostic Mesenteric Angiography

Diagnostic angiography has been discussed in detail in Chap. 2 (Fig. 13.3). Diagnostic angiography is most often done immediately prior to a planned intervention, either through the femoral or brachial approach. Access is established using ultrasound guidance and 0.035 in guidewire system. A 5 Fr sheath is positioned in the external iliac artery, and 5 Fr diagnostic flush catheter is advanced to T12 level over a 0.035 in guidewire. Modest intravenous heparinization (40 units/kg) is recommended prior to selective catheterization of the mesenteric arteries. Low-osmolar contrast agent (e.g., Visipaque®) minimizes abdominal discomfort during selective injections. Choice of catheter shape is dependent upon access site, angle of origin, and individual preference. MPA catheter is ideal for selective catheterization via brachial approach, whereas a secondary curve catheter (e.g., SOS or Simmons) or a catheter with more acute curve (e.g., Cobra 2) can be used for interventions done via femoral approach (Fig. 13.4). A complete study includes abdominal aortogram with anterior-posterior and lateral views to define the location, severity, and extent of visceral artery involvement and to identify concomitant lesions in the aorta, renal,

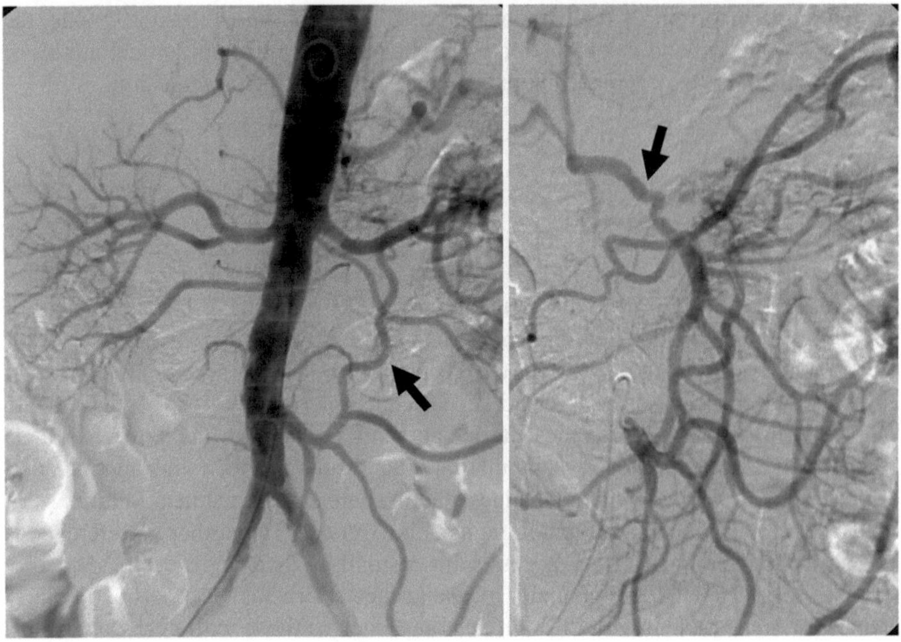

Fig. 13.3 Abdominal aortogram with right anterior-oblique view demonstrates large patent inferior mesenteric artery (IMA). Selective IMA angiography confirms collateralization to the superior mesenteric artery via arc of Riolan (*arrow*) and collateralization to the celiac axis via gastroduodenal artery (*arrow*)

or iliac arteries. The optimal projection to display the proximal CA and SMA is a lateral view, and for the origin of the IMA, it is a 15° right lateral-oblique view. Selective angiography is necessary to confirm the severity of disease and to identify tandem lesions and collateral patterns. In patients with questionable lesions, pressure gradients can be measured using pressure wire, "pull-back," or simultaneous pressure measurement technique [26].

Selective Catheterization

Selective catheterization requires systemic heparinization (80 mg/kg), which should be administered prior to catheter manipulations in order to achieve an activated clotting time over 250 s. Using the brachial artery access, a 6 or 7 Fr 90 cm hydrophilic sheath is positioned in the descending thoracic aorta above the CA origin. A 5 Fr MPA catheter is ideal for selective catheterization of the mesenteric arteries using the brachial approach, whereas a SOS or VS1 catheter can be used from the femoral approach. The initial selective angiography should demonstrate the origin of the vessel from the aortic wall and the severity of the stenosis and should document the distal branches for comparison with post-intervention views.

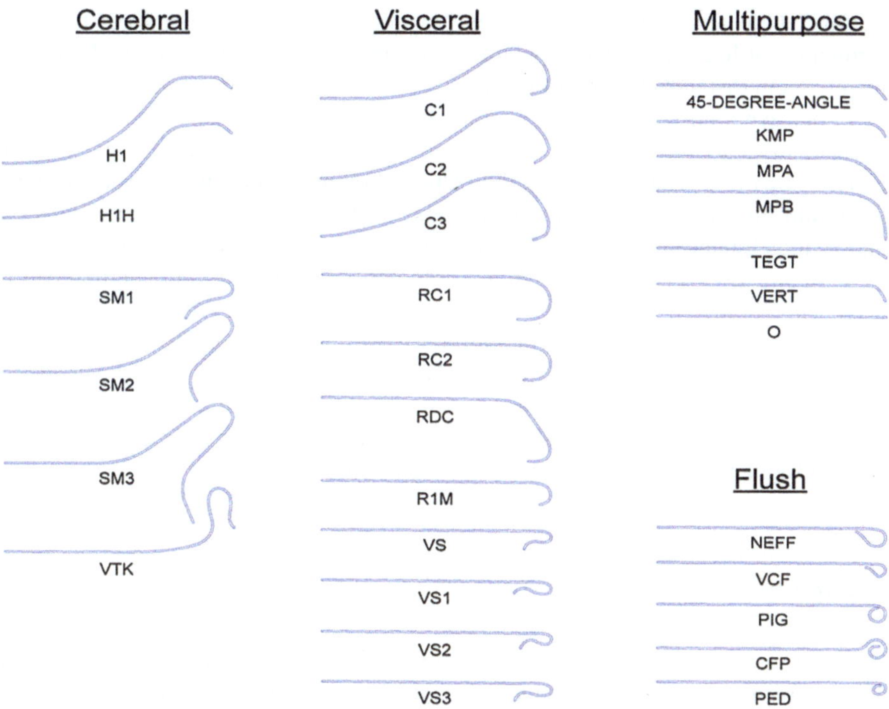

Fig. 13.4 Catheter shapes frequently utilized for mesenteric interventions

The target lesion is initially crossed using a 0.035 in soft angled glidewire, which is exchanged for the interventional wire of choice after confirmation of true lumen access. The authors' preference is to use a small profile (0.014 or 0.018 in) stiff guidewire for most interventions. The tip of the guidewire should be visualized and positioned within the main trunk of the SMA, rather than within small jejunal branches, which are prone to perforate or dissect.

Embolic Protection Devices

The use of embolic protection devices is highly controversial. The potential advantage is limiting or preventing distal embolization, which has been described as a known intraprocedural complication and cause of death after mesenteric interventions. Limitations include the added cost and the potential risk of arterial damage by the filter basket. In addition, there is limited information on which is the ideal filter device and where it should be placed within the mesenteric vessel. The Mayo Clinic group has reviewed the anatomy of the SMA to identify diameter and number of jejunal branches. Most patients have an average of 13 major jejunal branches, and >90 % of these branches originate >5 cm distal to the aortic origin of the SMA. The average diameter of the SMA in this location is 5–6 mm. Therefore, the most frequently utilized filter device would be a 7-mm filter basket positioned approximately 5 cm distal to the SMA origin.

In our experience, embolic protection devices are used selectively. Patients with acute or subacute mesenteric ischemia have a component of fresh in situ thrombosis and may be more prone to distal embolization. Among patients with chronic lesions, we found higher embolization rates in those with occlusions, severe calcification, and lesions longer than 30 mm. The author recommends use of embolic protection in these situations [22]. Our preference is to use a 320 cm working length 0.014 in filter wire (Spider RX, Covidien, Plymouth, MN; Fig. 13.5). Alternatively, Brown and associates described the use of temporary balloon occlusion and aspiration with GuardWire (Medtronic, Minneapolis, MN) [27]. If a 0.035 in stent is selected, a two-wire technique can be used by combining a 0.014 in filter wire with a 0.018 in "buddy wire." The stent is introduced via both wires for better support and to facilitate subsequent retrieval of the embolic protection device.

Choice of Stent

The vast majority of patients (>90 %) are treated using balloon-expandable stents. These have the advantages of wide range of length, precise deployment, and radial force. Because mesenteric lesions mimic renal artery lesions and are ostial and

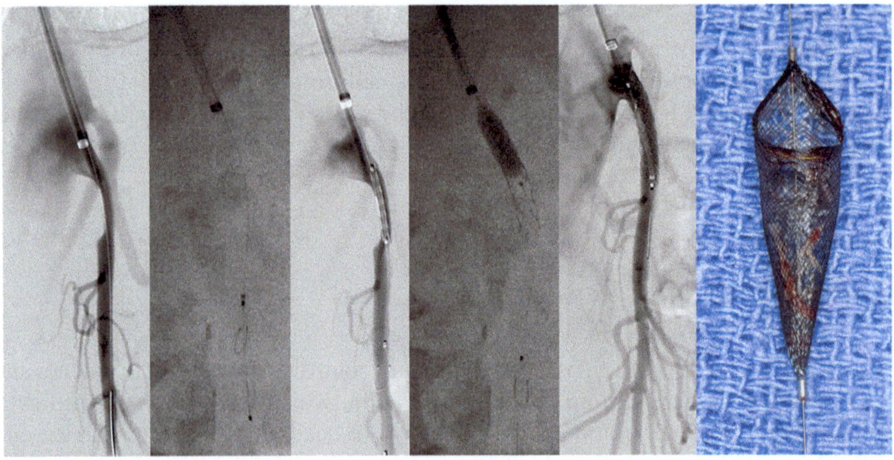

Fig. 13.5 Angioplasty and stenting of a focal stenosis of the superior mesenteric artery (SMA) stenosis using brachial approach. After selective angiography, the lesion is crossed, and a 0.014 in Spider Rx filter wire (Covidien, Plymouth MN) is deployed in the main trunk of the SMA, avoiding jejunal branches. The entire lesion is treated by balloon-expandable stent, which is extended 1–2 mm into the aorta and flared proximally. Completion angiography demonstrates patency of the stent without embolization or dissection. Appearance of a filter basked with moderate amount of debris

highly calcified, precise deployment and radial force are major advantages. Nonetheless, longer lesions affecting the bend of the SMA or those in tortuous segments may not be ideally suited for balloon-expandable stents. In these cases a short self-expandable stent may be used. If the lesion is long, it is not uncommon to combine a balloon-expandable stent for the ostia of the lesion with a self-expandable stent distally. Finally, we have recently shifted our practice to use preferentially covered balloon-expandable stents, which are resistant to intimal hyperplasia and have higher patency rates compared to bare metal stents. Covered stents are avoided in segments with critical side branches, which need to be preserved.

Angioplasty and Stenting of Mesenteric Stenosis

The primary goal of percutaneous treatment is to restore antegrade flow into at least one of the three mesenteric arteries, preferentially the SMA. First reports described successful results with balloon angioplasty alone, but elastic recoil and restenosis have limited its utility when used for ostial lesions [18, 28–37]. Although there are no prospective comparisons between angioplasty alone and primary stenting, most agree that routine stenting is indicated given that mesenteric lesions resemble renal artery stenoses [21, 27, 38–51]. Although there are no randomized comparisons between SMA and celiac stent placement, retrospective studies suggest that celiac stenting is associated with more recurrences in the first year after treatment [21]. In patients with compression of the CA by the median arcuate ligament, there is risk of stent fracture and compression. The role of two-vessel stenting remains controversial. Two retrospective studies by the MGH group and by Silva and colleagues have shown a nonsignificant trend towards less recurrence with two-vessel stenting [43, 46]. Malgor and colleagues from the Mayo Clinic reported nearly identical recurrence rates at 2 years in patients treated by SMA stents (78 %) compared to two-vessel stenting of the SMA and CA (60 %). Two-vessel mesenteric interventions may have a role in select patients with severe gastric ischemia and who do not have good collateral network between the CA and SMA. However, there is no proven benefit that routine two-vessel stenting provides more durable relief, and a second intervention adds cost and potential risk of complications.

CA intervention may be considered in higher-risk patient who fails attempted recanalization of the SMA or in those where an SMA intervention is felt to have a low yield for success due to excessive calcification or long-segment occlusion. In these patients, celiac stenting may be considered a "bridge" to open bypass or retrograde SMA stenting [52]. Angioplasty of the IMA in our experience carries a higher risk of rupture, dissection, or embolization, and is not advised with rare exceptions.

A brachial artery approach is preferred for patients with very angulated origin of the aorta and in those with occlusions or longer lesions. The author's preference is to use brachial artery approach whenever possible (Fig. 13.5). This offers excellent support with small profile system and precise stent deployment in patients with acute SMA angle. Although the risk of puncture-related complications is higher using total percutaneous technique, one option is to use a small 1–2 cm incision under local anesthesia to expose and repair of the brachial artery; less frequently, radial approach has been used.

Percutaneous access is established with a 0.018 in micropuncture set using ultrasound guidance, after which the system is exchanged to 0.035 in. Full systemic heparinization (80 mg/kg) is administered prior to catheter manipulations to achieve an activated clotting time of >250 s. A 6 or 7 Fr 90 cm hydrophilic sheath is positioned in the descending thoracic aorta above the CA origin. A 5 Fr MPA catheter is ideal for selective catheterization of the mesenteric arteries using the brachial approach, whereas a SOS or VS1 catheter can be used from the femoral approach. The initial selective angiography should demonstrate the origin of the vessel from the aortic wall and the severity of the stenosis and should document the distal branches for comparison with post-intervention views. The target lesion is initially crossed using a 0.035 in soft angled glidewire, which is exchanged for the interventional wire of choice after confirmation of true lumen access. The author's preference is to use a small profile (0.014 or 0.018 in) stiff guidewire for most interventions. Most recently, our practice has changed to covered stents, based on a recent report which indicates superior patency rates compared to bare metal stents [53]. The tip of the guidewire should be visualized and positioned within the main trunk of the SMA, rather than within small jejunal branches, which are prone to perforate or dissect (Fig. 13.6). Embolic protection may be useful in select patients with occlusions, long lesions (>30 mm length), severe calcification, thrombus, and acute or subacute symptoms; the author's preference is to use a 320 cm working length 0.014 in filter wire (Spider RX, Covidien, Plymouth MN). Alternatively, Brown and associates described the use of temporary balloon occlusion and aspiration with GuardWire (Medtronic, Minneapolis, MN) [27]. If a 0.035 in stent is selected, a two-wire technique can be used by combining a 0.014 in filter wire with a 0.018 in "buddy wire"; the stent is introduced via both wires for better support and to facilitate subsequent retrieval of the embolic protection device (Fig. 13.5). Pre-dilatation is recommended for tight stenosis, occlusions, severe calcification, and to size stents. A balloon-expandable stent with diameters ranging from 5 to 8 mm is used in >95 % of cases, allowing precise deployment and greater radial force. The stent is positioned under protection of the sheath, covering slightly more than the entire length of the lesion. Positioning the stent in the aortic lumen is critical to avoid missing the proximal portion of the lesion. It is important to position the stent 1–2 mm into the aortic lumen (Fig. 13.5). Ideally, the stent should be flared gently into the aorta, which prevents missing the ostia and facilitates re-catheterization if needed. Occasionally a self-expandable stent is needed to treat a non-ostial lesion or segments with excessive tortuosity, extending beyond the angulated portion of the SMA.

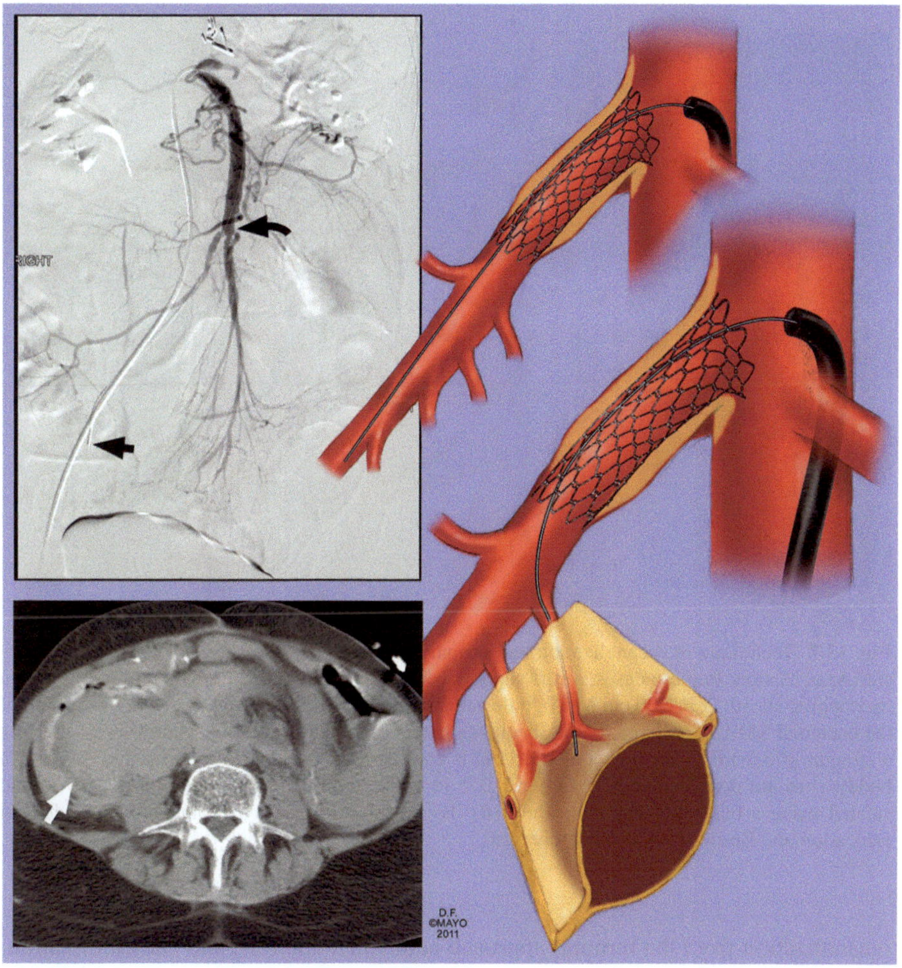

Fig. 13.6 An important technical point is to visualize the tip of the guidewire during the intervention and to position the guidewire in the main trunk of the superior mesenteric artery (*curved black arrow*) as opposed to distal jejunal branches (*black straight arrow*) which are prone to perforation resulting in mesenteric hematoma (*white straight arrow*) (By permission of Mayo Foundation for Medical Education and Research. All rights reserved)

Specific Situations

Recanalization of Mesenteric Occlusions

The technique is slightly modified in patients with difficult occlusions. In these cases it is of paramount importance to use the brachial approach and a stiff support system, which is accomplished by combining a 7 Fr sheath, 7 Fr MPA guide catheter, and 5 Fr MPA catheter (Fig. 13.7). In the author's opinion attempting a difficult

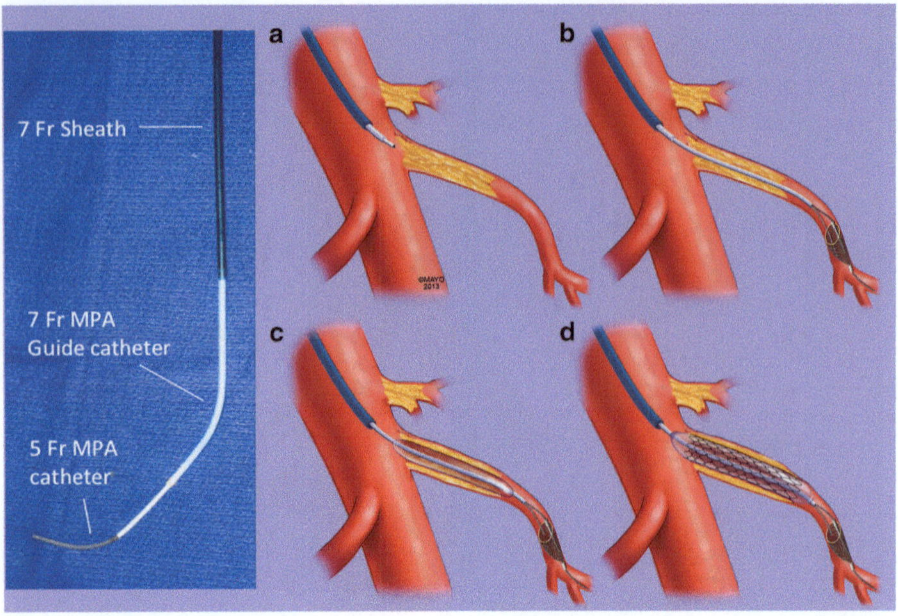

Fig. 13.7 Technique of recanalization and primary stenting of a total superior mesenteric artery (SMA) occlusion. In these cases, a stiff support system is build with combination of a 7 Fr 90 cm hydrophilic sheath, 7 Fr 100 cm MPA guide catheter and 5 Fr 125 cm MPA catheter. The stump of the occluded SMA is engaged by the sheath–catheter combination (**a**); the lesion is crossed using a straight glidewire. After true lumen access is confirmed, a 0.014 in filter wire and a 0.018 in buddy wire are deployed into SMA via 0.035 in catheter (**b**); the lesion is pre-dilated (**c**) and stented using a balloon-expandable stent (**d**) (By permission of Mayo Foundation for Medical Education and Research. All rights reserved)

recanalization from the femoral approach adds time, contrast, and catheter manipulations and is fraught with exceedingly high failure rates. Ideally the tip of the MPA catheter is used to engage the stump of the occluded SMA (Fig. 13.8), and sufficient support is provided by the combination of the sheath and guide catheter. The lesion is crossed using a straight tip, hydrophilic, soft 0.035 in glidewire but also using 0.018 in or 0.014 in guidewires if needed. It is ideal to avoid the subintimal plane, which is best achieved by using straight tip guidewires. A Quick-Cross (Spectranetics, Colorado Springs CO) or an alternative support catheter or even a small coronary balloon may be needed to cross a tight lesion. Once the lesion is crossed, access into the true lumen should be confirmed. Our preference has been to use embolic protection device (e.g., Spider RX, Covidien, Plymouth, MN) with two-wire technique routinely in cases of total occlusion.

Following deployment and flaring of the stent, the embolic protection device is retrieved with careful attention to avoid entrapment into the stent. The basket is examined for debris. A formal completion angiography should be obtained, including a focal magnified view of the stent with the sheath into the aorta to demonstrate

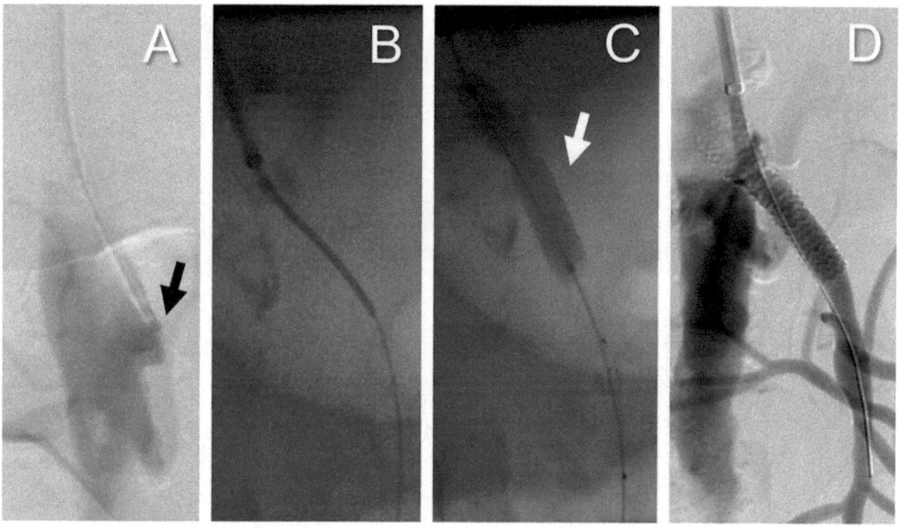

Fig. 13.8 Recanalization of superior mesenteric artery (SMA) occlusion utilizing the technique described in Fig. 13.7. After the stump is engaged by the catheter, guide catheter, and sheath (**a**, *black arrow*), the lesion was crossed (**b**) and stented using embolic protection (**d**). Note that the balloon is used to flare the proximal part of the stent (**c**, *white arrow*). Completion angiography shows a flared widely patent SMA stent (**d**)

the vessel origin and a panoramic view of the entire SMA and its branches to rule out embolization or perforation. The stiff guidewire should be retracted, and nitroglycerin may be administered via the sheath to minimize spasm or kinks caused by the guidewire tip. It is particularly important to note the presence of distal embolization, dissection, thrombus, or branch perforation. These complications occur in 5–10 % of patients and remain a major source of morbidity and mortality if not immediately recognized [22].

Orbital Atherectomy

A number of adjunctive techniques can be used to optimize results of mesenteric stents in patients with complex lesions, but the author acknowledges that these techniques are anecdotal or supported by a limited number of case reports. The presence of acute and subacute symptom presentation suggests fresh thrombus or complicated plaque. In these cases local administration of t-PA into the diseased segment 20–30 min prior to stent placement may improve technical success. For eccentric, calcified lesions, percutaneous atherectomy (Fig. 13.9) has been carefully used in very select cases [54]. Orbital atherectomy is used as a debulking tool prior to stent placement (Figs. 13.10 and 13.11). It is critical to have an appreciation of the limitations of this technique when applied as off-label use in the mesenteric arteries.

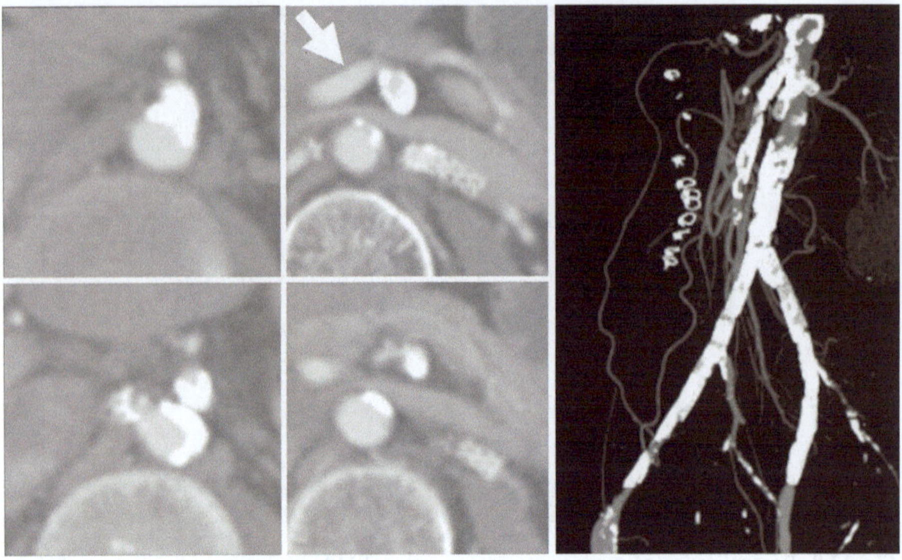

Fig. 13.9 Patient with severe eccentric calcifications and a replaced right hepatic artery (arrow)

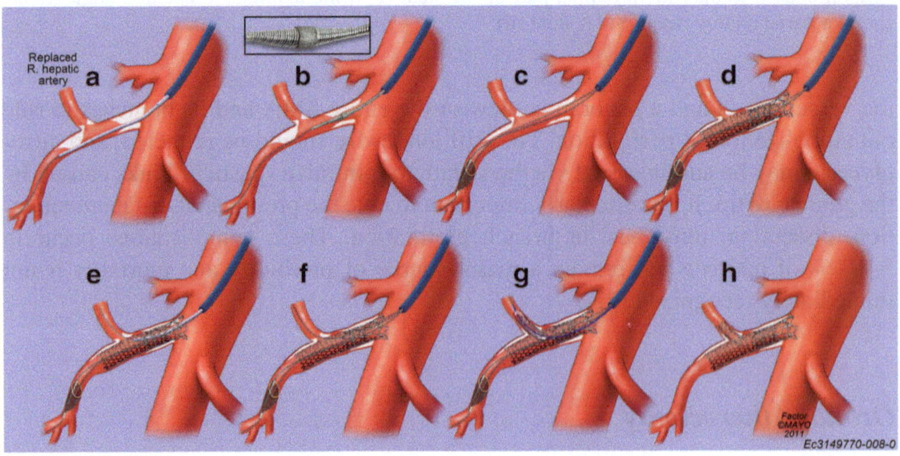

Fig. 13.10 Technique of orbital atherectomy and bifurcated stent. After the calcified lesion is crossed using a 0.014 in wire (**a**), orbital atherectomy is utilized for debulking (**b**). The wire is exchanged for a double-wire technique with embolic protection (**c**), followed by placement of balloon-expandable stent for the ostia and self-expandable stent for the distal SMA lesion (**d**). A cell of the stent is catheterized, (**e**) and a buddy 0.014 in wire is advanced to the replaced hepatic artery through the cell of the self-expandable stent (**f**). The replaced hepatic artery is stented with a balloon-expandable stent (**g**). The embolic protection device is retrieved (**h**) (By permission of Mayo Foundation for Medical Education and Research. All rights reserved)

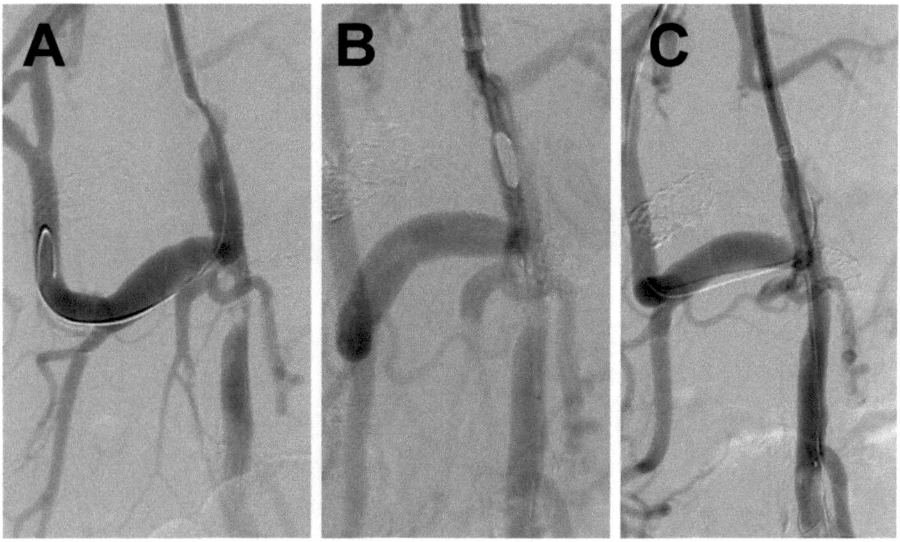

Fig. 13.11 Note eccentric calcifications in the proximal SMA (**a**) treated by orbital atherectomy (**b**) with significant luminal improvement (**c**)

Bifurcated Stents

Patients with longer lesions affective bifurcations (celiac axis or replaced hepatic artery) may benefit from bifurcated stent techniques (Fig. 13.12). These can be performed by combining a self-expandable stent for the mesenteric lesion and a smaller balloon-expandable stent for the side branch (Figs. 13.13 and 13.14), which is deployed via the cell of the self-expandable stent.

Retrograde Hybrid Revascularization

A hybrid approach using a midline laparotomy to expose the SMA and endovascular technique to place a retrograde SMA stent has been reported by Milner and colleagues from the University of Pennsylvania and Dartmouth Group [55, 56]. This option avoids the need for extensive dissection, vein harvesting, and use of a prosthetic graft. It may be selected in patients with extensive aortoiliac disease and no good source of inflow or in those with acute mesenteric ischemia, bowel gangrene, and contamination (Fig. 13.15).

The SMA is dissected below the pancreas as previously described. Several jejunal branches are controlled with silastic vessel loops and occluded prior to manipulation to avoid distal embolization. Retrograde SMA access is established using a micropuncture set with 0.018 in guidewire. This is exchanged for a 0.035 in guidewire system and a 6 to 7 Fr sheath is advance to the SMA. Retrograde angiography is obtained, and the SMA occlusion or stenosis is crossed, pre-dilated, and stented with

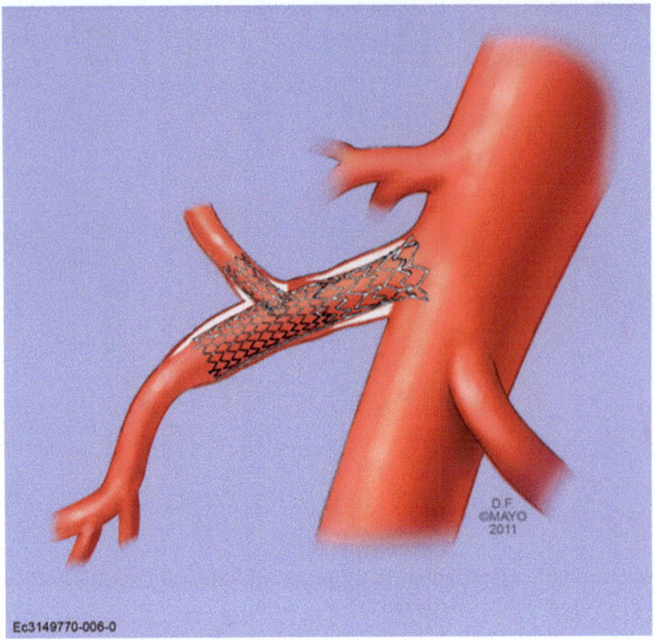

Fig. 13.12 Bifurcated stent technique (By permission of Mayo Foundation for Medical Education and Research. All rights reserved)

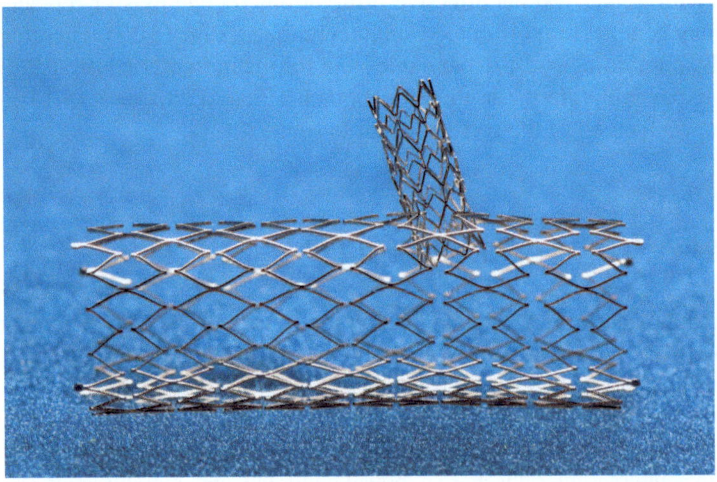

Fig. 13.13 A balloon-expandable stent is placed through the cell of a self-expandable stent

a balloon-expandable stent. Prior to restoring antegrade flow to the SMA, the sheath is flushed to prevent distal embolization. The puncture site may be closed with interrupted sutures or opened longitudinally and closed over a patch if severely diseased.

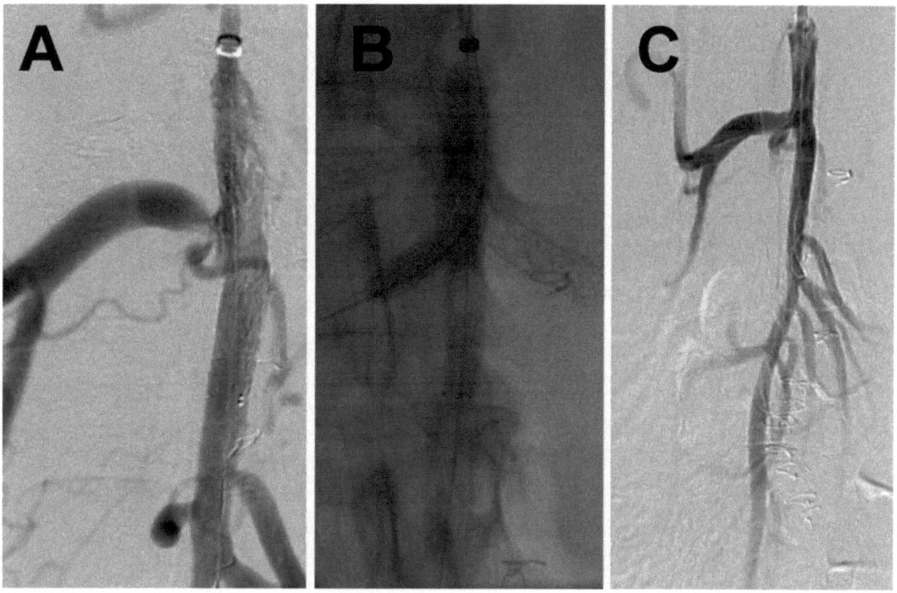

Fig. 13.14 After placement of a self-expandable stent (**a**), the cell is catheterized and a balloon-expandable stent is placed in the replaced hepatic artery (**b**). Completion angiography revealed widely patent SMA and replaced hepatic artery (**c**)

In-Stent Stenosis

Multiple approaches have been used to treat in-stent stenosis. Innovative techniques to maintain an "endovascular first approach" have included balloon angioplasty with cutting or cryoplasty balloons, redo stenting with bare metal or drug-eluting stents, and atherectomy [54, 57]. The latter has been used either as primary therapy or as an adjunct to debulk areas of neointimal hyperplasia prior to angioplasty or stenting. To date, none of these approaches has been shown any benefit as compared to standard angioplasty alone.

Despite the high rates of restenosis after mesenteric stenting, clinical data on outcomes of re-interventions is scarce. Tallarita and associates reported outcomes of 30 patients treated for in-stent restenosis [23]. The type and location of restenosis were also analyzed using contrast angiography. Intimal hyperplasia within the stented segment accounted for 43 % of the 30 cases of restenosis, while 57 % of patients had restenosis affecting arterial segments proximal or distal to the stent edge. Importantly, in 43 % of the patients, the area of restenosis coincided with technical imperfections noted on review of the index completion angiography performed at the time of the first intervention. This finding emphasizes how critical it is to pay attention to detail at the time of the first mesenteric intervention. Furthermore, some "restenosis" reported on post-intervention ultrasound imaging may actually represent incomplete or inadequate treatment, rather than progression of disease or development of neointimal hyperplasia. Technical imperfections include inadequate stent length or treatment segment or poor stent expansion due to unfavorable anatomy, such as with highly calcified or eccentric lesions. Our preference has been to treat restenosis with a covered balloon expandable stent (Fig. 13.16).

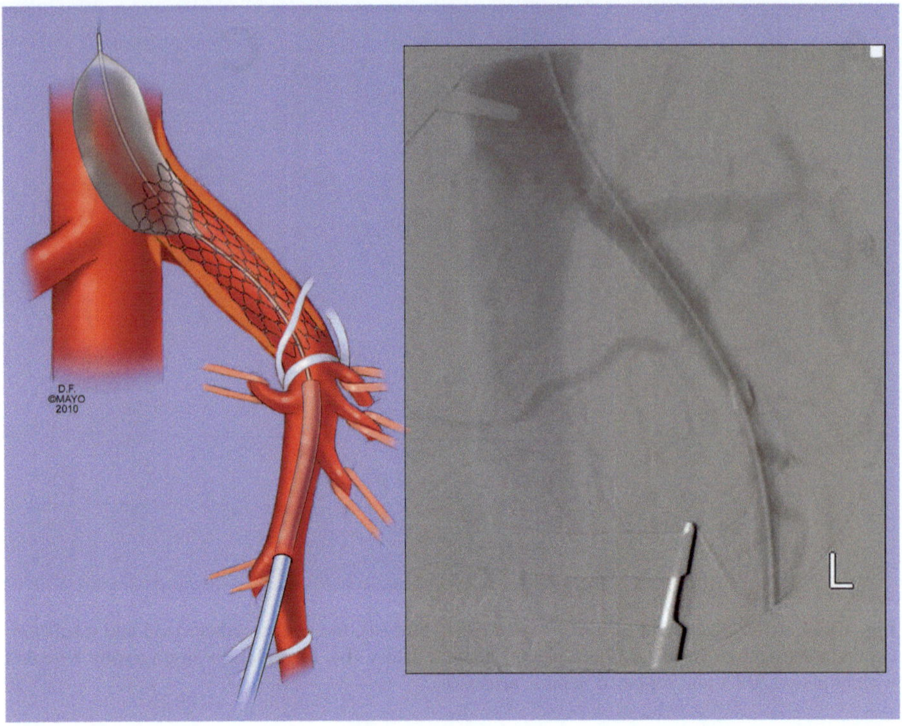

Fig. 13.15 Hybrid revascularization with retrograde stenting of the superior mesenteric artery via midline laparotomy (By permission of Mayo Foundation for Medical Education and Research. All rights reserved)

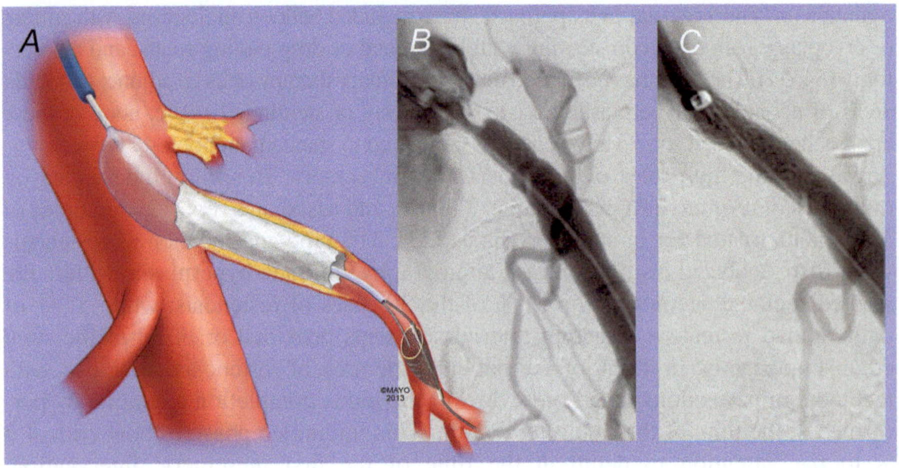

Fig. 13.16 Treatment of in-stent restenosis with placement of covered balloon-expandable stent (**a**). Pre-deployment angiography demonstrates a high-grade stenosis in the proximal aspect of the stent (**b**). After placement of a covered balloon expandable stent (**c**), there is no residual stenosis (By permission of Mayo Foundation for Medical Education and Research. All rights reserved)

Complications

The most common causes of death after mesenteric stenting are cardiac events, gastrointestinal bleeding, and bowel ischemia. The latter is typically associated with intraprocedural complications such as distal embolization, thrombosis, or dissection. Distal embolization occurs in 8 % of patients treated by SMA stents without embolic protection, with higher rates among patients with subacute symptoms, occlusion, long lesions (>30 mm), and severe calcification [24]. Therefore, there may be a role for selective use of embolic protection in these patients. The most commonly reported complications are access-related problems in 2–15 %, renal insufficiency in 5–12 %, acute bowel ischemia in 1–5 %, gastrointestinal bleeding in 1–4 %, cardiac events in 1–3 %, and respiratory complications in 3 %.

Post-procedure Management

The post-procedure care after mesenteric interventions is comparable to that of other peripheral endovascular procedures. All patients are admitted for observation overnight. Worsening abdominal pain after the procedure is unusual and warrants evaluation to rule out thrombosis, embolization, or a mesenteric hematoma from jejunal branch perforation (Fig. 13.6). Patients are allowed to resume a regular diet within six to eight hours. Antiplatelet therapy is typically started prior to the intervention with acetylsalicylic acid and continued indefinitely thereafter. Clopidogrel is started the day of the intervention with a loading dose of 300 mg and continued for six to eight weeks as a dual antiplatelet agent, after which patients are kept on acetylsalicylic acid alone. The author's preference is to obtain a duplex ultrasound scan prior to discharge or within the first few days after the procedure to serve as a baseline for future comparison. The presence of elevated velocity on duplex ultrasound may be due to inadequate stenting with missed lesion proximal or distal to the stent. Follow-up includes clinical examination and duplex ultrasound every 6 months during the first year and annually thereafter.

Conclusion

Endovascular revascularization has become the first treatment option in most patients with occlusive mesenteric artery disease. Patient selection is critical to achieve good anatomical and clinical result. The most suited lesions are focal stenosis with limited amount of calcification, but endovascular approaches have been widely applied to more challenging lesions.

References

1. Mikkelsen WP. Intestinal angina: its surgical significance. Am J Surg. 1957;94(2):262–7; discussion 267–9.
2. Carrick RP, et al. Chronic mesenteric ischemia resulting from isolated lesions of the superior mesenteric artery–a case report. Angiology. 2005;56(6):785–8.
3. Oderich GS, et al. Open versus endovascular revascularization for chronic mesenteric ischemia: risk-stratified outcomes. J Vasc Surg. 2009;49(6):1472–9. e3.
4. van Petersen AS, et al. Open or percutaneous revascularization for chronic splanchnic syndrome. J Vasc Surg. 2010;51(5):1309–16.
5. Mueller C, Borriello R, Perlov-Antzis L. Parenteral nutrition support of a patient with chronic mesenteric artery occlusive disease. Nutr Clin Pract. 1993;8(2):73–7.
6. Rheudasil JM, et al. Surgical treatment of chronic mesenteric arterial insufficiency. J Vasc Surg. 1988;8(4):495–500.
7. Thomas JH, et al. The clinical course of asymptomatic mesenteric arterial stenosis. J Vasc Surg. 1998;27(5):840–4.
8. Oderich GS, Gloviczki P, Bower TC. Open surgical treatment for chronic mesenteric ischemia in the endovascular era: when it is necessary and what is the preferred technique? Semin Vasc Surg. 2010;23(1):36–46.
9. Schermerhorn ML, et al. Mesenteric revascularization: management and outcomes in the United States, 1988–2006. J Vasc Surg. 2009;50(2):341–8. e1.
10. Assar AN, Abilez OJ, Zarins CK. Outcome of open versus endovascular revascularization for chronic mesenteric ischemia: review of comparative studies. J Cardiovasc Surg (Torino). 2009;50(4):509–14.
11. Atkins MD, et al. Surgical revascularization versus endovascular therapy for chronic mesenteric ischemia: a comparative experience. J Vasc Surg. 2007;45(6):1162–71.
12. Biebl M, et al. Surgical and interventional visceral revascularization for the treatment of chronic mesenteric ischemia – when to prefer which? World J Surg. 2007;31(3):562–8.
13. Gupta PK, et al. Chronic mesenteric ischemia: endovascular versus open revascularization. J Endovasc Ther. 2010;17(4):540–9.
14. Indes JE, et al. Outcomes of endovascular and open treatment for chronic mesenteric ischemia. J Endovasc Ther. 2009;16(5):624–30.
15. Kasirajan K, et al. Chronic mesenteric ischemia: open surgery versus percutaneous angioplasty and stenting. J Vasc Surg. 2001;33(1):63–71.
16. Oderich GS, Malgor RD, Ricotta 2nd JJ. Open and endovascular revascularization for chronic mesenteric ischemia: tabular review of the literature. Ann Vasc Surg. 2009;23(5):700–12.
17. Rawat N, Gibbons CP. Surgical or endovascular treatment for chronic mesenteric ischemia: a multicenter study. Ann Vasc Surg. 2010;24(7):935–45.
18. Rose SC, Quigley TM, Raker EJ. Revascularization for chronic mesenteric ischemia: comparison of operative arterial bypass grafting and percutaneous transluminal angioplasty. J Vasc Interv Radiol. 1995;6(3):339–49.
19. Sivamurthy N, et al. Endovascular versus open mesenteric revascularization: immediate benefits do not equate with short-term functional outcomes. J Am Coll Surg. 2006;202(6):859–67.
20. Zerbib P, et al. Endovascular versus open revascularization for chronic mesenteric ischemia: a comparative study. Langenbecks Arch Surg. 2008;393(6):865–70.
21. Malgor RD, et al. Results of single- and two-vessel mesenteric artery stents for chronic mesenteric ischemia. Ann Vasc Surg. 2010;24(8):1094–101.
22. Oderich GS, et al. Mesenteric artery complications during angioplasty and stent placement for atherosclerotic chronic mesenteric ischemia. J Vasc Surg. 2012;55(4):1063–71.
23. Tallarita T, et al. Reinterventions for stent restenosis in patients treated for atherosclerotic mesenteric artery disease. J Vasc Surg. 2011;54(5):1422e1–9e1.

24. Oderich GS et al. Anatomic measurements and factors associated with embolic events during superior mesenteric artery stenting: implications for use of embolic protection devices. Abstract book of the 37th Society for Clinical Vascular Surgery Annual Symposium, 2009.
25. Oderich GS, et al. RR26. Natural history of mesenteric artery stent restenoses and clinical and anatomic predictors for re-intervention in patients with chronic mesenteric ischemia. J Vasc Surg. 2009;49(5):e1–2. Supplement.
26. Hannawi B, Lam WW, Younis GA. Pressure wire used to measure gradient in chronic mesenteric ischemia. Tex Heart Inst J. 2012;39(5):739–43.
27. Brown DJ, et al. Mesenteric stenting for chronic mesenteric ischemia. J Vasc Surg. 2005;42(2):268–74.
28. Allen RC, et al. Mesenteric angioplasty in the treatment of chronic intestinal ischemia. J Vasc Surg. 1996;24(3):415–21; discussion 421–3.
29. Hackworth CA, Leef JA. Percutaneous transluminal mesenteric angioplasty. Surg Clin North Am. 1997;77(2):371–80.
30. Hallisey MJ, et al. Angioplasty for the treatment of visceral ischemia. J Vasc Interv Radiol. 1995;6(5):785–91.
31. Levy PJ, Haskell L, Gordon RL. Percutaneous transluminal angioplasty of splanchnic arteries: an alternative method to elective revascularisation in chronic visceral ischaemia. Eur J Radiol. 1987;7(4):239–42.
32. Maspes F, et al. Percutaneous transluminal angioplasty in the treatment of chronic mesenteric ischemia: results and 3 years of follow-up in 23 patients. Abdom Imaging. 1998;23(4):358–63.
33. Matsumoto AH, et al. Percutaneous transluminal angioplasty of visceral arterial stenoses: results and long-term clinical follow-up. J Vasc Interv Radiol. 1995;6(2):165–74.
34. McShane MD, et al. Mesenteric angioplasty for chronic intestinal ischaemia. Eur J Vasc Surg. 1992;6(3):333–6.
35. Nyman U, et al. Endovascular treatment of chronic mesenteric ischemia: report of five cases. Cardiovasc Intervent Radiol. 1998;21(4):305–13.
36. Odurny A, Sniderman KW, Colapinto RF. Intestinal angina: percutaneous transluminal angioplasty of the celiac and superior mesenteric arteries. Radiology. 1988;167(1):59–62.
37. Roberts Jr L, et al. Transluminal angioplasty of the superior mesenteric artery: an alternative to surgical revascularization. Am J Roentgenol. 1983;141(5):1039–42.
38. Aksu C, et al. Stent implantation in chronic mesenteric ischemia. Acta Radiol. 2009;50(6):610–6.
39. Daliri A, et al. Endovascular treatment for chronic atherosclerotic occlusive mesenteric disease: is stenting superior to balloon angioplasty? Vasa. 2010;39(4):319–24.
40. Fioole B, et al. Percutaneous transluminal angioplasty and stenting as first-choice treatment in patients with chronic mesenteric ischemia. J Vasc Surg. 2010;51(2):386–91.
41. Kougias P, et al. Management of chronic mesenteric ischemia. The role of endovascular therapy. J Endovasc Ther. 2007;14(3):395–405.
42. Kougias P, Huynh TT, Lin PH. Clinical outcomes of mesenteric artery stenting versus surgical revascularization in chronic mesenteric ischemia. Int Angiol. 2009;28(2):132–7.
43. Silva JA, et al. Endovascular therapy for chronic mesenteric ischemia. J Am Coll Cardiol. 2006;47(5):944–50.
44. Matsumoto AH, et al. Percutaneous transluminal angioplasty and stenting in the treatment of chronic mesenteric ischemia: results and long-term followup. J Am Coll Surg. 2002;194(1 Suppl):S22–31.
45. Gibbons CP, Roberts DE. Endovascular treatment of chronic arterial mesenteric ischemia: a changing perspective? Semin Vasc Surg. 2010;23(1):47–53.
46. Peck MA, et al. Intermediate-term outcomes of endovascular treatment for symptomatic chronic mesenteric ischemia. J Vasc Surg. 2010;51(1):140–7. e1–2.
47. Sarac TP, et al. Endovascular treatment of stenotic and occluded visceral arteries for chronic mesenteric ischemia. J Vasc Surg. 2008;47(3):485–91.

48. Schaefer PJ, et al. Stent placement with the monorail technique for treatment of mesenteric artery stenosis. J Vasc Interv Radiol. 2006;17(4):637–43.
49. Schaefer PJ, et al. Chronic mesenteric ischemia: stenting of mesenteric arteries. Abdom Imaging. 2007;32(3):304–9.
50. Schoch DM, et al. Management of chronic mesenteric vascular insufficiency: an endovascular approach. J Am Coll Surg. 2011;212(4):668–75; discussion 675–7.
51. Sharafuddin MJ, et al. Endovascular recanalization of total occlusions of the mesenteric and celiac arteries. J Vasc Surg. 2012;55(6):1674–81.
52. Biebl M, et al. Endovascular treatment as a bridge to successful surgical revascularization for chronic mesenteric ischemia. Am Surg. 2004;70(11):994–8.
53. Oderich GS, et al. SS14. Comparison of covered stents versus bare metal stents for treatment of chronic atherosclerotic mesenteric arterial disease. J Vasc Surg. 2012;55(6):23S.
54. Manunga JM, Oderich GS. Orbital atherectomy as an adjunct to debulk difficult calcified lesions prior to mesenteric artery stenting. J Endovasc Ther. 2012;19(4):489–94.
55. Milner R, Woo EY, Carpenter JP. Superior mesenteric artery angioplasty and stenting via a retrograde approach in a patient with bowel ischemia – a case report. Vasc Endovascular Surg. 2004;38(1):89–91.
56. Wyers MC, et al. Retrograde mesenteric stenting during laparotomy for acute occlusive mesenteric ischemia. J Vasc Surg. 2007;45(2):269–75.
57. Visconti G, Taranto D, Briguori C. Recalcitrant in-stent restenosis of the celiac trunk treated by drug-eluting stent. Catheter Cardiovasc Interv. 2008;72(6):873–6.

Chapter 14
Results of Endovascular Mesenteric Revascularization

Timur P. Sarac

History

The first description of mesenteric vascular occlusion is attributed to Antonio Beniviene from Florence in the fifteenth century [1]. The correlation of mesenteric artery occlusive disease with symptoms of postprandial abdominal pain did not occur until the late 1800s when councilman identified a patient with abdominal pain and discovered mesenteric occlusive disease at autopsy [2]. This was soon corroborated by Schinzler, who in 1901 reported on a patient with a long history of abdominal pain and occlusive mesenteric thrombus of the superior mesenteric artery [1]. The final proof came in 1936 when Dunphy [3] performed an autopsy of a patient with bowel infarction, abdominal pain, and weight loss and found all three mesenteric vessels were occluded.

It was 64 years later that someone first took the leap to treat chronic mesenteric ischemia. In 1958 Shaw and Maynard [4] reported the first open mesenteric revascularization by transaortic endarterectomy. Shortly thereafter, in 1961 Morris [5] reported the first bypass by doing a retrograde bypass using a Dacron graft. In 1972, Stoney and Wylie introduced transaortic visceral thromboendarterectomy and described their results with this and aortomesenteric bypass [6, 7].

Soon after, minimally invasive techniques began to be explored to treat occluded blood vessels, and the technology began to take off in the latter half of the twentieth century. The German born cardiologist Andreas Gruentzig was the first to perform

T.P. Sarac, MD (✉)
Section of Vascular Surgery, Heart and Vascular Institute,
Yale University School of Medicine, New Haven, CT, USA
e-mail: Timur.sarac@yale.edu

G.S. Oderich (ed.), *Mesenteric Vascular Disease*,
DOI 10.1007/978-1-4939-1847-8_14

Table 14.1 Angioplasty alone for mesenteric occlusive disease

Author	Year	*N*	Clinical success (%)	Patency (%)	30 day mortality	Complications (%)
Odurney	1988	10	50	30	NR	10
Matsumoto	1995	15	80	53	NR	16
Allen	1996	18	79	89	6 %	6
Maspes	1998	41	77	86	0	5

NR not reported

balloon angioplasty of an artery in 1977 in Zurich, Switzerland, when he opened a blocked coronary artery [8]. Three years later Furrer extended this technology to the mesenteric vessels, as he was the first to report the first percutaneous angioplasty of the superior mesenteric artery [9].

Many investigators reported their results of celiac and sma angioplasty over the ensuing years, with variable outcomes in the pre-stent era. (Table 14.1) [10–14]. One initial report by Odurney had only 50 % clinical success and 30 % primary patency. Matsumoto reported on 19 patients who had percutaneous therapy. The immediate technical failure rate was 37 %, but of those that were successful, there was 83 % clinical improvement of symptoms. Allen et al. had good clinical success achieving 79 % symptom relief and 89 % patency, and Maspes reported similar results in 41 patients. Nevertheless, standardized documentation of technical success, clinical success, objective patency, and morbidity and mortality was not consistent and lacked uniformity.

Early Mesenteric Stent Results

From what was reported, angioplasty alone did have some benefit, but there was a real need for improvement in immediate- and longer-term results. In an effort to improve these, Ivancev's group described the first sma stent, which included not only stenting the sma but also recanalizing a chronic total occlusion (CTO) [15]. They reported continued patency 9 months after the intervention, which was documented by angiography. Since the time of early reports, balloon angioplasty and stenting of mesenteric occlusive disease were slow to be adopted. However, with refinement in techniques, lower-profile devices, and extended training of multiple subspecialties, soon many case series described the success of PTA and stenting of the visceral vessels [16] (Table 14.2). Sheeran et al. looked at their results of PTA and stent in 12 patients, 3 of whom were chronic total occlusions. Their initial technical success was 92 %, including 3 patients with chronic occlusions. One patient died within 30 days of the procedure (mortality 8.3 %) due to bowel infarction, despite a patent stent. Primary and primary-assisted patency was 74 % and 83 % respectively, and secondary patency was 83 %. All three patients with chronic occlusions had relief of clinical signs and symptoms at a mean follow-up of 22 months. Chahid et al. reported their results after treating 14 patients [17]. Their technical success and initial clinical success was 100 %. Long-term relief of

Table 14.2 Early PTA and stent results

Author	Year	*N*	Clinical success (%)	Primary patency	30 day mortality	Complications
Linblad	1996	1	100	100 % at 9 months	0	0
Sheeran	1999	12	92	74 %	8.3 %	8.3
Chahid	2004	14	79	86 %	0	14.3 %
Matsumoto	2002	33	83.3	83.3 %	0	13 %
Sharruddin	2003	25	88	92 % at 6 months	4 %	12 %

symptoms was 79 %, and two patients underwent repeat angioplasty for an absolute patency rate 86. Two major complications were observed: one hematoma and one false aneurysm occurring at the brachial puncture site (14.3 %).

Matsumoto reported one of the first larger series of patients [18]. He reviewed their experience of PTA and stenting in a group of 33 patients. Twenty-one patients underwent PTA alone and 12 PTA and stenting. Technical success occurred in 81 % of patients with PTA and 100 % PTA and stent. The long-term clinical success was 83.3 %, and assisted clinical success was 96.6 % as four patients underwent repeat angioplasty. Patency rates were not reported. The complication rate was 13 % and 30 day mortality 0 %. Another large series was published by Sharrudin et al. [19] They evaluated their results of mesenteric stenting in 25 patients, 21 of whom were done for chronic mesenteric ischemia. Their reported technical success was 96 %, and clinical outcomes showed primary and primary-assisted clinical benefits at 11 months of 85 % and 91 %. He also was the first to report actuarial Kaplan Meier patencies, which were both 92 % at six months. Major complications occurred in three patients for a rate of 12 %.

Mesenteric Intervention vs. Open Surgery

As minimally invasive techniques started receiving a ground swell of enthusiasm, people soon began to compare the results to the gold standard open surgery (Table 14.3). Although mesenteric bypass' results were improving, there was still significant morbidity and mortality [20]. The first large series reported was that from the Cleveland Clinic [21]. Kasirajan et al. compared outcomes of endovascular versus open surgery; outcomes were compared between 28 patients treated with PTA and stent and 85 patients who underwent open mesenteric revascularization. Of the patients who underwent PTA and stent, 18 % had angioplasty alone and 82 % angioplasty plus stent. Of the patients who had open surgery, 71 % had bypass, 22 % transaortic endarterectomy, and 7 % local endarterectomy and patch angioplasty. Fewer vessels were revascularized per patient in the PTA and stent group (1.1) compared with the OS group (1.5). There was no difference noted in the early in-hospital complications (17.9 % vs. 32.9 %) or mortality rate (10.7 % vs. 8.2 %).

Table 14.3 PTA and stent vs. open surgery

Author	Year	Open					Endovascular				
		N	Clinical success (%)	1° patency (%)	30 day mortality (%)	Major morbidity (%)	*N*	Clinical success (%)	1° patency (%)	30 day mortality %	Major morbidity (%)
Kasirajan	2001	85	87	24[a]	8	33	28	66	27[a]	11	18
Atkins	2007	49	77	90	2.4	4.1	31	78	59	3.2	12.9
Oderich	2009	146	96	88	2.7	36	83	92	41	2.4	18

[a]Restenosis rates

However, there was a trend towards reduced length of hospital stay in the PTA stent (5 days vs. 13 days). The 3-year cumulative recurrent stenosis rates also were not different (27 % vs. 24 %), but recurrent symptoms were significantly higher in the PTA stent vs. open surgery (34 % vs. 13 %). The end result was that while PTA and stents were improving, they had not yet met the gold standard.

Refinement in techniques, improved devices, better patient selection, and patient preference continued to promote use of endovascular procedures. Atkins reported the Massachusetts General experience of 80 patients [22]. PTA and stent were performed in 31 patients and open surgery in 49 patients. The open revascularization procedures consisted of bypass grafting in 63 %, transaortic endarterectomy in 14 %, patch angioplasty in 8 %, or combined in 15 %. Mean follow-up was 15 months in the PTA/stent group and 42 months in the open surgery cohort. The PTA/stent group had fewer vessels revascularized (1.5 vs. 1.8 vessels). Hospital length of stay was less for the PTA/stent group (5.6 vs. 16.7 days). No difference was noted in in-hospital major morbidity (13 % vs. 4 %) or mortality (1/31 vs. 1/49). Two-year survival was similar between the groups (88 % PTA/stent vs. 74 % open), as was recurrent symptoms (23 % vs. 22 %) or radiographic recurrence (32 % vs. 37 %). Radiographic primary patency (58 % vs. 90 %) and primary-assisted patency (65 % vs. 96 %) at 1 year were lower in the PTA/stent group compared with open surgery. There was no difference in second procedures as 16 % PTA/stent patients compared with 22 % open repair. The end results still were not convincing in favor of PTA and stent, but the pendulum began to swing.

Soon thereafter, Oderich and colleagues from the Mayo Clinic compared their results of open surgery to PTA and stent for symptomatic mesenteric ischemia [23]. They compared 229 consecutive patients treated for CMI with open surgery (146 patients) or PTA/stent (83 patients). Those who underwent PTA/stent were significantly older, had higher risk, and fewer vessels revascularized (1.3 vs. 1.8). There was no difference in mortality in the open group vs. PTA/stent (2.7 % vs. 2.4 %). Open repair had significantly more complications (36 % vs. 18 %) and longer hospitalization (12 vs. 3 days). At 5 years, open surgery had improved recurrence-free survival (89 % vs. 51 %) and primary (88 % vs. 41 %) and secondary patency rates (97 % vs. 88 %). Symptom improvement was not different between open and PTA/stent (96%vs. 92 %).

The end results of all three studies found that mesenteric stenting has a high re-intervention rate but reduced length of stay and reduced morbidity and mortality

Contemporary Mesenteric Stent Results

The next generation of stents and catheters included smaller devices, and large-volume centers became more aggressive in treating more complex lesions. Sarac et al. described the Cleveland Clinic experience that included a cohort of patients who had chronic total occlusions (CTO) [24]. The first report of recanalizing a CTO for mesenteric ischemia was in the 1996 by Linblad [14], but there was a general fear of being too aggressive in treating CTOs as several reports indicated that these lesions were off limits for fear of dissection and distal embolization. However, this myth was demystified as Sarac et al. from the Cleveland Clinic reported their results on 65 patients treated by PTA and stent for chronic mesenteric ischemia (Table 14.4). Completely occluded vessels were treated in 28 %, and greater than 60 % stenosis was treated in 72 %. Cumulative 1-year results were primary patency 65 %, primary-assisted patency 97 %, secondary patency 99 %, and survival 89 %. The endovascular treatment of visceral artery occlusion was not associated with diminished patency or survival, irrespective of stent size or number. One-year primary patency was worse among patients who had femoral access. Re-intervention rates remained high.

Peck et al subsequently reported the Massachusetts General in results in 49 patients [25]. Initial symptom relief was noted in 89.8 % with no change in 5 patients. The 30-day mortality rate was 2.0 %, and major complications occurred in 16.3 %. Restenosis on follow-up imaging occurred in 65 %, and 29 % developed recurrent symptoms with 13 requiring a re-intervention. Actuarial 36-month freedom from symptomatic recurrence was 61 % %. Two-vessel treatment was protective against symptom recurrence and re-intervention. Primary patency at 36 months was 64 %.

The next major report came from Turba et al. [26], who reported on 166 patients treated over 28 years. The technical success rate of stenting (99.4 %) was higher than for percutaneous transluminal angioplasty (86 %). Immediate clinical improvement was seen in 146 out of 166 (88.2 %). Soon after, another longer-term study was published by Abu Rahma 2013 [27]. They reported on 83 patients and found a procedure related morbidity of only 2 % and 2 % mortality. The primary late clinical success rate was 59 %, and the late 70 % in-stent stenosis rate was 51 % at a mean follow-up of 31 months (range 1–124). Freedom from late recurrent symptoms at 1, 2, 3, 4, and 5 years was 83, 77, 70, 70, and 65 %, respectively. Survival rates at the same intervals were 88, 82, 70, 64, and 51 %. Primary patency rates for the whole series were 69, 48, 39, 28, and 19 % at 1, 2, 3, 4, and 5 years, respectively. There was no difference in patency rates between celiac versus sma PTA and stent.

In an attempt to improve on the poor primary patency rates, Oderich and his colleagues from Mayo Clinic looked at using ePTFE-covered balloon-expandable stents instead of bare metal stents [28]. They compared outcomes of mesenteric angioplasty and stenting using iCAST-covered stents to uncovered stents in 225 patients. In the primary intervention group, patients treated by CS had higher freedom from restenosis (92 % vs. 53 %; $P = .003$), symptom recurrence (92 % vs. 50 %), re-intervention (91 % vs. 56 %), and better primary patency at 3 years (92 % vs. 52 %) than for BMS. The re-intervention group had similar results.

Conclusions

The treatment of symptomatic mesenteric arterial occlusive disease has undergone dramatic changes over the past century. While the results of open surgery remain good, improvement in technique, devices, training, and patient preference have

Table 14.4 Contemporary PTA and stent results

Author	Year	*N*	Pta or ptas	Vessels treated	Clinical success (%)	1°, 1°assisted, & secondary patency	Major morbidity (%)	30 day mortality (%)
Sarac	2008	65	ptas	87	85	65, 97, 99	20	7.7
Peek	2010	49	ptas	66	81	78, 95, NR	14	2.0
Turba	2012	166	Pta/ptas	221	81	85, 97, 100	10	3
Abu Rama	2013	83	ptas	105	96	69, 80, NR	2	2
Oderich[a]	2013	42	ptas (covered)	79	91	92, NR, 100	12	0

PTA percutaneous angioplasty alone, *ptas* percutaneous angioplasty and stent, *NR* not reported

[a]2 centers and covered cohort only

lead to PTA and stenting to be the preferred treatment of choice for mesenteric arterial occlusive disease. However, primary patency rates with bare metal stents are less than desirable, and covered stent grafts appear to have improved primary patency rates.

References

1. Glebova NO, Freischlag JA. Management of acute and chronic mesenteric ischemia. In: Ascher E, Veith F, editors. Haimovici's vascular surgery. 6th ed. Hoboken: Wiley Blackwell; 2012. p. 639.
2. Councilman WT. Three cases of occlusion of the superior mesenteric artery. Boston Med Surg J. 1894;130:410–1.
3. Dunphy JE. Abdominal pain of vascular origin. Am J Med Sci. 1936;192:109–13.
4. Shaw RS, Maynard III EP. Acute and chronic thrombosis of mesenteric arteries associated with malabsorption. A report of two cases successfully treated by thromboendarterectomy. N Engl J Med. 1958;258:874.
5. Morris GC, Crawford ES, Cooley DA, Debakey ME. Revascularization of the celiac and superior mesenteric arteries. Arch Surg. 1962;84:95–107.
6. Stoney RJ, Wylie EJ. Recocognition and Surgical Management of Visceral Ischemic Syndrome. Ann Surg. 1966;164:714.
7. Stoney RJ, Ehrenfeld WK, Wiley EJ. Revascularization medthods in chronic visceral ischemia caused by atherosclerosis. Ann Surg. 1977;186:468–76.
8. Gruentzig AR, Senning A, Siegeuthaler WE. Non-operative dilatation of coronary artery stenosis. Percutaneous transluminal coronary angioplasty. N Engl J Med. 1979;301:61–8.
9. Furrer J, Gruntzig A, Kugelmeier J, et al. Treatment of abdominal angina with percutaneous dilatation of an arteria mesenterica superior stenosis: preliminary communication. Cardiovasc Intervent Radiol. 1980;3:43–4.
10. Matsumoto AH, Tegtmeyer CJ, Fitzcharles EK, Bayne Selby J, Tribble CG, Angle JF, Kron I. Percutaneous transluminal angioplasty of visceral arterial stenoses: results and long-term clinical follow-up. J Vasc Intervent Rad. 1995;6:165–74.
11. Odurney A, Sniderman KW, Colapinto RF. Intestinal angina: percutaneous transluminal angioplasty of the celiac and superior mesenteric arteries. Radiology. 1988;167:59–63.
12. Oderich GS, Malgor D, Ricotta JJ. Open and endovascular revascularization for chronic mesenteric ischemia: tabular review of the literature. Ann Vasc Surg. 2009;5:700–12.
13. Maspes F, Gandini R, Innocenzi L, Barzi F, Simonetti G, Mazzetti di Pietralta G. Percutaneous transluminal angioplasty in the treatment of chronic mesenteric ischemia: results and 3 year follow up in 23 patients. Abdom Imaging. 1998;23:358–63.
14. Allen RC, Martin GH, Rees CI, Rivera FJ, Talkington CM, Garrett WV, Smith BL, Pearl GL, Diamond NG, Lee SP, Thompson JE. Mesenteric angioplasty in the treatment of chronic mesenteric ischemia. G J Vasc Surg. 1996;24:415–23.
15. Linblad B, Lind M, Chuter T, Ivnacec K. Superior mesenteric artery occlusion treated with PTA and stent placement. Euro J Vac Endovasc Surg. 1996;11:493–5.
16. Sheeran SR, Murphy TP, Khwaja A, Sussman SK, Hallisey MJ. Stent placement for treatment of mesenteric artery stenoses or occlusions. Vasc Interv Radiol. 1999;10(7):861–7.
17. Chahid T, Alfidja AT, Biard M, et al. Endovascular treatment of chronic mesenteric ischemia: results in 14 patients. Cardiovasc Intervent Radiol. 2004;27(6):637–42.
18. Matsumoto AH, Angle JF, Spinosa DJ, Hagspiel KD, Cage DL, Leung DA, Kern JA, Tribble CG. Percutaneous transluminal angioplasty and stenting in the treatment of chronic mesenteric ischemia: results and long-term follow up. J Am Coll Surg. 2002;194:S22–31.

19. Sharafuddin MJ, Olson CH, Sun S, Kresowik TF, Corson JD. Endovascular treatment of celiac and mesenteric arteries stenoses: applications and results. J Vasc Surg. 2003;38:692–8.
20. Jimenez JG, Huber TS, Ozaki CK, Flynn TC, Berceli SA, Lee WA, Seeger JM. Durability of antegrade synthetic aortomesenteric bypass for chronic mesenteric ischemia. J Vasc Surg. 2002;35(6):1078–84.
21. Kasirajan K, O'Hara PJ, Gray BH, Hertzer NR, Clair DG, Greenberg RK, Krajewski LP, Beven EG, Ouriel K. Chronic mesenteric ischemia: open surgery versus percutaneous angioplasty and stenting. J Vasc Surg. 2001;33(1):63–71.
22. Atkins MD, Kwolek CJ, LaMuraglia GM, Brewster DC, Chung TK, Cambria RP. Surgical revascularization versus endovascular therapy for chronic mesenteric ischemia: a comparative experience. J Vasc Surg. 2007;45(6):1162–71.
23. Oderich GS, Bower TC, Sullivan TM, et al. Open versus endovascular revascularization for chronic mesenteric ischemia: risk-stratified outcomes. J Vasc Surg. 2009;49(6):1472–9.
24. Sarac TP, Altinel O, Kashyap VS, Bena J, Lyden S, Srivastava S, Eagleton M, Clair D. Endovascular treatment of stenotic and occluded visceral arteries for chronic mesenteric ischemia. J Vasc Surg. 2008;47:485–91.
25. Peck MA, Conrad MF, Kwolek CJ, LaMuraglia GM, Paruchuri V, Cambria RP. Intermediate-term outcomes of endovascular treatment for symptomatic chronic mesenteric ischemia. J Vasc Surg. 2010;51:140–7.
26. Turba UC, Saad WE, Arslan B, Sabri SS, Trotter S, Angle JF, Hagspiel KD, Kern JA, Cherry KJ, Matsumoto AH. Chronic mesenteric ischaemia: 28-year experience of endovascular treatment. Eur Radiol. 2012;22:1372–84.
27. AbuRahma AF, Campbell JE, Stone PA, Hass SM, Mousa AY, Srivastava M, Nanjundappa A, Dean S, Keiffer T. Perioperative and late clinical outcomes of percutaneous transluminal stentings of the celiac and superior mesenteric arteries over the past decade. J Vasc Surg. 2013;57:1052–61.
28. Oderich GS, Erdoes LS, LeSar C, Mendes BC, Gloviczki P, Cha S, Duncan AA, Bower TC. Comparison of covered stents versus bare metal stents for treatment of chronic atherosclerotic mesenteric arterial disease. J Vasc Surg. 2013;58:1316–24.

Part III
Acute Mesenteric Ischemia

Chapter 15
Clinical Presentation, Etiology, and Diagnostic Considerations

Ramoncito A. David, Young Erben, and Manju Kalra

Introduction and History

Acute mesenteric ischemia (AMI) was first described by Antonio Benivieni, a Florentine physician who is known for his work, *De Abditis Morborum Causis* (*The Hidden Causes of Disease*), which describes his discoveries as a pioneer in postmortem dissection. The first successful treatment of AMI is attributed to Elliott, who successfully resected infarcted bowel from a patient with AMI in 1895. Following this, further progress in management leading to an improvement in outcomes was extremely slow. The next breakthroughs did not occur until 1950 when Klass performed the first superior mesenteric artery (SMA) embolectomy and 1980 when Furrer performed the first percutaneous angioplasty of the SMA. Today, AMI continues to be an uncommon clinical problem, comprising 1–2 per 1,000 hospital admissions [1] and remains an extremely challenging clinical problem to diagnose. The mortality rate of AMI has declined very modestly from 80–90 % in the 1970s to 60–70 % in the 1980s and 1990s. This improvement in outcomes is likely attributable to a higher index of suspicion among clinicians, advances in radiographic diagnosis, and an aggressive surgical approach with better perioperative care [2, 3]. Over the last decade, endovascular surgery has been touted as the preferred treatment for chronic and, to some extent, acute mesenteric ischemia due to the obvious advantages of a minimally invasive approach [4–9]. The major drawback of relying solely on an endovascular strategy is the lack of widespread availability and a

R.A. David, MD • Y. Erben, MD
Division of Vascular and Endovascular Surgery, Department of Surgery, Mayo Clinic, Rochester, MN, USA
e-mail: David.ramoncito@mayo.edu; erben.young@mayo.edu

M. Kalra, MBBS (✉)
Professor of Surgery, Division of Vascular and Endovascular Surgery, Department of Surgery, Mayo Clinic, Rochester, MN, USA
e-mail: kalra.manju@mayo.edu

G.S. Oderich (ed.), *Mesenteric Vascular Disease*,
DOI 10.1007/978-1-4939-1847-8_15

potential delay in assessment of intestinal viability. Too often, AMI is suspected only when peritoneal signs are found in conjunction with leukocytosis and acidosis, leading to delayed diagnosis, septic shock, multisystem organ failure, death, or short gut syndrome secondary to extensive resection of infarcted bowel [10].

Etiology

Most patients present in their sixth or seventh decade of life and often have significant predisposing factors and concomitant medical comorbidities. From most to least common, the causes of AMI include arterial embolism, arterial thrombosis, nonocclusive mesenteric ischemia (NOMI), and mesenteric venous thrombosis (MVT) [11]. The major risk factors and presentation of patients with AMI differ depending on the etiology of the patient's ischemia (Table 15.1). Arterial embolism is often associated with arrhythmia (atrial fibrillation or atrial flutter), recent myocardial infarction, cardiomyopathy, congestive heart failure, ventricular aneurysm, rheumatic valve disease, thoracic aortic thrombus, and/or peripheral arterial embolic disease. Given the acute nature of an embolic occlusion, this will often present with abrupt onset of severe abdominal pain. In contrast, a history of postprandial abdominal pain, anorexia, and weight loss over a period of months with insidious progression to severe abdominal pain is more suggestive of acute or chronic mesenteric arterial thrombosis. This slower progression of disease allows for more collateral vasculature to develop, which would explain the better prognosis for AMI patients with arterial thrombosis versus arterial embolism [12]. The highest mortality rates

Table 15.1 Major risk factors and presentation of AMI differ depending on etiology

Etiology	Presentation	Risk factors
Arterial embolism	Acute catastrophe	Arrhythmia
		MI/cardiomyopathy
		Ventricular aneurysm
		Rheumatic valve disease
		Thoracic aortic thrombus
Arterial thrombosis	Acute/insidious, progressive	Atherosclerosis
		Prolonged hypotension
		Hypovolemia
		Hypercoagulable state
Nonocclusive mesenteric ischemia	Acute/subacute	Hypovolemia/hypotension
		Low cardiac output state
		Alpha-adrenergic agonists, digoxin
Mesenteric venous thrombosis	Subacute	Hypercoagulable state
		Malignancy
		Inflammatory bowel disease
		H/O DVT

in patients with AMI are seen in patients with NOMI. This entity is often seen in critically ill patients who have had recent episodes of severe hypotension causing ischemic insult to the bowel. Other risk factors include hypovolemia, hypotension, low cardiac output, and recent use of alpha-adrenergic agonists or digoxin. Patients at highest risk for NOMI include cardiac surgery and hemodialysis patients, a population that is also at highest risk for multisystem organ failure. Lastly, MVT is a rare cause of AMI that is seen in patients with a hypercoagulable state, malignancy, or inflammatory bowel disease. Smoking was also found to be a strong risk factor for MVT and is likely a risk factor for all forms of AMI [13]. These patients often present with fever, abdominal pain, distention, nausea, vomiting, and bloody stools. An abnormal D-dimer level, while nonspecific, is almost always seen in patients with MVT.

Clinical Presentation

The hallmark of clinical presentation of a patient with AMI is abrupt onset, severe, nonlocalized abdominal pain out of proportion to physical signs; however, a more subacute/chronic presentation may be seen in patients with atherosclerotic disease of the mesenteric vessels. In some patients, there may be a total lack of physical findings in the early stages. Identifying risk factors and important clues in the clinical history is extremely important and can help make a timely diagnosis. Postprandial pain, unintentional weight loss, and food fear are all symptoms of chronic mesenteric ischemia which can progress to acute on chronic mesenteric ischemia. Patients may also present with a recent history of gastrointestinal issues including treatment of a small bowel obstruction or persistent abdominal discomfort after undergoing a cholecystectomy within the past year. Other associated complications that should be considered include ileus, peritonitis, pancreatitis, and GI bleeding that may mask the underlying AMI. A delay in diagnosis and treatment will invariably lead to bowel ischemia which can then develop into irreversible bowel necrosis, multisystem organ failure, and death.

Diagnostic Considerations and Imaging Studies

Once the diagnosis of AMI is suspected, it is often only confirmed with radiographic or intraoperative findings. Laboratory findings are nonspecific in the early stages of AMI and are for the most part noncontributory in making the diagnosis. By the time a patient is found to have leukocytosis, metabolic acidosis, elevated amylase levels, elevated liver function tests, or elevated lactate levels, the patient will have already developed bowel ischemia with frank peritonitis manifested as rebound tenderness and abdominal guarding on exam. In an experimental rat model, it has been suggested that the D-dimer level obtained two hours after an insult may correlate with the presence of AMI [14]. Further, plasma and urine levels of intestinal fatty acid-binding protein (FABP) have also been linked to bowel infarction in humans and have been suggested as tools in the early diagnosis of AMI [15–18].

Historically, *plain X-rays* of the abdomen were used to rule out other causes of acute abdomen, but in contemporary practice, these are of little use in making decisions regarding the definitive management of AMI. *Computerized tomographic angiography (CTA)* with intravenous contrast is now widely available and has replaced mesenteric arteriography as the definitive diagnostic tool in contemporary practice [19, 20]. It is a fast, effective, and noninvasive way to rule out more common causes of acute abdomen, confirm the diagnosis of AMI, and potentially identify the etiology [21]. In a patient that is stable, computerized tomographic angiography (CTA) has become the standard of care in diagnosing and guiding the treatment of AMI.

Mesenteric angiography was previously considered the "gold standard" due to the possibility of being both diagnostic and therapeutic. Its role has diminished as less invasive tests such as duplex ultrasonography, magnetic resonance angiography (MRA), and CTA have continued to improve in quality and availability. Over the past decade, the use of mesenteric angiography in the management of acute mesenteric ischemia in our experience decreased from 97 to 53 % of cases. Concomitantly, there was a rise in the use of CTA and MRA from 55 to 88 % and 12 to 33 %, respectively [22]. A major disadvantage of mesenteric angiography is that it can cause a delay in heparinization and definitive treatment of a patient presenting with severe AMI. Angiography is now indicated mostly in the treatment of in situ mesenteric arterial thrombosis with angioplasty with or without stenting, injection of intra-arterial vasodilators, thrombolysis, and aspiration thrombectomy. As a diagnostic modality, it may still be useful in select patients with extensive calcification, small vessels, or prior stents in place resulting in suboptimal imaging quality with noninvasive tests.

Duplex ultrasonography is an effective screening test for patients presenting with symptoms of chronic mesenteric ischemia. For example, if a patient presenting with subacute postprandial abdominal pain has a good quality duplex study with negative findings, the diagnosis of mesenteric ischemia can be ruled out. One study showed that duplex ultrasonography can be relatively reliable in identifying a greater than 50 % stenosis in the mesenteric vessels with a sensitivity, specificity, and accuracy of 93, 100, and 95 %, respectively, for the celiac trunk and 90, 91, and 91 %, respectively, for the SMA [23]. In order to obtain the most optimal images with duplex ultrasonography, patients are asked to undergo a 6–8-h fast prior to the test. Thus, in an acute setting, duplex is not often useful because abdominal tenderness and gaseous bowel distension impede the ultrasound technologist's ability to visualize the mesenteric vessels. In addition to being heavily operator dependent, the patient's body habitus can greatly affect the quality of the images obtained.

Gadolinium-enhanced magnetic resonance imaging (MRA) is another option for imaging of the mesenteric vessels as well as the surrounding viscera. It was previously the preferred mode of imaging for patients with chronic kidney disease; however, more recent reports of gadolinium-related systemic fibrosis have curtailed its use in these patients. Nevertheless, it is a reliable imaging modality for identifying stenosis in the visceral vessels with a sensitivity of 92 %, specificity of 84 %, PPV of 65 %, NPV of 97 %, and accuracy of 86 % [24]. When compared with CTA, the main advantage of MRA is that the patient is not exposed to ionizing radiation. The drawbacks of MRA include lower spatial resolution and potential artifacts from previously placed stents which can limit its ability to identify clinically relevant mesenteric vessel stenosis [25]. Furthermore, longer acquisition times and limited availability make MRA a less practical option for patients presenting acutely with mesenteric ischemia.

Computerized tomography angiography (CTA) with intravenous iodinated contrast has many of the same advantages of the other noninvasive studies discussed but is a more effective test for ruling out other common causes of acute abdomen, confirming the diagnosis, and potentially identifying the etiology of AMI [26]. CTA has become more widely available and is now the standard of care as the definitive diagnostic tool in contemporary practice [27, 28]. In one study comparing duplex ultrasonography, CTA, and MRA to conventional angiography, CTA was found to have the highest mean image quality and concordance rate with findings on digital subtraction angiography. Sensitivity, specificity, positive predictive value (PPV), negative predictive value (NPV), and accuracy for identifying a relevant stenosis in the celiac trunk (defined as greater than 50 % in this study) were highest for CTA with 100, 95, 86, 100, and 96 %, respectively [24]. In addition, CTA may also assist in identifying the etiology of mesenteric ischemia and in planning an appropriate intervention. With this in mind, a biphasic scan with arterial and venous phase would be the optimal study for discerning between mesenteric arterial occlusion and venous thrombosis. While the arterial phase may reveal arterial flow disruption secondary to thrombosis, embolus, dissection, or an aneurysm, the venous phase would be needed to show venous thrombosis. Regardless of findings, all patients diagnosed with AMI on CTA should receive appropriate resuscitation with intravenous fluids and broad-spectrum antibiotics simultaneously. Further course of treatment is guided by the etiology identified and the acuity of presentation.

Overview of Management by Etiology

Critical patients with suspicion of acutely ischemic bowel or signs of peritonitis should be taken to the operating room directly for exploratory laparotomy regardless of the underlying etiology. Bowel viability is assessed at exploration, nonviable bowel is resected, equivocally viable bowel is preserved, and the causative pathology of AMI is addressed. This is performed simultaneously with resuscitation with IV fluids and antibiotics.

Noncritical patients with slower symptom progression and no peritoneal signs should be treated with initial mesenteric revascularization by endovascular means, surgical intervention, or systemic anticoagulation based on the etiology of AMI identified. Subsequently the ischemic bowel can be addressed with close observation, laparoscopy, or laparotomy depending on outcome and progression.

Arterial Embolism

Arterial embolism is the most common etiology of AMI and accounts for 40–50 % of patients with AMI. The thrombus usually originates in the heart of a patient with atrial fibrillation, recent myocardial infarction, congestive heart failure, left ventricular aneurysm, or valvular heart disease and lodges in the superior mesenteric artery (SMA) a few centimeters distal to the orifice near the origin of the middle colic artery. On CTA the proximal SMA is often patent and without calcification with a filling defect seen at the site of the embolus (Fig. 15.1). Thus, the affected area of bowel is often limited to the distribution of the occluded vessel with clear demarcation that will often spare the proximal jejunum. Bowel wall findings on CTA may include increased thickening, dilatation, and attenuation. Pneumatosis intestinalis, portal venous air, mesenteric edema, and ascites are other CTA findings associated with bowel ischemia. At exploratory laparotomy, the entire bowel is inspected carefully. Visual inspection of normal color and peristalsis alone is sometimes misleading and other modalities to assess bowel viability include palpable pulses in the mesentery, dopplerable arterial signals on the antimesenteric border of the bowel, bleeding from the cut ends, inspection for perfusion under a Wood's lamp after fluoroscein injection, surface oximetry, and laser tissue flowmetry [29]. Balloon catheter thromboembolectomy is performed with removal of the thrombus from the SMA, and flow is restored to the bowel. Segments of obviously necrotic bowel are resected, and bowel continuity is restored only after revascularization is

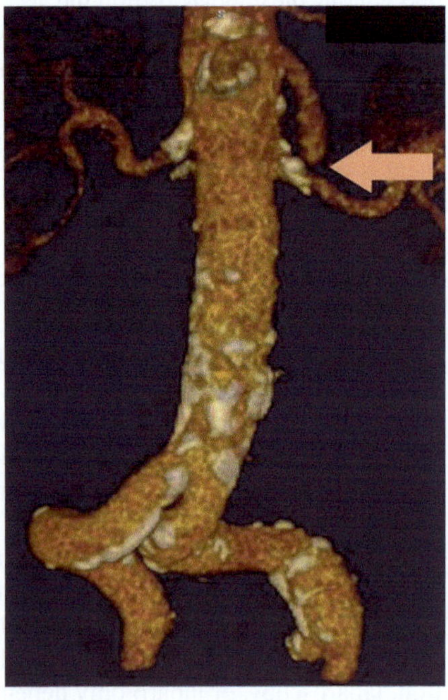

Fig. 15.1 Three-dimensional reconstruction of a CT angiogram demonstrating an occlusive acute arterial embolus in the SMA

completed and vascularity of the ends has been determined to be satisfactory. In most instances, it is prudent to preserve all equivocal segments of bowel for reassessment at a second look laparotomy in 24–48 h.

Acute Arterial Thrombosis

Acute arterial thrombosis superimposed on preexisting severe atherosclerotic disease and preexisting mesenteric arterial stenoses is the second most common cause of AMI, accounting for 25–30 % of cases [30]. Prior symptoms of chronic mesenteric ischemia can be elicited in 25–50 % of patients. Patients frequently present with a slower progression of symptoms, and the acuity and severity of the situation depend on the extent of preexisting arterial stenoses and degree of collateralization. Bowel infarction is more insidious in onset because extensive collaterals are able to maintain viability until there is final closure of a critically stenotic vessel or collateral. In fact, the natural history of mesenteric artery stenosis in the general population is benign, as described by Wilson et al. [31]. Asymptomatic mesenteric artery stenosis is not associated with either death or adverse cardiovascular events unless there is a history of prior bowel resection, which could result in loss of collaterals. As with arterial embolism, severely symptomatic patients with an acute abdomen should be taken directly to the operating room with the same strategy outlined above. Patients stable enough to undergo a CTA should have the study done; in acute mesenteric arterial thrombosis this will usually reveal ostial SMA occlusion in a calcified artery. In this setting, there is no sparing of the proximal jejunum, because the thrombosis extends to the origin of the SMA and across the proximal jejunal branches (Fig. 15.2). In the patients presenting with subacute symptoms and well-developed collateral vessels on CTA, mesenteric arteriography with stenting of the SMA is a viable option with potentially lower morbidity and mortality [4]. This approach is less optimal in severely symptomatic AMI patients due to the unavoidable delay in assessment of the bowel for possible necrosis. Intraoperative mesenteric bypass or retrograde stenting of the SMA during laparotomy are viable options in this situation, the latter being easier and superior especially when bowel resection is necessary [32, 33].

Nonocclusive Mesenteric Ischemia

Nonocclusive mesenteric ischemia (NOMI) is characterized by hypoperfusion of the mesenteric vessels without occlusion of the arteries, and it comprises 20–30 % of cases of AMI. NOMI is associated with the highest mortality rates due to associated comorbidities, incomplete understanding of the pathophysiology, and, commonly, a delay in diagnosis. Tolerance to ischemia of the intestine is limited and becomes critical after 3–6 h. In the early stage of NOMI, the intestinal mucosa is not

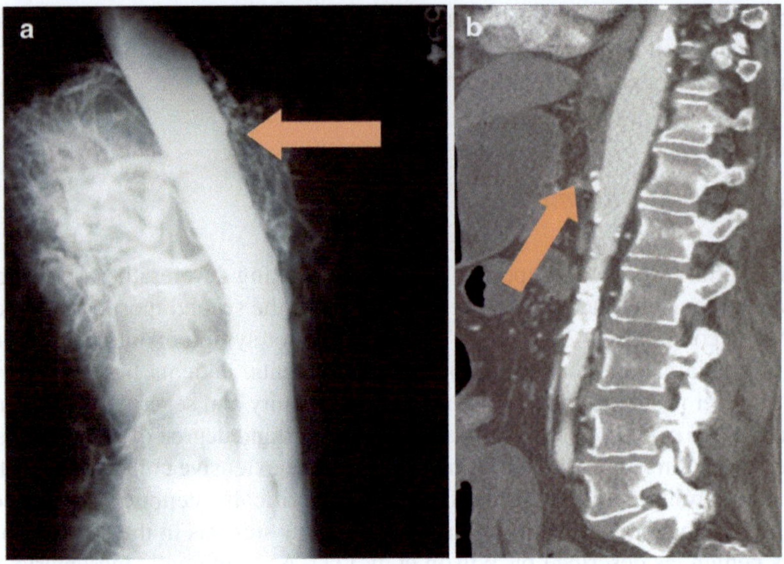

Fig. 15.2 (**a**) Mesenteric angiogram demonstrating occlusion of the SMA at its origin. (**b**) Sagittal cut of a CT angiogram showing acute arterial thrombosis at the origin of the SMA

yet necrotic, so reperfusion is the primary therapeutic option. The most common causes of NOMI are cardiac disease, shock, septicemia, dehydration, and hypotension following dialysis and any other major surgery [34]. A high index of suspicion is essential to improve outcomes as no diagnostic evaluation can confirm the diagnosis. At most, CTA can be used to rule out proximal SMA occlusion and other abdominal pathology [35]. When a low-flow state is suspected, the patient should be taken to angiography. Selective SMA arteriography will often reveal spasm and low flow with a "chain of sausages" appearance (Fig. 15.3). Treatment is with intra-arterial papaverine infusion until relief of symptoms or confirmation of relief of spasm on repeat arteriography is seen. Avoidance of vasopressors and aggressive management of the underlying pathology is paramount in addressing all of the complications from the low-flow state. Laparotomy and bowel assessment are recommended if peritoneal signs develop and bowel viability is suspected.

Mesenteric Venous Thrombosis

Mesenteric venous thrombosis (MVT) comprises 6–9 % of all cases of AMI. MVT still carries a significant mortality and may be either primary or secondary to other conditions such as cancer, hypercoagulable states, abdominal trauma or surgery,

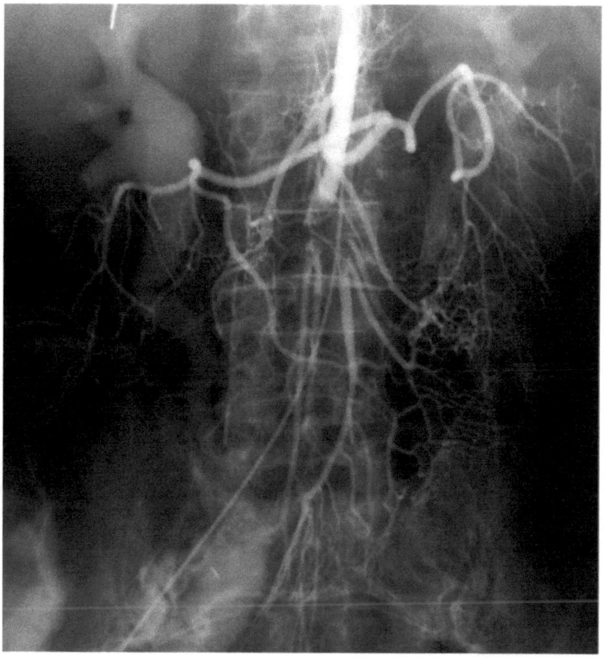

Fig. 15.3 Mesenteric angiogram demonstrating "chain of sausages" appearance of nonocclusive mesenteric ischemia

polycythemia, trauma, pancreatitis, and inflammatory bowel disease [36, 37]. Mesenteric venous thrombosis impairs venous return from the bowel, resulting in venous engorgement and ischemia. With abrupt occlusion of mesenteric veins, transmural bowel infarction may occur. The transition from normal to ischemic bowel is gradual, and arterial spasm secondary to venous engorgement may occur with resulting irreversible bowel ischemia. CTA findings may include venous engorgement or a "target sign" in the superior mesenteric vein, which is described as a thrombus in the center of the lumen surrounded by contrast peripherally (Fig. 15.4). Systemic anticoagulation is the treatment of choice and leads to an improvement in the majority of patients. The goals of treatment are to prevent extension of the thrombus and intestinal infarction in the short term and to prevent recurrent of thrombosis in the long term. Anticoagulation in the form of heparin should be administered as soon as the diagnosis is made. Once improvement is noted and invasive procedures no longer likely, warfarin therapy is initiated. Surgery, endovenous treatment, thrombectomy, and thrombolysis have not proved to be advantageous when attempted [38]. The duration of anticoagulation is about six months for patients with known reversible conditions but lifelong in patients with prothrombotic states and without any identifiable etiology. Anticoagulation helps recanalize the thrombosed vein [39]. Laparotomy is performed in cases with suspected bowel infarction.

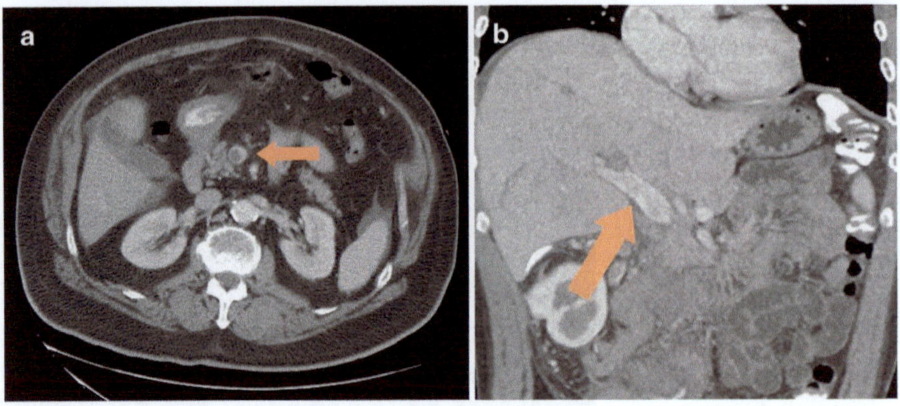

Fig. 15.4 CT venogram of mesenteric venous thrombosis. (**a**) Axial image demonstrating the "target sign" appearance of a nonocclusive thrombus within the superior mesenteric vein. (**b**) Coronal image demonstrating propagation of the thrombus into the portal vein

References

1. Stoney RJ, Cunningham CG. Acute mesenteric ischemia. Surgery. 1993;114(3):489–90.
2. Kougias P, et al. Determinants of mortality and treatment outcome following surgical interventions for acute mesenteric ischemia. J Vasc Surg. 2007;46(3):467–74.
3. Mamode N, Pickford I, Leiberman P. Failure to improve outcome in acute mesenteric ischaemia: seven year review. Eur J Surg. 1999;165(3):203–8.
4. Arthurs ZM, et al. A comparison of endovascular revascularization with traditional therapy for the treatment of acute mesenteric ischemia. J Vasc Surg. 2011;53(3):698–705.
5. Schermerhorn ML, et al. Mesenteric revascularization: management and outcomes in the United States, 1988–2006. J Vasc Surg. 2009;50(2):341–8. e1.
6. Oderich GS, et al. Open versus endovascular revascularization for chronic mesenteric ischemia: risk-stratified outcomes. J Vasc Surg. 2009;49(6):1472–9. e3.
7. Kasirajan K, et al. Chronic mesenteric ischemia: open surgery versus percutaneous angioplasty and stenting. J Vasc Surg. 2001;33(1):63–71.
8. Atkins MD, et al. Surgical revascularization versus endovascular therapy for chronic mesenteric ischemia: a comparative experience. J Vasc Surg. 2007;45(6):1162–71.
9. Peck MA, et al. Intermediate-term outcomes of endovascular treatment for symptomatic chronic mesenteric ischemia. J Vasc Surg. 2010;51(1):140 e1-2–7 e1-2.
10. Klempnauer J, et al. Long-term results after surgery for acute mesenteric ischemia. Surgery. 1997;121(3):239–43.
11. Oldenburg WA, et al. Acute mesenteric ischemia: a clinical review. Arch Intern Med. 2004; 164(10):1054–62.
12. Lock G. Acute intestinal ischaemia. Best Pract Res Clin Gastroenterol. 2001;15:83–98.
13. Al-Thani H, El-Mabrok J, El-Menyar A, Al-Sulaiti M, Tabeb AH, Hajaji K, Elgohary H, Asim M, Latifi R. Clinical presentation and outcome of mesenteric vein thrombosis: a single-center experience. Angiology. 2014 [Epub ahead of print].
14. Kurt Y, et al. D-dimer in the early diagnosis of acute mesenteric ischemia secondary to arterial occlusion in rats. Eur Surg Res (Europaische chirurgische Forschung Recherches chirurgicales europeennes). 2005;37(4):216–9.
15. Gollin G, Marks C, Marks WH. Intestinal fatty acid binding protein in serum and urine reflects early ischemic injury to the small bowel. Surgery. 1993;113(5):545–51.

16. Kanda T, et al. Intestinal fatty acid-binding protein is a useful diagnostic marker for mesenteric infarction in humans. Gastroenterology. 1996;110(2):339–43.
17. Thuijls G, et al. Early diagnosis of intestinal ischemia using urinary and plasma fatty acid binding proteins. Ann Surg. 2011;253(2):303–8.
18. Acosta S, Nilsson T. Current status on plasma biomarkers for acute mesenteric ischemia. J Thromb Thrombolysis. 2012;33(4):355–61.
19. Rastan AJ, Tillmann E, Subramanian S, Lehmkuhl L, Funkat AK, Leontyev S, et al. Visceral arterial compromise during intra-aortic balloon counterpulsation therapy. Circulation. 2010;122:S92–9.
20. Hechtman JF, Lento PA. Scordi-bello I, Ischemic bowel due to embolization from an isolated mobile thrombus of the ascending aorta: a case report and review of the literature. J Thromb Thrombolysis. 2011;32:238–41.
21. Zhang WW, Kulaylat MN, Anain PM, Dosluoglu HH, Harris LM, Cherr GS, Dayton MT, Dryjski ML. Embolization as cause of bowel ischemia after endovascular abdominal aortic aneurysm repair. J Vasc Surg. 2004;40:867–72.
22. Ryer EJ, et al. Revascularization for acute mesenteric ischemia. J Vasc Surg. 2012;55(6): 1682–9.
23. Zwolak RM, Fillinger MF, Walsh DB, et al. Mesenteric and celiac duplex scanning: a validation study. J Vasc Surg. 1998;27:1078–87.
24. Schaefer P, et al. Comparison of noninvasive imaging modalities for stenosis grading in mesenteric arteries. Rofo. 2013;185(7):628–34.
25. Shih MC, Angle JF, Leung DA, et al. CTA and MRA in mesenteric ischemia: part 2, normal findings and complications after surgical and endovascular treatment. Am J Roentgenol. 2007;188:462–71.
26. Furukawa A, et al. CT diagnosis of acute mesenteric ischemia from various causes. Am J Roentgenol. 2009;192(2):408–16.
27. Ofer A, et al. Multidetector CT angiography in the evaluation of acute mesenteric ischemia. Eur Radiol. 2009;19(1):24–30.
28. Aschoff AJ, et al. Evaluation of acute mesenteric ischemia: accuracy of biphasic mesenteric multi-detector CT angiography. Abdom Imaging. 2009;34(3):345–57.
29. Ballard JL, et al. A critical analysis of adjuvant techniques used to assess bowel viability in acute mesenteric ischemia. Am Surgeon. 1993;59(5):309–11.
30. Mansour MA. Management of acute mesenteric ischemia. Arch Surg. 1999;134(3):328–30; discussion 331.
31. Wilson DB, et al. Clinical course of mesenteric artery stenosis in elderly americans. Arch Intern Med. 2006;166(19):2095–100.
32. Wyers MC, et al. Retrograde mesenteric stenting during laparotomy for acute occlusive mesenteric ischemia. J Vasc Surg. 2007;45(2):269–75.
33. Sonesson B, et al. Hybrid recanalization of superior mesenteric artery occlusion in acute mesenteric ischemia. J Endovas Ther (An Official Journal of the International Society of Endovascular Specialists). 2008;15(1):129–32.
34. Trompeter M, et al. Non-occlusive mesenteric ischemia: etiology, diagnosis, and interventional therapy. Eur Radiol. 2002;12(5):1179–87.
35. Bailey RW, et al. Protection of the small intestine from nonocclusive mesenteric ischemic injury due to cardiogenic shock. Am J Surg. 1987;153(1):108–16.
36. Singal AK, Kamath PS, Tefferi A. Mesenteric venous thrombosis. Mayo Clin Proc. 2013; 88(3):285–94.
37. Rhee RY, et al. Mesenteric venous thrombosis: still a lethal disease in the 1990s. J Vasc Surg. 1994;20(5):688–97 [Review] [39 refs].
38. Brunaud L, et al. Acute mesenteric venous thrombosis: case for nonoperative management. J Vasc Surg: Official publication, the Society for Vascular Surgery [and] International Society for Cardiovascular Surgery, North American Chapter. 2001;34(4):673–9.
39. Plessier A, et al. Acute portal vein thrombosis unrelated to cirrhosis: a prospective multicenter follow-up study. Hepatology. 2010;51(1):210–8.

Chapter 16
Technique of Open Mesenteric Catheter Embolectomy

Young Erben and Manju Kalra

The arterial perfusion of the gastrointestinal tract is provided by the celiac, superior mesenteric, and the inferior mesenteric arteries. The celiac artery (CA) supplies arterial blood flow to the foregut, the spleen, and the hepatobiliary system. The superior mesenteric artery (SMA) supplies the jejunum, ileum, and ascending and transverse colon. The inferior mesenteric artery (IMA) supplies the hindgut from the transverse colon to the rectum. Robust collaterals between each vessel (superior and inferior pancreaticoduodenal arteries and arch of Riolan respectively) allow for stenosis and occlusion of one or even two of these main arteries without sequelae in the setting of chronic mesenteric ischemia (CMI), where the mesenteric vasculature has had the time to adapt to the reduced blood flow in the usual antegrade manner (Fig. 16.1). However, sudden occlusion of one of the mesenteric arteries without prior development of the collateral network leads to profound ischemia of the bowel. Acute mesenteric ischemia (AMI) is a surgical emergency with a well-documented high in-hospital mortality between 59 and 93 % [1]. The pathophysiology of the situation leading to compromise of the mesenteric circulation and development of AMI can be arterial embolism, arterial thrombosis, nonocclusive mesenteric ischemia (NOMI), and mesenteric venous thrombosis. The focus of this chapter will be the management of AMI secondary to arterial embolism.

Arterial embolism has been reported as the most common mechanism accounting for 40–50 % of cases of AMI; it accounted for >50 % of cases treated at our institution over the last two decades [2, 3]. The acute takeoff of the SMA from the aorta

Y. Erben, MD
Vascular Surgery Fellow, Division of Vascular and Endovascular Surgery, Department of Surgery, Mayo Clinic, Rochester, MN, USA
e-mail: erben.young@mayo.edu

M. Kalra, MBBS (✉)
Professor of Surgery, Division of Vascular and Endovascular Surgery, Department of Surgery, Mayo Clinic, Rochester, MN, USA
e-mail: Kalra.manju@mayo.edu

G.S. Oderich (ed.), *Mesenteric Vascular Disease*,
DOI 10.1007/978-1-4939-1847-8_16

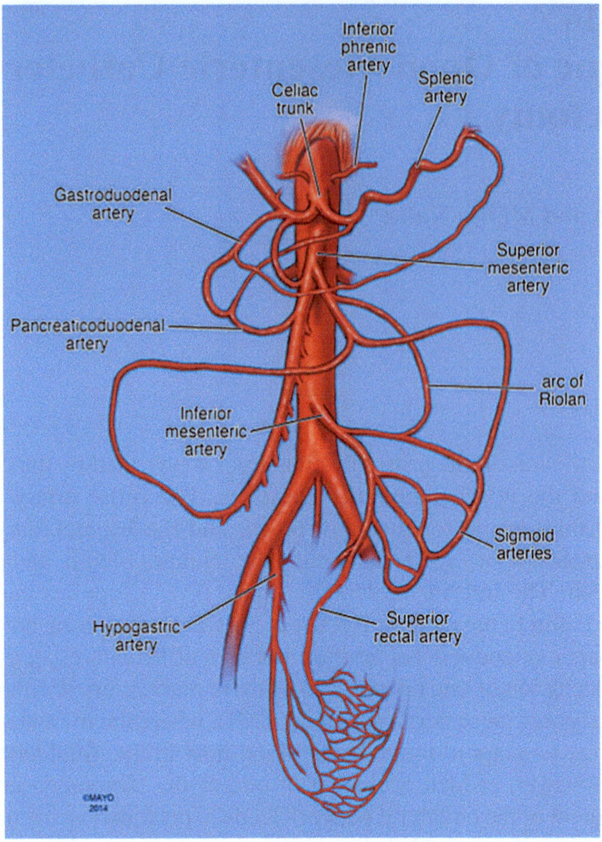

Fig. 16.1 Anatomy of the mesenteric vessels with rich collateral network (By permission of Mayo Foundation for Medical Education and Research. All rights reserved)

makes it the most vulnerable vessel to embolization, most frequently an embolus arising upstream in the arterial circulation, typically the heart or the thoracic aorta. The majority of emboli originate from thrombi in the left atrium in the setting of atrial fibrillation, in the left ventricle secondary to hypokinesis/aneurysm following myocardial infarction or upon cardiac valvular lesions/synthetic valves. The typical patient may have an acute change in his/her cardiac status including an episode of atrial tachyarrhythmia, congestive heart failure, myocardial infarction, ventricular aneurysm, or failure to maintain a therapeutic anticoagulation status with a known chronic tachyarrhythmia [4, 5]. Aortic thromboembolism is a less frequent source of AMI, arising from thrombus atop ulcerative atherosclerotic plaques. It may occur spontaneously; however, the commonest predisposing factor is an endovascular procedure in the aorta (arteriography, intra-aortic balloon placement). It can also occur during open procedures with placement of a high aortic clamp on a diseased, shaggy aorta [6–11].

Diagnosis of Mesenteric Embolism

Patient Population

The hallmark of clinical presentation of a patient with AMI is abrupt onset, severe, nonlocalized "abdominal pain out of proportion to physical signs." Identifying important clues and risk factors in the clinical history can often help make a timely diagnosis. These include: atrial fibrillation (AF), recent myocardial infarction, congestive heart failure, and prior embolic events. Not infrequently anticoagulation is interrupted in an elderly patient with chronic AF for an invasive procedure or due to fall risk [12]. In addition, a history of symptoms suggestive of chronic mesenteric ischemia (postprandial pain, weight loss, "food fear"), previous venous thromboembolic events, hypercoagulable states, and vasopressor therapy can point to a different etiology of the AMI.

Preoperative Testing

There is no laboratory study that confirms the presence of mesenteric ischemia. Furthermore, laboratory findings are often nonspecific and unaltered in the early stages, and delaying diagnostic imaging till results of laboratory tests are available in a suspected patient significantly decreases survival [13]. In the later stages, there is evidence of hemoconcentration from sequestration of fluid in the bowel wall including leukocytosis and elevated serum lactate and amylase. By the time these occur, there has usually already been compromise of bowel viability. Experimentally in a rat model, it has been suggested that the D-dimer level after two hours from insult may correlate with the presence of AMI [14]. Further, plasma and urine levels of intestinal fatty acid-binding protein (FABP) have been linked to bowel infarction and have been suggested as tools in the early diagnosis of AMI [15–17].

Preoperative Imaging

Computed tomography angiography (CTA) with intravenous contrast is now widely available and has replaced mesenteric arteriography as the definitive diagnostic tool in contemporary practice [18, 19]. It is a fast, effective, and noninvasive way to rule out commoner causes of acute abdomen, confirm the diagnosis of AMI, and potentially identify the etiology [20]. In addition, CTA differentiates between *acute mesenteric thrombosis* when an ostial occlusion of a calcified SMA is usually seen and *acute arterial embolism* when a more distal SMA occlusion of a noncalcified SMA is demonstrated. Typically emboli lodge at a branch point in the vascular tree, usually 1–2 cm distal to the origin of the vessel, most often at the takeoff of the middle colic artery branch, which results in the typical sparing of the proximal

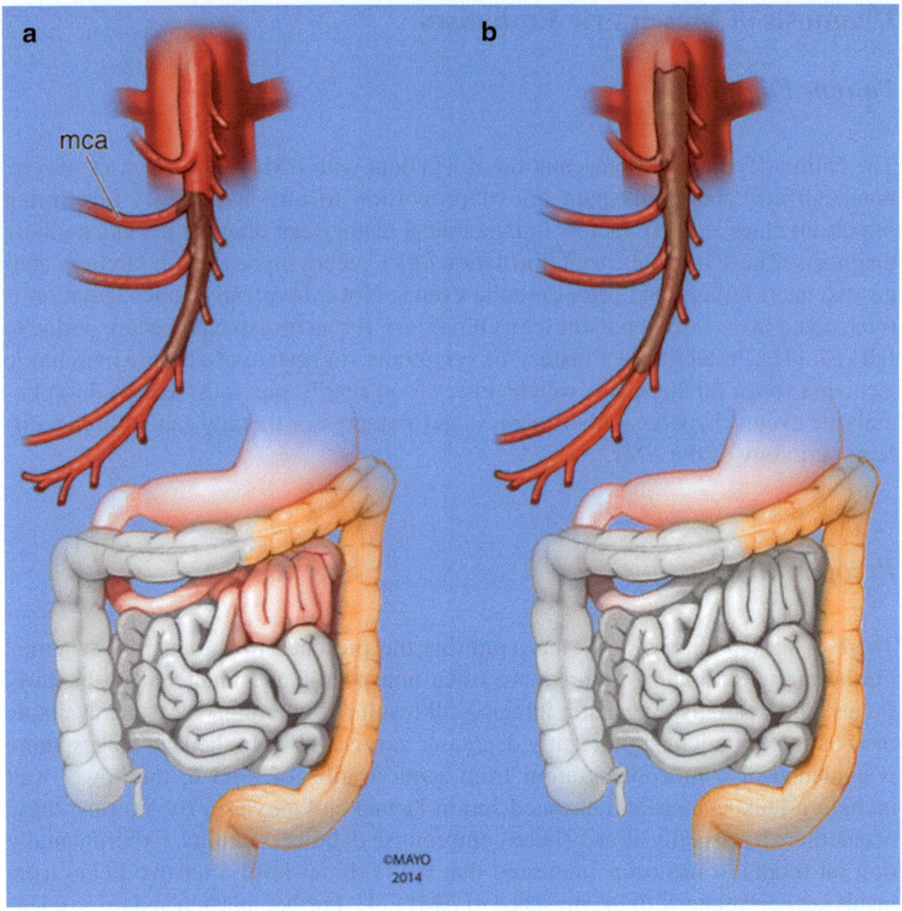

Fig. 16.2 Diagrammatic representation of typical location of embolic (**a**) and thrombotic (**b**) occlusion of the SMA with corresponding pattern of extent of bowel ischemia. (**a**) Embolic occlusion of the SMA at the branching point of the middle colic artery (*mca*). (**b**) In situ thrombosis of the SMA starting at the ostium (By permission of Mayo Foundation for Medical Education and Research. All rights reserved)

jejunum and distal transverse colon (Fig. 16.2). No one CTA finding is diagnostic of AMI; however, a combination of pneumatosis intestinalis, superior mesenteric artery occlusion, portomesenteric venous gas, or portomesenteric venous thrombosis together yields a positive predictive value of 100 % and a negative predictive value of 96 %, respectively. CTA is considered today the gold standard in diagnosis of AMI and should be the one and only imaging study ordered [19, 21].

The role of *mesenteric arteriography*, long held as the "diagnostic gold standard" has evolved to therapeutic indications mostly in the treatment of in situ mesenteric arterial thrombosis with angioplasty with or without stenting [2, 22]. Additional applications include injection of intra-arterial vasodilators, thrombolysis, and aspiration thrombectomy [23, 24].

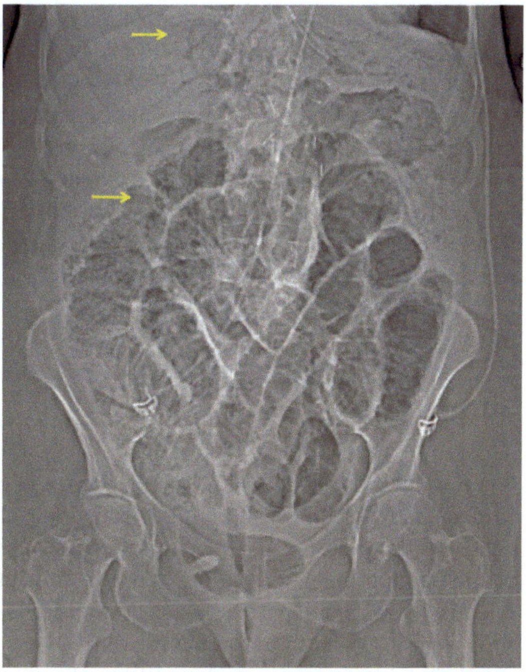

Fig. 16.3 Plain abdominal radiograph with evidence of portal venous gas and pneumatosis intestinalis (*arrow*)

Additional noninvasive imaging modalities traditionally useful in the elective setting do not have a significant role to play in the diagnosis of AMI, where time is of the essence. *Plain abdominal radiography* is usually nondiagnostic; it only demonstrates signs of mesenteric ischemia when the process is very advanced, such as pneumatosis intestinalis and portal venous gas (Fig. 16.3) that herald a very poor prognosis in this setting [25].

Duplex ultrasonography is a very useful screening tool to identify stenosis of the mesenteric vessels in the elective setting [26, 27]. However, it is virtually useless in the acute setting due to poor visualization of the mesenteric vessels as a result of bowel gas from distention combined with significant patient discomfort. Similarly, *magnetic resonance angiography (MRA)* is theoretically appealing because of lack of the potential nephrotoxicity and allergic reaction associated with intravenous iodinated contrast for CTA; however, it is too uncomfortable and time consuming for a patient with significant abdominal pain to provide meaningful visualization of the mesenteric vasculature [28].

Preoperative Considerations

Prompt operative intervention is necessary for the treatment of acute mesenteric ischemia. Ideally, however, resuscitative efforts should be started as soon as the diagnosis is suspected and continued in the operating room. The initial management is threefold, including optimization of oxygen delivery with supplemental oxygen, intubation and mechanical ventilation, and transfusion of red blood cells to achieve a hematocrit of 30 %. Secondly, preservation of intestinal blood flow in the form of dynamic goal-directed fluid resuscitation, systemic heparinization titrated to a partial thromboplastin time of 60–80s and the use of selective vasoactive and inotropic agents to improve cardiac output. Lastly, initiation of treatment of sepsis by administering broad-spectrum antibiotics to treat bacterial translocation [29]. Further, at the time of induction of anesthesia, the patient should undergo adjunctive invasive monitoring including arterial line, central venous line, and Foley catheter placement [4].

Surgical Treatment

Once a diagnosis of AMI has been made, occlusion of the SMA has been confirmed, and the etiology of this occlusion determined, urgent bowel evaluation needs to be undertaken. All patients with suspicion of threatened bowel require prompt abdominal exploration. With the advent of minimally invasive techniques, one might suggest laparoscopy as an option. However, this has been only successfully demonstrated in a porcine model [30]. Sauerland et al. in 2006 clearly delineated that laparoscopy in the setting of an acute abdomen resulting from AMI offers very limited therapeutic benefit. Further, a limited view of the entire abdomen does not guarantee adequate recognition of ischemia [31]. Prior to midline laparotomy, the surgeon should be prepared for multiple modes of treatment of SMA occlusion, including: SMA thromboembolectomy, bypass, or retrograde stenting depending upon the final assessment. The patient should be prepped for possible great saphenous vein harvest (GSV) for an interposition graft/patch angioplasty. During laparotomy, the entire small and large bowel should be evaluated for signs of ischemia, by direct observation and peristalsis, assessment of pulses in the bowel mesentery by Doppler, and/or the use of fluorescein and ultraviolet light (Fig. 16.4) [32]. The latter technique has been reported to have a sensitivity of 96 % and a specificity of 95 % in the recognition of small bowel compromise [33]. It is recommended that revascularization be achieved prior to any bowel resection unless perforation causes significant spillage of enteric contents. Further, any necessitated small bowel resection should be limited to only necrotic segments. All segments with ischemic changes and equivocal viability should be preserved because once revascularization is achieved, these "questionable" bowel segments may recover. In the rare event that the entire small bowel demonstrates necrotic changes as a result of profound ischemia, neither further exploration nor revascularization should be undertaken as complete necrosis of the small bowel is not compatible with meaningful life. The abdomen should be closed and comfort care measures instituted.

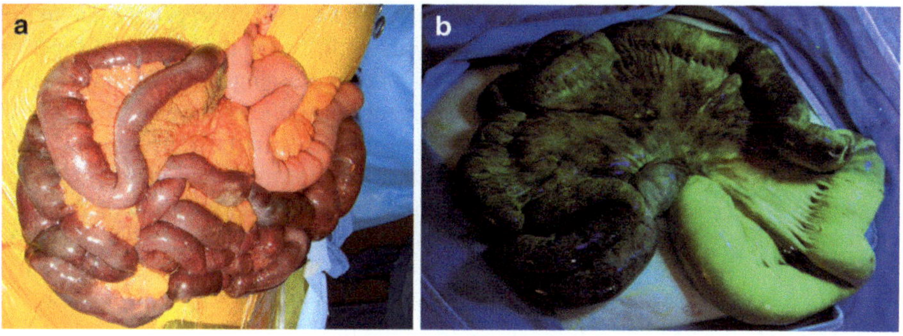

Fig. 16.4 Evaluation of small bowel during abdominal exploration. (**a**) Direct visualization and exploration facilitates the assessment of viability of the small bowel; note the sparing of the proximal jejunum. (**b**) Same patient as in (a). Assessment of the small bowel using fluorescein and ultraviolet light (Wood's lamp)

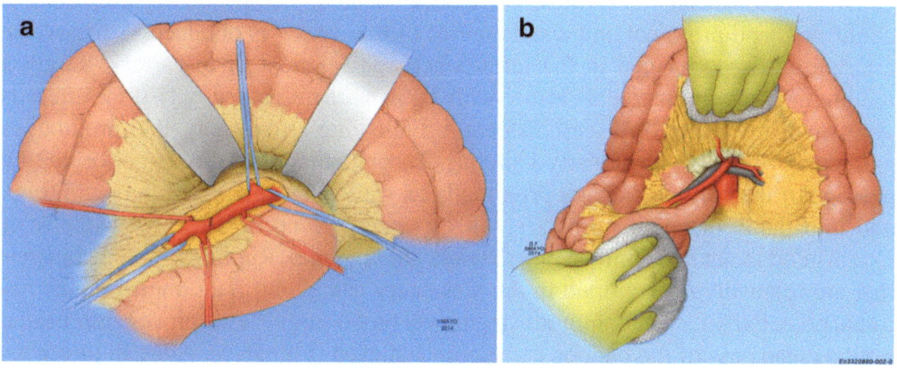

Fig. 16.5 Exposure of the superior mesenteric artery. (**a**) Anterior exposure of superior mesenteric artery. (**b**) Lateral exposure of superior mesenteric artery (By permission of Mayo Foundation for Medical Education and Research. All rights reserved)

Embolectomy of the Superior Mesenteric Artery

Once the bowel has been appropriately addressed, SMA revascularization is undertaken. The SMA can be exposed from an anterior and/or a lateral approach, both being equally effective. The *anterior approach* (Fig. 16.5a) ideally suited for embolectomy is performed through the base of the transverse mesocolon at the root of the mesentery without mobilization of the ligament of Treitz. To expose the main trunk of the SMA, the transverse colon is retracted cephalad and the small bowel caudad, which will allow for palpation of the vessel at the root of the mesentery, along the inferior margin of the pancreas especially if pulsatile or calcified. The peritoneum overlying it is next incised at the base of the transverse mesocolon, and careful dissection is carried down to the artery. It can often be difficult to expose due to the lack of pulsatility and significant mesenteric edema. It lies to the left of the superior mesenteric vein, and multiple small venous tributaries crossing the SMA may require ligation and division to facilitate exposure. The middle colic artery can also serve as a landmark to identify the SMA. It can be identified easily in the transverse mesocolon and traced proximally to its origin from the superior mesenteric artery. Careful dissection is necessary to not damage lymphatics, autonomic nerve fibers, the pancreas superiorly, and the delicate proximal jejunal branches coming off the SMA. If more proximal exposure of this vessel is necessary, this can be judiciously performed by carefully retracting the inferior pancreatic border cephalad. The *lateral approach* (Fig. 16.5b) to the SMA involves taking down the ligament of Treitz and mobilizing the entire small bowel to the right side of the abdomen. This provides access to an adequate length of the main trunk of the artery for direct revascularization without easy access for embolectomy of the distal branches. It is ideally suited for revascularization of the SMA with antegrade bypass from the supraceliac aorta or retrograde bypass from the infrarenal aorta or either iliac artery to treat in situ thrombosis.

Once the SMA and its branches have been isolated, therapeutic heparinization is confirmed, and proximal and distal control of this vessel is obtained. A transverse arteriotomy is performed in the infra-pancreatic segment of the artery. Rarely a longitudinal arteriotomy and closure with a patch are necessary, only if the artery is very small in caliber or diseased/stenotic. Following arteriotomy, the thrombus is extracted with 3–4 mm Fogarty balloons. Thromboembolectomy is performed by passage of the balloon catheter proximally as well as distally down the main trunk and into the branches if necessary, with special care not to force the catheter or overdistend the balloon and disrupt the delicate branches. Rupture of these branches that are relatively unsupported in the mesentery can result in an impressive hematoma, potentially further compromising bowel blood supply. This process is repeated until a clean pass of the balloon catheter is achieved (Fig. 16.6). After all thrombus has been removed, appropriate forward and backward bleeding followed by careful flushing with heparinized saline (10 units of heparin per mL) is performed. The arteriotomy is then closed primarily with interrupted 6–0 Prolene sutures, or with a GSV/bovine pericardium patch, and flow is restored (Fig. 16.7). At this point, reassessment of the bowel is recommended using a handheld Doppler, checking signals along the mesenteric and anti-mesenteric border of the bowel. Once SMA revascularization has been achieved and confirmed, obviously necrotic areas of bowel are resected but bowel continuity is not restored at this stage. Again, all equivocally viable bowel is preserved for reassessment at a later stage, and temporary abdominal closure is performed.

Embolectomy of the Celiac Artery

The CA and its branches are exposed through the lesser sac by opening the gastrohepatic ligament and exposing the area over the aorta just inferior to segments 2 and 3 of the liver (Fig. 16.8). Exposure and embolectomy of the CA is rarely required

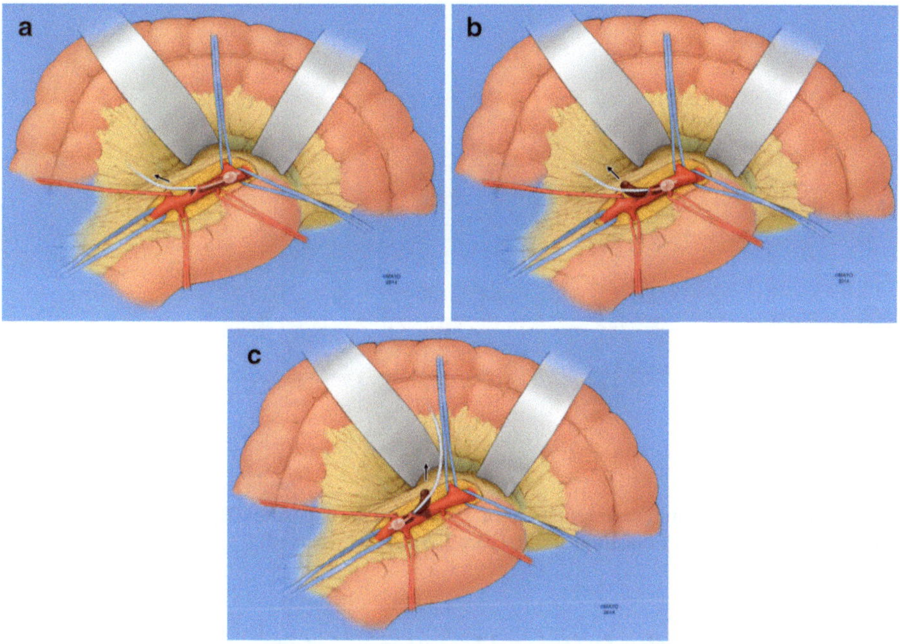

Fig. 16.6 (**a–c**) Balloon catheter embolectomy of the SMA, proximal and distal (By permission of Mayo Foundation for Medical Education and Research. All rights reserved)

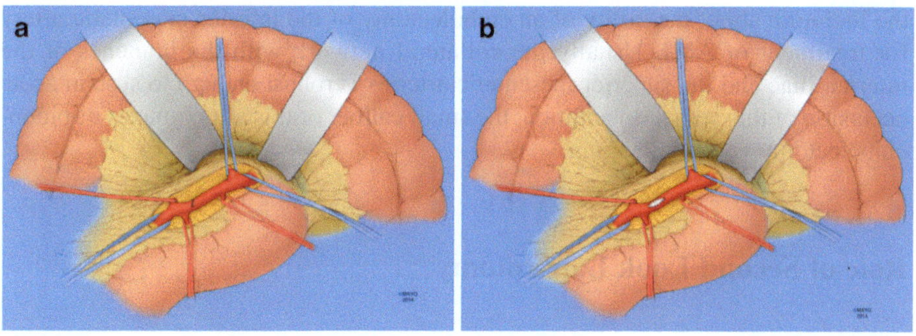

Fig. 16.7 (**a** and **b**) Arteriotomy closure, either primary or using a patch (By permission of Mayo Foundation for Medical Education and Research. All rights reserved)

and has only been reported in the literature as case reports [34]. Luther and colleagues described a case of AMI in whom they noted persistently ischemic liver and stomach following initial embolectomy of the SMA and successful revascularization of the small bowel. The CA was exposed and significant thrombus was noted to be present in all three branches of the artery. Flow to the liver and stomach was reestablished by thrombectomy of the hepatic and left gastric arteries, with only partial thrombectomy of the splenic artery.

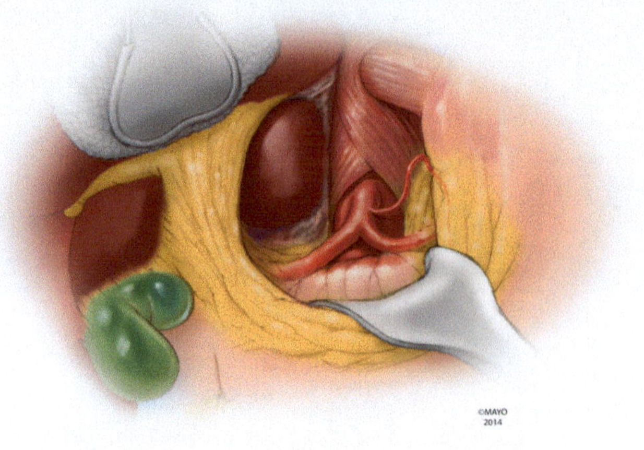

Fig. 16.8 Diagrammatic representation of celiac artery exposure (By permission of Mayo Foundation for Medical Education and Research. All rights reserved)

Embolectomy of the Inferior Mesenteric Artery

The inferior mesenteric artery is located along the anterolateral area of the infrarenal aorta at the base of the left colon mesentery (Fig. 16.9). No data is available in the literature about the utility of an embolectomy of the inferior mesenteric artery for treatment of AMI. Usually the collateral network with the branches of the internal iliac and the superior mesenteric arteries is robust enough to sustain acute occlusion of this vessel. In addition, the small caliber of this artery makes thromboembolectomy very challenging.

Role of Second Look Laparotomy

The benefits of a temporary abdominal closure in an acute situation were initially validated in the trauma literature and subsequently extended for use in the setting of vascular catastrophes [35–37]. These benefits include ability to reassess the small bowel with or without resection after allowing time for hemodynamic resuscitation subsequent to the revascularization. The expeditious "closure" of the abdominal cavity allows for further resuscitation and support of the patient in the intensive care unit with the plan to reanastomose segments of bowel on a different day, as well as the ability to reassess bowel anastomoses in tenuous tissues prior to final abdominal closure. In our experience, the use of this technique has increased in the most recent decade (2000–2010) from 48 to 80 % with concomitant decrease in overall mortality from 27 to 17 % from the previous decade (1990–1999) [2].

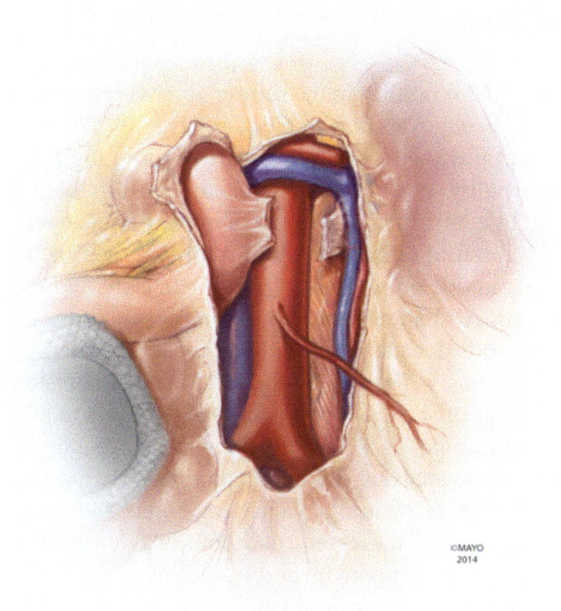

Fig. 16.9 Typical location of inferior mesenteric artery (By permission of Mayo Foundation for Medical Education and Research. All rights reserved)

Other Surgical Options

Recently, alternative treatment of SMA embolus has been described by using percutaneous mechanic-chemical thrombectomy (AngioJet®) and thrombolysis. Ballehaninna and colleagues demonstrated that this noninvasive technique was effective and successful in the treatment of an embolic event in the setting of atrial fibrillation [38]. Initial removal of the thrombus by mechanical thrombectomy (Angiojet®) was complimented with subsequent thrombolysis to treat residual thrombus identified by a filling defect on the angiogram. Complete clearance of this was confirmed on angiogram 24 h later with wide patency of the SMA and no residual stenosis. The obvious advantages of this minimally invasive technique include a lack of a general anesthetic and laparotomy. However, the latter may be a drawback as well in patients with more advanced ischemia as a lack of early bowel assessment could negatively impact outcome. It may be reasonable to defer evaluation of the bowel in patients with more subacute presentation in the setting of AMI secondary to mesenteric thrombosis, however, is almost mandatory in patients with SMA embolism due to the high likelihood of bowel compromise in the absence of preformed collaterals. The technique may be applicable in the setting of SMA embolism in very selective patients with early ischemia and significant medical comorbidities precluding laparotomy.

Surgical Outcomes: Short and Long Term

Overall, morbidity and mortality in the setting of AMI remain high (30–65 %) [39]. Although advances in endovascular techniques have offered a wide variety of potential intervention options that could help improve these high rates of negative outcomes, both morbidity and mortality remain similar between the open and endovascular era. In a retrospective review of our experience with surgically treated AMI secondary to arterial embolism and thrombosis over the last two decades [2, 3], a trend towards improved mortality from 27 to 17 % and morbidity from 73 to 63 % was observed. All patients with SMA embolism underwent laparotomy and thrombectomy in both decades with endovascular intervention being performed only for SMA thrombosis. The one factor that changed between the decades compared was the number of second-look operations (from 48 to 80 %), which aided in the diagnosis of additional 28 % of patients with necrotic bowel requiring further resection. On univariate analysis, factors predicting early mortality were SVS clinical score, serum creatinine, residing in a nursing home, and congestive heart failure. In contrast, having chronic mesenteric ischemia was protective against mortality. Our contemporary results compare favorably with other reports of large tertiary care centers. Three recent series of open revascularization for AMI from large volume centers reported mortality rates of 31–62 % [40–42]. A common theme among these reports, as well as ours, is that advanced age and visceral ischemia are predictors of poor outcome, especially in the older, sicker patients with SMA embolism who continue to be a challenge. The Cleveland Clinic reported their experience with treatment of AMI [43]. Although they adopted an endovascular first approach to patients with SMA thrombosis with significantly lower mortality (36 %) compared to open interventions (50 %), no such benefit was demonstrated in patients with SMA embolism who were mostly treated with laparotomy and thromboembolectomy. Similarly, Schermerhorn and colleagues reported on results of treatment for acute and chronic mesenteric ischemia from the Nationwide Inpatient Sample. The incidence of open surgery in the setting of acute ischemia remained unchanged over a decade (1995–2006) with the number endovascular interventions performed for mesenteric thrombosis gradually increasing. This rise was, however, very modest compared to the explosion in endovascular intervention in the setting of chronic mesenteric ischemia over the same period. The incidence of embolectomy in the setting of open surgery was 49 %, and mortality in these patients was also the highest at 49 %, proportional to the higher incidence of bowel resection (37 %) [44].

AMI with an embolic etiology continues to be a challenging problem. The patients presenting with this problem continue to get older with significant cardiac comorbidities. Regardless, a high index of suspicion, prompt diagnosis, and appropriate expeditious treatment with early assessment of bowel viability regardless of revascularization modality selected remain the keys to improving outcomes of this grave problem. The importance of liberal use of second-look laparotomy cannot be overemphasized.

References

1. Kassahun WT, Schulz T, Richter O, Hauss J. Unchanged high mortality rates from acute occlusive intestinal ischemia: six year review. Langenbecks Arch Surg. 2008;393:163–71.
2. Ryer EJ, Kalra M, Oderich GS, Duncan AA, Gloviczki P, Cha S, et al. Revascularization for acute mesenteric ischemia. J Vasc Surg. 2012;55:1682–9.
3. Park WM, Gloviczki P, Cherry Jr KJ, Hallett Jr JW, Bower TC, Panneton JM, et al. Contemporary management of acute mesenteric ischemia: factors associated with survival. J Vasc Surg. 2002;35:445–52.
4. Cronenwett JL, Johnston KW, editors. Rutherford's vascular surgery. Philadelphia: Saunders; 2010.
5. Wasilewska M, Gosk-Bierska I. Thromboembolism associated with atrial fibrillation as a cause of limb and organ ischemia. Adv Clin Exp Med. 2013;22:865–73.
6. Saric M, Kronzon I. Aortic atherosclerosis and embolic events. Curr Cardiol Rep. 2012; 14:342–9.
7. Rastan AJ, Tillmann E, Subramanian S, Lehmkuhl L, Funkat AK, Leontyev S, et al. Visceral arterial compromise during intra-aortic balloon counterpulsation therapy. Circulation. 2010; 122:S92–9.
8. Hechtman JF, Lento PA, Scordi-bello I. Ischemic bowel due to embolization from an isolated mobile thrombus of the ascending aorta: a case report and review of the literature. J Thromb Thrombolysis. 2011;32:238–41.
9. Zhang WW, Kulaylat MN, Anain PM, Dosluoglu HH, Harris LM, Cherr GS, et al. Embolization as cause of bowel ischemia after endovascular abdominal aortic aneurysm repair. J Vasc Surg. 2004;40:867–72.
10. Jarvinen O, Laurikka J, Sisto T, Tarkka MR. Intestinal ischemia following surgery for aorto-iliac disease. A review of 502 consecutive aortic reconstructions. Vasa. 1996;25:148–55.
11. Pfeifer M, Kogel H. Heymer B [Cholesterol crystal embolization, a rare cause of postoperative ischemic colitis]. Vasa. 1990;19:54–8.
12. Inui TS, Parina R, Chang DC, Coimbra R. Mortality after ground-level fall in the elderly patient taking oral anticoagulation for atrial fibrillation/flutter: a long-term analysis of risk versus benefit. J Trauma Acute Care Surg. 2014;76:642–9; discussion 9–50.
13. Renner P, Kienle K, Dahlke MH, Heiss P, Pfister K, Stroszczynski C, et al. Intestinal ischemia: current treatment concepts. Langenbecks Arch Surg. 2011;396:3–11.
14. Kurt Y, Akin ML, Demirbas S, Uluutku AH, Gulderen M, Avsar K, et al. D-dimer in the early diagnosis of acute mesenteric ischemia secondary to arterial occlusion in rats. Eur Surg Res. 2005;37:216–9.
15. Gollin G, Marks C, Marks WH. Intestinal fatty acid binding protein in serum and urine reflects early ischemic injury to the small bowel. Surgery. 1993;113:545–51.
16. Kanda T, Fujii H, Tani T, Murakami H, Suda T, Sakai Y, et al. Intestinal fatty acid-binding protein is a useful diagnostic marker for mesenteric infarction in humans. Gastroenterology. 1996;110:339–43.
17. Thuijls G, van Wijck K, Grootjans J, Derikx JP, van Bijnen AA, Heineman E, et al. Early diagnosis of intestinal ischemia using urinary and plasma fatty acid binding proteins. Ann Surg. 2011;253:303–8.
18. Ofer A, Abadi S, Nitecki S, Karram T, Kogan I, Leiderman M, et al. Multidetector CT angiography in the evaluation of acute mesenteric ischemia. Eur Radiol. 2009;19:24–30.
19. Aschoff AJ, Stuber G, Becker BW, Hoffmann MH, Schmitz BL, Schelzig H, et al. Evaluation of acute mesenteric ischemia: accuracy of biphasic mesenteric multi-detector CT angiography. Abdom Imaging. 2009;34:345–57.
20. Furukawa A, Kanasaki S, Kono N, Wakamiya M, Tanaka T, Takahashi M, et al. CT diagnosis of acute mesenteric ischemia from various causes. Am J Roentgenol. 2009;192:408–16.
21. Schieda N, Fasih N, Shabana W. Triphasic CT in the diagnosis of acute mesenteric ischaemia. Eur Radiol. 2013;23:1891–900.
22. Pisimisis GT, Oderich GS. Technique of hybrid retrograde superior mesenteric artery stent placement for acute-on-chronic mesenteric ischemia. Ann Vasc Surg. 2011;25:132. e7-11.

23. Meilahn JE, Morris JB, Ceppa EP, Bulkley GB. Effect of prolonged selective intramesenteric arterial vasodilator therapy on intestinal viability after acute segmental mesenteric vascular occlusion. Ann Surg. 2001;234:107–15.
24. Savassi-Rocha PR, Veloso LF. Treatment of superior mesenteric artery embolism with a fibrinolytic agent: case report and literature review. Hepatogastroenterology. 2002;49:1307–10.
25. Bausch D, Hopt UT, Obermaier R. [Of what relevance is the diagnosis of "pneumatosis intestinalis" and portal gas for the surgeon?]. Zentralbl Chir. 2009;134:203–8.
26. Bowersox JC, Zwolak RM, Walsh DB, Schneider JR, Musson A, LaBombard FE, et al. Duplex ultrasonography in the diagnosis of celiac and mesenteric artery occlusive disease. J Vasc Surg. 1991;14:780–6; discussion 6–8.
27. Moneta GL. Screening for mesenteric vascular insufficiency and follow-up of mesenteric artery bypass procedures. Semin Vasc Surg. 2001;14:186–92.
28. Carlos RC, Stanley JC, Stafford-Johnson D, Prince MR. Interobserver variability in the evaluation of chronic mesenteric ischemia with gadolinium-enhanced MR angiography. Acad Radiol. 2001;8:879–87.
29. Vitin AA, Metzner JI. Anesthetic management of acute mesenteric ischemia in elderly patients. Anesthesiol Clin. 2009;27:551–67, table of contents.
30. Paral J, Ferko A, Plodr M, Raupach J, Hadzi-Nikolov D, Dolezal D, et al. Laparoscopic diagnostics of acute bowel ischemia using ultraviolet light and fluorescein dye: an experimental study. Surg Laparosc Endosc Percutan Tech. 2007;17:291–5.
31. Sauerland S, Agresta F, Bergamaschi R, Borzellino G, Budzynski A, Champault G, et al. Laparoscopy for abdominal emergencies: evidence-based guidelines of the European Association for Endoscopic Surgery. Surg Endosc. 2006;20:14–29.
32. Lange KBL. The use of fluorescein to determine the adequacy of the circulation. Med Clin North Am. 1942;26:943–52.
33. Gorey TF. The recovery of intestine after ischaemic injury. Br J Surg. 1980;67:699–702.
34. Luther B, Schwilden ED, Raichle H. [Successful embolectomy of the main branches of the celiac trunk and the superior mesenteric artery]. Chirurg. 1993;64:741–3.
35. Navsaria P, Nicol A, Hudson D, Cockwill J, Smith J. Negative pressure wound therapy management of the "open abdomen" following trauma: a prospective study and systematic review. World J Emerg Surg. 2013;8:4.
36. Cheatham ML, Safcsak K. Is the evolving management of intra-abdominal hypertension and abdominal compartment syndrome improving survival? Crit Care Med. 2010;38:402–7.
37. Boele van Hensbroek P, Wind J, Dijkgraaf MG, Busch OR, Goslings JC. Temporary closure of the open abdomen: a systematic review on delayed primary fascial closure in patients with an open abdomen. World J Surg. 2009;33:199–207.
38. Ballehaninna UK, Hingorani A, Ascher E, Shiferson A, Marks N, Aboian E, et al. Acute superior mesenteric artery embolism: reperfusion with AngioJet hydrodynamic suction thrombectomy and pharmacologic thrombolysis with the EKOS catheter. Vascular. 2012;20:166–9.
39. Kougias P, Lau D, El Sayed HF, Zhou W, Huynh TT, Lin PH. Determinants of mortality and treatment outcome following surgical interventions for acute mesenteric ischemia. J Vasc Surg. 2007;46:467–74.
40. Mamode N, Pickford I, Leiberman P. Failure to improve outcome in acute mesenteric ischaemia: seven-year review. Eur J Surg. 1999;165:203–8.
41. Edwards MS, Cherr GS, Craven TE, Olsen AW, Plonk GW, Geary RL, et al. Acute occlusive mesenteric ischemia: surgical management and outcomes. Ann Vasc Surg. 2003;17:72–9.
42. Endean ED, Barnes SL, Kwolek CJ, Minion DJ, Schwarcz TH, Mentzer Jr RM. Surgical management of thrombotic acute intestinal ischemia. Ann Surg. 2001;233:801–8.
43. Arthurs ZM, Titus J, Bannazadeh M, Eagleton MJ, Srivastava S, Sarac TP, et al. A comparison of endovascular revascularization with traditional therapy for the treatment of acute mesenteric ischemia. J Vasc Surg. 2011;53:698–704; discussion –5.
44. Schermerhorn ML, Giles KA, Hamdan AD, Wyers MC, Pomposelli FB. Mesenteric revascularization: management and outcomes in the United States, 1988–2006. J Vasc Surg. 2009; 50:341–8. e1.

Chapter 17
Techniques of Open and Hybrid Mesenteric Revascularization for Acute Mesenteric Ischemia

Jason R. Moore, Sadaf Sadie Ahanchi, and Jean M. Panneton

Despite many advances in technology and treatment of vascular disease over the last decade, acute mesenteric ischemia (AMI) continues to carry significant morbidity and mortality [1]. Over the last two decades there has been a significant increase in the use of endovascular therapy for the treatment of AMI [2]. However, the 2005 and 2011 combined American College of Cardiology/American Heart Association guidelines recommend open surgery (class I, level of evidence B) as treatment for AMI, relative to endovascular therapy which was given a class IIb recommendation (level of evidence C) [3]. Thus, while endovascular therapy is increasingly utilized for AMI at major centers, open surgical revascularization remains the predominant treatment across the United States [2].

Diagnosis

Long-term outcomes for patients with AMI strongly depend on the timeliness of diagnosis and treatment, the etiology of the underlying lesion, and their associated cardiovascular status. Survival is worst (20 % at 5 years) in patients with mesenteric arterial thrombosis, and survival is best in patients with emboli or nonocclusive ischemia (about 70 % at 5 years) [4]. Any diagnosis requires prompt recognition and treatment as delay in diagnosis dramatically increases morbidity and mortality, emphasizing the importance of a timely diagnosis.

J.R. Moore, MD • S.S. Ahanchi, MD • J.M. Panneton, MD, FACS, FRCSC (✉)
Division of Vascular Surgery, Department of Surgery, Eastern Virginia Medical School, Norfolk, VA, USA

Sentara Heart Hospital, Norfolk, VA, USA
e-mail: moorejr@evms.edu; ssahanch@sentara.com; pannetjm@evms.edu

G.S. Oderich (ed.), *Mesenteric Vascular Disease*,
DOI 10.1007/978-1-4939-1847-8_17

The classic manifestation is a patient with acute, severe abdominal pain that is out of proportion to their physical findings. However, this finding may be present in as little as 35 % of patients with AMI [5]. Peritonitis may initially be absent, but may develop as the disease progresses. Vomiting and diarrhea may also be present, and occult gastric or rectal bleeding may be identified in as many as 25 % of patients [6].

CT angiography is considered the gold standard for diagnosing AMI with a sensitivity of 96 % and a specificity of 94 % [7]. The use of CTA along with history, physical exam, and serum markers can all clarify a diagnosis.

Initial Treatment and Resuscitation

If there is clinical suspicion of AMI, treatment and resuscitation should begin immediately. Patients who present with evidence of toxicity and high clinical suspicion of AMI need to be resuscitated expeditiously, and surgical intervention should not be delayed. Initial treatment of AMI includes volume resuscitation, correction of acidosis, administration of appropriate antibiotics, and surgical correction. Aggressive fluid resuscitation of a patient with AMI should begin with isotonic crystalloid solution and continue with blood, if necessary. Adequate fluid resuscitation is essential in the management of AMI secondary to the fluid shifts that occur with bowel ischemia. Electrolyte imbalances, particularly hyperkalemia, should be monitored and corrected aggressively. Invasive monitoring needs to be started early to ensure optimization before intravenous contrast administration or operative exploration. Broad-spectrum antibiotics should be administered to guard against translocated bacteria and sepsis. If there are no contraindications, therapeutic anticoagulation with intravenous heparin should also be started. A nasogastric tube also can be placed to decrease the chance of aspiration. Once it is determined that surgery is indicated, there should be no hesitation, and the patient should proceed immediately to the operating room.

Considerations

There are several considerations when planning for surgical intervention. The primary goals of any open and/or hybrid surgical procedure for AMI are to reestablish pulsatile inflow, to ensure adequate perfusion to viable bowel, and to resect nonviable bowel. In the case of an open surgical intervention, the patient should be placed supine on the operating table. The abdomen and both legs are prepared and draped, for possible need of vein conduit. During abdominal exploration, intestinal viability and the status of mesenteric blood flow should be evaluated to determine the appropriate management. Be ready and able to complete both revascularization and bowel resection.

The intraoperative appearance of bowel can be misleading. Bowel that is approaching irreversible ischemia and necrosis can appear normal; conversely, bowel that looks gray and flabby without peristalsis or has other ischemic changes may in fact be viable after revascularization. Thus, in most cases it is best to proceed with revascularization before resection of any intestine, unless faced with frank necrosis or perforation and peritoneal contamination. In those cases, the affected bowel should be resected without reanastomosis and the spilled content contained rapidly, before revascularization. Revascularization may be withheld at surgeon's discretion in extreme cases when the patient is in extremis and has diffusely necrotic bowel.

The distribution of ischemic changes provides valuable information about the cause of the ischemia. SMA thrombosis often results in ischemia to the entire small bowel, with the stomach, the duodenum, and the distal colon spared; in severe cases, however, the entire foregut may be ischemic [8]. Some patients with prolonged intestinal ischemia may have diffuse bowel necrosis. In this situation, revascularization usually proves to be futile, and this situation almost always proves fatal; therefore attempts at revascularization are not warranted. In comparison, embolization to the SMA generally spares the stomach, the duodenum, and the proximal jejunum because the emboli tend to lodge more distally at the level of the middle colic artery rather than at the origin of the SMA [9]. The choice of operation for revascularizing the bowel depends on the underlying causative condition and the status of the bowel and the patient. Thromboendarterectomy, retrograde open mesenteric stenting, and mesenteric bypass are indicated for thrombotic occlusion.

Exposure of SMA

Open and hybrid procedures will typically begin with the same exposure and initial evaluation of the peritoneal contents. A local thromboendarterectomy will be performed if possible, and then the decision to end the procedure or proceed with bypass or retrograde stenting must be made.

Start with a midline laparotomy and abdominal exploration. Elevate the temperature in the operating room. Keep the bowel warm and moist to minimize heat loss and vasoconstriction. Expose the SMA by dividing the ligament of Treitz at the base of the transverse colon mesentery. Retract the duodenum and the small bowel to the patient's right. Follow this by incising the visceral peritoneum above the ligament of Treitz, superior to the third portion of the duodenum. The SMA should now be palpable as it traverses over the duodenum. Continue the dissection until proximal and distal control of the SMA is obtained (Fig. 17.1). Administer a systematic weight-based heparin bolus, and clamp the vessel proximally and distally.

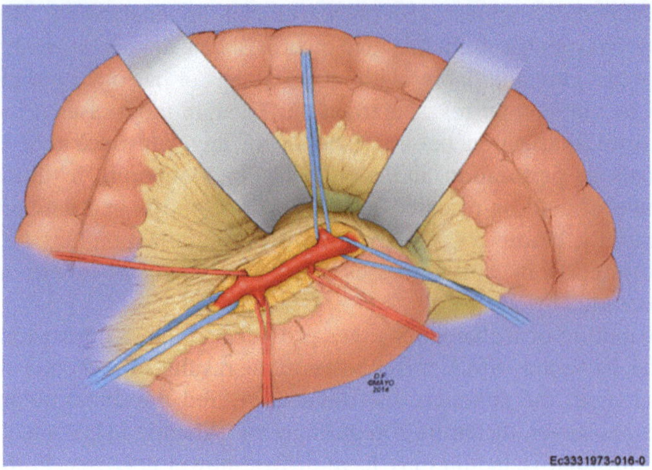

Fig. 17.1 Superior mesenteric artery exposed with proximal and distal control (By permission of Mayo Foundation for Medical Education and Research. All rights reserved)

Exposure and Control of the Supraceliac Aorta

In some cases it may be necessary to obtain some level of proximal control at the level of the supraceliac aorta. This should generally be avoided if possible, but when necessary it should be performed through a midline laparotomy and transperitoneal approach to allow for evaluation of the bowel at the same time. First, pack the abdominal contents inferiorly, and retract the left lobe of the liver superiorly and to the patient's right. To increase exposure it might be helpful to divide the left triangular ligament. Next, enter the lesser sac by incising the gastrohepatic ligament to the right of the esophagus. When extending this incision, be aware that a replaced or accessory left hepatic artery may be present, and care should be taken to avoid injury to this vessel. The esophagus and stomach are then retracted to the left to expose the right crus of the diaphragm. Incise the posterior peritoneum, and separate the right crus to expose the anterior supraceliac aorta. Clear the walls of both sides of the aorta with blunt finger dissection. To complete the exposure perform a vertical incision extending cephalad into the thoracic cavity, through the median arcuate ligament and the right crus, anterior to the anterior aorta. Once there is adequate clearance both medially and laterally, a curved aortic clamp can be placed.

Thromboendarterectomy

After proximal and distal control is gained, a longitudinal arteriotomy is made on the anterior wall of the SMA. The endarterectomy is begun with a plaque elevator. The optimal endarterectomy plane is that between the inner and outer medial layers.

The proximal endpoint is obtained by endarterectomy of the plaque as close to the origin of the SMA as possible. In most cases, atherosclerotic disease involves the ostia, and it can be very difficult if not impossible to adequately perform an endarterectomy of the origin from this location. This needs to be considered if an endarterectomy is intended to be the sole procedure as it will be prone to failure and should include either retrograde stenting or bypass if the origin has significant involvement.

The plaque is then elevated under full vision while the endarterectomy is continued distally. When branches of the SMA are encountered, eversion endarterectomy of those branches is performed. At the distal arteriotomy, the plaque is either feathered so that a smooth taper is achieved in transition to normal distal intima or sharply transitioned and tacked down with Prolene suture. After completion of the endarterectomy, all residual debris and medial fibers are excised because of their potential contribution to embolization or hyperplastic restenosis. The endarterectomy surface is irrigated with heparinized saline to facilitate visualization and removal of all debris.

The management of acute SMA thrombosis caused by underlying atherosclerotic lesions with simple surgical thrombectomy is unlikely to be durable [10]; however, in some selected high-risk patients that would not tolerate a long revascularization procedure, it may be the best option.

If no bypass is planned, the arteriotomy should be closed with a patch. The patch may be constructed from a piece of vein or synthetic material. If there is significant peritoneal soilage, a vein patch is preferred. The patch should be cut to the appropriate size. The ends should be rounded, to avoid narrowing. Next a double-armed, nonabsorbable monofilament suture is used for the repair. The needle is passed from inside of the artery to outside, through all layers of the wall, to avoid creating an intimal flap. Starting at one end, pass one needle through the patch and through the artery and secure with a knot on the outside of the artery. Suturing is continued around the artery, starting at the far wall, with the needle passing outside-in on the graft and inside-out on the artery. Use an assistant to follow, making sure to keep appropriate tension on the suture line. Handle the artery with care, especially the intima. This reduces the risk of late thrombosis. When halfway around with each needle, repeat the process at the opposite apex with another double-ended suture, meeting in the middle. Before closing the arteriotomy, inflow and outflow are released to remove any clot, and the artery is flushed with heparinized saline. The sutures are then tied on the sides of the repair.

Superior Mesenteric Artery Bypass

Patients with SMA thrombosis will typically have severe atherosclerotic plaque at the orifice of the SMA. Those patients who are identified early and have no or limited intestinal necrosis may undergo SMA bypass grafting with a prosthetic conduit. Some of these patients may have fluid within the peritoneal cavity. This finding is not necessarily a contraindication to the use of a prosthetic graft. However, if the patient has perforation with significant spillage, use of autologous vein as conduit is preferred. A good-quality vein is mandatory; if the saphenous vein is inadequate, the femoral vein may be used instead [11].

These patients are often critically ill, so it is imperative to perform the operation rapidly and efficiently. In the acute setting, bypass to the SMA alone (single-vessel bypass) is strongly preferred [12, 13]. Inflow for mesenteric bypass grafts may be derived either above or below the renal arteries. The graft is antegrade if it originates cephalad to the celiac artery. The graft is retrograde if it originates from the infrarenal aorta or a common iliac artery. An antegrade bypass has definite advantages, mainly improved hemodynamics, and also a straighter graft configuration that minimizes graft kinking. Typically, there is also reduced atherosclerotic calcification in the supraceliac aorta [14]. One of the main disadvantages of an antegrade bypass is the need to clamp the supraceliac aorta for the proximal anastomosis. Use of side-biting clamps may be possible but not always practical. Clamping the supraceliac aorta carries an increased risk of cardiac events, embolization, and ischemia. It is essential to ensure that the supraceliac aorta can safely be clamped, prior to proceeding with an antegrade bypass. It should be acknowledged that reoperation and attempts to reexpose the supraceliac aorta are much more difficult the second time around and generally riskier.

Antegrade Mesenteric Bypass

Supraceliac aorta–superior mesenteric artery bypass is performed through a midline incision and transperitoneal approach. Begin the dissection by dividing the gastrohepatic ligament and retracting of the left lobe of the liver to the right. This is followed by incision of the diaphragmatic crus and exposure of the anterior aspect of the aorta. For more details see section on Exposure and Control of the Supraceliac Aorta. In most cases Dacron grafts or reinforced expanded polytetrafluoroethylene (ePTFE) is preferred. If the use of a prosthetic graft is combined with resection of necrotic bowel, Dacron should be used, and it should be soaked in rifampin. Soak the graft for 15 min in a 1 mg/ml saline solution of rifampin at 37 °C [15] prior to implantation. After implantation the graft should be excluded with the omentum prior to performing enterectomy [5]. Autologous vein grafts are usually reserved for severely contaminated cases. The femoral vein is an excellent conduit for mesenteric arterial bypass [11]. The SMA is typically the mesenteric vessel involved; however, if the celiac artery needs to be revascularized, consider an end-to-side anastomosis to the aorta, followed by an end-to-side distal anastomosis to the common hepatic artery. When revascularizing the SMA, it is usually necessary to tunnel the graft behind the pancreas. Use caution when creating the retropancreatic tunnel. If the area appears narrow or is scarred from previous pancreatic inflammation, consider a tunnel anterior to the pancreas to ensure that it is not compressed and to avoid causing bleeding from disrupted pancreatic veins [16]. When an anterior tunnel is needed, consider using vein conduit because the graft will lie posterior to the stomach. After creation of the tunnel, either anterior or posterior, perform an end-to-side anastomosis to the SMA at that level.

Retrograde Mesenteric Bypass

There are several combinations of graft orientation that may be used for a retrograde bypass, and there are several types of conduit to choose from. The choice of orientation and conduit is largely influenced by the adequacy of the potential inflow vessels and by the presence or absence of peritoneal soilage. Foley et al. have reported the use of the distal infrarenal aorta or the infrarenal aorta–right common iliac artery junction as the preferred sites for the inflow anastomosis. There does not appear to be a significant difference in long-term patency between antegrade and retrograde bypasses (primary patency of 93 % and 95 % at 36 months, respectively) [17]. An advantage to the retrograde bypass is that most surgeons are more comfortable with the approach to the infrarenal aorta. Another advantage is that dissection and clamping of the infrarenal aorta carries less physiologic risk than dissection and clamping of the supraceliac aorta. The main disadvantage is the potential for graft kinking. Kinking is less likely to occur if Dacron or reinforced ePTFE is used and if the right common iliac is used as the site for distal anastomosis. The key to avoiding graft elongation, angulation, or kinking of the graft is to cut it to length with the SMA in a nearly anatomic position [13].

Our preference for retrograde graft orientation is the "reverse C-loop" configuration, with its origin from the right common iliac artery (Fig. 17.2). This way aortic clamping is avoided. It also provides a good lie for the graft and theoretically decreases the chance of it kinking. Similar C-loop grafts can be used for other inflow sources, such as the left iliac or distal infrarenal aorta if the right common iliac artery is not adequate. The lie of C-loop grafts tends to be improved by slightly increasing graft length and by performing an end-to-end anastomosis with the SMA. If none of those inflow vessels are suitable for bypass, a very short retrograde

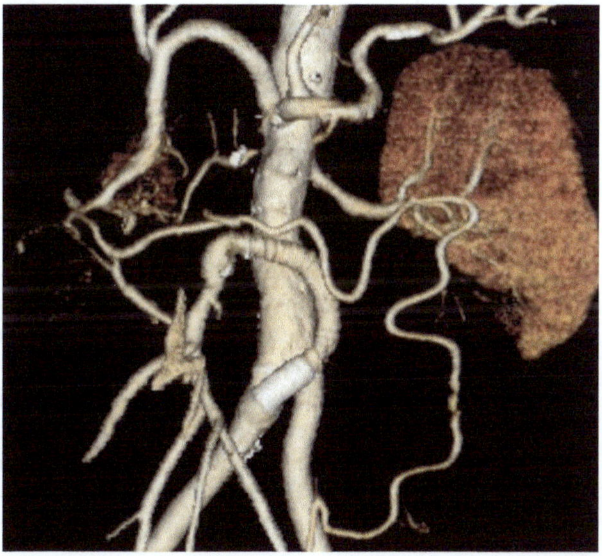

Fig. 17.2 Superior mesenteric artery bypass with a synthetic graft in a "reverse C-loop" configuration

bypass using a larger diameter graft (8–10 mm) can be performed from the proximal infrarenal aorta. Keep in mind that there is a higher potential for graft kinking with shorter grafts.

The SMA and distal aorta are dissected out and isolated in a similar manner to the techniques described earlier. In addition, the fourth portion of the duodenum needs to be fully mobilized for a more lateral approach to the SMA to facilitate the retrograde bypass. The retroperitoneum is divided distally along the aorta to a point just beyond the level of the aortic bifurcation. Assess both the distal aorta and common iliac arteries to determine the optimal inflow vessel for the proximal anastomosis. Typically, grafts made of Dacron or of ringed, reinforced ePTFE are the preferred conduits. The use of autologous vein has the potential to cause kinking when the viscera are replaced. However, if there is significant peritoneal contamination, consideration must be made to their use. When a retrograde vein bypass is performed, the graft may be brought straight up from the right iliac artery so that it lies between the aorta and the duodenum and then anastomosed to the posteromedial wall of the SMA. This is done to decrease the chance of kinking. Care must then be taken to check for kinking after the viscera have been repositioned.

The junction of the aorta with the right common iliac artery is the preferred site for the proximal anastomosis. Grafts originating from the midportion of the infrarenal aorta are prone to kinking when the viscera are returned to their normal position. The graft to the SMA is passed cephalad, turned anteriorly and inferiorly 180°, and anastomosed to the anterior wall of the SMA just beyond the inferior border of the pancreas [16]. If performed correctly, a gentle "C-loop" should be formed by the graft, and this will decrease the chance the graft will kink when the viscera are restored to their anatomic position after retractor removal. The ligament of Treitz and peritoneum are closed over the graft to exclude it from the peritoneal cavity.

Hybrid Technique: Retrograde Open Mesenteric Stenting (ROMS)

Milner et al. [18] reported the first technically successful ROMS, a hybrid approach for the treatment of acute atherosclerotic SMA thrombosis that involves a less invasive mesenteric revascularization without compromising important general surgical principles. They experienced no ROMS-related complications or morbidity. Wyers [19] and coauthors from Dartmouth reported similar findings in their report on 6 patients. In a well-stocked operating suite, with readily available fluoroscopy, ROMS should take less time than a saphenous vein harvest and bypass procedure and is probably quicker than synthetic bypass as well. It maintains sound surgical principles of thorough abdominal exploration while minimizing physiologic stress and may prevent a prosthetic graft infection in the face of bowel perforation or resection. In addition, a patient with mesenteric ischemia likely has aortoiliac disease compromising inflow into the bypass graft. Cross-clamping of an aorta that is heavily diseased and suturing to a heavily diseased graft donor vessel expose the

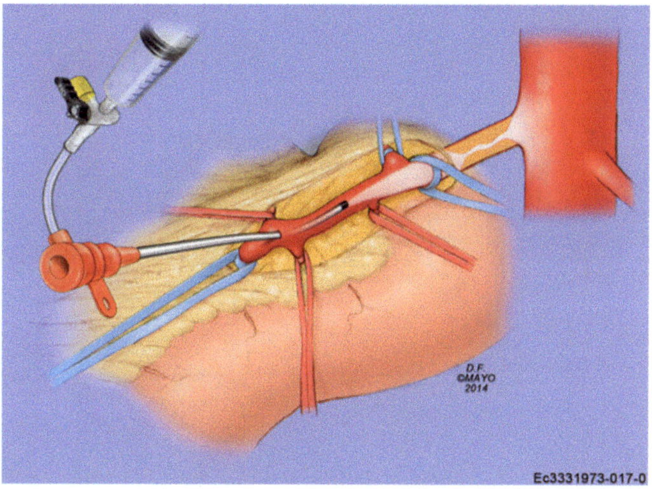

Fig. 17.3 Retrograde angiogram performed through SMA arteriotomy to visualize occlusion (By permission of Mayo Foundation for Medical Education and Research. All rights reserved)

hypotensive and acidotic patient to hazardous changes in hemodynamics and potential injury to atherosclerotic and calcified vessels. All of these potential problems with mesenteric bypass are avoided with ROMS. If the endovascular procedure proves difficult or impossible, converting to a bypass operation is easy with the exposure being half complete.

Our technique and early experience were previously reported by our group in 2010 [20]. After exposing the SMA, the infrapancreatic SMA is isolated and punctured with either a micropuncture needle or an 18-gauge needle. Then, over a wire, a 6 or 7-French sheath is placed. A local thromboendarterectomy through a longitudinal arteriotomy and placement of a patch angioplasty, as previously described, may be necessary prior to placement of wire and sheath. In some instances a transverse arteriotomy and embolectomy with an embolectomy catheter (4 Fr proximally and 3 Fr distally) may be needed to thrombectomize the proximal SMA prior to placement of a wire and sheath. After placement of a wire and sheath, a retrograde angiogram is performed to confirm the SMA occlusion proximally (Fig. 17.3). Appropriate wire and catheter selection is important when attempting to cross these lesions. We prefer a Berenstein catheter (Cordis, Inc, Warren, NJ) and soft-angled glidewire (Terumo Interventional Systems, Somerset, NJ) to maneuver through the occlusion. Once wire and catheter have crossed the lesion, an aortogram is performed (Fig. 17.4). If there is any question as to appropriate sizing for the mesenteric vessel, intravascular ultrasound is a valuable tool. The wire is then exchanged for a lower profile 0.018- or 0.014-in. platform. The lesion, if necessary, can then be predilated with a 3- or 4-mm angioplasty balloon. A 6–8-mm balloon expandable stent should be deployed partially into the aorta and flared (Fig. 17.5). More than one stent may be required to cross the entire length of the lesion. Completion angiography in the

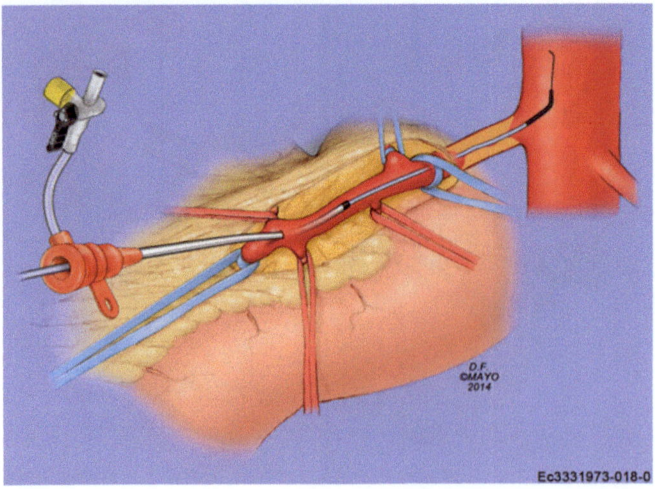

Fig. 17.4 Wire and catheter crossing the SMA lesion (By permission of Mayo Foundation for Medical Education and Research. All rights reserved)

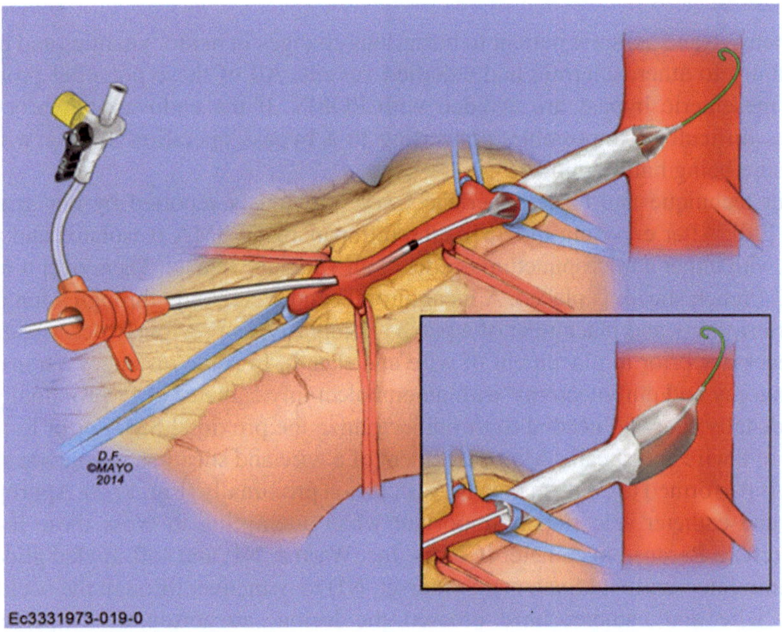

Fig. 17.5 Balloon expandable stent being deployed in SMA and partially into the aorta and flared (By permission of Mayo Foundation for Medical Education and Research. All rights reserved)

anteroposterior and lateral projections with or without pressure measurements is performed across the lesion to confirm patency. The arteriotomy is closed with a patch angioplasty with nonabsorbable monofilament sutures (Fig. 17.6). Small bowel viability is reassessed at the end of the operation.

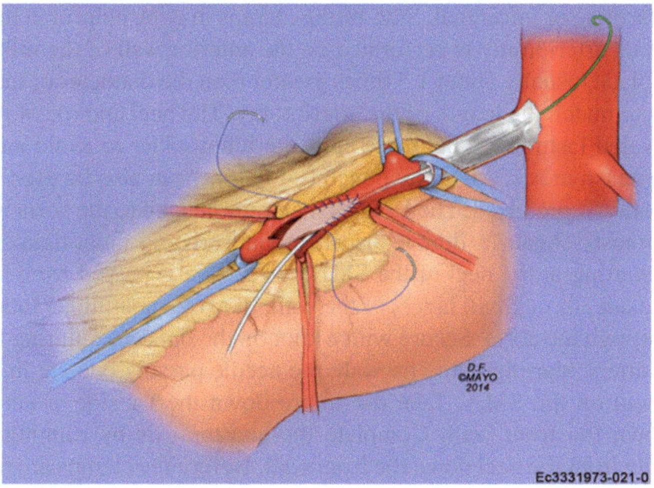

Fig. 17.6 Arteriotomy closed with patch angioplasty and nonabsorbable monofilament suture (By permission of Mayo Foundation for Medical Education and Research. All rights reserved)

Recurrent stenosis after ROMS is a possibility, as mesenteric artery in-stent restenosis occurs frequently [21–23] after mesenteric interventions. It is recommended to perform duplex surveillance for the first month and every 6 months thereafter. Most patients with recurrent stenosis can be re-treated with a percutaneous approach as outpatients. Many of these patients remain poor operative candidates and have limited life expectancies because of severe comorbidities [24]. In this situation, repeated SMA dilatations are a viable, safe option. For patients who make a good recovery and are nutritionally sound, a more durable operative bypass may be considered [25].

SMA Reimplantation

In the case of bowel necrosis and severe peritoneal contamination, SMA reimplantation can avoid the use of prosthetic graft. In 1990, Kieny et al. [26] reported on their success of SMA reimplantation to the juxtarenal aorta. Only seven of their 90 patients were for AMI, and their long-term follow up was limited. This procedure may be useful in patients who would not do well with prosthetic graft and do not have a suitable vein. Care should be taken when considering this as a possibility because this procedure is only possible in patients with very proximal disease and short focal occlusion of the diseased artery.

Following medial visceral rotation, the SMA is identified above the renal vein. Proximal and distal control is obtained. The SMA is transected. It is imperative to ensure adequate dissection of the SMA from the mesentery to allow for sufficient length for reimplantation. The proximal stump is sutured close with a nonabsorbable monofilament suture in two layers. The aorta is then clamped. Aortic clamping can be supraceliac or infrarenal. Side-biting clamps may be helpful in this situation. A longitudinal arteriotomy is performed on the anterior wall of the infrarenal aorta with an 11 blade, usually about 1.5 times greater than the diameter of the SMA. The SMA is cut to match the length of the arteriotomy. The heel and toe of the SMA are cut in a beveled fashion so that these ends are blunt/wider to avoid narrowing the ends of the anastomosis. An aortic punch (~4–6 mm) can also be used to complete the arteriotomy, if preferred. The SMA is then reimplanted to the aorta in an end-to-side anastomosis. Again a double-armed, nonabsorbable monofilament suture is preferred. Starting at the heel of the SMA, the needle is passed from inside of the artery to outside, through all layers of the wall, to avoid creating an intimal flap; do the same through the aorta. Secure with a knot on the outside. Suturing is continued around the artery, starting at the far wall, the needle passing outside-in on the aorta and inside-out on the SMA. Take the suture down the far side around the toe to halfway down the front wall. Complete the anastomosis by running the second armed needle from the heel down the front wall. Before the clamps are removed and the suture is tied, the proximal and distal ends are flushed.

Bowel Viability

When flow is restored, the bowel is re-inspected for persistent regions of ischemia [27]. If possible, 20–30 min of reperfusion should be permitted while retractors are being repositioned before making a decision about viability [28]. Segments that previously demonstrated equivocal viability may improve with revascularization, and resection may be avoided; lengths of bowel that are obviously nonviable must be removed. Initial clinical evaluation of the bowel consists of assessment of pulses in the mesentery, appearance and color of the serosa, any bleeding from cut surfaces, and peristalsis. These are subjective findings and are therefore prone to inaccuracy. Using clinical evaluation alone, bowel viability can be determined with a sensitivity of only 82 % and a specificity of 91 % [29].

The absence of pulsatile signals on the antimesenteric border of the intestine when using continuous wave Doppler implies a nonviable segment [30]. Use of this technique in conjunction with surgical judgment has been demonstrated in multiple studies [28, 31, 32]. However, continuous wave form Doppler ultrasound alone should not be used for determining bowel viability [33]. The use of fluorescein and a Wood's lamp is another adjunct to consider when evaluating bowel for ischemia. The ultraviolet light from the Wood's lamp shows a fine reticular vascular pattern in the viable bowel and has been shown to be sensitive in determining irreversible bowel ischemia when used with clinical judgment [29].

Ultimately, accurate determination of intestinal viability is the product of clinical judgment, adjunct diagnostic techniques, and timely reevaluation. The need to preserve bowel length should deter the surgeon from being overly aggressive in resecting any questionably viable bowel. Bowel continuity can be restored primarily, or stomas may be exteriorized if the patient is unstable. In most instances, a "second-look" operation should be performed within 24–36 h to reassess the bowel and the effect of reperfusion [34]. Planning for re-exploration allows the surgeon to minimize the bowel resected primarily and to ensure that bowel anastomoses are performed with viable bowel.

Complications

Complications occur frequently (~68 %) in these patients [5]. Major complications such as death, repeat bowel ischemia, stroke, acute renal failure requiring hemodialysis, MI, cardiac arrest, and respiratory failure requiring tracheostomy occur in ~47 % of patients. The most frequent complications are respiratory failure and multisystem organ failure [24].

Postoperative Care

Therefore, it is extremely important to continue care in the intensive care unit in the immediate perioperative and postoperative period in order to optimize the patient's cardiac and respiratory status. It is not uncommon to see a significant decrease in hepatic function postoperatively with transaminases rising 90- to 100-fold [35].

Hepatic impairment and associated coagulopathy are usually temporary, returning to normal within 7–10 days. Total parenteral nutrition should be considered and started early in the postoperative period in patients who underwent significant bowel resection, and it may need to be continued for months in patients with short gut syndromes.

Outcomes

Though patency rates remain high regardless of operation performed, more recent studies still tend to report poor overall patient outcomes in AMI. Perioperative mortality for arterial thrombosis remains high, at 39 % [5]. The mortality remains relatively high when compared to chronic mesenteric ischemia in part because of delayed diagnosis, the extensive nature of the bowel ischemia, and the need for complex surgical revascularization. Long-term survival for this patient population remains abysmal at 32 % at 3 years [24].

In some of these small series published on the less invasive approach of ROMS [18–20], the technical success rate can be as high as 100 %, and mortality ranges from 0 to 17 %. This suggests that retrograde open mesenteric stenting for acute mesenteric ischemia is a viable alternative to bypass surgery. More data will be needed before any conclusions about superiority can be made, but this hybrid strategy of combining open surgery with endorevascularization may become the surgeon's go-to procedure for revascularization in the setting of AMI.

References

1. Kougias P, Lau D, El Sayed HF, et al. Determinants of mortality and treatment outcome following surgical interventions for acute mesenteric ischemia. J Vasc Surg. 2007;46:467–74.
2. Schermerhorn ML, Giles KA, Hamdan AD, et al. Mesenteric revascularization: management and outcomes in the United States, 1988–2006. J Vasc Surg. 2009;50:341–8.
3. Hirsch AT, Haskal ZJ, Hertzer NR, et al. ACC/AHA 2005 Guidelines for the Management of Patients With Peripheral Arterial Disease (Lower Extremity, Renal, Mesenteric, and Abdominal Aortic): A Collaborative Report from the American Association for Vascular Surgery/Society for Vascular Surgery, Society for Cardiovascular Angiography and Interventions, Society for Vascular Medicine and Biology, Society of Interventional Radiology, and the ACC/AHA Task Force on Practice Guidelines (Writing Committee to Develop Guidelines for the Management of Patients With Peripheral Arterial Disease). J Am Coll Cardiol. 2006;47:e1–192.
4. Klempnauer J, Grothues F, Bektas H, et al. Long-term results after surgery for acute mesenteric ischemia. Surgery. 1997;121:239–43.
5. Ryer EJ, Kalra M, Oderich GS, et al. Revascularization for acute mesenteric ischemia. J Vasc Surg. 2012;55(6):1682–9.
6. Ottinger LW. The surgical management of acute occlusion of the superior mesenteric artery. Ann Surg. 1978;188:72L.
7. Kirkpatrick ID, Kroeker MA, Greenberg HM. Biphasic CT with mesenteric CT angiography in the evaluation of acute mesenteric ischemia: initial experience. Radiology. 2003;229:91–8.
8. Kaleya RN, Sammartano RJ, Boley SJ. Aggressive approach to acute mesenteric ischemia. Surg Clin North Am. 1992;72:157–82.
9. Boley SJ, Feinstein FR, Sammartano R, et al. New concepts in the management of emboli of the superior mesenteric artery. Surg Gynecol Obstet. 1981;153:561–9.
10. Whitehill T, Rutherford R. Acute mesenteric ischemia caused by arterial occlusions: optimal management to improve survival. Semin Vasc Surg. 1990;3:149–55.
11. Modrall JG, Sadjadi J, Joiner DR, et al. Comparison of superficial femoral vein and saphenous vein as conduits for mesenteric arterial bypass. J Vasc Surg. 2003;37:362–6.
12. Gentile AT, Moneta GL, Taylor Jr LM, et al. Isolated bypass to the superior mesenteric artery for intestinal ischemia. Arch Surg. 1994;129(9):926–31; discussion 931–2.
13. Foley MI, Moneta GL, Abou-Zamzam Jr AM, et al. Revascularization of the superior mesenteric artery alone for treatment of intestinal ischemia. J Vasc Surg. 2000;32(1):37–47.
14. Murray SP, Ramos TK, Stoney RJ. Surgery of the celiac and mesenteric arteries. In: Ascher E, editor. Haimovici's vascular surgery. Malden: Blackwell; 2004. p. 861.
15. Goëau-Brissonnière O, Leport C, Bacourt F, et al. Prevention of vascular graft infection by rifampin bonding to a gelatin-sealed Dacron graft. Ann Vasc Surg. 1991;5(5):408–12.
16. Taylor LM, Moneta GL, Porter JM. Treatment of chronic visceral ischemia. In: Rutherford RB, editor. Vascular surgery. Philadelphia: WB Saunders; 2000. p. 1532.
17. McMillan WD, McCarthy WJ, Bresticker MR, et al. Mesenteric artery bypass: objective patency determination. J Vasc Surg. 1995;21:729–40.
18. Milner R, Woo EY, Carpenter JP. Superior mesenteric artery angioplasty and stenting via a retrograde approach in a patient with bowel ischemia – a case report. Vasc Endovasc Surg. 2004;38:89–91.
19. Wyers MC, Powell RJ, Nolan BW, Cronenwett JL. Retrograde mesenteric stenting during laparotomy for acute occlusive mesenteric ischemia. J Vasc Surg. 2007;45(2):269–75.
20. Stout CL, Messerschmidt CA, Leake AE, et al. Retrograde open mesenteric stenting for acute mesenteric ischemia is a viable alternative for emergent revascularization. Vasc Endovascular Surg. 2010;44(5):368–71.
21. Tallarita T, Oderich GS, Macedo TA, et al. Reinterventions for stent restenosis in patients treated for atherosclerotic mesenteric artery disease. J Vasc Surg. 2011;54(5):1422–9.
22. Kasirajan K, O'Hara PJ, Gray BH, et al. Chronic mesenteric ischemia: open surgery versus percutaneous angioplasty and stenting. J Vasc Surg. 2001;33:63–71.

23. Brown DJ, Schermerhorn ML, Powell RJ, et al. Mesenteric stenting for chronic mesenteric ischemia. J Vasc Surg. 2005;42:268–74.
24. Park WM, Gloviczki P, Cherry Jr KJ, et al. Contemporary management of acute mesenteric ischemia: factors associated with survival. J Vasc Surg. 2002;35:445–52.
25. Biebl M, Oldenburg WA, Paz-Fumagalli R, et al. Endovascular treatment as a bridge to successful surgical revascularization for chronic mesenteric ischemia. Am Surg. 2004;70:994–8.
26. Kieny R, Batellier J, Kretz JG. Aortic reimplantation of the superior mesenteric artery for atherosclerotic lesions of the visceral arteries: sixty cases. Ann Vasc Surg. 1990;4(2):122–5.
27. Horgan PG, Gorey TF. Operative assessment of intestinal viability. Surg Clin North Am. 1992;72:143.
28. Kazmers A. Operative management of acute mesenteric ischemia. Ann Vasc Surg. 1998;12: 187–97.
29. Bulkley GB, Zuidema GD, Hamilton SR, et al. Intraoperative determination of small intestinal viability following ischemic injury: a prospective, controlled trial of two adjuvant methods (Doppler and fluorescein) compared with standard clinical judgment. Ann Surg. 1981;193: 628–37.
30. Wright CB, Hobson 2nd RW. Prediction of intestinal viability using Doppler ultrasound technics. Am J Surg. 1975;129:642–5.
31. Cooperman M, Pace WG, Martin Jr EW, et al. Determination of viability of ischemic intestine by Doppler ultrasound. Surgery. 1978;83:705–10.
32. O'Donnell JA, Hobson 2nd RW. Operative confirmation of Doppler ultrasound in evaluation of intestinal ischemia. Surgery. 1980;87:109–12.
33. Dyess DL, Bruner BW, Donnell CA, et al. Intraoperative evaluation of intestinal ischemia: a comparison of methods. South Med J. 1991;84:966–74.
34. Lindbald B, Hakansson H. Rationale for second-look operation in mesenteric vessel occlusion. Acta Chir Scand. 1987;153:531.
35. Harward TR, Brooks DL, Flynn TC, et al. Multiple organ dysfunction after mesenteric artery revascularization. J Vasc Surg. 1993;18(3):459–67.

Chapter 18
Techniques of Endovascular Revascularization for Acute Mesenteric Ischemia

Timur P. Sarac

History for AMI

Litten gave the first description of acute mesenteric ischemia (AMI) in 1875 [1]. Since that time the condition of AMI has been viewed as one of the most serious surgical emergencies with significant morbidity and mortality. The true incidence of acute mesenteric ischemia (AMI) is unknown, as most reports quote the classic study from Stoney in 1993 [2]. The most recent report was from Malmo, Sweden, where AMI is reported to occur 12.9 per 100,000 person years over a 10-year period [3]. The etiology is most commonly attributed to in situ thrombosis in 60 % of patients, embolism from atrial fibrillation in 30 %, and nonocclusive mesenteric ischemia in 10 % [4]. The diagnosis of acute mesenteric ischemia is based on both physical examination and diagnostic imaging. The symptoms will include progressive abdominal pain, which is classically described as "pain out of proportion to physical findings." Additionally, the patients usually have a significant history of tobacco abuse and other peripheral vascular disease. Once other etiologies of abdominal pain have been excluded, most patients will have a computerized tomographic scan (CT), which will delineate the mesenteric vessel anatomy. Traditional treatment has been open surgical revascularization, which includes embolectomy, bypass, and endarterectomy [5–7]. However, the morbidity and mortality for open surgical revascularization remain unacceptably high, with rates reported as high as 70 %.

In an effort to improve on the poor results of open mesenteric revascularization for AMI, many clinicians began to explore other alternative therapies, most notably endovascular surgery [8, 9]. With improvement in training, newer devices, and less morbidity, endovascular treatment of acute mesenteric ischemia is now the first initial therapeutic choice of treatment if clinical conditions allow it.

T.P. Sarac, MD (✉)
Section of Vascular Surgery, Heart and Vascular Institute,
Yale University School of Medicine, New Haven, CT, USA
e-mail: timur.sarac@yale.edu

G.S. Oderich (ed.), *Mesenteric Vascular Disease*,
DOI 10.1007/978-1-4939-1847-8_18

Endovascular Techniques

Several endovascular treatment options exist to treat acute mesenteric ischemia. The decision of which option to use depends on the patient's immediate clinical condition. The patient's symptoms can be misleading, as they usually have significant abdominal pain, but an acute abdomen only happens when there is bowel perforation. If the patient has an acute abdomen or pneumatosis intestinalis is seen on the CT scan, the traditional approach has been combined open bowel resection and mesenteric revascularization. However, contemporary treatment has evolved, and an acute abdomen no longer precludes angioplasty and stenting, as surgical intervention can be done in a hybrid operating room, where both abdominal explorations can be performed either through exploratory celiotomy or laparoscopy in addition to angioplasty and stenting.

If the patient's lactate and liver function tests are normal and there is no evidence of an acute abdominal emergency or bowel infarction, our first treatment consists of diagnostic imaging in addition to the CT scan. In the setting of acute mesenteric ischemia, the most commonly involved vessel is acute occlusion of the superior mesenteric artery (SMA). In this circumstance, there is insufficient time to develop collaterals, and acute occlusion of the SMA can lead to bowel infarction. AMI is seen less commonly with acute celiac or inferior mesenteric artery (IMA) occlusion. Most patients will have undergone a CT angiogram delineating the anatomy (Fig. 18.1). This can give a good image of both orifice lesions and the distal extent of thrombosis. We then get both an anterior-posterior (AP) and lateral angiogram to determine the patency of all vessels (Fig. 18.2a, b), and it is not uncommon to see a large meandering mesenteric artery in the AP views (Fig. 18.3).

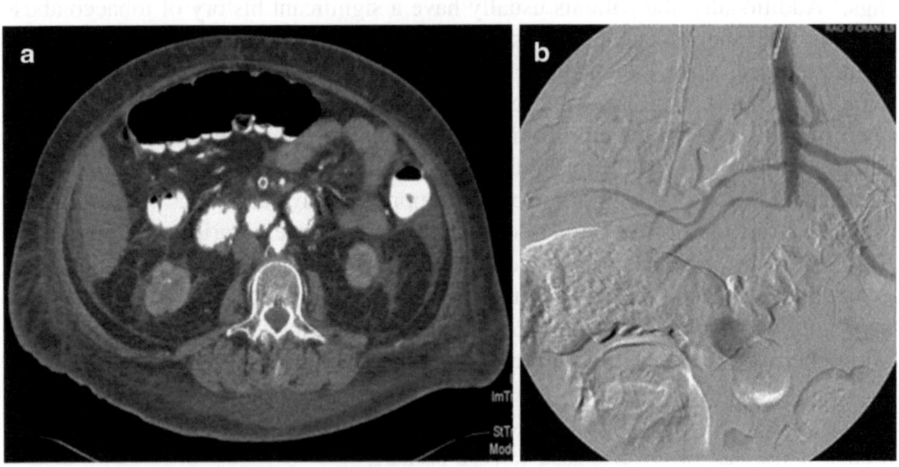

Fig. 18.1 (**a**) CT scan and (**b**) diagnostic angiogram of acute SMA occlusion

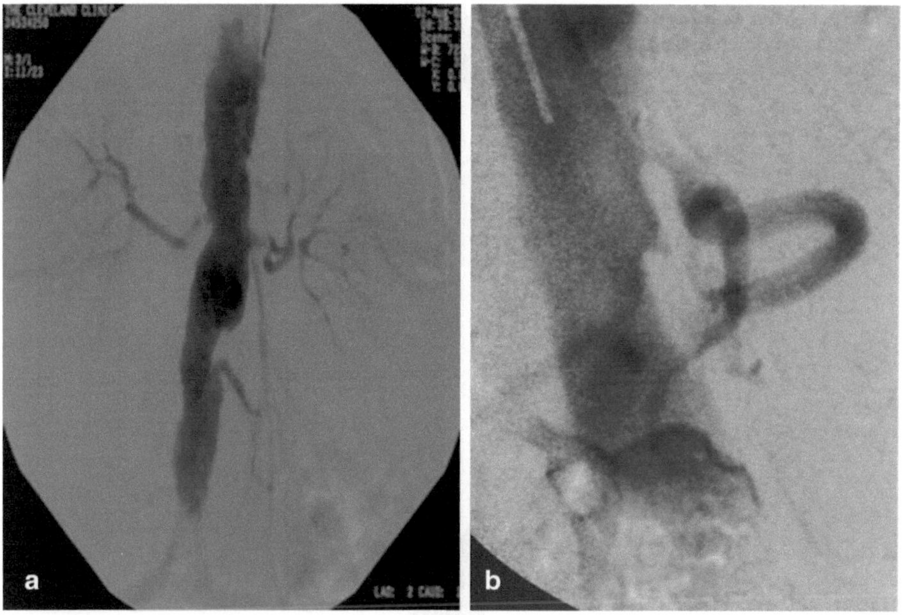

Fig. 18.2 (**a** and **b**) AP and lateral angiogram depicting visceral vessels

Fig. 18.3 Meandering mesenteric artery

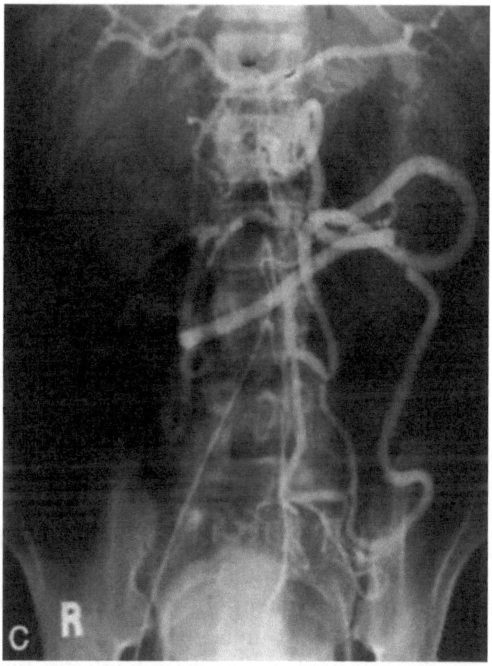

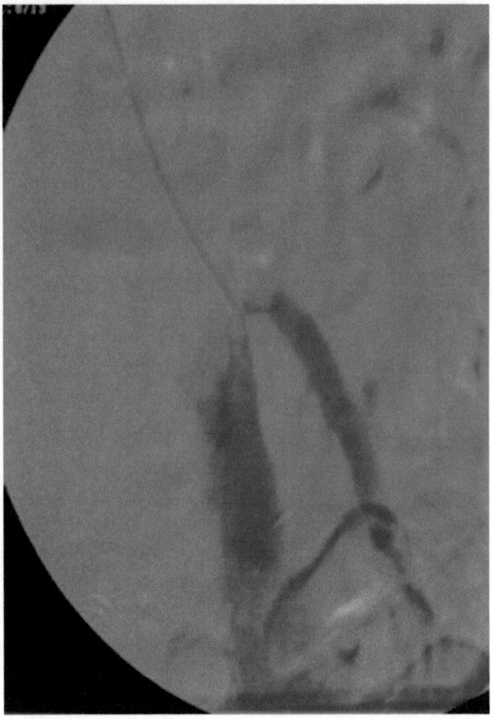

Fig. 18.4 MPA catheter with antegrade approach to the SMA

If the patient has complete occlusion of the superior mesenteric artery and their clinical condition will allow, we will attempt thrombolysis. Some contraindications to thrombolysis include severe hypertension, gastrointestinal bleeding, and embolism from atrial fibrillation. There are specific technical considerations to consider. The first step involves recanalizing and/or crossing the lesion. We usually use left brachial access as our initial approach as the angle makes it much easier to cross the lesion antegrade (Fig. 18.4). A long 5 F sheath (70–90 cm) usually is sufficient to provide adequate stability for tracking, as the final intervention will need to move to a 0.014 in wire. We usually use an MPA catheter and bury it into the stub of the occluded vessel, as it easily adapts to the curve of the aorta. Next I "drill" a 0.035 in stiff glide wire through the lesion, and then if possible pass the MPA catheter or a quick cross catheter through the lesion (Fig. 18.5). Once we have crossed the lesion, it is imperative to get an angiogram to confirm you are in the true lumen. If you have not reentered the true lumen, the catheter will need to be withdrawn and a new attempt should be made. If there is thrombus distal to the orifice and we have reentered and are not in a dissection plane, we will attempt thrombolysis with a short tip infusion catheter and/or wire [10]. The patient is then bolused with 2 mg of tissue plasminogen activator (TPA), and an infusion is started at 1 mg/h. We also keep the patient on a slightly higher dose of heparin that lower extremity ischemia, maintaining the activated partial thromboplastin time (APTT) near 40 s. If the patient's fibrinogen drops below 150 mg/dl, we then decrease the infusion rate to 0.5 mg/h.

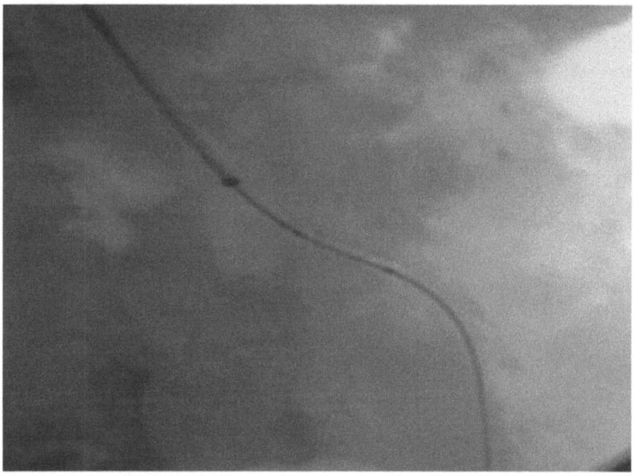

Fig. 18.5 Sheath and wire across occluded SMA

If the fibrinogen drops to 100 mg/dl, then we will either give cryoprecipitate or suspend the infusion depending on the patient's clinical condition. If the patient demonstrates any signs of increasing abdominal discomfort, rising lactic acidosis, or clinical deterioration, we then stop and prepare for open surgery. Repeat angiograph is performed every 12 h. Once the distal clot clears, we then proceed to definitive angioplasty and stenting. If there is spasm, we will use either 30–60 mg of papaverine or 200–400 μg of nitroglycerine. If the clot has not cleared within 36–48 h, we will attempt mechanical thrombectomy with the Possis mechanical thrombectomy catheter [11]. A 0.014 in wire is needed for 5 F and 0.035 in wire for 6 F. Additionally, I prefer to use an embolic protection filter to prevent embolization, as this has been reported as high as 19 % for peripheral pharmacomechanical thrombolysis [12].

The typical culprit lesion from in situ thrombosis usually occurs from extension of an orifice lesion. However, it is not uncommon for lesions of the superior mesenteric artery to extend further. If there is not distal thrombus, immediate revascularization with balloon angioplasty and stenting is warranted. For orifice lesions of the celiac, SMA, and IMA, we use a balloon expandable stent (Fig. 18.6), and for more distal lesions we will use a self-expanding stent to adapt to curves (Fig. 18.7). Occasionally, we will have to use a combination of a self-expanding stent distally and of a balloon expandable stent proximally. Recent data from the Mayo Clinic [13] now supports the use of an ePTFE-covered stent graft for chronic mesenteric ischemia, and we have extended this to AMI for thrombosis in situ. For patients with AMI from embolism, we will attempt percutaneous mechanical thrombolysis with the Possis thrombectomy catheter. If their clinical condition will allow it, we will get a transesophageal echocardiogram, and if there is no clot in the atrium, we will also offer them thrombolysis. If this is unsuccessful or there is suspected persistent atrial thrombus, we will either attempt stenting with a covered stent or proceed with open embolectomy.

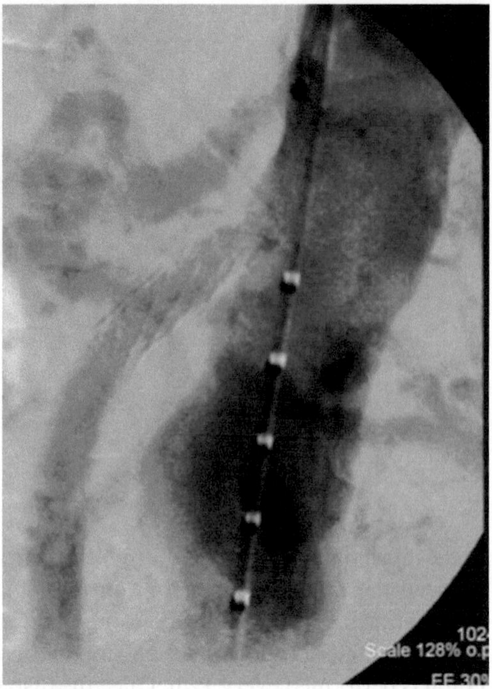

Fig. 18.6 Balloon expandable stent in orifice of the SMA

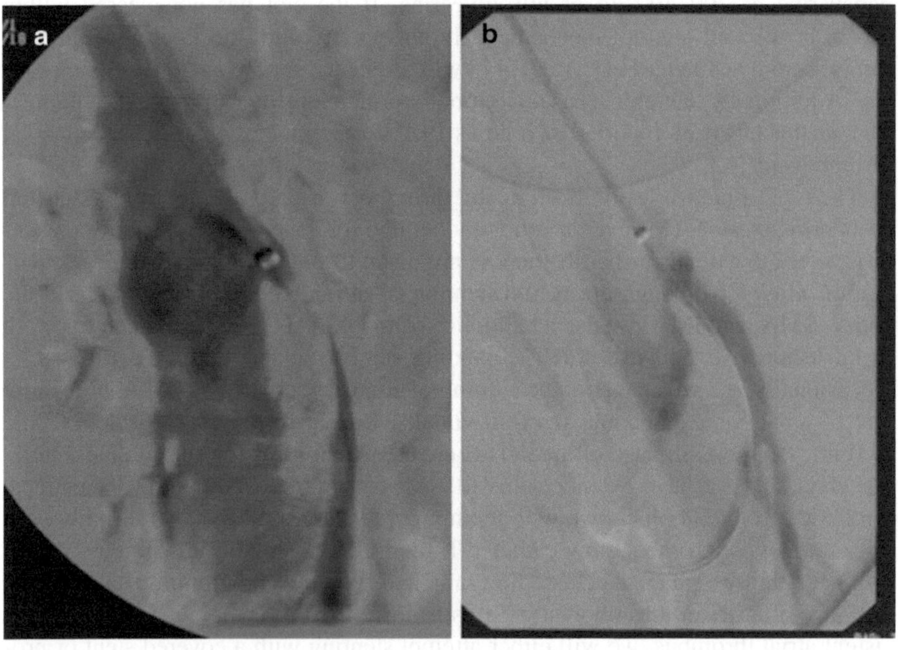

Fig. 18.7 (**a**) Selective SMA angiogram with disease beyond the orifice. (**b**) Self-expanding stent adapting to the curve

In circumstances where the patient's condition warrants emergent or urgent laparotomy, recent efforts have focused on a hybrid open surgery/stenting procedure [14, 15]. The technical details of this consist of performing the procedure in a hybrid operating suite and immediate exploration for control of sepsis and enteric spillage. We have been more inclined to use the brachial approach rather than the direct SMA cutdown if possible, as it allows more rapid revascularization. Nevertheless, there are advantages of the direct SMA cutdown as it will allow embolectomy. The procedure begins with dissecting the SMA out at the inferior margin of the pancreas or base of the transverse mesocolon. The artery is cannulated with a micropuncture needle, wire, and catheter, and then retrograde angiogram is performed. A 0.035 in wire is then used to exchange out for a 5 F sheath, and diagnostic imaging is performed. The lesion is crossed and the wire and a longer sheath are advanced into the aorta. Balloon angioplasty is frequently necessary before passing the sheath, and this usually requires exchanging out to a 0.014 in system. Retrograde stenting is done in the same fashion as antegrade which was previously described. It is not uncommon to have to perform a concomitant embolectomy, which can also be done with an over-the-wire balloon embolectomy catheter. On completion, the vessel is closed with either a vein or bovine pericardial patch angioplasty.

Less common etiologies of acute mesenteric ischemia include thoracoabdominal aortic dissection (TAAD), mesenteric venous thrombosis, and nonocclusive mesenteric ischemia. Acute mesenteric ischemia occurs in between 15 and 42 % of patients who suffer from TAAD [16]. Patient's symptoms include not only those severe of mid-thoracic back and chest pain but also abdominal pain. The diagnosis of AMI is entertained based on symptoms but also CT scan evidence of obstruction of the visceral vessels from the dissection flap (Fig. 18.8). Additionally, it is not uncommon in these circumstances for multiple visceral branch vessels to be involved.

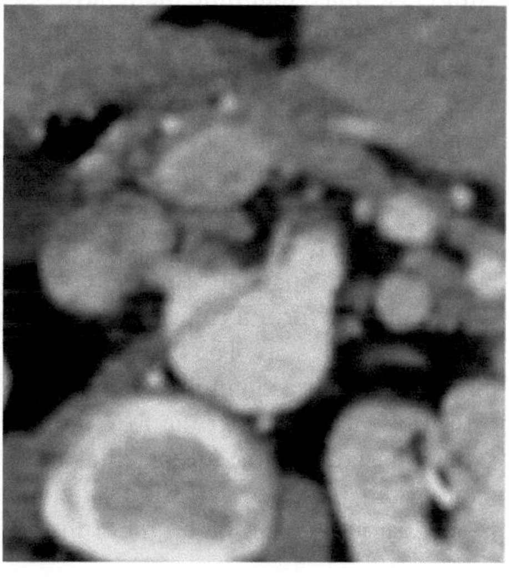

Fig. 18.8 CT scan depicting dissection flap in SMA

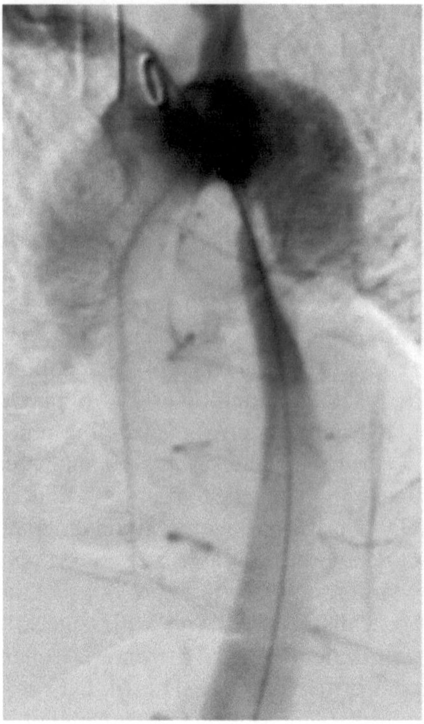

Fig. 18.9 Arch aortogram showing dissection at left subclavian artery

Symptoms can also be classified as subacute with waxing and waning of symptoms due to dynamic movement of the dissection flap. The morbidity and mortality with open surgical therapy have been previously described and remain as high as 50 % [16]. In 1999, Dake first described treatment for TAAD with a thoracic aortic stent graft [17]. Since that time there have been numerous studies documenting the success of endovascular therapy in treating malperfusion from TAAD [18–20]. Treatment in these circumstances consists of expansion of the true lumen with a thoracic stent graft, and occasionally an adjunctive self-expanding stent will need to be placed in the individual branch vessel. There are a number of technical details necessary to accomplish this, starting with preparation for bilateral femoral artery access, and be prepared to do an iliac conduit. Additionally, it is essential to have left brachial artery access, so the arterial line for blood pressure monitoring should be placed on the patient's right side. Intravascular ultrasound is a necessary adjunct. We usually perform a right femoral artery cutdown and obtain left brachial artery access from the start. The first step is to confirm you are in the true lumen, and here intravascular ultrasound is essential (Fig. 18.8). We then obtain an arch aortogram (Fig. 18.9) and exchange out for a 0.035 in stiff Lunderquist wire. A pigtail catheter is then placed from the left brachial artery into the aortic arch, which not only takes angiograms but also marks the subclavian artery. Often in an emergent setting, it is necessary to cover the origin of the left subclavian artery to cover the entry tear.

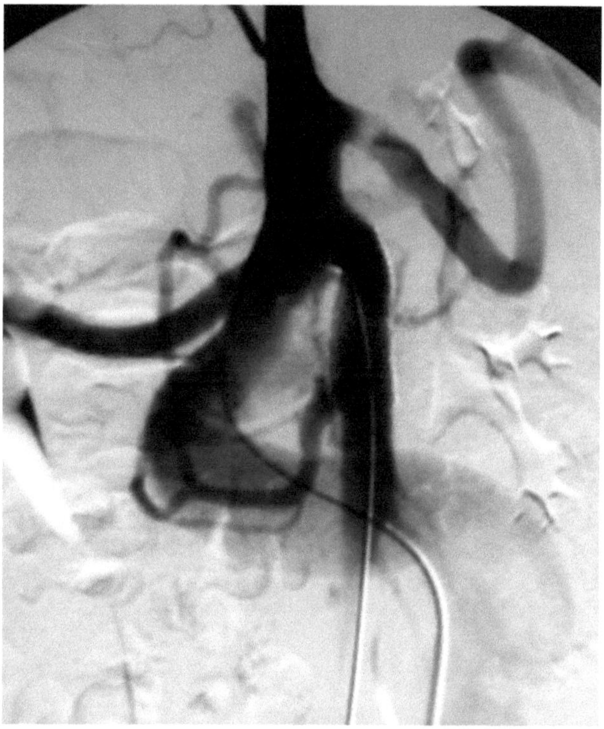

Fig. 18.10 Self-expanding stent in s=dissection

A subsequent emergent carotid subclavian bypass is necessary if there is not a normal size contralateral vertebral artery or if the patient is known to have an incomplete circle of Willis. Once the stent graft is placed, a distal angiogram is taken to confirm expansion of the aortic true lumen and evaluate the patency and flow of the visceral vessels. Occasionally, the dissection flap will necessitate the need to place a self-expanding stent into the branch vessel if flow remains compromised (Fig. 18.10).

Mesenteric venous thrombosis is another unusual cause of acute mesenteric ischemia, and the etiology usually is from a hypercoagulable state [21]. The mainstay of treatment usually consists of conservative management with systemic heparinization and conversion to oral anticoagulation, as long as there are no signs of an acute abdomen. However, if the patient's clinical condition deteriorates, several authors have reported success in improving symptoms by using intra-arterial thrombolysis through the SMA, and others have reported transhepatic venous success similar to TIPS [22]. Finally, nonocclusive mesenteric ischemia typically occurs from "low-flow states," such as cardiogenic or septic shock. The initial treatment involves supportive care for correcting the underlying condition. However, if the patient has persistent lactic acidosis, selective intra-arterial SMA perfusion with papaverine can correct the vasospasm (Fig. 18.11a and b).

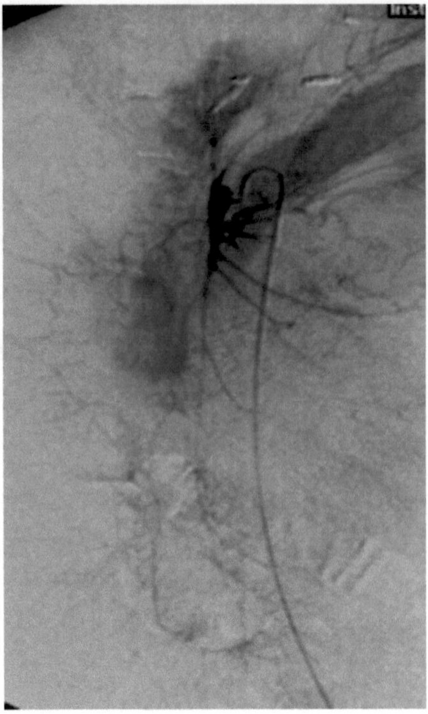

Fig. 18.11 Catheter in SMA infusing papaverine into a vessel with spasm

Results of Endovascular Therapy for Acute Mesenteric Ischemia

When analyzing new therapies, it is important to fully evaluate and compare the results to the traditional approach, here being open surgical revascularization for acute mesenteric ischemia. One recent series reporting the results of open surgical intervention came from Kougias et al. They evaluated 72 patients and found that the perioperative morbidity and mortality were 39 and 31 %, respectively [23]. As endovascular interventions became more popular, several authors reported their results. Arthurs et al. reported the Cleveland Clinic experience from 70 patients over 9 years [24]. Similar to almost all other studies, 65 % of the occlusions were thrombotic and 35 % embolic occlusions. Successful endovascular treatment resulted in a mortality rate of 36 % compared with 50 % with traditional open surgical therapy. Soon after Ryer et al. reported the Mayo Clinic experience over two decades [25]. They reported on 93 patients with AMI, 45 of who were treated during the 1990s and 48 during the 2000s. The majority of patients were treated with open revascularization. Endovascular therapy alone or as a hybrid procedure was used in 11 total patients, eight of which were treated in the last 10 years. Thirty-day mortality was 27 % in the 1990s and 17 % during the 2000s. Major adverse events occurred in

47 % of patients with no difference between decades and no significant difference in outcomes between open and endovascular revascularization.

Two separate reports evaluated and compared open to endovascular therapy using the National Inpatient Data Sampling during similar periods, with similar results. Beaulieu et al. [26] evaluated 23,744 patients presenting with AMI, 4665 underwent interventional treatment from 2005 through 2009, 679 patients underwent vascular intervention, 75.7 % underwent open surgery, and 24.3 % underwent endovascular treatment overall during the study period. The proportion of patients undergoing endovascular repair increased from 11.9 % of patients in 2005 to 30.0 % in 2009. Mortality was significantly more commonly associated with open revascularization compared with endovascular intervention (39.3 % vs 24.9 %); length of stay was also significantly longer in the patient group undergoing open revascularization (12.9 vs 17.1 days). They identified 6683 patients of which majority had an endovascular procedure (62.7 % vs 37.3) with an overall in-hospital mortality rate (IHM) of 17.4 %. Despite endovascular therapy having significantly lower in-hospital mortality (IHM) rates (15.3 % vs 21.2 %), over the 8-year period of study, there was no difference between open surgery and endovascular therapy.

Conclusions

Acute mesenteric ischemia has high mortality rates. However, with the incorporation of minimally invasive endovascular therapies, the rates have decreased. Prompt diagnosis and early treatment remains the mainstay of therapy.

References

1. Litten M. Uber die Folgen des Verschlusses der Arteria Mesaraica Superior. Arch Pathol Anat. 1875;63:289.
2. Stoney RJ, Cunningham CG. Acute mesenteric ischemia. Surgery. 1993;114:489–90.
3. Acosta S. Epidemiology of mesenteric vascular disease: clinical implications. Semin Vasc Surg. 2010;23:4–8.
4. Park WM, Gloviczki P, Cherry KJ, Hallett JW, Bower TC, Panneton JM, Schleck C, Ilstrup D, Harmsen WS, Noel AA. Contemporary management of acute mesenteric ischemia: factors associated with survival. J Vasc Surg. 2002;35:445–52.
5. Stoney RJ, Ehrenfeld WK, Wiley EJ. Revascularization methods in chronic visceral ischemia caused by atherosclerosis. Ann Surg. 1977;186:468–76.
6. Stoney RJ, Wylie EJ. Recognition and surgical management of visceral ischemic syndrome. Ann Surg. 1966;164:714.
7. Shaw RS, Maynard III EP. Acute and chronic thrombosis of mesenteric arteries associated with malabsorption. A report of two cases successfully treated by thromboendarterectomy. N Engl J Med. 1958;258:874.
8. Furrer J, Gruntzig A, Kugelmeier J, et al. Treatment of abdominal angina with percutaneous dilatation of an arteria mesenterica superior stenosis: preliminary communication. Cardiovasc Intervent Radiol. 1980;3:43–4.

9. Schermerhorn ML, Giles KA, Hamdan AD, Wyers MC, Pomposelli FB. Mesenteric revascularization: management and outcomes in the United States, 1988–2006. J Vasc Surg. 2009;50:341–8.
10. Björnsson S, Björck M, Block T, Resch T, Acosta S. Thrombolysis for acute occlusion of the superior mesenteric artery. J Vasc Surg. 2011;54:1734–42.
11. Heiss P, Loewenhardt B, Manke C, Hellinger A, Dietl KH, Schlitt HJ, et al. Primary percutaneous aspiration and thrombolysis for the treatment of acute embolic superior mesenteric artery occlusion. Eur Radiol. 2010;20:2948–58.
12. Kasirajan K, Gray B, Beavers FP, et al. Rheolytic thrombectomy in the management of acute and subacute limb-threatening ischemia. J Vasc Interv Radiol. 2001;12:413–21.
13. Oderich GS, Erdoes LS, LeSar C, Mendes BC, Gloviczki P, Cha S, Duncan AA, Bower TC. Comparison of covered stents versus bare metal stents for treatment of chronic atherosclerotic mesenteric arterial disease. J Vasc Surg. 2013;58:1316–24.
14. Milner R, Woo EY, Carpenter JP. Superior mesenteric artery angioplasty and stenting via a retrograde approach in a patient with bowel ischemia – a case report. Vasc Endovascular Surg. 2004;38:89–91.
15. Wyers MC, Powell RJ, Nolan BW, Cronenwett JL. Retrograde mesenteric stenting during laparotomy for acute occlusive mesenteric ischemia. J Vasc Surg. 2011;53:698–705.
16. Svensson LG, Kouchoukos NT, Miller DC, Bavaria JE, Coselli JS, Curi MA, et al. Expert consensus document on the treatment of descending thoracic aortic disease using endovascular stent-grafts. Ann Thorac Surg. 2008;85(1 Suppl):S1–41.
17. Dake MD, Kato N, Mitchell RS, et al. Endovascular stent-graft placement for the treatment of acute aortic dissection. N Engl J Med. 1999;340(20):1546–52.
18. Verhoye JP, Miller DC, Sze D, Dake MD, Mitchell RS. Complicated acute type B aortic dissection: midterm results of emergency endovascular stent-grafting. J Thorac Cardiovasc Surg. 2008;136(2):424–30.
19. White RA, Miller DC, Criado FJ, Dake MD, Diethrich EB, Greenberg RK, et al. Report on the results of thoracic endovascular aortic repair for acute, complicated, type B aortic dissection at 30 days and 1 year from a multidisciplinary subcommittee of the Society for Vascular Surgery Outcomes Committee. J Vasc Surg. 2011;53(4):1082–90.
20. Ryan C, Vargas L, Mastracci T, Srivastava S, Eagleton M, Kelso R, Lyden S, Clair D, Sarac TP. Progress in the management of visceral ischemia from type B aortic dissection. J Vasc Surg. 2013;57(5):1283–90. discussion 1290.
21. Acosta S, Alhadad A, Svensson P, Ekberg O. Epidemiology, risk and prognostic factors in mesenteric venous thrombosis. Br J Surg. 2008;95:1245–51.
22. Di Minno MN, Milone F, Milone M, Iaccarino V, Venetucci P, Lupoli R, et al. Endovascular thrombolysis in acute mesenteric vein thrombosis: a 3-year follow-up with the rate of short and long-term sequaelae in 32 patients. Thromb Res. 2010;126:295–8.
23. Kougias P, Lau D, El Sayed HF, Zhou W, Huynh TT, Lin PH. Determinants of mortality and treatment outcome following surgical interventions for acute mesenteric ischemia. J Vasc Surg. 2007;46:467–74.
24. Arthurs ZM, Titus J, Bannazadeh M, Eagleton MJ, Srivastava S, Sarac TP, Daniel G, Clair DG. A comparison of endovascular revascularization with traditional therapy for the treatment of acute mesenteric ischemia. J Vasc Surg. 2011;53:698–705.
25. Ryer EJ, Kalra M, Oderich GS, Duncan AA, Gloviczki P, Cha S, Bower TC. Revascularization for acute mesenteric ischemia. J Vasc Surg. 2012;55:1682–9.
26. Beaulieu RJ, Arnaoutakisn KD, Abularrage CJ, Efro DT, Schneider E, Black JH. Comparison of open and endovascular treatment of acute mesenteric ischemia. J Vasc Surg. 2014;59:159–64.

Chapter 19
Second-Look Laparotomy, the Open Abdomen, and Temporary Abdominal Closure in Acute Mesenteric Ischemia

Rishi Kundi and Todd E. Rasmussen

Planned, repeat laparotomy, also referred to as "second-look" laparotomy, is a recognized principle in the management of acute mesenteric ischemia. Re-exploration of the abdomen in the hours or days following the initial operation for acute mesenteric ischemia allows confirmation of patency of revascularization and viability of remaining bowel. In some scenarios, multiple, repeat laparotomies may be performed over a period of days to assure the surgeon that bowel perfusion is adequate and that any nonviable segments of the tract have been removed. Despite the importance of second-look procedures as part of the management of this challenging clinical scenario, inherent challenges and considerations must be understood in order to optimize its efficacy and reduce complications. The objective of this chapter is to review the reasoning and indications of second-look operations in the setting of acute mesenteric ischemia and describe techniques of the procedure. The compatibility of the second look with the open abdomen in the patient with acute mesenteric ischemia is also reviewed, and a summary of techniques used for temporary and definitive abdominal closure is provided.

R. Kundi, MD
Division of Vascular Surgery, Department of Surgery,
University of Maryland School of Medicine, Baltimore, MD, USA
e-mail: rishi.kundi@gmail.com

T.E. Rasmussen, MD (✉)
US Combat Casualty Care Research Program, Fort Detrick, MD, USA

Uniformed Services University, Bethesda, MD, USA
e-mail: todd.e.rasmussen.mil@mail.mil

G.S. Oderich (ed.), *Mesenteric Vascular Disease*,
DOI 10.1007/978-1-4939-1847-8_19

Rationale

Second-look surgery after exploratory laparotomy for acute mesenteric ischemia (AMI) was first described by Shaw et al. in 1965 [1]. Reexamination of the bowel 24–48 h after both restoration of perfusion and the initiation of resuscitation was promoted as a way of distinguishing between viable and nonviable bowel after correction of the inciting insult, a notoriously challenging prospect when attempted at the first surgery. On return to the operating room, Shaw reasoned, bowel that was irreversibly ischemic at the time of revascularization would have proven itself so and that which was merely stunned would be apparently vital. This strategy thus avoids both bowel necrosis and unnecessarily zealous resection leading to short gut syndrome.

This intuitive strategy is, in fact, supported by the pathophysiological mechanisms of the several etiologies of AMI. Acute embolic occlusion of mesenteric arteries causes, after several hours, a reflex vasoconstriction of neighboring patent arterioles with subsequent reduction in perfusion. This vasoconstriction of adjacent vasculature persists even once the embolus is removed and may, after sufficient ischemia, be irreversible [2]. In patients with a mixed, acute-on-chronic arterial mesenteric ischemia, the unpredictable anatomy and importance of collateral circulation make the ischemic consequences of segmental bowel resection equally unpredictable, and this uncertainty may make a second-look procedure necessary. Management of acute mesenteric venous thrombosis rarely involves laparotomy, but upon exploration, the edema of venous congestion, the diffuse pattern of occlusion, and the attendant arterial spasm make prediction of necrosis at the time of initial laparotomy challenging [3, 4]. Nonocclusive mesenteric ischemia is similarly diffuse in nature, and, given the variable response to the intra-arterial vasodilators that constitute the primary therapy of NOMI, it is unsurprising that in a series described by Ward et al., more than three quarters of patients with NOMI who underwent exploration were taken back for second look, and half of those underwent additional bowel resection [5].

The yield of second-look laparotomy as related by Ward et al. is consistent with published series, which report rates of positive relaparotomy ranging from 7 to 72 % (Table 19.1). This degree of variability is likely due to equally variable criteria for performing a second-look procedure. While tradition holds that the decision to take a patient back for a second look should be made at the first operation, the vast majority of literature is composed of retrospective, single-institution, multi-surgeon studies with undocumented criteria regarding that decision. Few studies have directly examined the role and technique of second-look laparotomy (Table 19.2). Of these, the positive yield has ranged from 14.6 to 50 % [6–8]. A single nonrandomized case–control study of planned versus clinically indicated relaparotomy demonstrated equivalent mortality despite a significantly higher rate of anastomotic leak and sepsis in the planned laparotomy group [9]. Few clear conclusions can be drawn from this single study, but relaparotomy, as any surgical procedure, has attendant risks that compel careful consideration of its technical aspects.

Table 19.1 Published studies on second-look operations for acute mesenteric ischemia

Author	Year	Number of patients	Number of second-look procedures	Number of positive findings from second-look procedure
Kaminsky [8]	2005	41	15	6
Yanar [15]	2007	71	14	1
Anadol [6]	2004	77	46	9
Bjorck [7]	2002	60	41	19
Park [39]	2002	58	23	11
Kougias [40]	2007	72	38	15
Freeman [41]	2005	20	12	7
Wadman [42]	2000	74	24	16
Edwards [43]	2003	76	34	17
Luther [44]	2002	64	29	21
Denecke [45]	1990	115	36	10

Adapted from Meng Meng X, Liu L, Jiang H. Indications and procedures for second-look surgery in acute mesenteric ischemia. Surg Today. 2010;40(8):700–5, with permission of Springer Science+Business Media

Table 19.2 Second-look operation versus no second look: differences in mortality

Author	Year	Number of patients	Number of second-Look procedures	Mortality after second look (%)	Number of non-second look	Mortality after non-second look (%)
Kaminsky [8]	2005	41	15	80	26	57.7
Anadol [6]	2004	54	23	34.8	31	48.4
Bjorck [7]	2002	60	41	51.2	19	52.6

Adapted from Meng Meng X, Liu L, Jiang H. Indications and procedures for second-look surgery in acute mesenteric ischemia. Surg Today. 2010;40(8):700–5, with permission of Springer Science+Business Media

Timing

The timing of the second-look laparotomy has traditionally been advocated as between 24 and 48 h after the initial surgery, a period advocated from the first description of the procedure [1]. Whatever the length, the goal of this interval is to allow the second look to be performed when the overall physiology of the patient has been optimized. This will ensure that any stunned bowel has been reperfused to the extent that it no longer exhibits ambiguous vitality, in addition to increasing the likelihood of anastomotic healing and decreasing the chance of fistula formation. Moreover, adequate resuscitation and physiological support increase the patient's tolerance of the second procedure.

Evidence supports the assertion that the 1- to 2-day intermission is sufficient to allow this optimization. In animal models, both serum and histopathological markers of intestinal ischemic injury are well past their peak by 24 h after perfusion is reestablished; by 48 h, they have returned to baseline [10]. This timeline is, of course, a guideline, and the clinical status of the patient should otherwise determine the schedule of treatment. After initiation of treatment and the primary laparotomy, an improvement in clinical parameters indicates progress toward optimization and resolution of any reperfusion injury. A lack of improvement or deteriorating clinical status, however, may indicate a missed bowel injury or the evolution of metabolically significant bowel necrosis and should compel re-exploration regardless of the length of time since the original surgery.

Technique

The technique of second-look laparotomy in AMI is entirely concerned with the inspection of the bowel. While ultrasonography, fluorescein, and angiography all have roles in the diagnosis of acute ischemia, their reliability in the prediction of intestinal viability is unacceptably low [11]. Clinical signs, such as absence of peristalsis, bowel wall edema, mucosal hemorrhage, and a lack of bleeding at cut bowel edges, are similarly poor predictors if employed at the time of the initial laparotomy. With a correction of the underlying vascular deficit, the patient's physiological parameters and time for ischemia–reperfusion damage to declare itself; however, the utility of these clinical indicators is reasonable in determining the need for additional resection.

In recent years, the advent of minimally invasive techniques in general surgery has prompted consideration of laparoscopy in place of second-look laparotomy. Its applicability in this context has yet to be defined, but the authors believe that laparoscopy is inadvisable for several reasons [6, 12–15]. The benefit of laparoscopy over second-look laparotomy is minimal. The patient already bears a midline incision and is not spared another. The procedure requires both general anesthesia and paralysis to a degree indistinguishable from that required for laparotomy. The limitations of laparoscopy over laparotomy are significant. Laparoscopy provides only visual assessment of the bowel and does not allow any tactile examination of signs of viability. That visual assessment is itself limited to the small field of vision of the laparoscope. Running the bowel laparoscopy is a technically challenging procedure that, in the best of cases, cannot visualize more than a few centimeters of bowel at any time.

The most compelling reason to avoid laparoscopy, however, is that the pneumoperitoneum that is the sine qua non of laparoscopy is physiologically inadvisable in the context of poor visceral perfusion. Physiological intra-abdominal pressure in the human being is approximately 10 mmHg. If this pressure is the context for acute mesenteric ischemia, raising it by 150–200 % cannot reasonably be expected to benefit the patient. Pneumoperitoneum requires intra-abdominal pressures that have been shown to impair visceral blood flow. In a rat model, pneumoperitoneum at pressures required for laparoscopy results in decreased intestinal perfusion and bacterial translocation [16]. Avoidance of intra-abdominal hypertension, in fact, not only makes second-look laparoscopy inadvisable but makes a planned open-abdomen strategy preferable.

The physiological effects of increased intra-abdominal pressure are well documented. The term intra-abdominal hypertension (IAH) is used to denote pressures higher than 10 mmHg [17]. In a dog model, IAH was shown to decrease splanchnic perfusion by a factor of 2 at intra-abdominal pressures of only 20 mmHg [18]. An identical pressure increase in a pig model resulted in a drop in intestinal perfusion of almost 40 % [19]. A pressure increase to only 15 mmHg – less than standard pneumoperitoneum, far less than would be required for the diagnosis of abdominal compartment syndrome, and only 5 mmHg above healthy controls – caused a drop in bowel tissue oxygenation of more than a quarter. A pressure of 25 mmHg, still less than generally regarded as abdominal compartment syndrome, dropped oxygenation to 50 % of the normal. In a rat model, a moderate degree of IAH caused not only a drop in mesenteric and intestinal perfusion but also resulted in bacterial translocation [20]. Increasing intra-abdominal pressure was directly related to markers of gut ischemia [19]. These findings of decreased perfusion, intestinal ischemia, and bacterial translocation occurred in the context of normal cardiac output and mean arterial pressure. The patient with acute mesenteric ischemia, already at a physiological disadvantage, is particularly vulnerable to the deleterious effects of increased abdominal pressure. The burgeoning ischemia of IAH, when relieved with second-look laparotomy, could lead to another cycle of ischemia–reperfusion injury that will not complete manifestation until 24–48 h after the relaparotomy, decreasing the utility of the second look and worsening bowel injury.

The AMI patient is not only particularly vulnerable to IAH but is particularly likely to develop the condition as is any patient undergoing emergency abdominal surgery – a third of whom will end up with the formal diagnosis of abdominal compartment syndrome [21]. The high prevalence of abdominal compartment syndrome (ACS) among acute care surgical patients is likely a consequence of the frequent need for fluid resuscitation in this population. Crystalloid volumes of 10 L or greater, rates of 250 mL/kg, or the administration of more than 6 L in 6 h have all been associated with a high risk of abdominal compartment syndrome [17]. In examining resuscitation to supranormal oxygen delivery parameters, Balogh et al. demonstrated a prevalence of either IAH or ACS of 58 % as well as an increase in visceral ischemia [22]. While the diagnosis of bowel ischemia predisposes the patient to IAH, intra-abdominal hypertension in the surgical patient has been associated with bowel necrosis at laparotomy [21, 23].

The clear benefits of second-look laparotomy, combined with the hazards posed by the development of intra-abdominal hypertension and the likelihood that such hypertension will develop, mandate careful consideration of maintenance of an open abdomen after laparotomy for acute mesenteric ischemia. Closure of the abdomen after laparotomy for AMI will increase the likelihood of intra-abdominal hypertension and worsened gut perfusion and possibly increase the subsequent necessity of additional bowel resection at second-look laparotomy. Delay of fascial closure until completion of the second-look laparotomy minimizes the probability of IAH-related gut ischemia, allows a more liberal resuscitation protocol, and facilitates second-look surgery.

The maintenance of an open abdomen after initial laparotomy for AMI is almost universally advantageous. Though the benefits of this strategy may be clear, the maintenance of the open abdomen and the eventual final closure are its attendant challenges. Despite the nomenclature, the open abdomen requires some method of temporary closure in the interval between the initial and final laparotomies, however separate in time those operations must be. Such temporary closure must accomplish several goals. First, it must provide coverage and protection of the viscera. Desiccation of the intra-abdominal contents must be prevented, particularly within the threatened bowel and anastomotic or staple lines. The obverse of this priority is the need to minimize insensible losses in the patient whose volume status is critical. Second, the temporary closure must allow for the maintenance of domain within the abdomen and prevent retraction of the fascial envelope. The preservation of domain as well as of the fascial edges is vital to eventual final closure. Retraction of fascial edges occurs rapidly. Without the use of fascial bridging, the chances of successful primary closure fall to zero after only 96 h [24].

Management of intra-abdominal fluid collection and stagnation with an eye to contamination control is an additional requirement and must be balanced with the need to avoid desiccation of the viscera. Finally, the temporary abdominal closure must avoid intra-abdominal hypertension and abdominal compartment syndrome. Though this risk seems obviated entirely by an open abdominal strategy, it is not [22].

Temporary and Permanent Abdominal Wall Closure

In the initial damage control experience, simple skin approximation was used for temporary abdominal closure; the resulting incidence of ACS led to the abandonment of this practice [25]. Aside from this, skin approximation is a suboptimal method of interval closure for other reasons. It does not prevent fascial retraction, nor does it avoid early loss of domain. Its watertight nature, in addition to enabling the development of ACS, does not allow control or drainage of contaminated intra-abdominal fluid and increases the risk of evisceration and skin necrosis. The complication rate of skin closure, no matter what the method, can be as high as 36 %, and so this technique is generally no longer used [25]. Skin interposition methods, such as the mesh silo and the Bogota bag, are not watertight and thus avoid the problems associated with fluid accumulation and stagnation such as ACS and infection. As these methods involve the sewing of an interposition material to the skin, and not the fascia, they do not prevent the latter from retracting. As such, rates of successful primary closure are generally poor.

The principle of interposition, however, may be applied to fascial apposition with significantly better results than found with skin closure as regards successful primary closure. The suturing of a mesh to the fascial edges will allow for relief of abdominal pressure while preventing fascial retraction. While each material used for interposition is accompanied by its own advantages and disadvantages, several characteristics are fundamental to the technique. Because the intra-abdominal volume will increase in the days after the initial laparotomy, the interposition mesh should initially be significantly redundant, allowing for expansion. As bowel edema resolves, the redundancy can be reduced with plication or, in the case of a Wittmann Patch, reclosed, as discussed below. Fascial separation can be addressed every 1–2 days until primary closure can be achieved. If multiple relaparotomies are performed, care must be taken to minimize trauma to the fascial edges, as weakening or fraying will make closure more difficult. With this in mind, relaparotomy is best performed by incision and subsequent reclosure of the mesh, rather than detachment and reattachment of the mesh to the fascia.

Initial mesh utilization was not to allow eventual primary closure but to encourage granulation over the viscera with eventual skin grafting. The massive ventral hernia was an accepted consequence of the method, which employed bioabsorbable mesh of either polyglactic or polyglycolic acid. These meshes were naturally very adherent to the adjacent bowel, and rates of enterocutaneous fistula with absorbable mesh have been reported as high as 26 % [26]. The use of polypropylene, a nonabsorbable mesh, improved the rate of primary closure but, being abrasive and adherent to visceral contents, failed to eliminate the formation of enterocutaneous fistula [27]. The use of these adherent meshes for temporary closure mandates interposition of the omentum between the mesh and the serosa, but this barrier does not eliminate the risk of either adherence or fistula [28]. Expanded polytetrafluoroethylene is relatively nonadherent and therefore allows repeat laparotomy and exploration, but has unacceptably high rates of infection when not immediately covered with tissue and is not advocated in this context [28].

The Wittmann Patch is a fascial interposition device that comes in two leaves with a "hook-and-loop" interface between the two. This allows both ease of re-exploration as well as ease of retightening, as the leaves come apart and readhere to each other easily. The Wittmann Patch is otherwise prone to the same complications as other interposition meshes, though with a substantially lower rate of fistula formation [29–33].

The creation of a vacuum pack dressing allows for control of intra-abdominal fluid while preventing bowel adherence and is intended to be a temporary measure to allow primary fascial closure. The vacuum pack, as originally described by Brock et al., involves a plastic sheet with vents cut into it that is positioned across the entire visceral block, from paracolic gutter to paracolic gutter laterally [34]. Above this plastic is placed a layer of porous material, whether composed of laparotomy pads, operative towels, or gauze dressing. Within this layer are drains that will apply suction to the entire dressing. Over the porous layer is an outer, biocclusive dressing that is secured to the skin of the flanks, chest, and pelvis. The drains are placed to continuous low suction. This dressing achieves a temporary closure of the abdomen that controls and drains fluid, allows for expansion, and protects the viscera. Adherence is prevented by the deepest plastic layer. The dressing can be rapidly removed and placed for re-exploration. Two years after first describing the negative-pressure closure, Smith et al. examined their four-year employment of the technique and found less than a 5 % incidence of fistula formation and abscess formation with a primary closure rate of almost 70 % [35].

The success of the negative-pressure method has spurred development of commercial abdominal dressings. These combine the components of the created dressing in fewer components, but fundamentally retain the three layers of nonadherent plastic barrier with a porous suction layer and an occlusive top layer. These systems have thus far demonstrated a successful primary closure rate of about 65 %, with a fistula rate of less than 3 % [36]. The best primary closure rates have been achieved with the use of fascial retention sutures. While the negative pressure has some purported ability to resist fascial retraction, there is no physical component of the dressing that actively opposes the process. The use of wide, low-tension retention sutures between fascial edges and above the deep plastic and porous layers but below the occlusive dressing compensates for this lack.

Once definitive surgical management of the intra-abdominal pathology has been accomplished, closure of the abdomen assumes primacy. The abdominal wall should be assessed at every dressing change for resolution of bowel edema and the ease with which the fascial edges may be approximated. The longer that an open abdomen is maintained, the less likely it is that primary closure will be achieved. At least half of all open abdomens will be able to be closed primarily with either one-stage or serial closures; the remainder will require a planned ventral hernia [37].

With rapid resolution of bowel edema, the ability to immediately close the abdomen may be possible. More often, serial closure must be pursued with delayed primary closure. This strategy involves stepwise approximation of fascial edges with sequential replacement of the initial mesh prosthesis with smaller bridges and eventual closure. Alternatively, as described above, the interposition mesh may be incised and reclosed in order to avoid repeat traumatization of the fascial edges. Excision and replacement of the mesh, however, possesses some advantages. With frequent removal and replacement, the adherence of the mesh to the underlying visceral block may be reduced. The short interval between excision and replacement negates the increased infection risk of expanded polytetrafluoroethylene, a mesh with excellent resistance to adhesion. The hook-and-loop design of the Wittmann Patch is specifically designed to enable frequent decreases in the size of the interposition graft without any trauma to the fascia. If a negative-pressure dressing is used with fascial retention sutures, any dressing change will require the removal of those sutures, which can be replaced in a manner that draws the fascial edges together in a serial manner. Finally, commercial systems employing "dynamic fascial closure" are available. These employ principles identical to serially replaced fascial retention sutures, but allow for redundancy to be eliminated without repeated trauma to fascial edges. If a negative-pressure dressing is used without any fascial retention technique, the options for delayed primary closure are limited.

If neither primary closure nor delayed primary closure is possible, closure with a planned ventral hernia is a strategy that allows rapid resolution of the open abdomen. An interposition mesh of suitable size is used as a base for granulation, and when a suitable granulation bed is achieved, split-thickness skin grafting is performed. A negative-pressure dressing can be used atop the mesh in order to speed granulation, as may wet-to-dry dressings with frequent dressing changes. Patients may be maintained with the intentional ventral hernia while they recover from the effects of the inciting abdominal pathology. Critical illness is, of course, inherently detrimental to nutritional status, and the catabolic response may persist for up to 2 years afterwards [38]. The nature of acute mesenteric ischemia and its treatment further predispose the patient to malnutrition. Repair of the ventral hernia, then, should be deferred until the patient is nutritionally robust in order to maximize the chances of success.

An alternative to delayed closure with planned ventral hernia is component separation in order to achieve delayed primary closure. This procedure allows for immediate fascial closure without the use of foreign material, reducing both the chance of infection and fistula. It is a more complex and involved operation than planned ventral hernia, but its advantages are significant. The operation involves raising subcutaneous flaps laterally and sagittal division of the external oblique fascia immediately lateral to the rectus sheath, after which the external oblique is dissected free of the underlying internal oblique as far laterally as possible. This allows for additional circumference, but if significant tension still exists cranial to the arcuate line, the posterior rectus sheath may be incised in a similar manner, and the rectus dissected away from it. Component separation can yield up to 20 cm of additional circumference and will often allow primary closure.

Conclusion

Despite significant advances in diagnostic methods and technology, acute mesenteric ischemia remains an unpredictable disease process with devastating consequences for missed progression. No greater method for determination of threatened or non-viable bowel and maximal preservation of bowel length has been found than second-look laparotomy. Taken together with the incidence and sequelae of intra-abdominal hypertension and abdominal compartment syndrome, the pursuit of an open-abdomen strategy in the management of acute mesenteric ischemia demonstrates significant utility. With careful use of temporary closure techniques, primary closure or delayed primary closure is possible in a majority of patients, and alternative methods enable closure in the remainder.

References

1. Mulholland JH, Ellison EH, Friesen SR. Current surgical management; a book of alternative viewpoints on controversial surgical problems. In: Mulholland JH, Ellison EH, Friesen SR, editors. Current surgical management. Philadelphia: Saunders; 1957. p. 1957–65.
2. Kozuch PL, Brandt LJ. Review article: diagnosis and management of mesenteric ischaemia with an emphasis on pharmacotherapy. Aliment Pharmacol Ther. 2005;21(3):201–15.
3. Boley SJ, Kaleya RN, Brandt LJ. Mesenteric venous thrombosis. Surg Clin North Am. 1992; 72(1):183–201.

4. Kumar S, Sarr MG, Kamath PS. Mesenteric venous thrombosis. N Engl J Med. 2001; 345(23):1683–8.
5. Ward D, et al. Improved outcome by identification of high-risk nonocclusive mesenteric ischemia, aggressive reexploration, and delayed anastomosis. Am J Surg. 1995;170(6):577–80. discussion 580–1.
6. Anadol AZ, et al. Laparoscopic "second-look" in the management of mesenteric ischemia. Surg Laparosc Endosc Percutan Tech. 2004;14(4):191–3.
7. Bjorck M, et al. Revascularization of the superior mesenteric artery after acute thromboembolic occlusion. Br J Surg. 2002;89(7):923–7.
8. Kaminsky O, et al. Does a second-look operation improve survival in patients with peritonitis due to acute mesenteric ischemia? A five-year retrospective experience. World J Surg. 2005;29(5):645–8.
9. Hau T, et al. Planned relaparotomy vs relaparotomy on demand in the treatment of intra-abdominal infections. The Peritonitis Study Group of the Surgical Infection Society-Europe. Arch Surg. 1995;130(11):1193–6. discussion 1196–7.
10. Guzman-de la Garza FJ, et al. Temporal relationship of serum markers and tissue damage during acute intestinal ischemia/reperfusion. Clinics (Sao Paulo). 2013;68(7):1034–8.
11. Ballard JL, et al. A critical analysis of adjuvant techniques used to assess bowel viability in acute mesenteric ischemia. Am Surg. 1993;59(5):309–11.
12. Seshadri PA, et al. Simplified laparoscopic approach to "second-look" laparotomy: a review. Surg Laparosc Endosc Percutan Tech. 1999;9(4):286–9.
13. Tola M, Portoghese A, Maniga AM. [Laparoscopic second-look in acute intestinal ischemia]. Minerva Chir. 1997;52(5):527–30.
14. Wang YZ. Staged second-look laparoscopy to evaluate ischemic bowel. J Soc Laparoendoscop Surg. 2009;13(4):560–3.
15. Yanar H, et al. Planned second-look laparoscopy in the management of acute mesenteric ischemia. World J Gastroenterol. 2007;13(24):3350–3.
16. Eleftheriadis E, et al. Gut ischemia, oxidative stress, and bacterial translocation in elevated abdominal pressure in rats. World J Surg. 1996;20(1):11–6.
17. CE RMaG. The open abdomen. In: BP Norton JA, Bollinger RR et al. editors. Surgery: basic science and clinical evidence. New York: Springer; 2013.
18. Caldwell CB, Ricotta JJ. Changes in visceral blood flow with elevated intraabdominal pressure. J Surg Res. 1987;43(1):14–20.
19. Diebel LN, Dulchavsky SA, Wilson RF. Effect of increased intra-abdominal pressure on mesenteric arterial and intestinal mucosal blood flow. J Trauma. 1992;33(1):45–8; discussion 48–9.
20. Diebel LN, Dulchavsky SA, Brown WJ. Splanchnic ischemia and bacterial translocation in the abdominal compartment syndrome. J Trauma. 1997;43(5):852–5.
21. McNelis J, et al. Abdominal compartment syndrome in the surgical intensive care unit. Am Surg. 2002;68(1):18–23.
22. Balogh Z, et al. Supranormal trauma resuscitation causes more cases of abdominal compartment syndrome. Arch Surg. 2003;138(6):637–42; discussion 642–3.
23. Williams M, Simms HH. Abdominal compartment syndrome: case reports and implications for management in critically ill patients. Am Surg. 1997;63(6):555–8.
24. Raeburn CD, et al. The abdominal compartment syndrome is a morbid complication of postinjury damage control surgery. Am J Surg. 2001;182(6):542–6.
25. Regner JL, Kobayashi L, Coimbra R. Surgical strategies for management of the open abdomen. World J Surg. 2012;36(3):497–510.
26. Bee TK, et al. Temporary abdominal closure techniques: a prospective randomized trial comparing polyglactin 910 mesh and vacuum-assisted closure. J Trauma. 2008;65(2):337–42; discussion 342–4.
27. Diaz Jr JJ, et al. The management of the open abdomen in trauma and emergency general surgery: part 1-damage control. J Trauma. 2010;68(6):1425–38.

28. Mayberry JC, et al. Prevention of abdominal compartment syndrome by absorbable mesh prosthesis closure. Arch Surg. 1997;132(9):957–61; discussion 961–2.
29. Hadeed JG, et al. Delayed primary closure in damage control laparotomy: the value of the Wittmann patch. Am Surg. 2007;73(1):10–2.
30. Keramati M, et al. The Wittmann Patch as a temporary abdominal closure device after decompressive celiotomy for abdominal compartment syndrome following burn. Burns. 2008; 34(4):493–7.
31. Tieu BH, et al. The use of the Wittmann Patch facilitates a high rate of fascial closure in severely injured trauma patients and critically ill emergency surgery patients. J Trauma. 2008;65(4):865–70.
32. Weinberg JA, et al. Closing the open abdomen: improved success with Wittmann Patch staged abdominal closure. J Trauma. 2008;65(2):345–8.
33. Wittmann DH, Aprahamian C, Bergstein JM. Etappenlavage: advanced diffuse peritonitis managed by planned multiple laparotomies utilizing zippers, slide fastener, and Velcro analogue for temporary abdominal closure. World J Surg. 1990;14(2):218–26.
34. Brock WB, Barker DE, Burns RP. Temporary closure of open abdominal wounds: the vacuum pack. Am Surg. 1995;61(1):30–5.
35. Smith LA, et al. Vacuum pack technique of temporary abdominal closure: a four-year experience. Am Surg. 1997;63(12):1102–7; discussion 1107–8.
36. Boele van Hensbroek P, et al. Temporary closure of the open abdomen: a systematic review on delayed primary fascial closure in patients with an open abdomen. World J Surg. 2009; 33(2):199–207.
37. Barker DE, et al. Vacuum pack technique of temporary abdominal closure: a 7-year experience with 112 patients. J Trauma. 2000;48(2):201–6; discussion 206–7.
38. Finnerty CC, et al. The surgically induced stress response. J Parenter Enteral Nutr. 2013;37 (5 Suppl):21s–9.
39. Park WM, et al. Contemporary management of acute mesenteric ischemia: Factors associated with survival. J Vasc Surg. 2002;35(3):445–52.
40. Kougias P, et al. Determinants of mortality and treatment outcome following surgical interventions for acute mesenteric ischemia. J Vasc Surg. 2007;46(3):467–74.
41. Freeman AJ, Graham JC. Damage control surgery and angiography in cases of acute mesenteric ischaemia. ANZ J Surg. 2005;75(5):308–14.
42. Wadman M, Syk I, Elmstahl S. Survival after operations for ischaemic bowel disease. Eur J Surg. 2000;166(11):872–7.
43. Edwards MS, et al. Acute occlusive mesenteric ischemia: surgical management and outcomes. Ann Vasc Surg. 2003;17(1):72–9.
44. Luther B, et al. [The acute mesenteric ischemia - not understood or incurable?]. Zentralbl Chir. 2002;127(8):674–84.
45. Denecke H, Stiegler H. Indications and results of second-look operation in acute mesenteric vascular occlusion. Langenbecks Arch Chir Suppl II Verh Dtsch Ges Chir, 1990. p. 311–5.

Chapter 20
Results of Open and Endovascular Revascularization for Acute Mesenteric Ischemia

Ramoncito A. David and Manju Kalra

Acute mesenteric ischemia (AMI) accounts for only 1–2 per 1,000 hospital admissions but continues to be a highly complex clinical problem with a relatively high mortality rate [1]. In a population-based autopsy study, the incidence of thromboembolic occlusion of the superior mesenteric artery with intestinal gangrene was 6.0 per 1,000 deaths, with the diagnosis carrying a mortality of 93 % [2]. The problem was suspected antemortem in only one-third of patients. The mortality rate from AMI has declined only very moderately from 80–90 % in the 1970s to 60–70 % in the 1980s. This was largely attributed to a higher index of suspicion among clinicians, advances in radiographic diagnosis, and an aggressive surgical approach with better perioperative care. However, following this, traditional treatment yielded no further improvement in mortality over the previous two decades [3, 4]. In order to further impact the grave outcome of AMI, an endovascular first treatment paradigm has been championed over the last decade. Indeed, endovascular treatment does offer some definite advantages and has been utilized very effectively in the more elective treatment of chronic mesenteric ischemia (CMI). While it is being increasingly used for revascularization in AMI, the main drawback is that it does not allow for immediate assessment of intestinal viability, limiting its applicability to select patients in whom immediate laparotomy is not indicated [5–7]. In addition, personnel with advanced endovascular skills and an extensive inventory of endovascular devices and equipment may not be readily available in many facilities. It is, therefore, more ideally suited for patients presenting somewhat subacutely and without peritoneal signs.

R.A. David, MD
Division of Vascular and Endovascular Surgery, Department of Surgery, Mayo Clinic, Rochester, MN, USA
e-mail: david.ramoncito@mayo.edu

M. Kalra, MBBS (✉)
Professor of Surgery, Division of Vascular and Endovascular Surgery, Department of Surgery, Mayo Clinic, Rochester, MN, USA
e-mail: kalra.manju@mayo.edu

G.S. Oderich (ed.), *Mesenteric Vascular Disease*,
DOI 10.1007/978-1-4939-1847-8_20

Contemporary Results of Open and Endovascular Revascularization

There are no randomized clinical trials of the treatment modalities for AMI, making it difficult to make valid comparisons. Because of the multiple confounding variables in the etiology, mode, and acuity of presentation and patient comorbidities, a systematic assessment of outcomes is not feasible. However, certain conclusions and treatment guidelines can be drawn from large single-center series as well as population-based registries in the literature.

Results from the US Nationwide Inpatient Sample

Based upon the data from the National Inpatient Sample (NIS) over the past decade, revascularization by endovascular means has surpassed open surgical bypass as the most frequently utilized method to treat CMI, while AMI continues to be treated with an open approach in most cases [8] (Fig. 20.1). In this study, Schermerhorn and associates reported a sevenfold increase in the number of mesenteric interventions

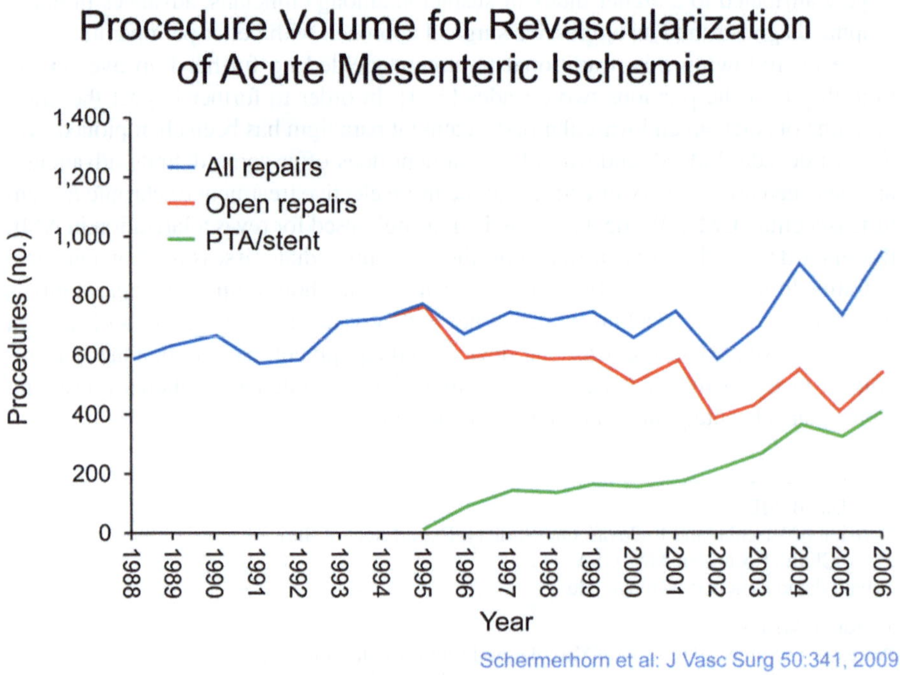

Fig. 20.1 Procedures performed for AMI from 1988 to 2006. Results from the US Nationwide Inpatient Sample (From Schermerhorn et al. [8], with permission)

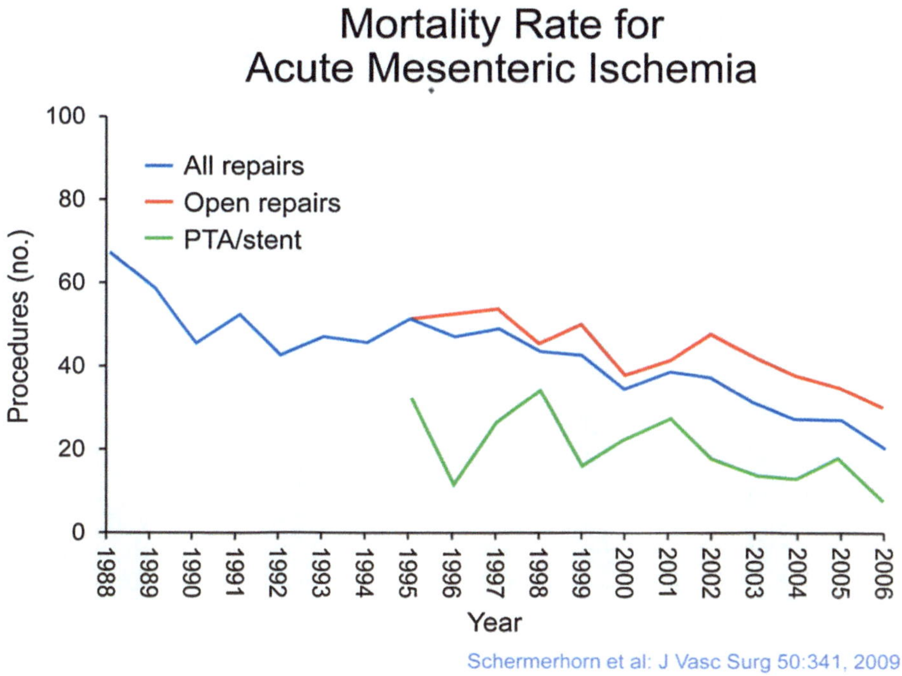

Fig. 20.2 Mortality rates by method of revascularization from 1988 to 2006. Results from the US Nationwide Inpatient Sample (From Schermerhorn et al. [8], with permission)

since 1988 and a remarkable reduction in mortality from 13 % with open bypass to 4 % with endovascular treatment for CMI and 28 % to 16 % for AMI respectively (Fig. 20.2). However, the significant shortcomings of this analysis include the inability to characterize patients with subacute vs AMI and primary vs secondary interventions. Overall the incidence of open surgery in the setting of acute ischemia remained unchanged during the time period from 1995 to 2006 while the number of endovascular procedures continued to increase gradually, further attesting to the fact that these additional patients undergoing endovascular treatment may have presented subacutely.

Among the patients undergoing open surgery, the incidence of embolectomy was 49 %, and the mortality rate was also highest in this group at 49 %. Mortality in the bypass patients was slightly lower at 44 % [8] (Fig. 20.3). The 37 % incidence of bowel resection in the open group was higher than the 28 % in the endovascular group. Since overall mortality was proportionate to the need for bowel resection, it is not surprising that mortality was lower in the endovascular group; however, this lower need for bowel resection may also be an indicator of the less acute/severe AMI in the endovascular group. In spite of the obvious benefits and equivalent clinical efficacy attributable to the minimally invasive approach, the longer experience with treatment of atherosclerotic CMI has revealed that endovascular treatment is

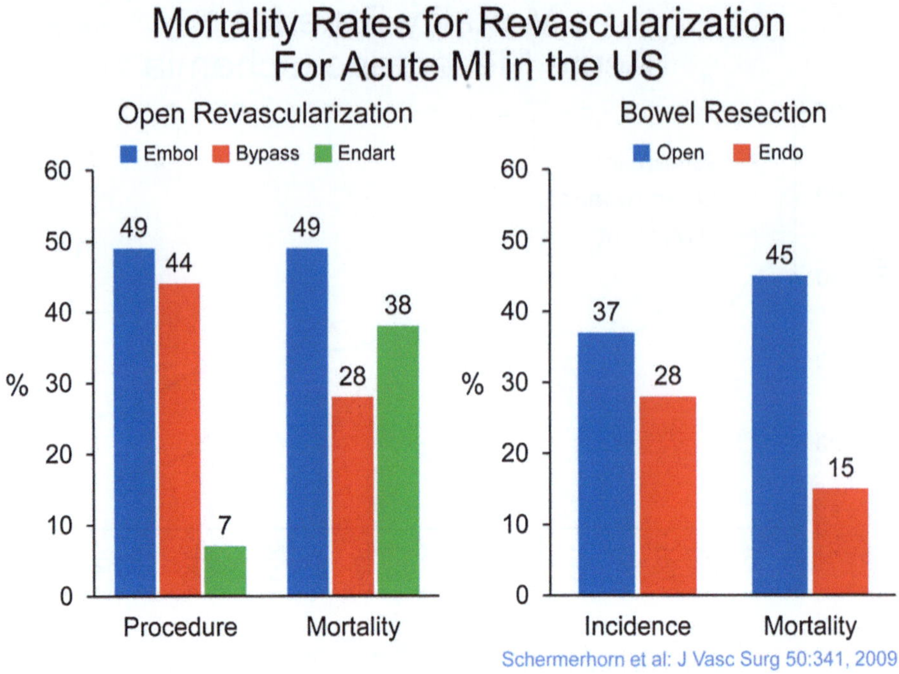

Fig. 20.3 Mortality rates by method of revascularization from 1988 to 2006. Results from the US Nationwide Inpatient Sample (From Schermerhorn et al. [8], with permission)

associated with similar mortality and more frequent restenoses, symptom recurrences, and re-interventions over time compared to open bypass, with up to one third of patients needing subsequent bypass [8–12].

Mayo Clinic Experience

Our experience at the Mayo Clinic over the last two decades (1990–2010) with treatment of acute mesenteric ischemia is comprised of 111 patients, 20 of whom were treated by endovascular means [13, 14]. Clinical presentation, treatment, and outcomes were compared over the two decades. A prior history of symptoms of CMI was obtained in ~40 % of patients presenting with AMI, unchanged over the two decades. The relative incidence of arterial embolism and thrombosis also remained unchanged over the two decades (Fig. 20.4). A greater proportion (26 %) of patients underwent endovascular intervention in the latter decade. Embolectomy of the SMA remained the commonest operative procedure in the open group (>50 %) followed by mesenteric bypass (40–45 %). In the endovascular group, 22 mesenteric vessels were treated: 18 superior mesenteric arteries (SMA) and 4 celiac

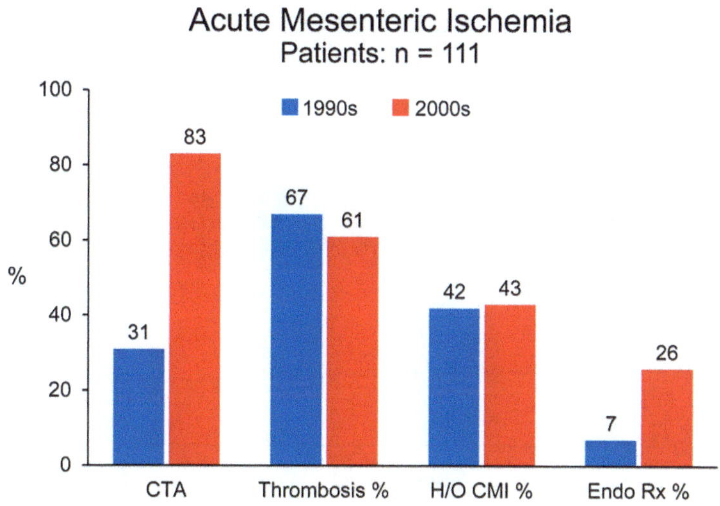

Fig. 20.4 Trends in the presentation, diagnosis, and treatment of AMI through the 1990s and 2000s. Mayo Clinic experience (From Ryer et al. [13], with permission)

arteries (CA), 18 with percutaneous angioplasty and stenting (PTA/S) and 4 with thrombolysis alone. Mechanical thrombectomy/thrombolysis was performed in four patients prior to PTA/S of the SMA. Femoral access was used in eight patients, brachial access in nine, and retrograde SMA access during laparotomy in three patients. As a testimony to the severity of AMI even in the endovascular group, 15 of 20 patients underwent concomitant or subsequent exploratory laparotomy, with bowel resection in 14. In two patients, this was delayed for 48–72 h after percutaneous SMA revascularization when peritoneal signs developed. Seven patients underwent a second-look laparotomy with further bowel resection in 29 % [13] (Fig. 20.5). The incidence of bowel resection was 41 % in the open group, with further resection at the second-look laparotomy in 22 %.

Our overall 30-day mortality rate from treatment of AMI over the last two decades improved slightly from 27 % in the 1990s to 17 % during the 2000s. Mortality following endovascular treatment was 25 % overall, 23 % in the recent decade, and 33 % in the preceding 10 years. This is not significantly different from an overall 20 % mortality in the 91 patients undergoing open revascularization over the same time period: 15 % in the 2000s and 26 % in the 1990s (Fig. 20.6). We hypothesize that the decrease in 30-day mortality is, at least in part, related to an increased use of second-look laparotomy. Comparing the two decades spanning this study, the number of patients undergoing a second-look operation has significantly increased from 48 to 80 % ($P=0.003$) in the contemporary cohort with ~28 % having necrotic bowel requiring resection at second look. This is in contrast to nationwide trends that show the number of patients undergoing a second-look operation has remained the same or has decreased, with only a fraction of patients operated on for AMI undergoing a second-look procedure [15, 16]. We feel strongly that the vast

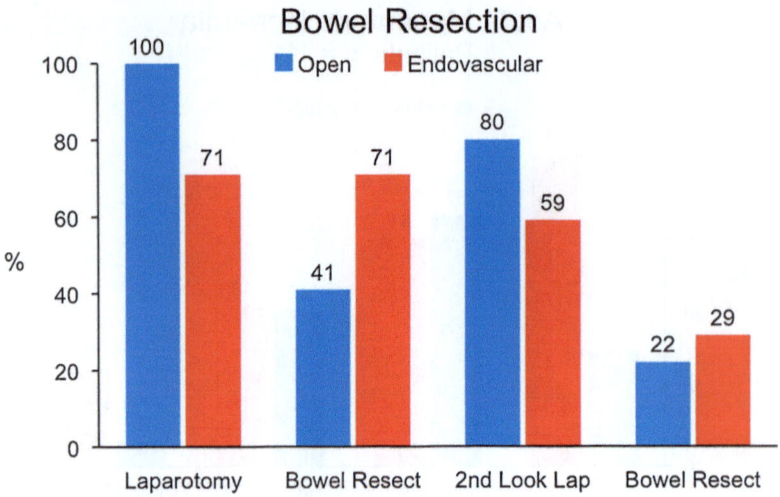

Fig. 20.5 Rates of laparotomy and bowel resection in open versus endovascular revascularization for AMI. Mayo Clinic experience (From Ryer et al.,[13], with permission)

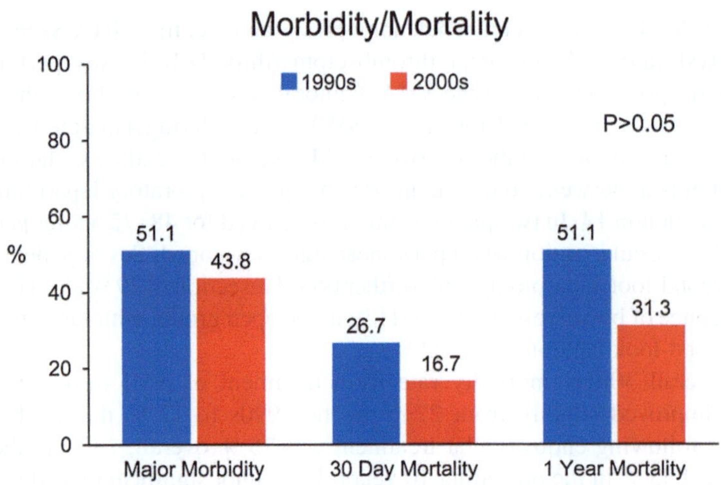

Fig. 20.6 Morbidity and mortality following revascularization for AMI. Mayo Clinic experience (From Ryer et al.,[13], with permission)

majority of patients should undergo a second-look laparotomy because assessment of the full extent of visceral ischemia is unreliable at the initial surgery, even when intraoperative Doppler ultrasonography and intravenous fluorescein are utilized (in this series both were utilized in ~28 % of cases). This is likely due to the fact that in AMI the serosa often appears viable despite infarction of the underlying intestinal mucosa [16]. Therefore, a second-look exploration is the only way to establish the full extent of nonviable bowel. Despite this small improvement in mortality, AMI-associated morbidity and length of hospitalization continued to be substantial. A major postoperative complication occurred in 47 % of patients, and average length of stay exceeded 20 days (mean 24 ± 17 days) with no significant improvement in either of these parameters throughout the 20-year period.

Contemporary Single-Center Series

Our contemporary results compare favorably with other reports from large tertiary care centers. For example, a recent report from Kougias et al. evaluated 72 patients who underwent open arterial revascularization by a variety of techniques. The 30-day mortality rate was 31 % and advanced age was predictive of mortality on multivariate analysis [17]. Similarly, Edwards et al. reviewed 41 patients with AMI undergoing traditional revascularization and two patients being treated with visceral angioplasty and stenting. They reported a 62 % perioperative mortality [18]. Lastly, Endean et al. [19] [17] reported on 43 patients with arterial AMI. All patients underwent traditional open revascularization with a reported 60 % perioperative mortality rate [20]. A common theme among these reports, as well as ours, is that advanced age and visceral ischemia with need for bowel resection are predictors of poor outcome. The lack of significant superiority of endovascular treatment in severe AMI is probably due to the often delayed presentation of these patients to tertiary referral centers with more prolonged ischemia time. The need for urgent assessment of intestinal viability and resection often renders endoluminal therapy alone less feasible. Undoubtedly, the number of endovascular interventions for AMI will continue to increase in the future. This fact is highlighted by a recent publication from Arthurs et al. in which 56 AMI patients underwent endovascular treatment with a high success rate (47/56) and a lower in-hospital mortality compared to open revascularization (36 % vs 50 %, $P < 0.05$), although overall mortality remained considerable [6]. This is explained by the high laparotomy rate following endovascular intervention, virtually identical to our rate of 71 %, attesting to the truly acute and not subacute presentation of patients in this series (Table 20.1).

Population-Based Registry Results

While the transition to a more endovascular-based approach to AMI has been slower to supplant open bypass as the standard of care in North America, studies based on the Swedvasc registry have shown a relatively positive experience. Block et al. identified all the patients from this registry who underwent SMA revascularization between 1999 and 2006 and found that at 28 hospitals, 121 open and 42 endovascular procedures were performed [19]. Overall, the trend has swayed

Table 20.1 Contemporary results for open and endovascular repair of AMI

	No. of patients		Mortality % (*p* value)	
Author (year)	Open	Endo	Open	Endo
Arthurs et al. (2011)	14	56	50	36 ($p<0.05$)
Ryer et al. (2011)	49	17	15	23 ($p>.05$)
Block et al. (2010)	121	42	42	28 ($p<.02$)
Wyers et al. (2007)	5	8 (6 hybrid)	80	100 (percutaneous)
				17 (hybrid)
Kougias et al. (2007)	72	0	31	–
Edwards et al. (2003)	41	2	62	–
Endean et al. (2001)	43	0	60	–

toward more endovascular revascularizations with a sixfold increase in the endovascular approach by the end of the study. When comparing the two groups of patients, it was noted that the endovascular group had a higher incidence of thrombotic occlusion ($P<.001$) and abdominal angina ($P=.042$), and the open group a higher incidence of atrial fibrillation ($P=.031$) and presumably embolic occlusion. As with the NIS study from the USA, the authors were not able to reliably differentiate between subacute and AMI and in fact noted that patients with symptoms of CMI were included if they presented with more acute onset of abdominal pain. Outcomes were better for the endovascular group with 30-day and 1-year mortality rates of 42 % versus 28 % ($P=.03$) and 58 % versus 39 % ($P=.02$) for open versus endovascular revascularization. Furthermore, rates of bowel resection ($P<.001$) and short bowel syndrome ($P=.009$; hazard ratio 2.6) were lower for the endovascular group compared with the open group, confirming the decreased severity of initial illness in the former [21]. For patients presenting with embolic SMA occlusion, the 30-day mortality rates after endovascular versus open revascularization were similar, 33 % versus 37 % respectively. On the contrary, for patients with thrombotic SMA occlusion, mortality was significantly lower following endovascular revascularization versus open surgery, 23 % versus 56 %. These results are likely a consequence of patient selection bias dependent upon differences in the severity of ischemia at the time of presentation as evidenced by the significantly lower rate of laparotomy (55 % vs 100%, $P<0.001$) and bowel resection (19 % vs 63 %, $P<0.001$) in the endovascular group overall. No doubt patients with severe ischemia and suspicion of bowel compromise underwent immediate laparotomy, while the ones with a more insidious presentation underwent endovascular intervention and selective laparotomy. As evidence to this fact, the same authors noted in an earlier communication that patients with embolic occlusion were intervened upon at a mean of 30 h from the onset of symptoms compared to 97 h in patients with SMA thrombosis [22].

Results of Newer Techniques

Thrombolysis for SMA Occlusion

Acosta et al. again reporting from the Swedvasc registry have demonstrated that thrombolysis can be an effective form of treatment in select patients with acute occlusion of the SMA. Between 1987 and 2009, 34 patients underwent thrombolysis of the mesenteric vessels. Out of these patients, none had presented with acute peritonitis, and most ($n=32$, 94 %) were diagnosed radiographically with a CT angiogram. Successful recanalization of the mesenteric vessels was achieved in 30 patients (88 %). Complications included bleeding in 6 patients, none of which required blood transfusions, cessation of thrombolysis, or surgical intervention. Ultimately, 13 exploratory laparotomies needed to be performed with 10 repeat laparotomies and 8 bowel resections. In-hospital mortality rate was 26 % ($n=9$). Of note, embolic occlusion made up the majority of the patients included in this study, accounting for 28 of the 34 patients (82 %) [23]. Though these results may not be applicable to all patients with AMI, patients with thrombotic SMA occlusion and those diagnosed early with acute embolic occlusion may be good candidates for thrombolysis especially if they would not tolerate an open procedure well [24].

Hybrid Mesenteric Revascularization

Finally, in patients with severe AMI requiring immediate revascularization and potential resection of nonviable bowel, a hybrid procedure with retrograde SMA intervention through the artery distal to the occlusion during laparotomy is an ideal approach. First reported by Wyers et al., it has the advantage of expeditious SMA stenting with technically much easier in-line retrograde access and no delay in attending to the bowel [25]. Some small series have published on this approach and reported up to 100 % technical success rates and mortality rates as low as 0–17 % [25–27]. It has become our preferred method of mesenteric revascularization in patients requiring immediate laparotomy, reserving the percutaneous approach for patients in whom a laparotomy can potentially be avoided. In order to validate this, we recently compiled a multicenter US experience with this treatment modality in 54 patients over 13 years and reported a technical success rate of 98 % and mortality of 41 % [28].

Long-Term Outcome

There is no doubt that in these patients with this grave problem and significant comorbidities, further mortality beyond 30 days is not insignificant. Long-term survival in our initial series was low at 43 % and 32 % at 1 and 3 years respectively

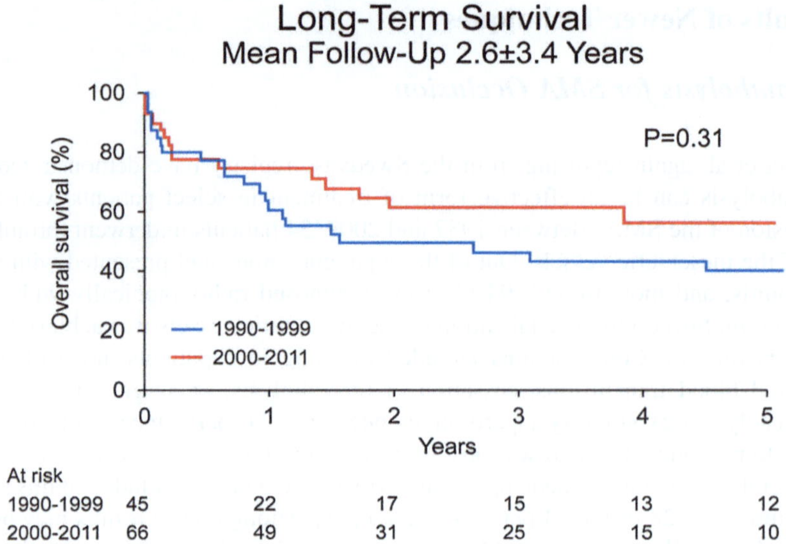

Fig. 20.7 Long-term survival following revascularization for AMI. Mayo Clinic experience (From Ryer et al. [13], with permission)

with further attrition due to short bowel syndrome early on [14]. This did show improvement in the subsequent decade to 51 % but did not reach statistical significance [13] (Fig. 20.7). Although there were 36 late deaths among 111 patients over a mean follow-up of 2.6 ± 3.4 years, the mean age at death was 70.9 ± 13 years and occurred 2.6 ± 2.4 years following their presentation with AMI. The exact cause of death could not be determined in two-thirds patients, but only one patient was known to have abdominal complaints at the time of death. In the Swedvasc registry, mid-term survival at 1 year after endovascular treatment was better than after open surgery (62 % vs 41 %; log rank, $P = 0.02$).

Conclusion

In summary, morbidity and mortality from acute mesenteric ischemia remain high. There has been a modest improvement in survival over the last two decades despite an aging patient population, likely due to the more liberal use of second-look laparotomy. Embolic etiology, bowel infarction at presentation, and markers of generalized atherosclerosis are predictors of poor outcome, while a history of chronic mesenteric ischemia is associated with better outcome. Revascularization by endovascular means has increased in the last decade and is promising, with further improvement anticipated with advances in technology, availability of a wider array of smaller profile devices with ability for rapid exchange, as well as embolic protection devices. Careful patient selection, procedure planning, and meticulous technique, as well as the liberal use of the hybrid technique with retrograde approach will likely lead to further improvements in the results of endovascular treatment of AMI. The key points for improving overall outcomes in the future are maintaining a high index of suspicion, prompt diagnosis and treatment by appropriate means, be this open or endovascular, and early and repeated assessment of the bowel.

References

1. Stoney RJ, Cunningham CG. Acute mesenteric ischemia. Surgery. 1993;114(3):489–90.
2. Acosta S, et al. Incidence of acute thrombo-embolic occlusion of the superior mesenteric artery – a population-based study. Eur J Vasc Endovasc Surg. 2004;27(2):145–50.
3. Kougias P, Lau D, El Sayed HF, Zhou W, Huynh TT, Lin PH. Determinants of mortality and treatment outcome following surgical interventions for acute mesenteric ischemia. J Vasc Surg. 2007;46(3):467–74.
4. Mamode N, Pickford I, Leiberman P. Failure to improve outcome in acute mesenteric ischaemia: seven-year review. Eur J Surg. 1999;165(3):203–8.
5. Fioole B, van de Rest HJ, Meijer JR, van Leersum M, van Koeverden S, Moll FL, et al. Percutaneous transluminal angioplasty and stenting as first-choice treatment in patients with chronic mesenteric ischemia. J Vasc Surg. 2010;51(2):386–91.
6. Arthurs ZM, Titus J, Bannazadeh M, Eagleton MJ, Srivastava S, Sarac TP, et al. A comparison of endovascular revascularization with traditional therapy for the treatment of acute mesenteric ischemia. J Vasc Surg. 2011;53(3):698–704.
7. Acosta S, Bjorck M. Modern treatment of acute mesenteric ischaemia. Br J Surg. 2014; 101(1):e100–8.
8. Schermerhorn ML, Giles KA, Hamdan AD, Wyers MC, Pomposelli FB. Mesenteric revascularization: management and outcomes in the United States, 1988–2006. J Vasc Surg. 2009;50(2):341–8 e1.
9. Peck MA, Conrad MA, Kwolek CJ, LaMuraglia GM, Paruchuri V, Cambria RP. Intermediate-term outcomes of endovascular treatment for symptomatic chronic mesenteric ischemia. J Vasc Surg. 2010;51(1):140-7 e1–2.
10. Oderich GS, Malgor RD, Ricotta 2nd JJ. Open and endovascular revascularization for chronic mesenteric ischemia: tabular review of the literature. Ann Vasc Surg. 2009;23(5):700–12.
11. Lee RW, Bakken AM, Palchik E, Saad WE, Davies MG. Long-term outcomes of endoluminal therapy for chronic atherosclerotic occlusive mesenteric disease. Ann Vasc Surg. 2008;22(4): 541–6.
12. Atkins MD, Kwolek CJ, LaMuraglia GM, Brewster DC, Chung TK, Cambria RP. Surgical revascularization versus endovascular therapy for chronic mesenteric ischemia: a comparative experience. J Vasc Surg. 2007;45(6):1162–71.
13. Ryer EJ, et al. Revascularization for acute mesenteric ischemia. J Vasc Surg. 2012;55(6): 1682–9.
14. Park WM, Gloviczki P, Cherry Jr KJ, et al. Contemporary management of acute mesenteric ischemia: factors associated with survival. J Vasc Surg. 2002;35(3):445–52.
15. Meng X, Liu L, Jiang H. Indications and procedures for second-look surgery in acute mesenteric ischemia. Surg Today. 2010;40(8):700–5.
16. Bradbury AW, et al. Mesenteric ischaemia: a multidisciplinary approach. Br J Surg. 1995; 82(11):1446–59.
17. Kougias P, et al. Determinants of mortality and treatment outcome following surgical interventions for acute mesenteric ischemia. J Vasc Surg. 2007;46(3):467–74.

18. Edwards MS, C GS, Craven TE, Olsen AW, Plonk GW, Geary RL, et al. Acute occlusive mesenteric ischemia: surgical management and outcomes. Ann Vasc Surg. 2003;17(1):72–9.
19. Endean ED, et al. Surgical management of thrombotic acute intestinal ischemia. Ann Surg. 2001;233(6):801–8.
20. Endean ED, Barnes SL, Kwolek CJ, Minion DJ, Schwarcz TH, Mentzer Jr RM. Surgical management of thrombotic acute intestinal ischemia. Ann Surg. 2001;17(1):801–8.
21. Block TA, Acosta S, Bjorck M. Endovascular and open surgery for acute occlusion of the superior mesenteric artery. J Vasc Surg. 2010;52(4):959–66.
22. Acosta S, Sonesson B, Resch T. Endovascular therapeutic approaches for acute superior mesenteric artery occlusion. Cardiovasc Intervent Radiol. 2009;32(5):896–905.
23. Bjornsson S, et al. Thrombolysis for acute occlusion of the superior mesenteric artery. J Vasc Surg. 2011;54(6):1734–42.
24. Heiss P, et al. Primary percutaneous aspiration and thrombolysis for the treatment of acute embolic superior mesenteric artery occlusion. Eur Radiol. 2010;20(12):2948–58.
25. Wyers MC, Powell RJ, Nolan BW, Cronenwett JL. Retrograde mesenteric stenting during laparotomy for acute occlusive mesenteric ischemia. J Vasc Surg. 2007;45(2):269–75.
26. Millner R, Woo EY, Carpenter JP. Superior mesenteric artery angioplasty and stenting via a retrograde approach in a patient with bowel ischemia – a case report. Vasc Endovasc Surg. 2004;38(1):89–91.
27. Stout CL, Messerschmidt CA, Leake AE, et al. Retrograde open mesenteric stenting for acute mesenteric ischemia is a viable alternative for emergent revascularization. Vasc Endovasc Surg. 2010;44(5):368–71.
28. Coelho Macedo RA, Oderich GS, Manju K, Stone D, Woo E, Panneton J, et al. Multicenter experience with retrograde open mesenteric artery stenting via laparotomy for treatment of acute and chronic mesenteric ischemia. J Vasc Surg. 2014;59(2):565–6.

Chapter 21
Medical Management of Short Bowel Syndrome and Nutritional Support

Jithinraj Edakkanambeth Varayil and Ryan T. Hurt

Acute mesenteric ischemia is a complex and difficult disease process. The results of ischemia are related to the presence of intestinal infarction and underlying causes of vascular compromise. Overall survival has not significantly changed in the past three decades with perioperative mortality being approximately 50 % [1]. In patients surviving multiple intestinal resections following the initial ischemic event, patients may develop short bowel syndrome (SBS). SBS can result in severe fluid, electrolyte, and vitamin deficiencies [2]. The most important factor in the care of patients with mesenteric ischemia and the resulting SBS is the management of their underlying comorbidities and nutritional deficiencies. Currently in the United States, the incidence of severe SBS is estimated to be 1–2 per 100,000 inhabitants per year [3, 4]. There is still some confusion about the long-term outcomes and management of SBS. Over the past few decades, several advances have been made in the field of total parenteral nutrition (TPN) and home parenteral nutrition (HPN) to improve the outcomes of these patients and improve their quality of life. The purpose of this chapter is to describe short bowel syndrome and discuss the medical management of SBS.

Definition of Short Bowel Syndrome

There is no consensus in the literature for the definition of SBS. The average length of the adult human small intestine is approximately 600 cm, as calculated from studies performed on cadavers [5]. SBS can be defined as a global malabsorption

J. Edakkanambeth Varayil, MD
Department of Internal Medicine, Mayo Clinic, Rochester, MN, USA

R.T. Hurt, MD, PhD (✉)
Division of General Internal Medicine, Mayo Clinic, Rochester, MN, USA
e-mail: hurt.ryan@mayo.edu

G.S. Oderich (ed.), *Mesenteric Vascular Disease*,
DOI 10.1007/978-1-4939-1847-8_21

syndrome due to insufficient absorptive capacity and/or disturbed gastrointestinal regulation resulting from extensive small bowel resections [5–7]. SBS may occur after resection of more than 50 % and is obligatory after resection of 70 % of the small intestine or if less than 100 cm of small bowel remains [8]. SBS is characterized by the inability to maintain protein-energy, fluid, electrolyte, or micronutrient balances when on a conventionally accepted, normal diet. SBS is not uniformly tied to a specific length of bowel, and the survival depends on the adaptability of the remaining small intestine [7, 9]. The successful clinical management of SBS requires a firm understanding of the pathophysiology of SBS. For example, the absolute length does not always correlate with the clinical scenario, and the amount of functional bowel might be much lower than the documented length.

Signs and Symptoms

Symptoms of SBS are mainly dependent on the anatomical site of the bowel resection. Irrespective of that, diarrhea and steatorrhea predominate in the early phase of SBS. Other possible symptoms may include weight loss, fatigue, edema (usually of the feet and legs), cramping, and bloating. Chronic diarrhea may result in dehydration which may present as light-headedness or dizziness, dry mouth, fatigue, dark-colored urine, and low blood pressure. Loss of the duodenum is associated with malabsorption of various macro- and micronutrients [10]. Proximal bowel is also the site of specific gastrointestinal hormone production such as gastrin, cholecystokinin (CCK), secretin, and motilin [11]. Secretin and CCK production have been shown to be decreased in severe cases of SBS further diminishing absorption. Diarrhea results from a reduction in the absorptive surface area, decreased transit time, increased osmolality, bacterial overgrowth, and fluid hypersecretion from the stomach and small and large intestine [6].

Types of Short Bowel Syndrome

In an average adult, the duodenum measures approximately 20 cm, jejunum 300 cm, and ileum is about 400 cm. The ileum has a functional length almost twice as that of the jejunum. Various diverse symptoms are produced when different areas are affected. Based on the location of ischemia and the length of the remaining bowel, SBS can be divided into three types: *type I* (end-jejunostomy), *type II* (jejunocolic anastomosis), and *type III* (jejunoileal anastomosis). The management of SBS depends on the type of SBS and the overall length of remaining small intestine. Compared with type I SBS, type II SBS anatomy is equivalent to approximately 30 cm of additional small intestine, and the type III anatomy is equivalent to having an additional 60 cm of small intestine (Fig. 21.1) [5]. Different types of SBS

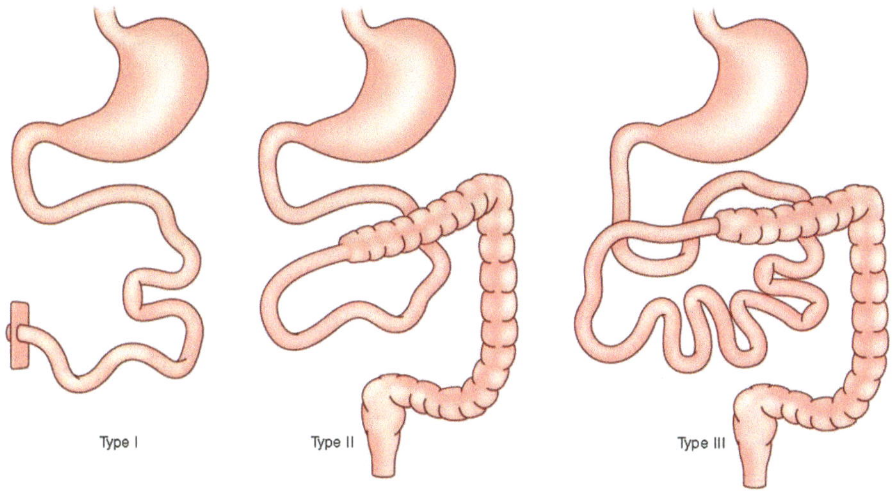

Fig. 21.1 The three types of SBS after surgical resection: type I (end-jejunostomy), type II (jejunocolonic anastomosis), and type III (ileocolonic anastomosis)

produce different symptoms and thus distinct consequences. Removal of the duodenum and jejunum causes defects in macronutrient and electrolyte absorption. This further reduces the secretion of mucosal hormones and results in pancreatic insufficiency. Removal of a significant part of the ileum affects bile acid absorption and leads to biliary diarrhea and also causes steatorrhea. The ileal resection affects absorption of various vitamins and macronutrients. Furthermore, ileal resection also shortens intestinal transit times, magnifying the absorptive defect. A combined resection of the small intestine and colon usually causes severe dehydration and sodium and potassium depletion because of decrease water absorption. Furthermore, colonic salvage, where bacterial fermentation of carbohydrate fiber produces short-chain fatty acids, can be helpful in the absorption properties of the remaining colon gaining up to 500 additional calories per day. Preservation of at least 50 % of the colon reduces morbidity and mortality after massive small intestinal resection.

Intestinal adaptation depends on multiple factors, including the extent and site of intestinal loss or dysfunction, the function of the remaining small bowel and associated digestive organs, the presence of the ICV and thus terminal ileum and colon, and the amount of time that has elapsed since resection. The adaptive process begins within 12–24 h after resection and continues for 1–2 years [5, 12, 13]. The process of adaptation involves the lengthening, dilation, growth of villi, deepening of the crypts, and enterocyte hyperplasia [14]. The combined effect of all of these mechanisms increases the surface area and enhances the absorption of nutrients and electrolytes (Fig. 21.2). Loss of the duodenum or the terminal ileum, in particular the ileocecal valve, impairs absorption much more than loss of other parts of the small bowel. Both the duodenum and the ileocecal region possess specific absorptive

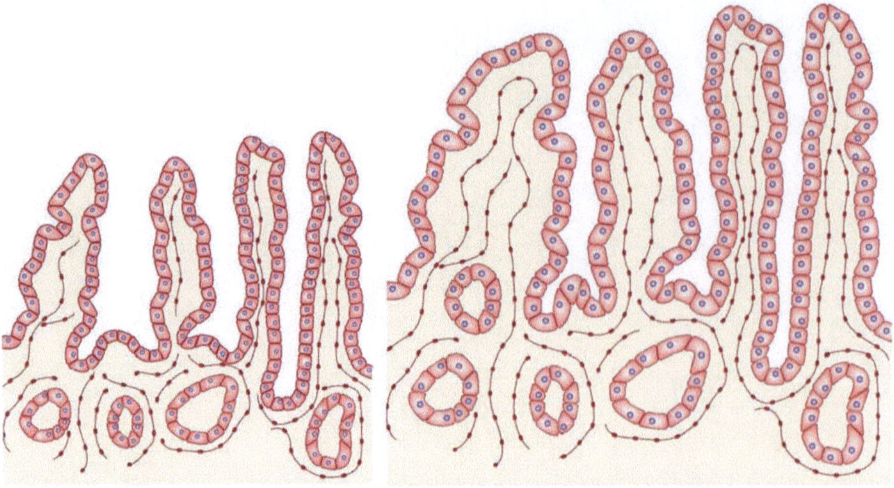

Fig. 21.2 This figure shows the lengthening, dilation, growth of villi, deepening of the crypts, and enterocyte hyperplasia during intestinal adaptation. The left side of the figure shows an intestinal epithelium before adaptation; the right side shows an intestinal epithelium after adaptation

functions and play a crucial role in the regulation and integration of postprandial gastrointestinal motility and secretion. The ileum better compensates for jejunal loss; the jejunum in contrast is less adaptable to the loss of the ileum [9–11, 15]. However, any adaptive mechanism can be overwhelming, and adaptation can be inadequate if too much small bowel is lost. Although length alone is not the only determining factor of complications related to small bowel resection, resection of up to 70 % of the small bowel is usually well tolerated if the terminal ileum and ileocecal valve are preserved.

Phases of Short Bowel Syndrome

The clinical phase of SBS can be divided into three phases: early phase, intermediate phase, and late phase. The early phase (first few days after the resection) is mainly characterized by watery diarrhea resulting in dehydration, hyponatremia, hypokalemia, hypocalcemia, and hypomagnesemia. An intermediate phase occurs from 1 week to approximately 1 year during which intestinal adaptation occurs. During the late phase, after maximal intestinal adaptation has been achieved, weight often stabilizes. After surgery, fluid losses may exceed 5 L/day, especially with concomitant colectomy [16, 17]. Gastric hypersecretion evokes intestinal mucosal damage, impaired micelle formation, and inhibition of pancreatic enzyme function.

Treatment of Short Bowel Syndrome

The management of SBS is different in the three phases. The management in the early phase involves intensive postoperative care and revolves around control and treatment of sepsis, maintenance of fluid and electrolytes, and nutritional support. The management in the intermediate phase is to initiate nutritional support (enteral, parenteral, and oral) with the goal of maximizing intestinal adaptation. During the late phase, no further improvement in nutrition can be achieved, and this time the goal is to provide adequate nutrition and prevent complications. The summary of management of SBS in all three phases is given in Table 21.1.

Nutritional Strategies

Optimizing and maintaining nutritional status is important for adaptation subsequent to surgery, and it is central to long-term survival. Most patients in the early phase require total parenteral nutrition (TPN). TPN and home parenteral nutrition (HPN) might be required in the intermediate and late phases too. Prior to the introduction of PN in the early 1970s, most patients with SBS died of severe malnutrition, dehydration, and weight loss. The 1- and 5-year survival of patients on TPN ranges from 91 % to 97 % in adults. Nutritional strategies include dietary modification, optimizing TPN and initiating enteral nutrition, and oral feeding when possible.

Table 21.1 Management strategies

Early phase
Treat postoperative complications
Diet modification to limit the output, diarrhea
ORS
Document the remaining bowel length
Assess the need for TPN/HPN
Intermediate phase
Pharmacotherapy (choice depends on the type of SBS)
Diet modification, ORS
Train for long-term TPN, set goals for weaning HPN
Assess bowel adaptation
Late phase
Monitor for QOL on HPN
Prevent complications on HPN
Other treatment options

Dietary Modifications

The proximal small bowel receives approximately nine liters of water and electrolytes daily from various sources, of which 90 % are reabsorbed. This reabsorption is significantly impaired in SBS patients. Thus, a substantial dietary modification is necessary in these patients to prevent diarrhea and dehydration [18]. It is a general opinion that polyphagia is required to meet the excess output from the gastrointestinal tract, but the authors propose that it is more important to choose the right type of food with low osmolarity to decrease the output. For most patients suffering from SBS, dietary strategies include small portions of frequent meals consisting of complex carbohydrates (40–60 % of the total energy requirement) and protein (20–30 % of the total energy requirement) while limiting simple sugars. In SBS patients, drinking regular water, juice, or sports drinks will also worsen the diarrhea. Liquids that have a high concentration of sugar and salt will cause osmotic fluid shift to the intestinal lumen. The additional fluid in the lumen will exacerbate the diarrhea and worsen the dehydration [6]. A list of food items and drinks that are recommended to be avoided by SBS patients is presented in Table 21.2. Proper guidance and recommendations should be provided to all patients with SBS to decrease diarrhea and improve symptoms. When a particular drink cannot be completely avoided, often diluting it with water can be recommended. For example, dilution of one cup of cranberry juice or regular soda with two cups of water can decrease the concentration of the drink considerably and provide a favorable osmolarity profile. Water, tea, coffee, and diet soda pop are considered as "free water" and should also be avoided by SBS patients. Because these fluids have small amounts of sodium, the sodium from the bloodstream moves into the intestinal lumen causing water to follow worsening diarrhea [6]. The diet requirements and recommendations may also vary with different types of SBS. SBS type II and type III patients with intact colon can be fed higher proportions of complex carbohydrates and medium-chain triglycerides. Oxalate restriction is also advised in these patients [19, 20]. SBS type I patients with the colon removed do not require an oxalate restriction and can be fed long-chain triglycerides and complex carbohydrates.

Table 21.2 List of common fluids that might exacerbate the fluid output in SBS patients

Fruit juices
Regular soda pop
Nutritional supplements such as Boost™, Boost Plus™, Boost Breeze™, Carnation Instant Breakfast™ (including sugar-free Carnation Instant Breakfast™) in powder form, Enlive™, Ensure™, Ensure Plus™, Glucerna Shake™, Resource™, Resource™ Fruit Beverage, Sportshake™
Fruit drinks such as Hi-C™, SunnyD™, Tang™
Sports drinks such as Gatorade™ or Powerade™

Oral Rehydration Solution

Oral rehydration solution (ORS) is a scientifically formulated blend of carbohydrates, salts, and water developed to treat dehydration. ORS works by effectively controlling the primary water absorption through osmosis. The effectiveness of ORS improved when the polymers of glucose in the ORS were replaced by various forms of simple glucose. Rice powder/rice syrup has been shown to effectively replace the standard glucose in ORS [6]. This change decreased the osmolarity of the ORS and increased the ratio of glucose to sodium. In the authors' clinical practice, ORS plays an integral part in the treatment of high stomal outputs of patients with SBS. Over the years, it has been realized that with adequate dietary strategies and improved ORS use, it is possible to avoid turning to parenteral solutions to maintain fluid. The details of the WHO recommended formula for preparing ORS is presented in Table 21.3. Electrolyte details and osmolarity of some of the commercially available ORS preparation are presented in Table 21.4. Despite these oral restrictions and recommendations, patients with severe SBS often still require parenteral rehydration with daily runs of intravenous saline.

Home Parenteral Nutrition

Total parenteral nutrition (TPN) is vital in the early phase of SBS treatment. TPN is also required in many SBS patients during the intermediate and late phases. If required during the intermediate and late SBS phases, patients can go home on PN [21]. It is essential that the home parenteral nutrition (HPN) is administered by a multidisciplinary team of nutrition experts. HPN aims both to prevent and restore nutritional deficits while minimizing the complications related to the therapy itself.

Table 21.3 Various electrolyte contents, sugar contents, and osmolarity of commercial ORS solution

Solution	Type of sugar	Carbohydrates (g/L)	Sodium (mEq/L)	Potassium (mEq/L)	Magnesium (mEq/L)	Osmolarity (mOsm)
WHO ORS	Glucose	20	90	20	0	330
Pedialyte®	Dextrose, acesulfame	25	45	20	0	250
CeraLyte 75®	Rice syrup solids, rice syrup	40	75	20	0	<250
CeraLyte 90®	Rice syrup solids, rice syrup	40	90	20	0	<275
DripDrop®	Sucrose, fructose, sucralose	33	60	20	13.7	235

Table 21.4 Modified WHO ORS recipe

Baking soda (sodium bicarbonate) – ½ teaspoon
Salt substitute (potassium chloride) – ¼ teaspoon
Table salt (sodium chloride) – ½ teaspoon
Sugar (sucrose) – 2 tablespoons
Tap water – add enough to make 1 l
Tip: patients can be recommended to flavor it with sugar-free drink mixes and artificial sweeteners to improve the taste

When sending a patient on HPN, it is essential to ensure that the benefits will outweigh the associated risks [21]. In addition, it is important to identify small intestine adaptation (e.g., less fluid and calorie requirements) and make necessary changes in the HPN infusate. One of the most important decisions with initiation of HPN is to determine duration of the intended therapy and taking necessary steps to reach this goal. This will guide the HPN team and patients in realistic expectations for a time frame for weaning off HPN. Furthermore, this can serve as a guide for providing proper training techniques and choice of central venous access devices. For short-term (6 weeks) TPN and eventually HPN, a peripherally inserted central catheter (PICC) can be used. Usually, when the HPN is required for more than 6 weeks, a single lumen Hickman® or implanted port is more ideal. PICC lines carry a greater risk of thrombosis and catheter-related blood stream infection probably due to multiple lumens, smaller diameter, and greater overall length. Some advantages of a port are minimal alteration in body image, no concern for accidental pulling or cutting of the device, and ability to swim in lakes. However, when removal is needed, ports have to be surgically removed. It is for this reason that many of the specialized centers managing HPN use single lumen Hickman® catheter.

Complicated cases of SBS that were previously thought to be terminal because of the extremely short bowel are now manageable with HPN. With the introduction of small portable pumps equipped with infusion rate monitors, it is now possible to administer HPN at night over shorter periods of time (12 h instead of 24 h), giving patients the freedom from being connected for 24 h. This has led to more independence with the ability to maintain employment, travel, and live at home instead of skilled nursing facilities. There is some difficulty in capturing and defining QOL in HPN patients. This is because it is difficult to determine the impact on QOL from symptoms related to the primary disease vs HPN. Although there are numerous complications of HPN (e.g., infection, thrombosis, liver disease, and metabolic bone disease), for many SBS patients it is lifesaving.

Pharmacologic Treatments

One of the main complaints in patients with SBS is diarrhea due to rapid transit. Pharmacological agents can be used in SBS patients to slow down the small intestine's transit time. These agents can be divided into subgroups based on their

Table 21.5 Various drugs, recommended maximum dosage, and adverse effects

Drug	Maximum recommended dosage	Adverse effects
Loperamide	32 mg/day	Nausea, toxic megacolon, angioedema
Diphenoxylate-atropine	30 mg/day	Confusion, dry mouth, lethargy, dizziness, drug dependence
Tincture of opium	0.24 ml/day	Dizziness, seizure, painful urination, nausea
Octreotide	1,500 mcg/day	Cholelithiasis, ascending cholangitis, pancreatitis, syncope
Clonidine	0.2–0.4 mg/day	Orthostatic hypotension, arrhythmias, angioedema, syncope, bradycardia
Glutamine	5 g, six times daily	Hepatotoxicity, nephrolithiasis, edema, nausea, insomnia
Teduglutide	0.05 mg/kg/day	Bowel obstruction, pancreatitis, nausea, headache, potential growth of existing neoplasms

mechanisms of action including antidiarrheals, antisecretory, and growth factors. A combination of these three general classes may be needed to achieve optimal results in SBS patients. A list of common drugs used in SBS patients, their recommended dosage, and common side effects is presented in Table 21.5.

Antidiarrheal Medications

Loperamide

Loperamide decreases rapid transit through reduction of circular and longitudinal muscle activity by activation of opioid receptors [22]. In addition, loperamide may decrease pancreatic and gastric acid secretions which might potentially reduce the intestinal fluid volume. Loperamide is normally absorbed through the enterohepatic circulation. Because the enterohepatic circulation can be altered in SBS, higher doses are often required to achieve the same effects compared to patients with normal gastrointestinal function [23]. SBS patients can take up to 4 capsules before meals and at bedtime (16 capsules = 32 mg). One strategy is to open the capsules and mix them with sugar-free applesauce 30 min prior to meals and at bedtime. The main side effect of loperamide in higher doses is nausea. Because of the low incidence of side effects, loperamide is typically the first medicine used to slow down the increased transit time in SBS.

Diphenoxylate-Atropine

Like loperamide, diphenoxylate-atropine is an antidiarrheal agent that decreases intestinal transit time through opioid receptors in the small bowel [24]. Diphenoxylate-atropine is commonly used alone or in combination with other medications (such as loperamide and tincture of opium) to help decrease stool output and thus transit time. The typically dosing for SBS patients is one to two tablets to be taken before meals and at bedtime with a maximum dose of 30 mg/day. Like loperamide, it is recommend that patients crush the tablets and mix them with applesauce 30 min prior to meals and at bedtime. This opening of capsules and crushing of tablets enhance the absorption of the medications. The main limiting factor with diphenoxylate-atropine is the anticholinergic central nervous side effects. These include but are not limited to confusion, dry mouth, lethargy, and dizziness. In addition to the central side effects, there is increased risk of dependence and overdose [25]. If diphenoxylate-atropine is abruptly stopped, some patients may experience symptoms of withdrawal. After SBS patients obtain maximum doses of loperamide (4 capsules 4 times a day = 32 mg), diphenoxylate-atropine may be added and titrated for effect.

Opioids

Opioids are the most potent antidiarrheal medications used in the treatment of SBS patients. Like other antidiarrheal medications, opioids will decrease gastrointestinal transit time. Examples of opioid-based narcotics used in SBS patients include paregoric, tincture of opium, and codeine phosphate [26]. The dosing of tincture of opium is 0.6 ml four times a day. Because of the poor taste, it can be mixed with orange juice. Codeine phosphate may be given as 30 mg tablets (1–2 tablets q 6 h as needed) [27]. Once SBS patients have reached maximum doses of loperamide and diphenoxylate-atropine, opioids can be added. There has been a synergistic effect reported between opioids and other antidiarrheals such as loperamide and diphenoxylate-atropine. The main side effects of these medications are central including nausea, dizziness, and drowsiness. The side effects of slowed transit time and constipation are how these medications offer a benefit in SBS patients [28]. These are controlled agents and there is risk of dependence and overdose. Ordering providers must be cautious and decrease doses as bowel adaptation and enhanced absorption occurs in SBS patients as small intestinal obstruction can occur.

Antisecretory Medications

Octreotide

Octreotide is a somatostatin analog which will inhibit serotonin, vasoactive inhibitory polypeptide (VIP), and gastrin to decrease stool output [29]. Use of octreotide in SBS patients reduces fluid and electrolyte output. Octreotide can be given subcutaneously or intravenously with the dosing being as high as 1,500 mcg/day (500 mcg TID) [30]. The main side effects of octreotide are cholelithiasis, ascending cholangitis, pancreatitis, and syncope [31]. These severe side effects in addition to the high cost have limited the use of octreotide in SBS. If it is used after antidiarrheal strategies have been maxed (loperamide, diphenoxylate-atropine, and tincture of opium), a short trial of octreotide (48 h) can be performed. If there is no additional benefit, then it can be discontinued as it is unlikely to be effective.

Clonidine

Clonidine, an alpha-adrenergic agonist, is commonly used as an antihypertensive agent. It has been shown to have antidiarrheal properties through the alpha-2 stimulation of the receptors on the enterocytes which promotes fluid and electrolyte absorption [32]. This can lead to reduced intestinal fluid loss by stimulating small bowel fluid absorption and inhibiting anion secretion. A dosing of 0.1–0.2 mg orally twice a day has been shown to decrease fluid loss in high output SBS patients. There is a transdermal form which has its advantages in SBS patients who have poor oral absorption of medications. The main side effects of clonidine are severe orthostatic hypotension (in patients already prone to dehydration), arrhythmias, angioedema, syncope, and bradycardia [33]. Caution should be observed when discontinuing clonidine as abrupt cessation can lead to withdrawal symptoms. The side effects have limited the use of clonidine in SBS patients.

Growth Factors

Glutamine and Growth Hormone

Glutamine and growth hormone were the first two growth factors studied in SBS patients. Glutamine is a primary energy source for the small bowel enterocyte and in surgical and trauma patients may aid in mucosal healing and increasing wound healing. In SBS patients, recombinant human growth hormone (rhGH) increases insulin-like growth factor (IGF-1), body weight, and free-fat mass [34]. There have been a number of clinical studies evaluating rhGH and GH in SBS with the results being variable. The combination of rhGH, glutamine, and high-carbohydrate, low-fat diet in SBS patients significantly increased protein absorption and decreased stool output [35]. Side effects of oral glutamine include hepatotoxicity, nephrolithiasis, edema, nausea, and insomnia. Side effects of rhGH include fatigue, lethargy, joint pain, and increased risk of diabetes [34]. Because of the lack of strong evidence in SBS patients, glutamine and rhGH is not routinely used.

Teduglutide

Teduglutide was recently FDA approved for use in SBS patients who are dependent on HPN and have failed other medical therapies. It is an analog of glucagon-like peptide 2 (GLP-2), which may be important in stimulating intestinal adaptation [36–38]. A decrease in fecal wet weight and fecal energy excretion while increasing villus height and crypt depth has been shown with the use of teduglutide. In a recent study, teduglutide has shown a significant reduction in HPN volume with teduglutide compared to placebo during 24 weeks of therapy [39]. In a subsequent trial of 52 subjects, teduglutide resulted in a ≥20 % decrease in volume of HPN and a reduction in one or more days of PN dependency in 68 % of subjects [40]. The conclusion from these trials was that the optimal dose of teduglutide in SBS patients is 0.05 mg/kg/day delivered subcutaneously. Some side effects include bowel obstruction, pancreatitis, nausea, and headache. Furthermore, because of the trophic effect on the intestinal mucosa, ileostomy stoma sites can increase dramatically in size. Since teduglutide promotes growth of intestinal epithelial cells in the GI tract, it could potentially promote growth of existing neoplasms and aggressive screening must be done for colorectal cancer. Despite these benefits of teduglutide, it is an extremely expensive medication (estimated >$200,000/year), and it is not clear if the adaptation is persistent or disappears with cessation of the medication. Like other medications there is a potential of enhanced absorption of other concomitant oral medications while on teduglutide, and reduction of doses should be made as needed.

Intestinal Transplantation/Small Bowel Transplantation

Small bowel transplantation (SBT) may become necessary in SBS patients who fail to achieve intestinal adaptation during the intermediate and late phases of treatment [41]. The Centers for Medicare and Medicaid Services (CMMS) recommends SBT as a standard of care for patients with irreversible intestinal failure who cannot be maintained on HPN [42]. SBT may be considered as a possible option in the following scenarios: failure of HPN, increased risk of mortality due to underlying disease, and intestinal failure with high morbidity and unwillingness to accept HPN. Patients who have significant fluid losses and frequent bouts of severe dehydration despite appropriate medical management may also be candidates for SBT. There are mainly three types of SBT: isolated intestinal transplantation, intestine and liver transplantation, and multivisceral transplantation. Each type has specific indications and associated risks. SBT poses a substantial immunologic challenge because the immune cells in the donor intestine are repopulated with recipient cells [43]. Despite improvement in patient and graft survival rates, it is associated with significant mortality and morbidity. Sepsis is the leading cause of death in 51.3 % patients [44], followed by graft rejection in 10.4 % SBT patients [44, 45]. Even though SBT can prolong the life of few patients with irreversible intestinal failure who can no longer be managed on HPN, the outcomes of SBT are inferior to those of HPN. Evidence suggests that SBT should only be used when HPN is no longer feasible.

References

1. Sise MJ. Acute mesenteric ischemia. Surg Clin North Am. 2014;94(1):165–81 [Review].
2. Bobadilla JL. Mesenteric ischemia. Surg Clin North Am. 2013;93(4):925–40. ix. [Review].
3. Cudnik MT, Darbha S, Jones J, Macedo J, Hiestand BC, Stockton SW. The diagnosis of acute mesenteric ischemia: a systematic review and meta-analysis. Acad Emerg Med. 2013;20(11): 1087–100.
4. DiBaise JK, Young RJ, Vanderhoof JA. Intestinal rehabilitation and the short bowel syndrome: part 1. Am J Gastroenterol. 2004;99(7):1386–95 [Review].
5. Nightingale JM. Management of patients with a short bowel. World J Gastroenterol. 2001;7(6): 741–51 [Review].
6. Kelly DG, Tappenden KA, Winkler MF. Short Bowel Syndrome: highlights of patient management, quality of life, and survival. JPEN J Parenter Enteral Nutr. 2014;38(4):427–37.
7. Buchman AL, Scolapio J, Fryer J. AGA technical review on short bowel syndrome and intestinal transplantation. Gastroenterology. 2003;124(4):1111–34 [Research Support, Non-U.S. Gov't Review].
8. Genton L, Nardo P, Huber O, Pichard C. Parenteral nutrition independence in a patient left with 25 cm of ileum and jejunum: a case report. Obes Surg. 2010;20(5):666–71 [Case Reports Research Support, Non-U.S. Gov't].
9. O'Keefe SJ, Buchman AL, Fishbein TM, Jeejeebhoy KN, Jeppesen PB, Shaffer J. Short bowel syndrome and intestinal failure: consensus definitions and overview. Clin Gastroenterol Hepatol. 2006;4(1):6–10 [Consensus Development Conference Research Support, Non-U.S. Gov't].
10. Hofmann AF, Borgstrom B. Hydrolysis of long-chain monoglycerides in micellar solution by pancreatic lipase. Biochim Biophys Acta. 1963;70:317–31.
11. Borgstrom B, Dahlqvist A, Lundh G, Sjovall J. Studies of intestinal digestion and absorption in the human. J Clin Invest. 1957;36(10):1521–36.
12. Jeong SH, Lee HJ, Bae HJ, Kim Y, Yoo MW, Yoon YK, et al. Factors affecting postoperative dietary adaptation in short bowel syndrome. Hepatogastroenterology. 2009;56(93):1049–52.
13. Vanderhoof JA, Langnas AN. Short-bowel syndrome in children and adults. Gastroenterology. 1997;113(5):1767–78 [Review].
14. Buccigrossi V, Armellino C, Tozzi A, Nicastro E, Esposito C, Alicchio F, et al. Time- and segment-related changes of postresected intestine: a 4-dimensional model of intestinal adaptation. J Pediatr Gastroenterol Nutr. 2013;56(1):40–5 [Research Support, Non-U.S. Gov't].
15. Nightingale JM, Lennard-Jones JE, Gertner DJ, Wood SR, Bartram CI. Colonic preservation reduces need for parenteral therapy, increases incidence of renal stones, but does not change high prevalence of gall stones in patients with a short bowel. Gut. 1992;33(11):1493–7 [Comparative Study].
16. Swaniker F, Guo W, Fonkalsrud EW, Brown T, Newman L, Ament M. Adaptation of rabbit small intestinal brush-border membrane enzymes after extensive bowel resection. J Pediatr Surg. 1995;30(7):1000–2. [Research Support, Non-U.S. Gov't]; discussion 3.
17. Nakayama H, Weser E. Adaptation of small bowel after intestinal resection: increase in the pentose phosphate pathway. Biochim Biophys Acta. 1972;279(3):416–23.
18. Kander R. SBS diet needs to address individual physiology. J Am Dict Assoc. 1999;99(5):529–30 [Comment Letter].
19. Hoppe B, Leumann E, von Unruh G, Laube N, Hesse A. Diagnostic and therapeutic approaches in patients with secondary hyperoxaluria. Front Biosci. 2003;8:e437–43 [Research Support, Non-U.S. Gov't Review].
20. Hoppe B, Langman CB. A United States survey on diagnosis, treatment, and outcome of primary hyperoxaluria. Pediatr Nephrol. 2003;18(10):986–91 [Research Support, Non-U.S. Gov't].
21. Barnadas G. Preparing for parenteral nutrition therapy at home. Am J Health Syst Pharm. 1999;56(3):270–2 [Review].
22. Awouters F, Niemegeers CJ, Janssen PA. Pharmacology of antidiarrheal drugs. Annu Rev Pharmacol Toxicol. 1983;23:279–301 [Review].

23. Nightingale J, Woodward JM. Guidelines for management of patients with a short bowel. Gut. 2006;55 Suppl 4:iv1–12 [Practice Guideline].
24. Coupar IM, De Luca A. Opiate and opiate antidiarrhoeal drug action on rat isolated intestine. J Auton Pharmacol. 1994;14(1):69–78 [In Vitro Research Support, Non-U.S. Gov't].
25. McGuigan M, Lovejoy Jr FH. Overdose of Lomotil. Br Med J. 1978;1(6118):990 [Letter].
26. Cruz-Correa M, Giardiello FM. Lymphocytic and Collagenous Colitis. Curr Treat Options Gastroenterol. 2000;3(3):243–8.
27. Kramer P. Effect of antidiarrheal and antimotility drugs on ileal excreta. Am J Dig Dis. 1977;22(4):327–32 [Clinical Trial Randomized Controlled Trial Research Support, U.S. Gov't, P.H.S.].
28. King RF, Norton T, Hill GL. A double-blind crossover study of the effect of loperamide hydrochloride and codeine phosphate on ileostomy output. Aust N Z J Surg. 1982;52(2):121–4 [Clinical Trial Comparative Study].
29. Ladefoged K, Christensen KC, Hegnhoj J, Jarnum S. Effect of a long acting somatostatin analogue SMS 201–995 on jejunostomy effluents in patients with severe short bowel syndrome. Gut. 1989;30(7):943–9 [Clinical Trial Controlled Clinical Trial Research Support, Non-U.S. Gov't].
30. Nehra V, Camilleri M, Burton D, Oenning L, Kelly DG. An open trial of octreotide long-acting release in the management of short bowel syndrome. Am J Gastroenterol. 2001;96(5):1494–8 [Clinical Trial Research Support, Non-U.S. Gov't Research Support, U.S. Gov't, P.H.S.].
31. Harris AG, O'Dorisio TM, Woltering EA, Anthony LB, Burton FR, Geller RB, et al. Consensus statement: octreotide dose titration in secretory diarrhea. Diarrhea Management Consensus Development Panel. Dig Dis Sci. 1995;40(7):1464–73 [Consensus Development Conference Research Support, Non-U.S. Gov't Review].
32. McDoniel K, Taylor B, Huey W, Eiden K, Everett S, Fleshman J, et al. Use of clonidine to decrease intestinal fluid losses in patients with high-output short-bowel syndrome. JPEN J Parenter Enteral Nutr. 2004;28(4):265–8 [Case Reports].
33. Buchman AL, Fryer J, Wallin A, Ahn CW, Polensky S, Zaremba K. Clonidine reduces diarrhea and sodium loss in patients with proximal jejunostomy: a controlled study. JPEN J Parenter Enteral Nutr. 2006;30(6):487–91 [Research Support, N.I.H., Extramural].
34. Seguy D, Vahedi K, Kapel N, Souberbielle JC, Messing B. Low-dose growth hormone in adult home parenteral nutrition-dependent short bowel syndrome patients: a positive study. Gastroenterology. 2003;124(2):293–302 [Clinical Trial Randomized Controlled Trial Research Support, Non-U.S. Gov't].
35. Scolapio JS, Camilleri M, Fleming CR, Oenning LV, Burton DD, Sebo TJ, et al. Effect of growth hormone, glutamine, and diet on adaptation in short-bowel syndrome: a randomized, controlled study. Gastroenterology. 1997;113(4):1074–81 [Clinical Trial Comparative Study Randomized Controlled Trial Research Support, Non-U.S. Gov't Research Support, U.S. Gov't, P.H.S.].
36. Jeppesen PB. Teduglutide for the treatment of short bowel syndrome. Drugs Today (Barc). 2013;49(10):599–614 [Review].
37. Vipperla K, O'Keefe SJ. Study of teduglutide effectiveness in parenteral nutrition-dependent short-bowel syndrome subjects. Expert Rev Gastroenterol Hepatol. 2013;7(8):683–7.
38. Storr M. Short bowel syndrome. GLP-2 analog teduglutide. Med Monatsschr Pharm. 2013; 36(9):343–5.
39. Jeppesen PB, Pertkiewicz M, Messing B, Iyer K, Seidner DL, O'Keefe SJ, et al. Teduglutide reduces need for parenteral support among patients with short bowel syndrome with intestinal failure. Gastroenterology. 2012;143(6):1473–81. [Clinical Trial, Phase III Multicenter Study Randomized Controlled Trial Research Support, Non-U.S. Gov't]. e3.
40. O'Keefe SJ, Jeppesen PB, Gilroy R, Pertkiewicz M, Allard JP, Messing B. Safety and efficacy of teduglutide after 52 weeks of treatment in patients with short bowel intestinal failure. Clin Gastroenterol Hepatol. 2013;11(7):815–23. [Multicenter Study Randomized Controlled Trial Research Support, Non-U.S. Gov't]. e1-3.

41. Minneci PC. Intestinal transplantation: an overview. Pathophysiology. 2014;21:119–22.
42. Services CfMaM. Department of Health and Human Services. Meeting your medicare needs. [guideline development]. 2014. [cited 1 Feb 2014]; Available from: http://apps.ngsmedicare.com/applications/Content.aspx?DOCID=20493&CatID=3&RegID=51&ContentID=34464.
43. Abu-Elmagd K, Reyes J, Todo S, Rao A, Lee R, Irish W, et al. Clinical intestinal transplantation: new perspectives and immunologic considerations. J Am Coll Surg. 1998;186(5):512–25. [Research Support, U.S. Gov't, P.H.S.]; discussion 25–7.
44. Health Quality Ontario. Small bowel transplant: an evidence-based analysis. Ont Health Technol Assess Ser. 2003;3(1):1–72.
45. Farmer DG, McDiarmid SV, Winston D, Yersiz H, Cortina G, Dry S, et al. Effectiveness of aggressive prophylactic and preemptive therapies targeted against cytomegaloviral and Epstein-Barr viral disease after human intestinal transplantation. Transplant Proc. 2002;34(3):948–9 [Research Support, Non-U.S. Gov't].

Part IV
Mesenteric Venous Thrombosis

Chapter 22
Clinical Presentation, Etiology, and Diagnostic Considerations

Michael G. Sarr, Shaun M. Gifford, and Patrick S. Kamath

When one thinks of mesenteric ischemia (and thus intestinal ischemia—the dreaded outcome), of course the focus becomes arterial compromise from inflow occlusion secondary to atherosclerosis, embolus, or other much less common causes such as arteritis (e.g., polyarteritis nodosa, Takayasu's disease, aortic dissection, etc.). But intestine ischemia can also occur from venous outflow occlusion. Indeed, mesenteric venous thrombosis (MVT) accounts for about 10 % of all cases of mesenteric-derived intestine ischemia.

When compared to arterial mesenteric ischemia, MVT represents a much different clinical picture, presentation, etiopathogenesis, and treatment. Indeed, arterial ischemia requires treatment primarily by the vascular surgeon and often/usually requires an emergent intervention (operative or endovascular). In contrast, MVT more commonly falls under the realm of the gastroenterologist/gastrointestinal surgeon and can usually (hopefully) be managed nonoperatively; indeed, the ultimate goal is to arrest the propagation of the thrombotic process, avoid irreversible intestinal ischemia, and then prevent further episodes in the future. As with arterial mesenteric ischemia, MVT can present as an acute or chronic event as well as what some have called a subacute event.

This chapter will deal with the etiopathogenesis of MVT and, more specifically, with the clinical presentation and diagnosis while also acknowledging much

M.G. Sarr, MD (✉)
Division of Subspecialty Surgery, Mayo Clinic, Rochester, MN, USA
e-mail: sarr.michael@mayo.edu; frank.deborah@mayo.edu

S.M. Gifford, MD
Division of Vascular Surgery, Department of Surgery, Mayo Clinic, Rochester, MN, USA
e-mail: Gifford.shaun@mayo.edu

P.S. Kamath, MD
Division of Gastroenterology and Hepatology, Department of Medicine,
Mayo Clinic, Rochester, MN, USA
e-mail: kamath.patrick@mayo.edu

G.S. Oderich (ed.), *Mesenteric Vascular Disease*,
DOI 10.1007/978-1-4939-1847-8_22

of the underlying coagulopathy/thrombophilia that serves as the underlying etiology of MVT. This chapter will focus on the clinical presentation and diagnosis of MVT for the clinician.

Mesenteric Venous Anatomy

A brief review of the pertinent mesenteric venous anatomy is prudent. Mesenteric venous drainage of the gut in many respects follows the mesenteric arterial inflow but differs in several respects. First, unlike the three levels of arterial inflow (celiac, superior mesenteric, and inferior mesenteric arteries), the venous drainage relevant in MVT has three different venous systems: superior mesenteric, inferior mesenteric, and splenic systems (Fig. 22.1). Although they all drain eventually into the portal system (portal vein), these three systems behave differently in the category of MVT. The superior mesenteric system drains the distal duodenum, all the small bowel, and the right and transverse colon. The inferior mesenteric system drains the descending and sigmoid colon as well as the proximal rectum. The splenic vein drains primarily the spleen and the body/tail of the pancreas. While these three systems have collateral connections between them that can develop over time, acute

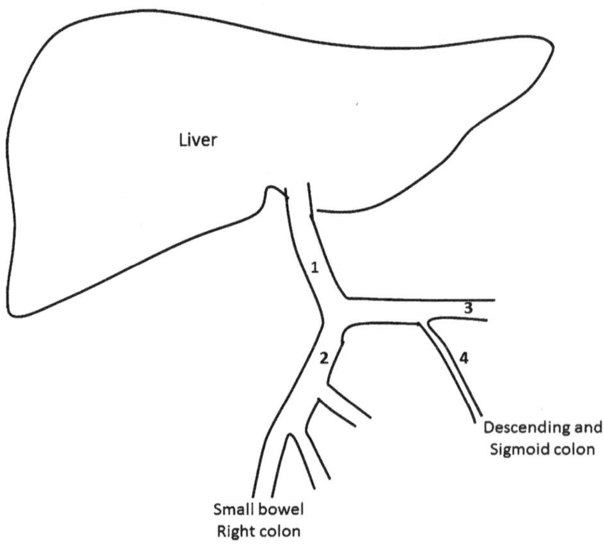

Fig. 22.1 Venous anatomy of MVT. *1* and *2* represent the portal and superior mesenteric veins involved predominately in portomesenteric venous thrombosis—usually acute and subacute MVT. *3* represents the splenic vein in the chronic MVT presentation of sinistral portal hypertension. *4* is the inferior mesenteric vein and is usually not involved in MVT. Chronic MVT can involve *1*, *2*, and *3* as extrahepatic venous occlusion leading to extrahepatic portal hypertension. Isolated thrombosis of *1* alone is usually not in the spectrum of MVT (By permission of Mayo Foundation for Medical Education and Research. All rights reserved)

occlusions in any one system usually cannot be well compensated for acutely by these venous collateral "anastomoses"; in this regard, this concept is quite similar to the arterial system. Over time, however, these collaterals can dilate, become collateral varicosities, and help to decompress in part a chronically developing obstruction—as, for instance, with portal hypertension, where the short gastric veins, the cardiac veins (right gastric vein), and the intramural gastric and esophageal veins dilate to become varices; similarly but less dramatically, the middle hemorrhoidal venous system helps to decompress, in part, the extrahepatic portal venous pressure as well. This venous decompression/collateral drainage (albeit partial) is possible, because, unlike in the systemic venous system, the mesenteric venous system has no venous valves; thus, patients with portal hypertension from primary liver parenchymal disease can develop quite bothersome anorectal hemorrhoids as well as the much more common and dangerous esophageal varices.

Interestingly, the majority of cases of acute and subacute MVT secondary to an underlying coagulopathy (see below) involve primarily the superior mesenteric venous system, less so the splenic venous system, and even less so the inferior mesenteric venous system. Indeed (and surprisingly), a syndrome of isolated inferior MVT is not apparent clinically. In contrast, the splenic venous system is more often involved secondary to local extravenous inflammatory effects (pancreatitis) or neoplastic etiologies (pancreatic cancers) that compress/occlude the splenic vein. Isolated portal venous, intrahepatic portal venous, or hepatic venous thrombosis is largely a different process and is usually not included under the clinical umbrella of MVT.

Similar in anatomic distribution to the small vessel arteriopathies of arterial mesenteric ischemia (vasculitis, etc.), MVT can start in the small veins (vena rectae) of the venous drainage arcades of the small intestine and propagate proximally to involve the larger, more central veins. Similarly, the thrombotic process can start more centrally (superior mesenteric vein or large primary tributary) and propagate distally. As will be seen below and in Chap. 24, the primary focus of treatment of MVT is not to relieve the obstruction with a thrombectomy or venous "bypass" as with arterial mesenteric ischemia, but rather to *prevent* any further propagation of the thrombotic process.

Etiopathogenesis

Pathogenesis

As with most disorders of the vasculature, the origin of the disorder arises from either presumed changes in blood flow within the lumen, extrinsic effects from local inflammation, pressure, etc., or the most common cause—some form of "injury" to the endothelium (either local or "global") (Table 22.1).

Table 22.1 Etiologies of MVT

Intraluminal effects (changes in blood flow)
Stasis
Cirrhosis with intrahepatic venous obstructions
Congestive heart failure—advanced
Extraluminal effects
Gastrointestinal inflammatory conditions (local or distant)
Acute/chronic pancreatitis
Diverticulitis
Inflammatory bowel disease
Appendicitis
Peritonitis
Trauma
Gastrointestinal surgery
Splenectomy
Laparoscopic surgery
Inflammatory bowel disease
Blunt mesenteric trauma
Neoplasms—extrinsic obstruction
Pancreatic cancer most common
Thrombophilic states[a]
Acquired
Non-hematologic
Oral contraceptives
Pregnancy
Nephrotic syndrome
Systemic malignancy (especially pancreatic)
Hyperhomocysteinemia
Hematologic
Polycythemia vera
Myelofibrosis
Thrombocythemia
Antiphospholipid antibodies
Paroxysmal nocturnal hemoglobinuria
JAK 2 gene sequence variation[b]
Inherited disorders
Protein S deficiency
Protein C deficiency
Antithrombin III deficiency
Factor V Leiden deficiency—homozygous[c]
Methylenetetrahydrofolate reductase gene sequence variation

Adapted from Singal et al. [6] and Kumar et al. [7], with permission

[a]See Chap. 24 for in-depth discussion of thrombophilia

[b]Janus Kinase gene (JAK2V617F)—a diagnostic criterion of a latent myeloproliferative neoplasm

[c]The heterozygous state not considered high risk for thrombophilia

Another approach to considering the etiopathogenesis is to think of either *primary* (so-called idiopathic) MVT when an underlying cause is not evident and *secondary* when the cause is evident (Table 22.1). The idiopathic category/classification shrinks each year as our understanding of the different forms of coagulopathies and thrombophilias expand.

Intraluminal Causes: Changes in Flow Characteristics

Changes in the dynamics of flow can lead to venous thrombosis—evident, for instance, in arteriovenous grafts, where turbulence predisposes to in situ thrombosis. In MVT, cirrhosis with portal hypertension, reversal of flow (hepatofugal flow), and relative stasis all appear to predispose to MVT. Indeed, the presence of portal hypertension is a not uncommon clinical disorder in patients presenting with MVT. These local, intraluminal disturbances in blood flow with the associated turbulence appear to alter the endothelial microenvironment, acting functionally as a form of endothelial injury/dysfunction [1]; this dysfunction then sets up a thrombophilic microenvironment within the vein and especially at the endothelium that can progress to venous thrombosis. This process is much less well understood than for disorders in arterial flow dynamics. Congestive heart failure can lead to a functional, posthepatic portal hypertension, again associated with presumed portal stasis and disruption of normal flow dynamics.

Extraluminal Effects

Changes in the surrounding environment of the mesenteric veins can lead to in situ thrombosis. Probably the most common causes in this regard are local inflammatory conditions. While not common when considering a patient with MVT, one should always at least entertain the possibility of appendicitis, diverticulitis, and peritonitis when MVT involves the superior mesenteric venous system. Other noninfective inflammatory conditions affecting the superior mesenteric system may be related to blunt mesenteric trauma, operative trauma (especially laparoscopic) [2], or inflammatory bowel disease, which has an as yet unexplained pathogenesis of MVT; indeed, MVT is a well-known, albeit uncommon, complication of surgery for inflammatory bowel disease [3]. Probably the most common etiologies are acute and chronic pancreatitis, but these inflammatory conditions affect primarily the splenic vein to cause splenic vein thrombosis. Because the splenic vein is so intimately associated with the posterior pancreas, effects of the local acute inflammation or the chronic cicatricial, fibrotic occlusion of the splenic vein alters the luminal microenvironment of the endothelium or actually occludes the vessel leading to local thrombosis.

Thrombophilic Etiologies

Probably the most common causes of MVT are the thrombophilic disorders—some of which are "acquired" (both non-hematologic and hematologic) and others are "inherited" genomic abnormalities in the germ line. These will be discussed in depth in Chap. 24. For the purposes of this chapter for the clinician, we at least need to consider these possibilities in patients without an obvious etiology.

The *acquired,* non-hematologic thrombophilic states include use of birth control pills, the nephrotic syndrome, certain malignancies with a systemic state of thrombophilia (especially pancreatic and gastric cancers), and states of hyperhomocysteinemia. These coagulopathies are potentially reversible. The acquired hematologic thrombophilias are more serious and include polycythemia vera (PCV), myelofibrosis, certain states of thrombocythemia, antiphospholipid antibodies, and paroxysmal nocturnal hemoglobinuria (PNH) (JAK 2 mutation is a diagnostic marker for PCV and thrombocythemia).

The *inherited* disorders of thrombophilia are hematologic and genomic in origin. These more commonly appreciated disorders of coagulation include deficiencies in protein S, protein C, antithrombin III (the current appropriate terminology is "antithrombin"), and factor V Leiden mutations; the heterozygote state of factor V Leiden is relatively common, and most hematologists do not consider the heterozygote state alone as a meaningful thrombophilic state, but the homozygote state is clinically relevant. Other less common variants will be entertained in Chap. 24.

Clinical Presentation

The clinical presentation of MVT takes three rather distinct forms: acute MVT, subacute MVT, and chronic MVT.

Acute MVT

These patients present with acute, central abdominal pain, presumably from a recent in situ thrombosis with clinically relevant distal venous obstruction. The pain is usually constant, mostly periumbilical, and often somewhat colicky, but not like the classic colic of a small bowel obstruction [4]. The duration of the pain is usually >24 h and some patients may often present several days after the onset of symptoms. Associated symptoms include anorexia, nausea, vomiting, hematochezia, or rarely melena; occult hematochezia when looked for will be present in about half the patients and should heighten your suspicion for MVT.

Patients with acute MVT usually look acutely ill. Physical examination, like in arterial mesenteric ischemia, may be rather unimpressive if there is no severe gut ischemia. This state of pain out of proportion to the physical findings requires an open-minded index of suspicion to the possibility of MVT, especially when risk factors are present. With advanced states with established ischemia or transmural infarction, frank peritonitis may be present, and an emergent operation is indicated, but many, perhaps most cases of acute MVT, will not require immediate operative intervention, and most, if treated appropriately and in a timely manner, will not progress to irreversible venous ischemia of the gut requiring exploration; indeed, the therapeutic goal is to prevent further propagation of the thrombosis with the development of ischemic necrosis. Fever at an early stage may be indicative of pylephlebitis, but the presence of infected thrombus is exceedingly unusual unless associated with active diverticulitis or appendicitis, the symptoms of which will dominate the clinical picture—the MVT will be noted "incidentally." As with any acute inflammatory condition involving the gut, dehydration may be prominent due to third spacing, acute development of ascites, and volume loss (vomiting, diarrhea). Hemodynamic instability at presentation is less common (~5–30%) and, of course, heightens the worry of intestinal infarction; when combined with fever and peritoneal signs, the presence of infarction should be assumed and aggressive resuscitation for emergent operation planned.

Subacute MVT

The clinical spectrum for subacute MVT involves a much more gradual onset, less severe, nagging, persistent pain than with acute MVT, often being present for several days or even several weeks. Although the subacute form may progress to transmural infarction with the patient then presenting with severe acute or chronic pain, this scenario is much less common. More likely is the story of a progressive dull, nonspecific, generalized, mid-abdominal pain with some anorexia, nausea, and occasionally vomiting. Diarrhea may be a prominent complaint, but overt hematochezia is less common. Some ascites may be present depending on the extent and duration of the process, but ascites is not a prominent finding. A high index of suspicion is necessary to entertain the diagnosis unless there are obvious known predisposing factors (Table 22.2). In some cases, the patients have been seen before with no diagnosis arrived at. Indeed, these patients may look more chronically ill than acutely ill.

Chronic MVT

Unlike acute and subacute MVT, chronic MVT does not present with a history of abdominal pain, but rather with the signs and symptoms of portal hypertension, selective mesenteric venous hypertension, or splenic venous hypertension (so-called left-sided or sinistral portal hypertension). Here the history of abdominal pain, vomiting, and diarrhea is usually absent, and the findings of a more central, chronic

Table 22.2 Differential diagnosis of MVT

	No peritonitis	Peritonitis
Acute MVT	Arterial intestinal ischemia[a]	Ruptured appendicitis
	Embolus	Perforated peptic ulcer
	Thrombosis	Perforated acute diverticulitis
	Aortic dissection	Acute pancreatitis
	Aortic aneurysm	Vascular catastrophe
	Perforated viscous—elderly patient on steroids	Acute arterial ischemia
	MVT	Embolus
		Aortic dissection
		Cocaine abuse
		MVT

[a]Must be the first consideration in an acutely ill-appearing patient with unimpressive abdominal examination

venous thrombosis is often unexpected. Physical findings when present are those of extrahepatic portal hypertension with esophagogastric or gastric varices, splenomegaly, and sometimes ascites.

Diagnosis

The most important point concerning the *diagnosis* of all forms of MVT is the need for a high index of suspicion for the possibility of MVT. Indeed, most cases are only diagnosed after obtaining a cross-sectional imaging procedure or, for acute MVT, actually in the operating room. Realistic suspicion of MVT by the astute clinician may be stimulated in patients presenting with abdominal pain who have known coagulopathies or known thrombophilia, but otherwise the diagnosis is usually a surprise. The following discussion will address each of the three forms of MVT separately.

Acute MVT

After the history and physical examination, the differential diagnosis is that of an intra-abdominal inflammatory process or an acute intra-abdominal catastrophe. When diffuse peritonitis is present, the differential is broad and includes many abdominal catastrophes, the most common being ruptured appendicitis, perforated duodenal ulcer, acute perforated diverticulitis, acute pancreatitis, acute arterial mesenteric ischemia, and other causes of bowel ischemia/infarction. The lack of initial localizing signs that progress to generalized abdominal pain, such as right lower quadrant pain (acute appendicitis) and left lower quadrant pain (acute diverticulitis), can often exclude certain diagnoses, while the relatively acute nature of onset of the symptoms of mid-abdominal pain should lead the clinician to consider a different diagnostic spectrum. The presence of peritonitis requires an attempt to exclude any causes that would *prevent* the need for abdominal exploration, such as acute pancreatitis; otherwise, abdominal exploration (regardless of the cause) will be required. The presence of ascites, while usually not obvious on physical examination, would change the clinical focus of possible causes and should increase one's suspicion of acute MVT.

In contrast, in acute MVT without transmural bowel infarction, when peritonitis is absent, the differential diagnosis is quite different, and the ultimate diagnosis is more difficult. The absence of impressive physical findings on abdominal examination in the patient who otherwise looks acutely ill should immediately initiate the possibility of some vascular catastrophe, such as acute arterial (superior mesenteric artery) mesenteric ischemia (embolus, acute atherosclerotic occlusion, aortic dissection), ruptured abdominal aortic aneurysm, and finally MVT. In this setting, i.e., unimpressive physical findings in the presence of diffuse abdominal pain in a patient who looks sick, MVT should at least be entertained and, just as with acute arterial mesenteric ischemia, timely diagnosis is crucial.

The patient's history can be of considerable help in differentiating arterial from venous mesenteric ischemia. The presence of cardiac abnormalities, such as atrial fibrillation, recent acute myocardial infarction, prosthetic cardiac valves, a very recent coronary angiography, or cocaine abuse, should steer the clinician toward an arterial etiology. In contrast, in patients with a known personal or family history of a coagulopathy or history of peripheral deep vein thrombosis (present in about one third of patients), the suspicion of thrombophilia steers the diagnosis a bit away from arterial ischemia [5]. But, arterial ischemia must be excluded definitively, because its treatment is so different than for MVT and timely intervention is crucial (see Chap. 15).

Laboratory Investigation

Routine laboratory tests are usually not helpful. Changes in hemoglobin are nonspecific unless the hemoglobin is greater than normal values which would suggest PCV. A markedly increased platelet count $>10^6$ may be indicative of a predisposing thrombocytosis. The white blood cell count (WBC) again is nonspecific and will be increased in most abdominal disorders being considered. When peritonitis is not present in acute MVT, the WBC should not be markedly increased (>15,000), and there should not be left shift. In contrast, when peritonitis is present, an increased WBC with a shift to the left is unhelpful when considering the differential diagnosis. The more sophisticated tests of a coagulopathy would probably not be entertained at this time, and the more routine tests (international ratio [INR] or partial thromboplastin time) would not be helpful. The other routine screening tests, such as electrolytes, liver function tests, etc., are of no discriminative value.

Imaging

The hallmark of the diagnosis of acute MVT is cross-sectional imaging—computed tomography (CT) or magnetic resonance imaging (MRI). Plain abdominal radiographs may help the astute clinician to suspect MVT by showing thickened small bowel with a nonspecific bowel pattern of early ileus with mildly dilated loops of small bowel. The classic signs of "thumb printing" from mucosal edema are rarely present (<5 %), however, and difficult to see. The presence of ascites is not recognized readily on plain film, and other signs of intestinal infarction, such as pneumatosis intestinalis, portal venous gas, or rarely free air, only serve to support a diagnosis of intestinal infarction from any cause. Therefore, cross-sectional imaging becomes the key to diagnosis.

Contrast-Enhanced Computed Tomography

CT is the most common diagnostic test and the test of choice when MVT is suspected. Its accuracy is >90 % but varies with the site of thrombosis—the larger the vein(s), the greater the accuracy. Typical features of MVT on CT include a central lucency within the vein with a sharply defined wall and dilation of the vessel. Findings of MVT on CT also include bowel wall thickening of >3 mm associated with local mesenteric thickening/inflammation, indistinct margins of adjacent bowel loops, and, when present, ascites. While these findings are suggestive but not diagnostic, the presence of thrombosis in the mesenteric vein(s) clinches the diagnosis. When the thrombotic process is limited to the small vena rectae in the more peripheral mesentery, recognition of the thrombosed veins may be less obvious, but when the process propagates into major branches off the superior mesenteric vein or more proximally, the CT becomes diagnostic. As will be seen in Chap. 23, this finding should initiate immediate anticoagulation to prevent propagation of the venous thrombosis.

Magnetic Resonance Imaging

Although there is much less experience with MRI than with CT, the findings are similar. MRI will clearly demonstrate central venous thrombosis, but thromboses in the smaller vena rectae are difficult to see. Ascites and bowel wall and mesenteric thickening (edema) are well visualized with MRI.

Other Cross-Sectional Imaging

Transabdominal ultrasonography is an excellent test to detect ascites, but bowel gas usually prevents adequate imaging of the bowel and/or the mesentery. Doppler ultrasonography may be able to show abnormal venous flow in the large central veins but is severely limited in visualizing the smaller vena rectae of the mesentery. Nuclear scintigraphy is of little use due to its nonspecific resolution. Mesenteric angiography, though usually diagnostic, is seldom needed when the patient has had a prior CT; one might imagine a role for mesenteric angiography in a patient in whom an arterial ischemic process cannot be excluded.

Subacute MVT

Unlike acute MVT, the clinical presentation of subacute MVT is less dramatic and the diagnosis even less obvious. These patients usually have a history of a nagging central abdominal pain for days to several weeks. Because acute bowel ischemia or infarction is not present, the pain is usually less severe and not cramping. There may be a history of diarrhea, on occasion bloody, but ascites is usually not obvious or advanced. The physical examination is usually unhelpful with findings of generalized abdominal discomfort. Unlike the patient with acute MVT, these patients do not look acutely ill and are usually not dehydrated. Indeed, the patient may not have been investigated by CT or MRI, and the diagnosis is often delayed and may require several visits to the physician or emergency room setting before a cross-sectional imaging procedure is ordered or the clinician thinks of MVT.

Laboratory Evaluation

Routine laboratory values, except possibly the increased hemoglobin of PCV and a severe thrombocytosis ($>10^6$), are of little diagnostic benefit. See Chap. 23 for more specific hematologic tests of thrombophilia.

Imaging

Findings on plain abdominal radiography are not helpful. CT is the procedure of choice and, unless there is a known coagulopathy or family history of such, the diagnosis is usually a surprise. With chronic MVT, the bowel wall thickening, though present, may not be as extreme as with acute MVT due to the formation of collateral drainage. But the thrombotic process should be more obvious on the contrast-enhanced views, because the thrombosis often has extended more proximally. As with acute MVT, the presence of this mesenteric venous thrombosis should initiate immediate systemic heparinization. Because of a more central venous thrombosis, Doppler ultrasonography may show changes in mesenteric venous flow, but the diagnosis and etiology may not be obvious, and the subsequent diagnosis is usually made by CT or MRI.

Chronic MVT

The diagnosis of the various forms of chronic MVT is made solely on cross-sectional imaging. Symptoms are those of complications of an otherwise asymptomatic, chronic portomesenteric or splenic venous hypertension. Variceal hemorrhage (esophageal, gastric, or much less commonly intestinal or hemorrhoidal) or findings of a watermelon stomach (portal hypertensive gastropathy) on gastroscopy in a patient without a history of hepatopathy usually initiate the imaging procedure. A prior history of severe acute pancreatitis, chronic pancreatitis, or symptoms of pancreatic cancer associated with prominent gastric varices and splenomegaly may heighten the suspicion of splenic vein thrombosis with resultant sinistral portal hypertension. Ascites is usually absent due to the chronic nature of the extrahepatic portal hypertension with an otherwise normal liver, but splenomegaly is present.

Laboratory Evaluation

This evaluation is consistent with extrahepatic portal hypertension usually with some extent of thrombocytopenia due to the splenomegaly. Myeloproliferative disorders may be missed, because in the presence of hypersplenism, the platelet count and hemoglobin are often decreased. The absence of abnormalities in the liver function tests points one away from the diagnosis of cirrhosis.

Imaging

Other than splenomegaly, plain abdominal radiographs are not helpful. CT or MRI makes the diagnosis and shows clearly the central venous clot(s) as well as the resultant varices throughout the stomach and small bowel mesentery. Doppler ultrasonography will show marked changes in venous flow, but may be of little actual help in diagnosis, management, and treatment.

Conclusions

The diagnosis of MVT is often overlooked and delayed either until operative exploration for intestinal ischemia or until a cross-sectional imaging procedure is performed. One key to the diagnosis of MVT is clinical suspicion, but CT and MRI are the primary diagnostic modalities. A prior history or family history of a coagulopathy should heighten clinical suspicion. The key to treatment is a rapid diagnosis and systemic anticoagulation to prevent further propagation of the thrombosis.

References

1. Tripodi A, Mannucci PM. The coagulopathy of chronic liver disease. N Engl J Med. 2011; 365(2):147–56.
2. Goitein D, Matter I, Raziel A, Keidar A, Hazzan D, Rimon U, et al. Portomesenteric thrombosis following laparoscopic bariatric surgery: incidence, patterns of clinical presentation, and etiology in a bariatric patient population. JAMA Surg. 2013;148(4):340–6.
3. Landman C, Nahon S, Cosnes J, Bouhnik Y, Brixi-Benmansour H, Bouguen G, et al. Portomesenteric vein thrombosis in patients with inflammatory bowel disease. Inflamm Bowel Dis. 2013;19(3):582–9.
4. Rhee RY, Gloviczki P, Mendonca CT, Petterson TM, Serry RD, Sarr MG, et al. Mesenteric venous thrombosis: still a lethal disease in the 1990s. J Vasc Surg. 1994;20(5):688–97.
5. Brandt LJ, Boley SJ. AGA technical review on intestinal ischemia. American Gastrointestinal Association. Gastroenterology. 2000;118(5):954–68.
6. Singal AK, Kamath PS, Tefferi A. Mesenteric venous thrombosis. Mayo Clin Proc. 2013; 88(3):285–94.
7. Kumar S, Sarr MG, Kamath PS. Mesenteric venous thrombosis. N Engl J Med. 2001; 345(23):1683–8.

Chapter 23
Thrombophilia Testing in Splanchnic Vein Thrombosis

Robert D. McBane II and Waldemar E. Wysokinski

The splanchnic venous system is comprised of confluent venous segments including the superior and inferior mesenteric veins and the splenic vein which together empty into the portal venous system to supply the liver [1]. The hepatic veins drain the liver into the inferior vena cava just caudal to the right atrium (Fig. 23.1). When considering the splanchnic venous circulation, it is important to recognize the many unique physiologic features beyond mere anatomy compared to venous segments elsewhere in the body. These differences may impact the thrombotic process and are therefore worthy of contemplation [2–4]. First, mesenteric venous blood is rich in both nutrients and intestinal elements such as microbial flora and both senescent and damaged cells. Second, marked variations in mesenteric blood flow and viscosity occur depending on the time of day, nutrition intake, physical activity, emotional stress, diarrheal illness, and dehydration. Third, the splanchnic circulation is richly innervated by the sympathetic nervous system and responds to a variety of vasoactive stimuli including epinephrine, norepinephrine, angiotensin II, and vasopressin. Furthermore, this circulation is subject to a number of blood-borne gastrointestinal peptides such as glucagon, VIP, and cholecystokinin which may further impact hemostasis and blood flow [3]. Fourth, the splanchnic circulation serves as an important blood reservoir containing approximately 80 % of the blood volume and is thus designated a "capacitance venous system." As such, there is tremendous variation in blood stasis within this system [3]. Fifth, the splanchnic venous circulation is not known to contain venous valves, at least not in the larger channels [2]. Valves have been identified in smaller venous tributaries of the stomach and colon but only in infants.

R.D. McBane II, MD • W.E. Wysokinski, MD (✉)
Department of Medicine, Division of Cardiovascular Diseases,
Gonda Vascular Center, Mayo Clinic, Rochester, MN, USA
e-mail: mcbane.robert@mayo.edu; Wysokinski.Waldemar@mayo.edu

G.S. Oderich (ed.), *Mesenteric Vascular Disease*,
DOI 10.1007/978-1-4939-1847-8_23

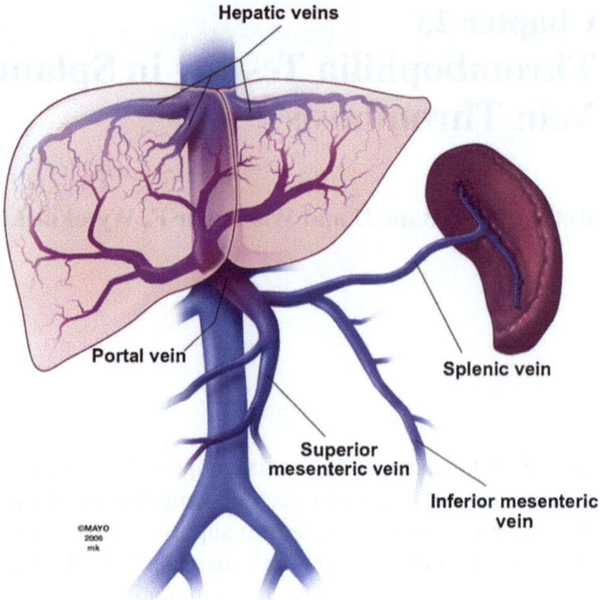

Fig. 23.1 Splanchnic veins (By permission of Mayo Foundation for Medical Education and Research. All rights reserved)

This is important whereby venous thrombi occurring in the deep veins of the leg are thought to originate in the valve pockets. Sixth, venous blood within this system may be enriched with inflammatory cells, such as dendritic cells, monocytes, and macrophages, and various antibodies. The splenic vein, in particular, serves as an important element of the reticuloendothelial system. Seventh, each organ within the splanchnic circulation may be impacted by a variety of malignant, infectious, and inflammatory processes. For example, the spleen can be a site for metastatic diseases in addition to lymphoproliferative, myeloproliferative, or hematologic malignancies. The liver is a common and important site of metastatic disease. Finally, the complexity and interrelationship of the splanchnic circulation is such that thrombosis of one venous segment alters blood flow within the entire system. Altered blood flow within the local prothrombotic milieu increased the propensity for thrombus propagation into other adjoining venous segments, common to this disease. For these combined reasons, the splanchnic venous circulation is entirely unique. Thrombosis occurring within this system should therefore be considered as a distinctive entity requiring special consideration and evaluation beyond simply an event occurring in an unusual venous location.

Splanchnic venous thrombosis is an uncommon disease with an incidence of 2.7–4.5 per 100,000 person-years [5, 6]. This disease may result in considerable morbidity and mortality [1]. Determining the underlying cause of thrombosis can help guide management including the duration of anticoagulant therapy [1, 7]. For most patients with splanchnic vein thrombosis, the underlying mechanism is readily apparent. In contrast to typical deep vein thrombosis or pulmonary embolism, splanchnic vein thrombosis generally results from organ pathology of the venous segment involved. For some patients, however, the underlying cause may not be clear. For these individuals, a thorough assessment of underlying congenital or acquired thrombotic propensity should be considered.

The intent of this chapter is to review the acquired and congenital causes of thrombosis within the splanchnic venous circulation and to provide a framework useful for the evaluation of thrombotic mechanisms in patients with this disorder. This framework will help to discern which patients are most likely to benefit from thrombophilia testing, define an appropriate thrombophilia test panel, and discuss how test results might impact management.

Acquired Provoking Factors for Splanchnic Vein Thrombosis

Identifying causal factors underlying splanchnic vein thrombosis is central to the clinical assessment. These factors may be broadly categorized into those which are inherited and therefore intrinsically permanent and those which are acquired. The acquired conditions may be categorized as transient, correctable, or permanent. Examples of transient acquired factors include oral contraception, pregnancy, surgery, and trauma. In general, provoked thromboembolic events attributed to transient or correctable acquired risk factors have a sufficiently low risk of recurrence such that prolonged anticoagulant therapy is neither necessary nor advisable [8]. For unprovoked thrombotic events or for those with acquired and non-correctable risk factors, the risk of recurrence is deemed sufficiently high as to warrant prolonged secondary prevention with anticoagulants assuming the risk of major bleeding is mild to moderate. This distinction can be particularly important for splanchnic vein thrombosis where portal and mesenteric venous hypertension are associated with varix formation, which can greatly augment the bleeding risk [1, 7, 8].

Thrombosis involving the splanchnic veins results predominantly from acquired pathology of the organ drained by the involved venous segment or by inflammation and injury of adjacent organs. As part of the initial evaluation, it is therefore important to scrutinize the history, physical examination, cross-sectional imaging, and laboratory data for clues to organ pathology as a potential acquired cause for the splanchnic vein thrombosis. If identified, the laboratory assessment for an acquired or congenital thrombophilia is not likely warranted [8, 9]. A number of acquired conditions contributing to splanchnic vein thrombosis have been identified including a prevalence estimate from published cohorts (Table 23.1) [10–14]. In a series of 832 patients with splanchnic vein thrombosis, the most common underlying pathology was malignancy, present in 43 % of the cohort [14]. These cancers included solid tumors (27 %), hematologic malignancies (5 %), and myeloproliferative neoplasms (11 %). The three most common solid tumors were pancreatic (38 %), hepatobiliary (32 %), and gastrointestinal (19 %). When multiple splanchnic venous segments are involved, cancer was present in nearly half of patients. Moreover, cancer was associated with a higher prevalence of thrombosis in specific venous segments. For example, nearly half of patients with either splenic or portal vein thrombosis had an

Table 23.1 Demographic characteristics and underlying etiology of acquired thrombosis

Author	N	MPD (%)	Trauma (%)	PNH (%)	IBD (%)	APL Ab (%)	Cancer (%)	Pancreatitis (%)	Infection	Surgery	Hormones	Cirrhosis
Janssen et al. [10]	135	21	2	2	4	2	2	7	8	28 %	17 %	16 %
Plessier et al. [11]	102	21	1	–	1	8	–	8	11	–	22 %	–
Deltenre et al. [12]	61	51	–	–	–	15	–	–	–	–	–	–
Sutkowska et al. [13]	341	11	1	–	8	6	11	–	–	17 %	3 %	–
Thatipelli et al. [14]	832	11	–	1	6	–	32	13	10	10 %	6 %	24 %

MPD myeloproliferative disorder, *PNH* paroxysmal nocturnal hemoglobinuria, *IBD* inflammatory bowel disease, *APL Ab* antiphospholipid antibody syndrome, *Hormone* oral contraception, hormone replacement, pregnancy underlying malignancy. By comparison, hepatic vein thrombosis was associated with a solid tumor in 13 % of patients and a myeloproliferative neoplasm in 22 %. These high percentages mandate a thorough search for an underlying malignancy in all patients with documented splanchnic vein thrombosis.

A recent meta-analysis reported that the prevalence of myeloproliferative neoplasms may account for one third of patients with splanchnic vein thrombosis [15]. This compares to only 1 % for patients with conventional venous thromboembolism. In fact splanchnic vein thrombosis may be the initial clinical manifestation of myeloproliferative neoplasms in some patients. Myeloproliferative neoplasms, including polycythemia vera, essential thrombocythemia, and primary myelofibrosis, are an important consideration in the search for underlying mechanism of splanchnic vein thrombosis [1, 10, 14, 16–18]. These disorders represent a stem cell-derived clonal myeloproliferation [16–19]. Polycythemia vera results in an increased number of red cells, white cells, and platelets with limited bone marrow fibrosis. Essential thrombocythemia involves primarily platelet expansion. Primary myelofibrosis may be primary or reflect transformation of the polycythemia vera and essential thrombocythemia and is characterized by progressive fibrosis of the bone marrow. Although the most dramatic outcome is transformation to myeloid leukemia, the most common clinical manifestation and cause of death is thrombosis related [18]. These disorders result from an acquired mutation within JAK2, a member of the Janus kinase family of cytoplasmic tyrosine kinases associated with growth factor receptors [17]. This mutation involves a replacement of valine for phenylalanine in position 617 (V617F) of the JAK2 protein resulting in growth factor-independent proliferation of various cell lines [20]. This mutation may explain 90 % of cases of polycythemia vera and up to 50 % of cases of essential thrombocythemia. Screening for this mutation is therefore appropriate in the initial evaluation of patients suspected of having these disorders [20]. In a large series of patients with splanchnic vein thrombosis, myeloproliferative disorders were a prominent cause of both hepatic vein thrombosis (22 %) and multisegmental splanchnic vein thrombosis (17 %) [14]. In other series, investigators performed bone marrow biopsies on 128 patients with splanchnic vein thrombosis [21, 22]. Of these, 4 % carried a diagnosis of MPD prior to development of splanchnic vein thrombosis. An additional 33 % met criteria based on the bone marrow biopsy results.

Acute pancreatitis was also an important cause of splanchnic vein thrombosis accounting for 7–13 % of cases [10, 11, 14]. In one series, acute pancreatitis explained nearly half of all patients with splenic vein thrombosis [14]. This diagnosis should be relatively straight forward to confirm or exclude based on the acute presentation, clinical risk factors, examination, imaging, and commonly available laboratory testing. Cirrhosis is an important association, present in 16–24 % of cases. In particular, cirrhosis may account for up to one third of cases of portal vein thrombosis. This is an important diagnosis to confirm given the complexity of anticoagulant management in such patients. Recent abdominal surgery may explain 10–28 % of cases, particularly procedures involving splenectomy or liver transplantation [14]. Other important associations include sepsis of intra-abdominal origin (8–11 %), inflammatory bowel disease (1–8 %), and connective tissue diseases (up to 6 %).

Table 23.2 Demographic characteristics and underlying etiology

Variable (%)	Total (n=832)	Hepatic (n=45)	Portal (n=329)	Mesenteric (n=76)	Splenic (n=62)	Multiple (n=320)
Age (Mn ± SD)	53 ± 17	45 ± 17	54 ± 18	59 ± 16	56 ± 16	51 ± 17
Female (%)	42	67	38	37	29	45
Idiopathic	15	9	16	22	5	15
Cancer	27	13	31	20	36	24
Cirrhosis	24	16	34	8	10	22
Pancreatitis	13	4	9	12	45	13
Myeloproliferative	11	22	5	5	5	17
Surgery	10	11	9	12	5	11
Infection	10	7	13	18	5	7
Inflammatory bowel disease	6	11	8	3	2	6
OCP/HRT	6	13	4	7	5	8
Connective tissue disease	6	9	5	5	2	8
Leukemia/ lymphoma	5	0	6	4	2	5

Adapted from Thatipelli et al. [14], with permission
OCP oral contraception pill, *HRT* hormone replacement therapy

Paroxysmal nocturnal hemoglobinuria is a rare but serious disorder involving clonal expansion of hematopoietic stem cells which lack the glycosylphosphatidylinositol membrane protein which anchors important proteins to the cell surface [22, 23]. Of these, complement-inhibiting proteins, CD55 and CD59, are particularly important for inhibition of complement fixation and mediated cellular lysis. Clinical manifestations of this disease include hemolytic anemia and both venous and arterial thromboembolism. Patients with this disease have been reported to suffer splanchnic vein thrombosis. Indeed, up to 10 % of patients with hepatic vein thrombosis may have this disease as an underlying mechanism. In large series, the prevalence of PNH in splanchnic vein thrombosis may account for 1–2 % of underlying causes [9, 14]. This disorder can be readily detected using flow cytometry and antibodies against CD55 and CD59 surface antigens.

Acquired risk factors for splanchnic vein thrombosis can be further stratified by thrombus location, which may be helpful to address the risk for specific cases (Table 23.2) [14]. Although splanchnic vein thrombosis can be viewed as a composite of venous segments, thrombosis within each individual venous segment contains unique features in terms of underlying etiology, risk of recurrence, and long-term prognosis [14]. Cancer is a prominent cause of thrombosis in each of the splanchnic venous segments and particularly when multiple venous segments are involved. Beyond cancer, hepatic vein thrombosis, for example, affects primarily younger women and has myeloproliferative disorder, cirrhosis, and oral contraception as prominent causes. Portal vein thrombosis, the most common within the splanchnic territory, has poor survival because of the relatively high incidence of cirrhosis. Isolated splenic vein thrombosis is uncommon, mainly occurs in middle-aged males with pancreatitis, and has a strong association with pancreatitis. Infection and recent abdominal surgery are common among patients with mesenteric vein thrombosis. For mesenteric vein thrombosis, a relatively high percentage of patients without an identifiable underlying etiology was evident.

In summary, the effective evaluation of patients with splanchnic vein thrombosis must begin with a thorough history and physical examination supported by appropriate laboratory testing and cross-sectional imaging. This evaluation should focus on the exclusion of underlying cancers including solid tumors, myeloproliferative neoplasms, and hematologic malignancies as well as other abdominal pathologies. This search will help to determine which patients are most likely to benefit from thrombophilia testing.

Thrombophilia Testing

When considering thrombophilia testing, it is important to discern which patients to test, when to perform the testing, and what tests to include in the panel. Identifying those patients most likely to benefit from thrombophilia testing is an important first step for several reasons. First, indiscriminate thrombophilia testing in unselected patients with incident venous thrombosis is neither indicated nor cost-effective [9]. Second, thrombophilia test results have been shown to neither influence the initiation nor the intensity of anticoagulant therapy. Both the initiation and intensity of anticoagulation are the same irrespective of thrombophilia status. For example, heparin therapy in patients with antithrombin deficiency results in a therapeutic failure in only a small minority of patients [24]. Warfarin skin necrosis is very rare even in those patients with protein C or protein S deficiencies [25, 26]. High-intensity warfarin (INR 3.1–4.0) has not been shown to be superior to standard warfarin (INR goal 2.0–3.0) in patients with antiphospholipid antibodies and previous thrombosis [27]. Third, thrombophilia testing in unselected patients has not been shown to reduce thrombosis recurrence [28–30]. In a case-control study of patients from the MEGA cohort, the odds ratio for venous thrombosis recurrence was similar for those patients undergoing thrombophilia testing compared to those who were not tested [28]. In a separate cohort of 570 otherwise unselected patients with first objectively proven venous thrombosis, testing for thrombophilia did not aid in the prediction of venous thrombosis recurrence at 2 years [29]. Similar results were noted in a prospective study of 474 consecutive patients from the Leiden Thrombophilia Study [30]. Whereas the majority of patients with splanchnic vein thrombosis have clearly identified provoking factors, the role of thrombophilia testing should therefore be pursued with constraint [23]. Within large cohorts of patients with splanchnic vein thrombosis, only between 15 and 20 % lacked an identifiable provoking cause [9, 12, 13]. This percentage of unprovoked venous thrombosis is lower than has been observed for leg DVT/PE which has been reported at 26 % [13]. It is therefore our practice to reserve thrombophilia testing for patients with idiopathic or unprovoked venous thromboembolism.

Table 23.3 Thrombophilia risk factors for mesenteric venous thrombosis

Inherited thrombophilias
Activated protein C resistance and factor V Leiden mutation
Antithrombin deficiency
Elevated factor VIII
Protein C deficiency
Protein S deficiency
Prothrombin G20210A mutation
Hyperhomocysteinemia
Acquired or secondary thrombophilias
Disseminated intravascular coagulation (DIC)
Heparin-induced thrombocytopenia[a]
Lupus anticoagulant and antiphospholipid antibody syndrome
Paroxysmal nocturnal hemoglobinuria[a]

[a]Indicates testing reserved for selective patients

When pursued, the thrombophilia test panel should be comprehensive and should include testing for both congenital and acquired thrombotic diatheses (Table 23.3) [23]. This ensures that specific thrombotic variables are not overlooked including the rare instance of combined abnormalities. While factor V Leiden and prothrombin G20210A mutations are the most common thrombophilias, it is our practice to include testing for all of the known congenital and acquired thrombophilias. Although rare, entities such as protein C, protein S, and antithrombin deficiency carry high thrombotic propensity, impact anticoagulant management, and therefore are important not to overlook. In addition to the conventional panel, heparin platelet factor 4 testing (for diagnosing heparin-induced thrombocytopenia) and red cell flow cytometry measures of GPI (glycosylphosphatidylinositol)-linked proteins (for diagnosing paroxysmal nocturnal hemoglobinuria) can be considered in selected patients [31, 32]. When feasible, this test panel ought to be performed once the patient has recovered from the acute thrombotic event, anticoagulation therapy has been discontinued, and hepatic dysfunction (if present) has resolved [23]. This last recommendation has both practical and economic implications. It can be difficult to interpret thrombophilia test results in the setting of anticoagulation therapy. For example, direct factor inhibitors and warfarin may lead to falsely positive lupus anticoagulant. Heparin therapy excludes lupus anticoagulant testing by the aPTT methodology thus decreasing test panel sensitivity and accuracy for this disorder. Acquired antithrombin deficiency is a common finding when drawn during heparin therapy. Warfarin is a well-known cause of both acquired protein C and protein S deficiencies. The oral direct thrombin inhibitor, dabigatran, is known to overestimate protein C and S levels and reduce the sensitivity of activated protein C resistant ratio testing [33]. The oral direct factor Xa inhibitor, rivaroxaban, can have variable effects on clot-based assays depending on the reagents and instruments used [34]. Hormonal therapy may result in an acquired protein S deficiency. Lastly, this testing is expensive and the requirement for repeat testing is not cost-effective. Therefore, the timing of test requisition is important. For these reasons, it is prudent to delay test acquisition until anticoagulants have been discontinued, the impact of the acute thrombotic event has resolved, and the organs (especially the liver) have recovered from the injury.

To date, thrombophilia testing in this clinical entity has been assessed by several authors with conflicting results. This may stem from differences in recruitment and ethnicity of cohorts [5, 9–12]. The prevalence of thrombophilia was assessed in 1,238 patients with venous thromboembolism including 119 with splanchnic vein thrombosis [35]. Of those patients with splanchnic vein thrombosis, factor V Leiden was present in 5 % which was not different relative to a sample of 1,304 individuals from the general population (4.6 %). The prothrombin G20210A mutation (8.4 % vs. 4.3 %) and compound heterozygous mutations (3.4 % vs. 0.1 %) were more prevalent in patients with splanchnic vein thrombosis compared to the general population sample. Of thc protcin dcficiencies, only protein C deficiency was noted in splanchnic vein thrombosis patients (3.4 %). In the series from Mayo Clinic, 341 cases of splanchnic vein thrombosis, thrombophilia prevalence was compared to 3,621 control patients with leg DVT [12]. Thrombophilia prevalence was assessed by thrombotic location (Table 23.4). As in other series, factor V Leiden mutation was the most common thrombophilia for splanchnic vein thrombosis. Yet, only a small percentage carries the homozygous mutation. Within the splanchnic circulation, factor V Leiden may be more common in one venous segment compared to others. In the Mayo Clinic series, this mutation was most common in those with splenic and mesenteric vein thrombosis [12]. Antiphospholipid antibody syndrome was the second most prevalent thrombophilia and was most frequent in patients with hepatic vein thrombosis. The prothrombin G20210A mutation was seen less frequently in most series accounting for approximately 5 % of cases particularly for patients with splenic and mesenteric vein thrombosis. In general, protein C, protein S, and antithrombin deficiencies were infrequent and account for 10 % of thrombophilias in total.

In a study comparing thrombophilia prevalence in patients with splanchnic vein thrombosis compared to lower extremity deep vein thrombosis, the prevalence of “strong thrombophilia” defined as deficiency of either antithrombin, protein C, or protein S, antiphospholipid antibody syndrome, homozygous factor V Leiden or prothrombin G20210A mutations, or compound heterozygous mutations of factor V Leiden and prothrombin G20210A [12] were more common in patients with splanchnic vein thrombosis (Table 23.5). This high prevalence was notably observed for patients with hepatic and mesenteric vein thrombosis. Whereas the finding of “strong” thrombophilia usually mandates long-term secondary anticoagulation prophylaxis, this finding is of practical importance.

Table 23.4 Inherited thrombophilia characteristics

Author	*N*	Factor V Leiden (%)	Prothrombin G20210A (%)	Protein C deficiency (%)	Protein S deficiency (%)	Antithrombin deficiency (%)
Janssen et al. [10]	135	13	4	7	1.5	1
Plessier et al. [11]	102	3	14	1	5	2
Deltenre et al. [12]	63	32	6	19	7	0
Sutkowska et al. [13]	341	11	4	0.3	4	1
Acosta et al. [5]	51	45	0	3	7	–

Table 23.5 Thrombophilia prevalence in patients with splanchnic vein thrombosis compared with lower extremity deep vein thrombosis

Test *n*, (%)	HVT *N*=22	PVT *N*=112	SVT *N*=11	MVT *N*=67	M-SpVT *N*=129	Total *N*=341	LE DVT *N*=3,621	*P*-value
Anticardiolipin antibodies[a] (ACLa)								
IgG	3 (16)	0	0	2 (3)	0	5 (1)	37 (1)	0.2337
IgM	1 (5)	2 (2)	0	1 (2)	1 (1)	5 (1)	45 (1)	0.4141
Lupus anticoagulant (LAC)	4 (18.2)	3 (2.7)	0	3 (4.5)	3 (2.3)	13 (3.8)	138 (3.8)	0.9991
LAC or ACLa (IgG or IgM)	5 (22.7)	5 (4.5)	0	6 (9.0)	4 (3.1)	20 (5.9)	189 (5.2)	0.6102
Factor V Leiden								0.0497
Heterozygous mutation	2 (9.1)	5 (4.5)	3 (27.3)	16 (23.9)	9 (7.0)	35 (10.3)	547 (15.1)	
Homozygous mutation	0	0	0	1 (1.5)	1 (0.8)	2 (0.6)	27 (0.7)	
Prothrombin G20210A								0.1901
Heterozygous mutation	0	3 (3.5)	1 (10.0)	4 (7.3)	4 (4.3)	12 (4.6)	154 (4.9)	
Homozygous mutation	0	0	0	1 (1.8)	0	1 (0.4)	1 (0.03)	
Homocystein, >20 mcmol/L	1 (5.6)	0	0	0	0	0	41 (1)	1.0000
Protein C deficiency	0	0	0	0	1 (0.8)	1 (0.3)	8 (0.2)	0.5555
Protein S deficiency	0	3 (2.7)	1 (9.1)	1 (1.5)	7 (5.4)	12 (3.5)	33 (0.9)	0.0003
Antithrombin deficiency	0	2 (1.8)	0	2 (3.0)	1 (0.8)	5 (1.5)	48 (1.3)	0.8036
Positive testing	7 (31.8)	18(16.1)	5 (45.5)	28 (41.8)	26 (20.2)	84 (24.6)	939 (25.9)	0.6004
Strong thrombophilias[b]	5 (22.7)	10 (8.9)	1 (9.1)	11 (16.4)	15 (11.6)	42 (12.3)	307 (8.5)	0.0168

Adapted from Sutkowska et al. [13], with permission

[a]Positive testing for IgG and IgM anticardiolipin antibodies does not include borderline and weakly positive titers.

[b]Strong thrombophilia was classified as the presence of: deficiency of either antithrombin, protein C, or protein S, positive testing for lupus anticoagulant, positive or highly positive testing for anticardiolipin antibodies, homozygous factor V Leiden mutation or prothrombin G20210A mutation, or compound heterozygous mutations of factor V Leiden and Prothrombin G20210A.

Management

The role of anticoagulant therapy for patients with splanchnic vein thrombosis is to inhibit thrombus propagation and promote venous recanalization and collateral formation in order to limit organ damage related to venous congestion such as acute mesenteric ischemia, portal hypertension, fulminant hepatic failure, and splenic infarction. Contrary to leg vein thrombosis, there is no direct risk of pulmonary embolism with the exception of hepatic vein thrombosis. Anticoagulation in this setting has been poorly studied with no randomized controlled trials to guide management. It is generally accepted that patients with splanchnic vein thrombosis should receive anticoagulant therapy in the absence of major contraindications [8]. Optimal duration of anticoagulation however has not been established and remains a topic of debate. This decision-making requires a balancing of the risk of recurrent venous thrombosis against the risk of major hemorrhage. Rates of major hemorrhage and recurrent venous thrombosis have been evaluated in several cohorts of patients with splanchnic vein thrombosis. In a large single-center cohort, the venous thromboembolism recurrence rate was 3.5/100 patient-years of follow-up [13]. The 10-year recurrence rate was lowest in those with splenic vein thrombosis (3 %) and highest in those with mesenteric vein thrombosis (40 %). Recurrence rates were higher in those patients with multisegment involvement (36 %) compared to those with isolated venous thrombosis (20 %). Of the recurrent events, only 34 % occurred within the splanchnic circulation. Recurrence rates were not influenced by anticoagulation strategy; however, the retrospective nature of these reports precludes inferences on anticoagulation efficacy. These recurrence rates are similar to those reported by other investigators [36]. Rates of major hemorrhage have varied from 6.9/100 patient-years to 12.5/100 patient-years [13, 36]. Gastroesophageal varices (HR 2.63, 95 % CI 1.72–4.03; $p<.001$) and warfarin therapy (HR 1.91, 95 % CI 1.25–2.92; $p=0.003$) have been identified as independent predictors of major hemorrhages [13]. In a multicenter consortium, treatment outcomes were assessed in 77 patients followed for a median of 36 months [37]. All patients received anticoagulant therapy. Recurrent venous thromboembolism occurred at a rate of 2.3/100 patient-years. Of these, five occurred after oral anticoagulants had been discontinued and two recurred despite continued warfarin. Bleeding events were uncommon occurring in only two patients.

Current anticoagulation guidelines for venous thromboembolism management define the treatment period as the initial 3 months of therapy. Thereafter, continued anticoagulation is termed “secondary prophylaxis” [23]. Expert opinion on the duration of anticoagulation varies between 3 and 6 months for reversible etiologies [7, 23, 24]. Prolonged secondary prophylaxis is generally recommended for patients with persistent “strong” prothrombotic conditions or events occurring without identifiable causes. Underlying malignancy, strong thrombophilias, and abnormal postthrombotic venous physiology augment the risk of recurrent thrombosis. Current guidelines recommend balancing the risk of recurrent thrombosis with the risk of major bleeding in this decision-making process [8]. Since gastrointestinal varices, hepatic synthetic dysfunction, and thrombocytopenia increase the potential for bleeding complications, prolonged secondary prophylaxis is generally not warranted for patients with these conditions [7, 23]. For those patients for whom prolonged anticoagulation secondary prophylaxis is contemplated, endoscopic surveillance and treatment of gastroesophageal varices may help guide anticoagulation decision-making and management [24]. In the absence of major bleeding complication, it has been our practice to provide patients with splanchnic thrombosis 6 months of anticoagulation therapy. For those patients with malignancy or a strong thrombophilia, we would provide continued secondary prophylaxis therapy as long as management has not been complicated by major bleeding.

Summary

Splanchnic vein thrombosis should be considered as a thrombotic entity unique from venous thrombosis involving the lower extremity veins or pulmonary emboli. This disease largely stems from organ pathology to injury within the splanchnic circulation. Clinical assessment should begin with a thorough evaluation to exclude such pathology. For approximately 20 % of individuals, a provoking risk factor will not be evident. For these individuals, thrombophilia testing for both inherited and acquired thrombotic variables is warranted. The timing of thrombophilia testing is also important to consider. Many clot-based thrombophilia assays will be influenced by the thrombotic process, anticoagulant therapy, or hepatic injury associated with the event. Delaying test acquisition until these variables are no longer present will maximize test performance and resource utilization. Although not specifically established by randomized controlled trials, the results of this testing can influence anticoagulant duration if a strong thrombophilia can be identified.

References

1. Singal AK, Kamath PS, Tefferi A. Mesenteric venous thrombosis. Mayo Clin Proc. 2013; 88:285–94.
2. Gilfillan RS. Anatomic study of the portal vein and its main branches. Arch Surg. 1950;61: 449–61.
3. Parks DA, Jacobson ED. Physiology of the splanchnic circulation. Arch Intern Med. 1985;145:1278–81.
4. Rothe CF. Physiology of venous return. An unappreciated boost to the heart. Arch Intern Med. 1986;146:977–82.
5. Acosta S, Alhadad A, Svensson P, Ekberg O. Epidemiology, risk and prognostic factors in mesenteric venous thrombosis. Br J Surg. 2008;95:1245–51.
6. Tafur AJ, Kalsi H, Wysokinski WE, McBane RD, Ashrani AA, Marks RS, Crusan DJ, Petterson TM, Bailey KR, Heit JA. The association of active cancer with venous thromboembolism location: a population-based study. Mayo Clin Proc. 2011;86:25–30.
7. McBane RD, Wysokinski WE. Treatment of venous thrombosis at unusual sites. Curr Treat Options Cardiovasc Med. 2008;10:136–45.

8. Kearon C, Akl EA, Comerota AJ, Prandoni P, Bounameaux H, Goldhaber SZ, Nelson ME, Wells PS, Gould MK, Dentali F, Crowther M, Kahn SR. Antithrombotic therapy for VTE disease. Antithrombotic Therapy for VTE: Antithrombotic Therapy and Prevention of Thrombosis, 9th ed: American College of Chest Physicians Evidence-Based Clinical Practice Guidelines. Chest. 2012;141(2_suppl):e419S–94.
9. Baglin T, Gray E, Greaves M, Hunt BJ, Keeling D, Machin S, Mackie I, Makris M, Nokes T, Perry D, Tait RC, Walker I, Watson H, British Committee for Standards in Haematology. Clinical guidelines for testing for heritable thrombophilia. Br J Haematol. 2010;149:209–20.
10. Janssen HL, Meinardi JR, Vleggaar FP, et al. Factor V Leiden mutation, prothrombin gene mutation, and deficiencies in coagulation inhibitors associated with Budd-Chiari syndrome and portal vein thrombosis: results of a case-control study. Blood. 2000;96:2364–8.
11. Plessier A, Darwish-Murad S, Hernandez-Guerra M, et al. Acute portal vein thrombosis unrelated to cirrhosis: a prospective multicenter follow-up study. Hepatology. 2010;51:210–8.
12. Deltenre P, Denninger MH, Hillaire S, et al. Factor V Leiden related Budd-Chiari syndrome. Gut. 2001;48:264–8.
13. Sutkowska E, McBane RD, Tafur AJ, Sutkowski K, Grill DE, Slusser JP, Wysokinski WE. Thrombophilia differences in splanchnic vein thrombosis and lower extremity deep venous thrombosis in North America. J Gastroenterol. 2013;48:1111–8.
14. Thatipelli MR, McBane RD, Hodge DO, et al. Survival and recurrence in patients with splanchnic vein thromboses. Clin Gastroenterol Hepatol. 2010;8:200–5.
15. Dentali F, Galli M, Gianni M, Ageno W. Inherited thrombophilic abnormalities and risk of portal vein thrombosis. A meta-analysis. Thromb Haemost. 2008;99:675–82.
16. De Stefano V, Teofili L, Leone G, Michiels JJ. Spontaneous erythroid colony formation as the clue to an underlying myeloproliferative disorder in patients with Budd-Chiari syndrome or portal vein thrombosis. Semin Thromb Hemost. 1997;23:411–8.
17. James C, Ugo V, Le Couedic JP, et al. A unique clonal JAK2 mutation leading to constitutive signaling causes polycythemia vera. Nature. 2005;434:1144–8.
18. Elliott MA, Tefferi A. Thrombosis and haemorrhage in polycythaemia vera and essential thrombocythaemia. Br J Haematol. 2004;128:275–90.
19. Finazzi G, Barbui T. How I, treat patients with polycythemia vera. Blood. 2007;109: 5104–11.
20. Tefferi A, Barbui T. bcr/abl negative, classic myeloproliferative disorders: diagnosis and treatment. Mayo Clin Proc. 2005;80:1220–32.
21. Chait Y, Condat B, Cazals-Hatem D, Rufat P, Atmani S, Chaoui D, Guilmin F, Kiladjian JJ, Plessier A, Denninger MH, Casadevall N, Valla D, Brière JB. Relevance of the criteria commonly used to diagnose myeloproliferative disorder in patients with splanchnic vein thrombosis. Br J Haematol. 2005;129:553–60.
22. Riva N, Donadini MP, Dentali F, Squizzato A, Ageno W. Clinical approach to splanchnic vein thrombosis: risk factors and treatment. Thromb Res. 2012;130 Suppl 1:S1–3.
23. Parker C, Omine M, Richards S, Nishimura J, Bessler M, Ware R, Hillmen P, Luzzatto L, Young N, Kinoshita T, Rosse W, Socié G, International PNH Interest Group. Diagnosis and management of paroxysmal nocturnal hemoglobinuria. Blood. 2005;106:3699–709.
24. Schulman S, Tengborn L. Treatment of venous thromboembolism in patients with congenital deficiency of antithrombin III. Thromb Haemost. 1992;68:634–6.
25. McGehee WG, Klotz TA, Epstein DJ, Rapaport SI. Coumarin necrosis associated with hereditary protein C deficiency. Ann Intern Med. 1984;101:59–60.
26. Sallah SA, Abdallah JMA, Gagnon GAB. Recurrent Warfarin-induced skin necrosis in kindreds with protein S deficiency. Pathophysiol Thromb Haemost. 1998;28:25–30.
27. Crowther MA, Ginsberg JS, Denburg J, et al. A comparison of two intensities of warfarin for the prevention of recurrent thrombosis in patients with the antiphospholipid antibody syndrome. N Engl J Med. 2003;349:1133–8.
28. Coppens M, Reijnders JH, Middeldorp S, Doggen CJ, Rosendaal FR. Testing for inherited thrombophilia does not reduce the recurrence of venous thrombosis. J Thromb Haemost. 2008;6:1474–7.

29. Baglin T, Luddington R, Brown K, Baglin C. Incidence of recurrent venous thromboembolism in relation to clinical and thrombophilic risk factors: prospective cohort study. Lancet. 2003; 362:523–6.
30. Christiansen SC, Cannegieter SC, Koster T, Vandenbroucke JP, Rosendaal FR. Thrombophilia, clinical factors, and recurrent venous thrombotic events. JAMA. 2005;293:2352–61.
31. Warkentin TE, Sheppard JI, Moore JC, Sigouin CS, Kelton JG. Quantitative interpretation of optical density measurements using PF4-dependent enzyme-immunoassays. J Thromb Haemost. 2008;6:1304–12.
32. Hall SE, Rosse WF. The use of monoclonal antibodies and flow cytometry in the diagnosis of paroxysmal nocturnal hemoglobinuria. Blood. 1996;87:5332–40.
33. Adcock DM, Gosselin R, Kitchen S, Dwyre DM. The effect of dabigatran on select specialty coagulation assays. Am J Clin Pathol. 2013;139:102–9.
34. Francart SJ, Hawes EM, Deal AM, Adcock DM, Gosselin R, Jeanneret C, Friedman KD, Moll S. Performance of coagulation tests in patients on therapeutic doses of rivaroxaban. A cross-sectional pharmacodynamic study based on peak and trough plasma levels. Thromb Haemost. 2014;111:1133–40.
35. Margaglione M, Brancaccio V, Ciampa A, Papa ML, Grandone E, Di Minno G. Inherited thrombophilic risk factors in a large cohort of individuals referred to Italian thrombophilia centers: distinct roles in different clinical settings. Haematologica. 2001;86:634–9.
36. Condat B, Pessione F, Helene Denninger M, et al. Recent portal or mesenteric venous thrombosis: increased recognition and frequent recanalization on anticoagulant therapy. Hepatology. 2000;32:466–70.
37. Dentali F, Ageno W, Witt D, Malato A, Clark N, Garcia D, McCool K, Siragusa S, Dyke S, Crowther M, WARPED consortium. Natural history of mesenteric venous thrombosis in patients treated with vitamin K antagonists: a multi-centre, retrospective cohort study. Thromb Haemost. 2009;102:501–4.

Chapter 24
Treatment of Mesenteric Venous Thrombosis

Shaun M. Gifford, Michael G. Sarr, and Patrick S. Kamath

The treatment of mesenteric vein thrombosis (MVT) is driven largely by whether the MVT is acute, subacute, or chronic, as well as the chronicity of the symptoms, the extent of confirmed venous thrombosis, and the presumed or confirmed status of the bowel involved. The prior Chap. 22 went into great detail concerning the clinical symptoms associated with MVT, as well as the diagnostic modalities available for differentiating true MVT from other etiologies of abdominal pain, the most likely presenting symptom. Once the diagnosis is presumed or confirmed, MVT has been managed in a variety of ways. For both acute and subacute MVT, anticoagulation to prevent further extension of the thrombosis is the hallmark of initial therapy with the ultimate goal directed at preventing progression of the thrombosis to avoid mesenteric ischemia. Various open surgical and endovascular options exist in lessening thrombus burden in the mesenteric venous system, but these aggressive maneuvers of thrombectomy are utilized less often in acute/subacute MVT and supported only by small case series. For chronic MVT, treatment depends on symptoms and complications of the chronic thrombosis—extrahepatic, mesenteric, splenic, and portal hypertension.

As discussed in the previous chapter and outlined in previous literature reviews, the clinical presentation of MVT is categorized into acute, subacute, or chronic, and although the presence of thrombus in the mesenteric and/or portal system is present

S.M. Gifford, MD
Division of Vascular Surgery, Department of Surgery, Mayo Clinic, Rochester, MN, USA
e-mail: Gifford.shaun@mayo.edu

M.G. Sarr, MD (✉)
Division of Subspecialty Surgery, Mayo Clinic, Rochester, MN, USA
e-mail: sarr.michael@mayo.edu

P.S. Kamath, MD
Division of Gastroenterology and Hepatology, Department of Medicine,
Mayo Clinic, Rochester, MN, USA
e-mail: kamath.patrick@mayo.edu

G.S. Oderich (ed.), *Mesenteric Vascular Disease*,
DOI 10.1007/978-1-4939-1847-8_24

in all, the clinical presentation and management varies [1]. This chapter will review treatment options for MVT, with a focus on directing therapy according to the presentation: acute, subacute, or chronic.

Acute Mesenteric Vein Thrombosis

As described in the previous chapter, clinical history determines the chronicity of the problem and categorizes the patient as having an acute event. Acute onset of severe abdominal pain is often first evaluated by the general surgeon or gastrointestinal specialist. Need for abdominal exploration based on the patient's status and physical examination is made quickly and usually by the presence of an obvious intra-abdominal catastrophe or frank peritonitis. Abdominal exploration may be undertaken in the absence of any cross-sectional imaging (computed tomography (CT), magnetic resonance imaging (MRI), even ultrasonography). In today's environment of high-speed, high-resolution CT capabilities in many emergency departments, most patients with severe enough acute abdominal pain undergo CT early in the evaluation, often prior to the patient even being seen by a surgeon (Fig. 24.1). The radiologist can evaluate bowel status and inflammatory changes, as well as the arterial and venous system. This information, in conjunction with the patient's

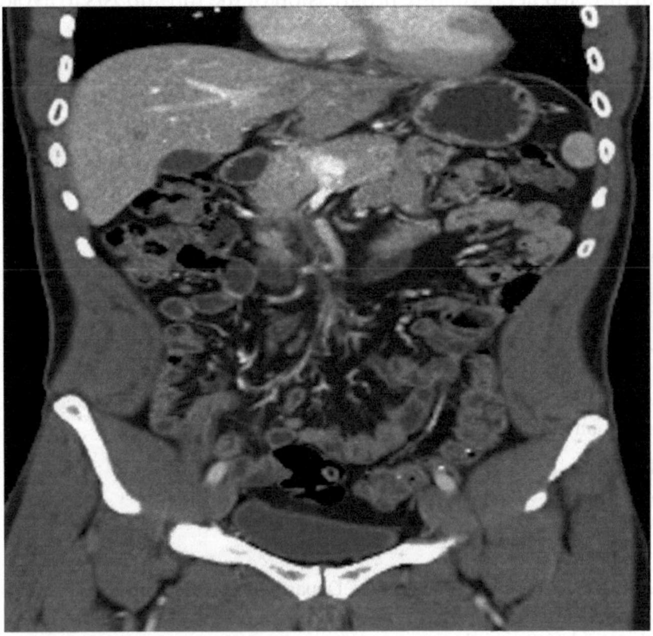

Fig. 24.1 CT showing thrombus in the superior mesenteric vein

clinical presentation and status, dictates operative intervention or conservative management in the patient with acute MVT. If the bowel is compromised and/or the patient has peritonitis, emergent exploration without further investigation is warranted and is recommended in various algorithms [2, 3]. Using the patient's clinical history, imaging, and laboratory and diagnostic studies, an etiology for the current problem should be sought actively. Several etiologies leading to secondary MVT are described in previous chapters. If these are present, the diagnosis of MVT is more likely, intervention can be individualized, and aggressive anticoagulation will be necessary.

From a strictly historic standpoint, interventions to "debulk" the thrombus, relieve the venous obstruction, and decrease venous hypertension have been described. Mergenthaler and Harris reported in 1967 a successful case of venous thrombectomy of an acutely thrombosed SMV during a planned pancreatoduodenectomy [4]. Inahara further reported on planned, open, surgical thrombectomy in 1971 and reviewed both clinical and experimental aspects of the treatment of MVT understood at the time. In his review, anticoagulation after intervention was required, and all patients with suspected diagnosis underwent an operation [5]. If bowel was compromised, the involved bowel was resected based on the clinician's judgment with the sole intent of preserving as much viable intestine as possible. Second look operations were often warranted; however, single resection procedures have been successful with comparable mortality when the demarcation of viable and nonviable bowel is obvious and when anticoagulation was timely. Prior to our better understanding of the diagnosis and treatment of acute MVT, mortality early on was exceedingly high, ranging from 40 to 70 % in some reports.

As our knowledge of the etiopathogenesis of MVT has matured, further evidence supported the use of immediate anticoagulation in the pre- and perioperative period to improve bowel salvage and decrease mortality. If the diagnosis of MVT has been made in a patient with acute onset abdominal pain, full anticoagulation should be started immediately (preferably preoperatively but if not, intraoperatively) to prevent further extension of thrombosis; no attempt should be made to delay full anticoagulation until after the abdomen is closed because further extension of the thrombosis can occur during the perioperative period of relative hypercoagulability (Fig. 24.2). This aggressive anticoagulation has been shown in several studies both to prevent progression and to improve survival [2, 6, 7]. Many of these reports utilize and recommend surgical exploration and resection of compromised bowel with or without a second-look operation. Mortality remained high (10–40 %) but has improved with this aggressive strategy of immediate anticoagulation.

Clinical experience of attempts at nonoperative management led to a retrospective assessment of clinical outcomes in two published series. These reports challenged the use of routine operative intervention in conjunction with anticoagulation. In the first study, Brunaud and colleagues evaluated their 12-year single-center experience [8]. They found that of the 26 patients treated, the overall morbidity was 35 % and mortality was 19 %. With further comparative analysis, the early group with treatment based on operative intervention ($n = 14$) and late treatment group of anticoagulation ($n = 12$) showed no difference in mortality between groups; indeed,

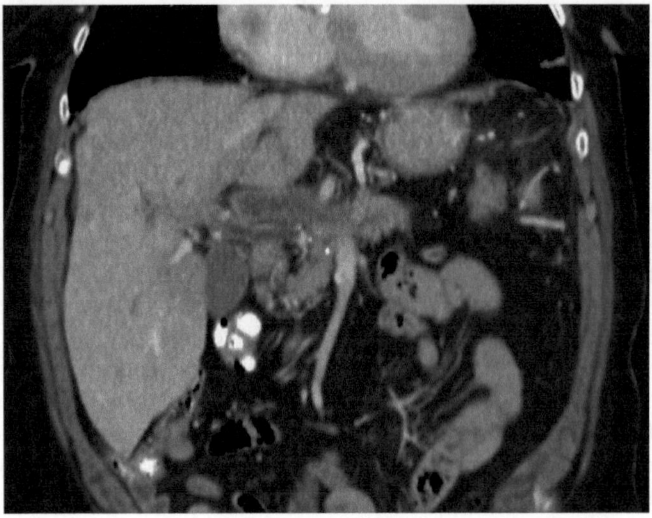

Fig. 24.2 CT showing thrombus extending up into the portal vein

nonoperative management was at least as good as open intervention. In review of the pathology reports of bowel resected in the operative group, these investigators found that 10 of 12 patients had only mucosal necrosis, begging the question of whether operative intervention and intestinal resection could have been avoided [8].

In a similar study, Zhang and colleagues were able to show a benefit of nonoperative management in many patients with acute MVT [9]. In their report, 41 patients were treated for acute MVT over a 25-year period. Again, a change in management occurred based on the observation that a nonoperative approach of anticoagulation and close observation could be successful. They found a 39 % mortality in the group undergoing early operation (13 patients) versus the results in the 28 patients treated initially by a nonoperative approach with anticoagulation first; 32 % of these patients treated with close observation eventually underwent operation because of progression of symptoms [9]. Clearly, in the absence of peritonitis or clinical instability, a trial of nonoperative management with anticoagulation is warranted in most patients without peritonitis.

Systemic anticoagulation with the addition of targeted thrombolytic strategies has also been tried, albeit with various success and complications. Systemic thrombolytic therapy has been shown to be of little benefit and is accompanied by an extensive list of contraindications, making its usefulness prohibitive. In contrast, local directed delivery of thrombolytics into the superior mesenteric artery or into the venous segment directly or from a transjugular approach has been shown to improve venous flow in selected cases [10]. Although several case reports suggest some success, concern remains about the overall usefulness and practicality of these interventional approaches in the setting of a condition often difficult to diagnose that is often delayed several days and can progress to the need for operative intervention because of compromised bowel. Opponents of thrombolytic therapy suggest that when providing lytic therapy directly into the superior mesenteric artery, there is no way to guarantee delivery to the segment of venous thrombosis, because the lytic agents may just sidestep through collaterals. In this setting, there is no benefit and only increased risk of bleeding. Contrary to the indirect route of lytic infusion, percutaneous access to the extrahepatic portal and mesenteric venous system is possible and may offer a more beneficial approach to the retrograde delivery of the lytic agents directly at the site of thrombus.

With advances in endovascular techniques, minimally invasive efforts to debulk venous thrombus or perform thrombectomy have been attempted in several reports [11–13]. Unlike peripheral venous thrombosis, percutaneous access to the superior mesenteric and portal venous system can be problematic but can usually be obtained through the liver (transhepatically or via a transjugular approach) in a fashion similar to that for transjugular intrahepatic portosystemic shunt (TIPS) procedures. Once access is established, directed lytic therapy or mechanical thrombectomy can be attempted. Wasselius et al. expanded this concept with an aggressive combined approach via the superior mesenteric artery, portal vein (partial), and proximal intrahepatic branches [13]. Simultaneous access of the common femoral artery and transjugular intrahepatic access to the portal venous system allowed a mechanical venous thrombectomy combined with intra-arterial and intravenous delivery of tissue plasminogen activator (TPA) at a dose of 1 mg/h. This aggressive approach led to thrombolysis of a main branch of the superior mesenteric vein with venous decompression of the bowel. Their patient avoided operation, resumed eating in 3 days, and was kept on low-molecular-weight heparin with no bleeding events or other complications [13].

Obviously, with these more aggressive scenarios, the patient must be assessed repeatedly for worsening of their clinical condition or development of peritonitis. Such deterioration demands immediate exploration and resection of compromised, irreversibly ischemic bowel. In the setting of partial systemic thrombolytic treatment, an increased risk of bleeding is present. In a report from Hollingshead and colleagues of transcatheter thrombolytic therapy of acute MVT, although 75 % of patients had improvement in their clot burden and 85 % had resolution of their MVT, 60 % experienced a major complication of which bleeding was the most common [14].

The proposed duration of anticoagulation is variable across reports and depends heavily on the underlying etiology, resolution of symptoms, and the risk of continued anticoagulation. In the absence of a hereditary or acquired thrombotic disorder, anticoagulation is recommended for 6–12 months. During systemic anticoagulation, the risk of bleeding is low, but recurrence is quite high and occurs most frequently in the first 30 days after operation and in the area of bowel resection or thrombosis [15, 16]. A large, single-series report from Rhee et al. demonstrated recurrence in 36 % of patients despite aggressive anticoagulation; three-quarters of the recurrences developed during the same hospitalization or within 30 days, highlighting the need for close postoperative follow-up, even after discharge, at least for the first month or two [2]. Residual thrombus in the mesenteric venous system acts as a nidus and may propagate into larger veins. Complete resection of involved bowel and prevention of

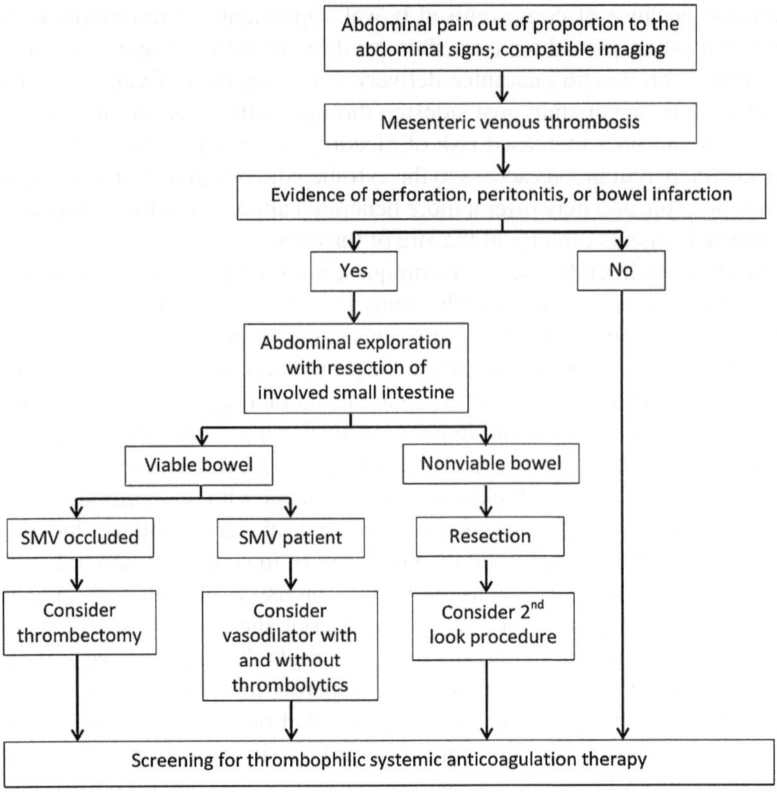

Fig. 24.3 Algorithm for the management of chronic mesenteric venous thrombosis. *TIPS* transjugular intrahepatic portosystemic shunt

propagation by maintaining the international ratio (INR) on warfarin therapy in the range of 2.0–3.0 appears to be the best course to limit recurrence. Both unfractionated and low-molecular-weight heparin have been used successfully to bridge to warfarin. The newer direct thrombin inhibitors, like Pradaxa and Xarelto, have not been evaluated in the setting of MVT and, therefore, cannot be recommended at this time until studied formally for this type of thrombosis. With all of these approaches to prevent propagation of thrombus and limit thrombus burden in the mesenteric venous system, currently mortality rates have decreased to 0–23 % [3]. An algorithm for management of acute MVT is proposed in Fig. 24.3.

Subacute Mesenteric Vein Thrombosis

Patients who have had symptoms present for days to weeks and thrombus in the mesenteric venous system are categorized as having subacute MVT. Some reports have combined the patients meeting these criteria with those patients with chronic

MVT [2]. Mostly likely, these patients had a mild, less acutely symptomatic MVT that extended to involve more venous drainage beds leading to exacerbation of pain and other symptoms. Because of the difficulty in diagnosis of subacute MVT, a strong history of clotting disorders both personal or within close family members should raise suspicion. Patients with subacute MVT often have had an extensive work-up with multiple studies and subspecialists involved. Ideally, once the diagnosis is made, anticoagulation should be initiated immediately to limit further extension of the thrombus.

As with acute MVT, the goal in treating subacute MVT is also to prevent extension of the thrombosis with systemic anticoagulation. Due to the nagging nature and progression of symptoms, it is unlikely that bowel is irreversibly ischemic, thus requiring resection. Often, these patients have not developed extensive collateral drainage or development of varices. This lack of effective collateral venous drainage is both good and bad—good in the sense that the sequelae of variceal bleeding are unlikely but bad in the sense that propagation of thrombus can lead to an acute change in status such that the bowel becomes ischemic due to lack of collateral flow. Once the presence of MVT is identified, these patients should be anticoagulated immediately. Hopefully, early recognition and initiation of systemic anticoagulation will prevent progression of the thrombosis and eventual innate thrombolysis. Although one might consider more aggressive endovascular interventions in this setting to prevent venous progression, such an aggressive approach is usually not necessary, and the most appropriate treatment consists primarily of anticoagulation.

Chronic Mesenteric Vein Thrombosis

Chronic MVT is usually recognized incidentally on imaging for another indication or secondary to the sequelae of chronically occluded veins (i.e., esophageal or gastric variceal hemorrhage, splenomegaly, or rarely ascites). Imaging may demonstrate various degrees of vein thrombosis, ranging from segmental branches to more commonly the larger veins. Collateral veins are present usually and are the reason for the lack of symptomatology (Fig. 24.4). The lack of abdominal pain suggests the occlusion occurred gradually over several months, with slow enlargement of collateral beds compensating for the venous hypertension resulting from the venous occlusion.

Management of chronic MVT is different and requires an in-depth discussion with the patient concerning any abdominal symptoms, predisposition for thrombosis in their personal or family history, and possible determination of when the thrombosis occurred. In the absence of any symptoms or underlying hypercoagulable state, it appears to be unnecessary to institute anticoagulation; indeed, anticoagulation would increase complication rates in the setting of variceal bleeding. The literature suggests that recanalization of the larger veins can occur in 50–80 % but is often of little importance because of the development of collateral drainage [17, 18]. Thrombectomy or venous bypass is usually futile, because these vessels are often scarred, the thrombus is well organized, and access through the engorged, thin-walled collateral beds

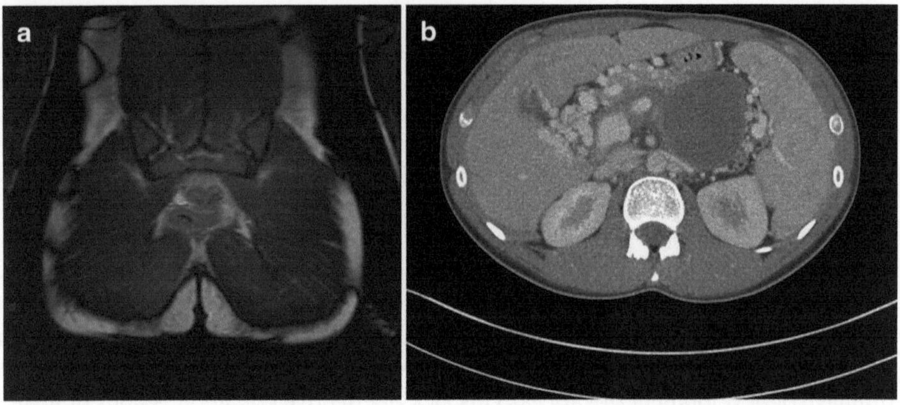

Fig. 24.4 CT of the progression of splenic vein thrombosis. (**a**) Thrombosis/obstruction of the mid-aspect of splenic vein. Note splenomegaly. (**b**) Extensive venous collaterals 18 months later

Fig. 24.5 Algorithm for the management of acute mesenteric venous thrombosis. *SMV* superior mesenteric vein

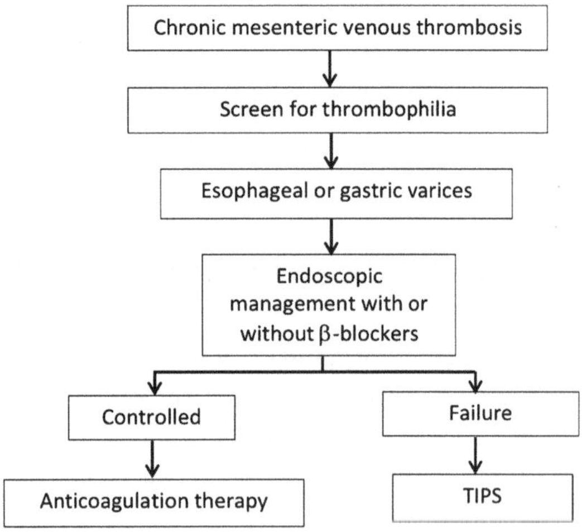

is prohibitive. The potential bleeding from gastroesophageal varices is usually the focus of treatment and prevention of further hemorrhage in this group of patients. Prophylaxis with propranolol, endoscopic therapeutic interventions, and portosystemic shunts are all possibilities for managing variceal bleeding [1], but conservative noninterventional measures are utilized first. Consideration for a portacaval shunt can be entertained, but only after in-depth discussion with patient about risks and adverse events associated with this procedure. If bleeding occurs, the treatment approach is that for the management of portal hypertension and is governed by patency of the extrahepatic venous anatomy. An algorithm for management of chronic MVT is shown in Fig. 24.5.

Special Situations

Thrombosis of the larger veins of the extrahepatic venous system can occur from other secondary causes that have a definite etiology. Thrombosis of the portal venous anastomosis after an orthotopic liver transplantation can occur rarely (<2 %), and if the liver graft is threatened, emergency operative thrombectomy either by operative approaches or by transhepatic endovascular techniques may be indicated [19–21]. Superior mesenteric venous/portal venous anastomosis or a bridging conduit from superior mesenteric vein to portal vein can also thrombose after a pancreatoduodenectomy with resection of the retropancreatic portal/superior mesenteric venous junction; should hepatic viability be jeopardized, operative thrombectomy can be performed [22–25], but this is a very uncommon situation. Similarly, extension of thrombus from the remnant splenic vein near the superior mesenteric venous/portal venous confluence can occur, but usually serious complete portal venous thrombosis is rare; management is usually anticoagulation. Rare cases of interventional approaches to portal vein thrombosis have been described as well [26].

Conclusion

Treatment for MVT depends on the clinical presentation of the patient. A high index of suspicion is needed to prevent delay in diagnosis in the acute or subacute setting; once the diagnosis of acute or subacute MVT is confirmed, all patients should be started immediately on full, systemic anticoagulation to prevent propagation of the thrombus. Operative intervention is reserved for those patients who present with signs, symptoms, or radiologic evidence of irreversible ischemia or in whom irreversible ischemia is highly suspect. Once resolution of the acute episode occurs, anticoagulation should be continued for at least 6 months. If an underlying hypercoagulable state is identified, anticoagulation should be continued indefinitely. In chronic MVT, therapy should be focused on preventing complications of the mesenteric venous hypertension. Long-term anticoagulation should be considered in select individuals.

References

1. Kumar S, Sarr MG, Kamath PS. Mesenteric venous thrombosis. N Engl J Med. 2001; 345:1683–8.
2. Rhee RY, Gloviczki P, Mendonca CT, et al. Mesenteric venous thrombosis: still a lethal disease in the 1990s. J Vasc Surg. 1994;20:688–97.
3. Singal AK, Kamath PS, Tefferi A. Mesenteric venous thrombosis. Mayo Clin Proc. 2013; 88:285–94.
4. Mergenthaler FW, Harris MN. Superior mesenteric vein thrombosis complicating pancreatoduodenectomy: successful treatment by thrombectomy. Ann Surg. 1968;167:106–11.

5. Inahara T. Acute superior mesenteric venous thrombosis: treatment by thrombectomy. Ann Surg. 1971;174:956–61.
6. Abdu RA, Zakhour BJ, Dallis DJ. Mesenteric venous thrombosis – 1911 to 1984. Surgery. 1987;101:383–8.
7. Mathews JE, White RR. Primary mesenteric venous occlusive disease. Am J Surg. 1971; 122:579–83.
8. Brunaud L, Antunes L, Collinet-Adler S, et al. Acute mesenteric venous thrombosis: case for nonoperative management. J Vasc Surg. 2001;34:673–9.
9. Zhang J, Duan ZQ, Song QB, et al. Acute mesenteric venous thrombosis: a better outcome achieved through improved imaging techniques and a changed policy of clinical management. Eur J Vasc Endovasc Surg. 2004;28:329–34.
10. Poplausky MR, Kaufman JA, Geller SC, et al. Mesenteric venous thrombosis treated with urokinase via the superior mesenteric artery. Gastroenterology. 1996;110:1633–5.
11. Rivitz SM, Geller SC, Hahn C, et al. Treatment of acute mesenteric venous thrombosis with transjugular intramesenteric urokinase infusion. J Vasc Interv Radiol. 1995;6:219–23; discussion 224–8.
12. Kim HS, Patra A, Khan J, et al. Transhepatic catheter-directed thrombectomy and thrombolysis of acute superior mesenteric venous thrombosis. J Vasc Interv Radiol. 2005;16:1685–91.
13. Wassélius J, Sonesson B, Elf J, et al. Treatment of mesenteric vein thrombosis with transjugular mechanical thrombectomy and subsequent simultaneous arterial and venous thrombolysis. J Vasc Surg Venous Lymphatic Dis. 2013;2(3):320–3.
14. Hollingshead M, Burke CT, Mauro MA, et al. Transcatheter thrombolytic therapy for acute mesenteric and portal vein thrombosis. J Vasc Interv Radiol. 2005;16:651–61.
15. Jona J, Cummins Jr GM, Head HB, et al. Recurrent primary mesenteric venous thrombosis. JAMA. 1974;227:1033–5.
16. Naitove A, Weismann RE. Primary mesenteric venous thrombosis. Ann Surg. 1965;161: 516–23.
17. Amitrano L, Guardascione MA, Scaglione M, et al. Prognostic factors in noncirrhotic patients with splanchnic vein thromboses. Am J Gastroenterol. 2007;102:2464–70.
18. Condat B, Pessione F, Helene Denninger M, et al. Recent portal or mesenteric venous thrombosis: increased recognition and frequent recanalization on anticoagulant therapy. Hepatology. 2000;32:466–70.
19. Duffy JP, Hong JC, Farmer DG, et al. Vascular complications of orthotopic liver transplantation: experience in more than 4,200 patients. J Am Coll Surg. 2009;208:896–903; discussion 903–5.
20. Itri JN, Heller MT, Tublin ME. Hepatic transplantation: postoperative complications. Abdom Imaging. 2013;38:1300–33.
21. Shi Z, Yan L, Zhao J, et al. Prevention and treatment of rethrombosis after liver transplantation with an implantable pump of the portal vein. Liver Transpl. 2010;16:324–31.
22. Zyromski NJ, Howard TJ. Acute superior mesenteric-portal vein thrombosis after pancreaticoduodenectomy: treatment by operative thrombectomy. Surgery. 2008;143:566–7.
23. Kanda M, Takeda S, Yamada S, et al. Operative treatment of thrombotic occlusion of the portal vein immediately after pancreatectomy with portal vein resection. Pancreas. 2010;39:265–6.
24. Ausania F, Jackson R, Tsirlis T, et al. Portal vein occlusion following pancreaticoduodenectomy and portal vein resection: treatment by percutaneous portal vein stent. Ann R Coll Surg Engl. 2013;95:299.
25. Sanabria JR, Hiruki T, Szalay DA, et al. Superior mesenteric vein thrombosis after the Whipple procedure: an aggressive, combined treatment approach. Can J Surg. 1997;40:467–70.
26. Liu FY, Wang MQ, Duan F, et al. Interventional therapy for symptomatic-benign portal vein occlusion. Hepatogastroenterology. 2010;57:1367–74.

Part V
Non-Occlusive Mesenteric Ischemia

Chapter 25
Clinical Presentation and Diagnosis

A.S. Bode, M. Dekkers, T.R. van Oudheusden, J.A. Teijink, and M.D. Luyer

Nonocclusive mesenteric ischemia (NOMI), a condition in which blood supply to the splanchnic circulation is hampered by a non-obstructive cause, accounts for approximately 20 % of all causes of acute mesenteric ischemia [1, 2]. Prevalence is highest in the intensive care setting in patients suffering from either cardiogenic or septic shock in which mesenteric circulation is compromised by hypotension and decreased cardiac output and with the subsequent use of vasopressors [1]. As a result, a lowered mesenteric flow causes intestinal hypoxia with watershed areas of critical mesenteric circulation. Early and adequate diagnosis is essential to prevent intestinal ischemia, necrosis, sepsis, and death. Although the widespread use of invasive hemodynamic monitoring has reduced the mortality of NOMI from almost 100 to 70 % [3–5], increased awareness of clinical symptoms in combination with novel diagnostic modalities may help us further reduce these dramatic mortality rates.

In this chapter an overview of etiology, clinical presentation, and diagnostic considerations of NOMI will be presented, after which treatment will be discussed in Chap. 26.

Etiology

Splanchnic hypoperfusion can be caused by different mechanisms but is primarily the result of a homeostatic mechanism to preserve cardiac and cerebral blood flow at the cost of mesenteric and peripheral circulation via disproportionate vasoconstriction. Intestinal mucosal damage is initiated at the villous tips because of their

A.S. Bode, MD, PhD • M. Dekkers, MSc • T.R. van Oudheusden, MD
J.A. Teijink, MD, PhD • M.D. Luyer, MD, PhD (✉)
Department of Surgery, Catharina Hospital Eindhoven, Eindhoven, The Netherlands
e-mail: misha.luyer@catharinaziekenhuis.nl

G.S. Oderich (ed.), *Mesenteric Vascular Disease*,
DOI 10.1007/978-1-4939-1847-8_25

relatively high oxygen requirement and results in irreversible necrosis after 2–3 h of hypoperfusion. Particularly elderly people are at risk because of limited compensatory hemodynamic strategies. Besides age, also pre-existing myocardial infarction, congestive heart failure, hypotension following dialysis, and recent major cardiovascular or abdominal surgery in combination with extensive enteric feeding have been described as risk factors for the development of NOMI [3, 6–8]. Furthermore, administration of pharmacological agents such as alpha-adrenergic agonists is responsible for an increased vasoconstriction and thus an increased resistance in peripheral splanchnic vessels.

Clinical Manifestation

Compared to the acute and severe abdominal pain in occlusive mesenteric ischemia, severity and location of abdominal pain in NOMI is more variable. Peritoneal signs of inflammation are often absent in the early phase; however, when ischemia progresses, bowel distension, rebound tenderness and guarding of abdominal musculature, hypotension, fever, decreased bowel sounds, nausea, vomiting, diarrhea, and anorexia are likely to be observed [9]. However, these symptoms may take days to develop and are not seldom precluded by intestinal perforation [10]. Conversely, 20–30 % of patients with NOMI do not report any abdominal pain at all. The clinical condition of these patients is often dominated by extensive comorbidities. Under these circumstances, intestinal ischemia may not be clinically evident until hours or days after the initial hemodynamic insult [8].

Diagnostic Considerations

According to the ACC/AHA Guideline for the management of patients with peripheral artery disease, NOMI should be suspected in (1) patients with low flow states or shock of any origin who develop abdominal pain, (2) patients receiving vasoconstrictor substances and medications (e.g., cocaine, vasopressin, norepinephrine) who develop abdominal pain, or (3) patients who develop abdominal pain after coarctation repair or after surgical revascularization for intestinal ischemia caused by arterial obstruction [10].

Rapid diagnosis of mesenteric ischemia is crucial in order to avoid intestinal necrosis and its sequela. Therefore, priority should be given to resuscitation when suspecting NOMI by improving cardiac output and correcting hypotension, hypovolemia, and cardiac arrhythmias. Subsequently, diagnostic procedures need to be performed as soon as possible to confirm or reject clinical suspicion. Nonetheless, early symptoms of NOMI are nonspecific and often result in delayed diagnosis. Several diagnostic tools are available in the workup of mesenteric ischemia, and in many cases a combination of the outcome of several diagnostic modalities confirms the diagnosis.

Laboratory Assays

Although laboratory findings are nonspecific for the detection of mesenteric ischemia, several tests have been investigated in the context of NOMI. Firstly, following intestinal dehydration, hematocrit increases. Secondly, the anaerobic glycolysis during hypoxia leads to lactate acidosis. Thirdly, due to intestinal cell death, lactate dehydrogenase (LDH) and creatine kinase will be released into the circulation. Moreover, leukocytosis can be considered another nonspecific associated reaction [11].

Given that mesenteric ischemia starts from the intestinal mucosa, two promising mucosal biomarkers have been identified: intestinal fatty-acid binding protein (I-FABP) and alpha-glutathione S-transferase (alpha-GST) [12]. I-FABP comprises a class of low molecular weight cytosolic proteins and can be found in tissues involved in uptake and consumption of fatty acids. It is highly expressed in cells on the luminal side of small intestinal villi and released into the circulation upon enterocyte membrane integrity loss. Urinary and plasma I-FABP levels are significantly elevated in patients with intestinal ischemia compared to healthy controls [13]. I-FABP has been reported as a specific and sensitive marker for postoperative intestinal necrosis [14]. A clinical trial demonstrated a high sensitivity (0.90) and specificity (0.89) for urinary I-FABP [15]. Alpha-GST is released by a variety of cells following cell membrane damage [16] and is known to be highly active both in the liver and the small intestine mucosa [17]. Alpha-GST has pooled sensitivity and specificity for diagnosing mesenteric ischemia of 0.68 and 0.85, respectively.

Angiography

The American Gastroenterological Association guideline of 2000 states that mesenteric angiography is the standard of reference for diagnosing mesenteric ischemia [18]. When a clinician is aware of possible mesenteric ischemia, angiography is accurate and increases survival [19]. In patients with NOMI, selective angiography can exclude a significant arterial lesion while demonstrating areas of narrowing and irregularity in major branches, decreased or absent flow in the smaller vessels, and an absent submucosal blush [1].

Moreover, the major benefit of performing a digital subtraction angiography (DSA) in patients suspected of NOMI is that immediate treatment by infusion of vasodilators through the angiographic catheter can be initiated to reverse the underlying condition causing the mesenteric vasoconstriction. Nevertheless, intra-arterial angiography is invasive and time consuming, and the unavailability of this diagnostic modality in some hospitals may lead to a critical delay in diagnosis. Therefore, over the last decade there has been a major shift toward computed tomography angiography (CTA) because it is less invasive, less time- and resource consuming, and more readily available.

Computed Tomography

CTA has replaced angiography as the standard of reference in diagnosing mesenteric ischemia with a sensitivity and specificity of 0.96 and 0.94, respectively [20, 21]. With a short examination time and the ability to rule out several other causes of acute abdominal pain, CTA provides a noninvasive method to adequately depict the abdominal aorta, the origin of the splanchnic arteries, their central parts, and its branches in diagnostic quality. During the examination vascular enhancement is achieved by administration of iodinated contrast agents in bolus techniques after which luminal narrowing of the splanchnic vasculature can be assessed and graded. Besides evaluation of contrast distribution during bolus injection, thickening of the bowel wall, absence of bowel wall enhancement, intramural hemorrhage, focal or diffuse intraperitoneal fluid collections, intestinal pneumatosis, portal venous gas collections, edematous wall thickening, or inhomogeneous contrast enhancement of the mucosa may be observed and have been associated with mesenteric ischemia. Unfortunately, all of the above have been considered nonspecific and are present in only 20–60 % of patients with mesenteric ischemia [22, 23].

Magnetic Resonance Imaging

Contrast-enhanced magnetic resonance angiography (CE-MRA) is considered a novel approach in the identification of mesenteric ischemia. CE-MRA of the splanchnic vessels is appealing because of its noninvasive character, and moreover it avoids the nephrotoxicity and allergic risks associated with iodinated contrast agents [21]. Although, to our knowledge, CE-MRA has not been used to evaluate NOMI in humans, non-occlusive emboli have been adequately visualized as filling defects, and it yielded a sensitivity and specificity of 0.95 and 1.00, respectively, in a clinical trial designed to diagnose severe stenosis or occlusion of the origins of the celiac axes and superior mesenteric artery [24]. Unfortunately, the use of CE-MRA is limited to identification of more proximal located occlusions and does not have the same spatial resolution and acquisition time as CTA [25]. If better spatial resolution becomes available in the future, CE-MRA has the potential to become the diagnostic modality of choice.

Summary

Considering the potential lethal consequences of non-occlusive mesenteric ischemia, timely and adequate diagnosis is of the utmost importance. Although elevated levels of hematocrit, LDH, lactate, and creatine kinase have been associated with the presence of NOMI, lack of specificity hampers routine clinical implementation.

Novel markers (I-FABP and alpha-GST) are currently investigated for their early diagnostic power and their feasibility for diagnosing mesenteric ischemia in an early stage. Angiography by means of either CTA or DSA for detection of arterial vasoconstriction is still considered the standard of reference for evaluation of NOMI. Future improvements in spatial resolution and acquisition time may result in MRA being the superior, noninvasive modality.

References

1. Menon NJ, Amin AM, Mohammed A, Hamilton G. Acute mesenteric ischaemia. Acta Chir Belg. 2005;105(4):344–54. PubMed PMID: 16184714.
2. Trompeter M, Brazda T, Remy CT, Vestring T, Reimer P. Non-occlusive mesenteric ischemia: etiology, diagnosis, and interventional therapy. Eur Radiol. 2002;12(5):1179–87. PubMed PMID: 11976865.
3. Acosta S, Ogren M, Sternby NH, Bergqvist D, Bjorck M. Fatal nonocclusive mesenteric ischaemia: population-based incidence and risk factors. J Intern Med. 2006;259(3):305–13. PubMed PMID: 16476108.
4. Minko P, Groesdonk H, Stroeder J, Miodek J, Graeber S, Bucker A, et al. A scoring system for the assessment of angiographic findings in non-occlusive mesenteric ischemia (NOMI). RoFo. 2012;184(9):805–9. PubMed PMID: 22618477.
5. Tendler DA. Acute intestinal ischemia and infarction. Semin Gastrointest Dis. 2003;14(2): 66–76. PubMed PMID: 12889581.
6. Vicente DC, Kazmers A. Acute mesenteric ischemia. Curr Opin Cardiol. 1999;14(5):453–8. PubMed PMID: 10500910.
7. Howard TJ, Plaskon LA, Wiebke EA, Wilcox MG, Madura JA. Nonocclusive mesenteric ischemia remains a diagnostic dilemma. Am J Surg. 1996;171(4):405–8. PubMed PMID: 8604831.
8. Oldenburg WA, Lau LL, Rodenberg TJ, Edmonds HJ, Burger CD. Acute mesenteric ischemia: a clinical review. Arch Intern Med. 2004;164(10):1054–62. PubMed PMID: 15159262.
9. Bassiouny HS. Nonocclusive mesenteric ischemia. Surg Clin North Am. 1997;77(2):319–26. PubMed PMID: 9146715.
10. Hirsch AT, Haskal ZJ, Hertzer NR, Bakal CW, Creager MA, Halperin JL, et al. ACC/AHA guidelines for the ,management of patients with peripheral arterial disease (lower extremity, renal, mesenteric, and abdominal aortic): a collaborative report from the American Associations for Vascular Surgery/Society for Vascular Surgery, Society for Cardiovascular Angiography and Interventions, Society for Vascular Medicine and Biology, Society of Interventional Radiology, and the ACC/AHA Task Force on Practice Guidelines (writing committee to develop guidelines for the management of patients with peripheral arterial disease) – summary of recommendation. J Vasc Intervent Radiol. 2006;17(9):1383–97; quiz 98. PubMed PMID: 16990459.
11. Kolkman JJ, Groeneveld AB. Occlusive and non-occlusive gastrointestinal ischaemia: a clinical review with special emphasis on the diagnostic value of tonometry. Scand J Gastroenterol Suppl. 1998;225:3–12. PubMed PMID: 9515745.
12. Evennett NJ, Petrov MS, Mittal A, Windsor JA. Systematic review and pooled estimates for the diagnostic accuracy of serological markers for intestinal ischemia. World J Surg. 2009;33(7):1374–83. PubMed PMID: 19424744.
13. Lieberman JM, Sacchettini J, Marks C, Marks WH. Human intestinal fatty acid binding protein: report of an assay with studies in normal volunteers and intestinal ischemia. Surgery. 1997;121(3):335–42. PubMed PMID: 9068676.

14. Iacobellis F, Berritto D, Somma F, Cavaliere C, Corona M, Cozzolino S, et al. Magnetic resonance imaging: a new tool for diagnosis of acute ischemic colitis? World J Gastroenterol. 2012;18(13):1496–501. PubMed PMID: 22509081. Pubmed Central PMCID: 3319945.
15. Thuijls G, van Wijck K, Grootjans J, Derikx JP, van Bijnen AA, Heineman E, et al. Early diagnosis of intestinal ischemia using urinary and plasma fatty acid binding proteins. Ann Surg. 2011;253(2):303–8. PubMed PMID: 21245670.
16. Khurana S, Corbally MT, Manning F, Armenise T, Kierce B, Kilty C. Glutathione S-transferase: a potential new marker of intestinal ischemia. J Pediatr Surg. 2002;37(11):1543–8. PubMed PMID: 12407536.
17. Acosta S, Nilsson T. Current status on plasma biomarkers for acute mesenteric ischemia. J Thromb Thrombolysis. 2012;33(4):355–61. PubMed PMID: 22081293.
18. Brandt LJ, Boley SJ. AGA technical review on intestinal ischemia. Am Gastrointestin Assoc Gastroenterol. 2000;118(5):954–68. PubMed PMID: 10784596.
19. Clark RA, Gallant TE. Acute mesenteric ischemia: angiographic spectrum. AJR Am J Roentgenol. 1984;142(3):555–62. PubMed PMID: 6141717.
20. Kirkpatrick ID, Kroeker MA, Greenberg HM. Biphasic CT with mesenteric CT angiography in the evaluation of acute mesenteric ischemia: initial experience. Radiology. 2003;229(1): 91–8. PubMed PMID: 12944600.
21. Wyers MC. Acute mesenteric ischemia: diagnostic approach and surgical treatment. Semin Vasc Surg. 2010;23(1):9–20. PubMed PMID: 20298945.
22. Franquet T, Bescos JM, Reparaz B. Noninvasive methods in the diagnosis of isolated superior mesenteric vein thrombosis: US and CT. Gastrointest Radiol. 1989;14(4):321–5. PubMed PMID: 2680738.
23. Perez C, Llauger J, Puig J, Palmer J. Computed tomographic findings in bowel ischemia. Gastrointest Radiol. 1989;14(3):241–5. PubMed PMID: 2731697.
24. Meaney JF, Prince MR, Nostrant TT, Stanley JC. Gadolinium-enhanced MR angiography of visceral arteries in patients with suspected chronic mesenteric ischemia. J Magn Reson Imaging. 1997;7(1):171–6. PubMed PMID: 9039611.
25. Schoots IG, Koffeman GI, Legemate DA, Levi M, van Gulik TM. Systematic review of survival after acute mesenteric ischaemia according to disease aetiology. Br J Surg. 2004;91(1): 17–27. PubMed PMID: 14716789.

Chapter 26
Management and Results

T.R. van Oudheusden, M. Dekkers, A.S. Bode, J.A. Teijink, and M.D. Luyer

Mesenteric ischemia is a severe disease that was associated with a 100 % mortality level up until the 1980s due to the frequent use of vasopressors in cardiac patients. Although the knowledge about this entity increased and improvements were made in diagnostic modalities, the mortality rate nowadays still remains above 40 % due to the unfavorable setting in which patients present themselves [1]. The subgroup of non-occlusive mesenteric ischemia (NOMI) accounts for approximately 20 % [2] of all mesenteric ischemia syndromes and is associated with a mortality rate of 70 % [3]. The increased mortality in NOMI is mainly caused by the critical state of patients preceding the NOMI event. Many patients developing NOMI often have a lot of comorbidities, are intubated and sedated and receive medication. These circumstances can result in a different clinical presentation and often lead to a delay in diagnosis and treatment. As in other types of mesenteric ischemia, a timely diagnosis of the disease is of the utmost importance. A delay of 24 h increases mortality by 20 % due to progression of the disease to an irreversible state to extensive transmural bowel infarction with peritonitis and severe sepsis [2, 4]. In this chapter an overview of the treatment goals for NOMI and possible treatment modalities will be presented.

T.R. van Oudheusden, MD • M. Dekkers, MSc • A.S. Bode, MD, PhD
J.A. Teijink, MD, PhD • M.D. Luyer, MD, PhD (✉)
Department of Surgery, Catharina Hospital Eindhoven, Eindhoven, The Netherlands
e-mail: misha.luyer@catharinaziekenhuis.nl

G.S. Oderich (ed.), *Mesenteric Vascular Disease*,
DOI 10.1007/978-1-4939-1847-8_26

Table 26.1 Key steps in treatment of possible acute mesenteric ischemia

1.	Aggressive resuscitation
2.	Electrolyte imbalance correction
3.	Invasive monitoring
4.	Broad spectrum antibiotics
5.	IV heparin (at least until diagnosis is confirmed)
6.	Surgical (in case of high suspicion of threatened bowel)

Treatment Goal

In NOMI patients, ischemia is caused by splanchnic hypoperfusion as a result of severe vasoconstriction, initiated to preserve cardiac and cerebral blood flow. Therefore, the primary goal in the treatment of NOMI should be the return of adequate blood flow to the splanchnic circulation. Furthermore, treatment of the underlying cause of the mesenteric vasospasm should be started as soon as possible. All patients under suspicion of acute mesenteric ischemia (AMI) should undergo general treatment steps while diagnosis has yet to be confirmed (Table 26.1). Treatment for NOMI however differs from the mesenteric ischemia cases caused by an arterial or venous occlusive event (OMI). In NOMI, gut serosa can still be viable despite the presence of infarcted mucosa, making it impossible to determine which bowel segments are affected and establish a diagnosis. Therefore, surgical intervention has no role in the initial phase, and a laparotomy should only be applied when high suspicion of threatened bowel is present.

Pharmacological Treatment

While the first part of the treatment focuses on the underlying cause to relieve the low-flow state, a more direct treatment can be initiated to return blood flow to the splanchnic circulation. It is important to mention that the low-flow state, which usually precedes NOMI, cannot be treated with vasoconstrictors, since they would only worsen the condition by increasing resistance in peripheral splanchnic vessels. Furthermore, even when the precipitating event is corrected, the mesenteric vasospasm may still persist, indicating the importance of treatment continuation for this phenomenon [5, 6].

Two different treatment modalities exist: the first being intra-arterial application of vasodilators, the second being intravenous prostaglandin E1 (PGE1) administration. In the early 1970s, Boley et al. used intra-arterial papaverine (30–60 mg/h max. 4 h), a phosphodiesterase inhibitor that increases blood flow through smooth muscle relaxation, to improve bowel salvage [4]. Their group was able to obtain mortality rates of only 40 % by performing laparotomy only in patients who did not respond to treatment. This technique was practical since intra-arterial angiography was already used to differentiate between NOMI and OMI, giving the opportunity to directly engage intra-arterial treatment. Since in these days intra-arterial angiography was also used to follow up these patients and monitor the release of the vasospasm, continuation of vasodilators was possible. Alternative vasodilators for papaverine are phenoxybenzamine, tolazoline, and laevodosine, although these are not commonly used nowadays. In patients with poor or unstable conditions, repeated selective mesenteric angiography with papaverine may not be possible due to its complexity and invasiveness sometimes leading to acute tubular necrosis, local hematomas, and catheter dislodgement, especially in older patients [7, 8].

As mentioned in Chap. 25, computed tomography angiography (CTA) has now replaced angiography as the standard of reference in diagnosing mesenteric ischemia [9]. Additionally, CTA has a short examination time and the ability to rule out other causes of acute abdominal pain in a noninvasive way [10]. Consequently, an alternative for intra-arterial vasodilator therapy was found by administrating a continuous high dose of intravenous PGE1. PGE1 improves blood flow due to relaxation of vascular smooth muscle and inhibits reactive oxygen production due to ischemia [11]. Recently, two groups have tried this approach showing promising results by preventing acute NOMI in three out of three and eight out of nine patients using a PGE1 dose of 0.01–0.03 μg/kg/min for a maximum of 5 days (until improvement of abdominal symptoms) [7, 12]. Only one laparotomy was performed, and PGE1 infusion was deemed to be a safe treatment option. However, PGE1 also inhibits platelet aggregation. Therefore, particular care must be taken in elderly patients who are at risk for hemorrhage.

Surgical Treatment

A laparotomy is only required when symptoms persist after initial treatment and/or when serum markers continue to increase. During surgery it is possible to use direct transcatheter infusion of papaverine into the superior mesenteric artery (SMA), which will restore blood flow within minutes. After restoration of blood supply, the bowel must be accurately reassessed. In order to do so, at least 20–30 min of reperfusion time should be allowed before viability can be determined via thorough exploration [13]. The bowel sections in which irreversible damage took place must then be resected [2]. It is important to realize that although blood flow may be restored with direct infusion of papaverine, the initial stimulus causing the ischemia still has to be treated to prevent further progression of ischemia.

Recommendations

Although mortality rates in NOMI are poor, significant improvements have been made in both diagnostic and treatment modalities. Early identification is of the utmost importance to initiate early treatment, focused on returning blood flow to the mesenteric circulation. Intra-arterial application of papaverine can resolve the vasospasm, although mesenteric angiography might not be possible in critical patients. A good alternative is administration of a high dose of intravenous PGE1, which should be continued until the spasm and the symptoms are relieved. Surgical intervention is only indicated when initial treatment fails, in which case bowel segments with irreversible damage should be resected.

References

1. Sise MJ. Mesenteric ischemia: the whole spectrum. Scand J Surg. 2010;99(2):106–10. PubMed PMID: 20679047.
2. Oldenburg WA, Lau LL, Rodenberg TJ, Edmonds HJ, Burger CD. Acute mesenteric ischemia: a clinical review. Arch Intern Med. 2004;164(10):1054–62. PubMed PMID: 15159262.
3. Schoots IG, Koffeman GI, Legemate DA, Levi M, van Gulik TM. Systematic review of survival after acute mesenteric ischaemia according to disease aetiology. Br J Surg. 2004;91(1): 17–27. PubMed PMID: 14716789.
4. Boley SJ, Sprayregan S, Siegelman SS, Veith FJ. Initial results from an aggressive roentgenological and surgical approach to acute mesenteric ischemia. Surgery. 1977;82(6):848–55. PubMed PMID: 929375.
5. Trompeter M, Brazda T, Remy CT, Vestring T, Reimer P. Non-occlusive mesenteric ischemia: etiology, diagnosis, and interventional therapy. Eur Radiol. 2002;12(5):1179–87. PubMed PMID: 11976865.
6. Gewertz BL, Zarins CK. Postoperative vasospasm after antegrade mesenteric revascularization: a report of three cases. J Vasc Surg. 1991;14(3):382–5. PubMed PMID: 1880846.
7. Mitsuyoshi A, Obama K, Shinkura N, Ito T, Zaima M. Survival in nonocclusive mesenteric ischemia: early diagnosis by multidetector row computed tomography and early treatment with continuous intravenous high-dose prostaglandin E(1). Ann Surg. 2007;246(2):229–35. PubMed PMID: 17667501. Pubmed Central PMCID: 1933563.
8. Tabriziani H, Frishman WH, Brandt LJ. Drug therapies for mesenteric vascular disease. Heart Dis. 2002;4(5):306–14. PubMed PMID: 12350243.
9. Bozlar U, Turba UC, Hagspiel KD. Nonocclusive mesenteric ischemia: findings at multidetector CT angiography. J Vasc Interv Radiol. 2007;18(10):1331–3. PubMed PMID: 17911529.
10. Wyers MC. Acute mesenteric ischemia: diagnostic approach and surgical treatment. Semin Vasc Surg. 2010;23(1):9–20. PubMed PMID: 20298945.
11. Cawello W, Schweer H, Muller R, Bonn R, Seyberth HW. Metabolism and pharmacokinetics of prostaglandin E1 administered by intravenous infusion in human subjects. Eur J Clin Pharmacol. 1994;46(3):275–7. PubMed PMID: 8070511.
12. Kamimura K, Oosaki A, Sugahara S, Mori S. Survival of three nonocclusive mesenteric ischemia patients following early diagnosis by multidetector row computed tomography and prostaglandin E1 treatment. Intern Med. 2008;47(22):2001–6. PubMed PMID: 19015617.
13. Kazmers A. Operative management of chronic mesenteric ischemia. Ann Vasc Surg. 1998; 12(3):299–308. PubMed PMID: 9588521.

Part VI
Median Arcuate Ligament Syndrome

Chapter 27
Clinical Presentation and Diagnostic Considerations

Audra A. Duncan

The syndrome of celiac artery compression by the median arcuate ligament (MAL) or possibly by fibrotic celiac ganglion was first described by Harjola in 1963 [1] and then by Dumbar et al. in 1965 [2]. Symptoms may vary from postprandial abdominal pain, similar to that seen with chronic mesenteric ischemia, to pain with exercise [3], nausea, vomiting, or weight loss. Diagnosis may be confounded by a vague and variable clinical presentation, as well as by the fact that celiac compression by the ganglion is a normal variant noted on imaging in asymptomatic patients [4–7]. In fact, extrinsic compression of the celiac artery may be found in 20–70 % of individuals undergoing imaging for possible abdominal disease [8].

Hypotheses regarding the etiology of median arcuate ligament syndrome (MALS) remain theoretical, as the pathophysiology has yet to be determined in the past 45 years. Some authors hypothesize that MALS is caused by intermittent mesenteric ischemia [4]. Ischemia may contribute to MALS symptoms, but it seems unlikely as the sole cause in the setting of patent superior mesenteric (SMA) and inferior mesenteric arteries (IMA). In fact, when the celiac artery is ligated in cases of tumor, trauma, or occlusion in the setting of thoracoabdominal aneurysm repair, the patients often remain unaffected. In addition, there are no reports of MALS causing intestinal infarction, which would be the natural expected outcome in severe cases.

Intermittent foregut ischemia, however, could play a role in MALS. This theory is supported by a series from Reilly et al. that identified that 70 % of the asymptomatic group had a patient celiac artery, whereas 76 % of symptomatic patients had an occluded artery at 9-year follow-up [5]. Other unproven theories [4] have entertained the idea that the SMA collateral arteries that develop with intermittent celiac stenosis or occlusion may cause a postprandial "steal" of blood from the midgut, although this has not proven true in canine models [6].

A.A. Duncan, MD (✉)
Division of Vascular and Endovascular Surgery, Department of Surgery, Mayo Clinic, Rochester, MN, USA
e-mail: duncan.audra@mayo.edu

G.S. Oderich (ed.), *Mesenteric Vascular Disease*,
DOI 10.1007/978-1-4939-1847-8_27

Other theories consider the role of ganglion nerve involvement in the MALS pain syndrome either from direct sympathetic pain fiber irritation or indirectly from splanchnic vascoconstriction [7]. This neurogenic hypothesis is supported by the results of celiac ganglion block, often used for diagnosis of MALS as discussed below [9]. In addition, a study demonstrating improvement of radionucleotide gastric emptying after surgical transection of celiac ganglion supports this theory [10].

MALS has been reported in patients with rapid weight loss causing loss of periaortic fat and changes in the anatomic relationship between the ligament and the aorta. This effect has been reported following bariatric gastric bypass [11].

History and Physical

Patients undergoing MALS evaluation have often had previous evaluations for other causes of abdominal pain and symptoms such as cholecystitis or gastroesophageal reflux. Because of the difficulty in identifying patients who will respond to celiac ganglion release, MALS is often a diagnosis of exclusion. Gastrointestinal evaluation may include upper endoscopy, colonoscopy, motility studies, computed tomography (CT) or magnetic resonance (MR) imaging. Up to 50 % of patients may have abdominal operations or procedures, including cholecystectomy, exploratory laparoscopy or laparotomy, and biliary/pancreatic sphincterotomy, before a diagnosis of MALS is made [9].

Typically women are diagnosed more frequently than men in a ratio of 2–3:1, with a typical age range of 30–50, although patients have been reported with MALS from ages 18–70 [4, 9]. Symptoms of chronic celiac axis compression most commonly include abdominal pain (80–90 %), postprandial abdominal pain (60–80 %), nausea and vomiting (50–60 %), weight loss (50 %), and bloating (40 %) [9]. In a smaller group of patients (8–20 %), pain may be triggered by exercise [3, 9].

Physical exam is frequently normal, and patients are often thin but not malnourished. Epigastric abdominal bruit may be present. Vague abdominal pain, either diffuse or epigastric, may be noted, as well as tenderness to palpation or mild distention. If peritonitis is suspected, however, a more emergent workup for intestinal ischemia caused by an alternative etiology should be considered. Secondary hypertension has been reported in a rare case report due to compression of the renal artery by the MAL [12].

Imaging Studies

Although diagnosing MALS preoperatively can be elusive because of the vague symptoms, imaging offers the best chance to delineate the anatomical features of MALS. Duplex ultrasound with inspiration and expiration may be a good screening study during initial evaluation of MALS if done by an experienced ultrasonographer. Celiac stenosis is defined as a peak systolic velocity >200 cm/s, but the

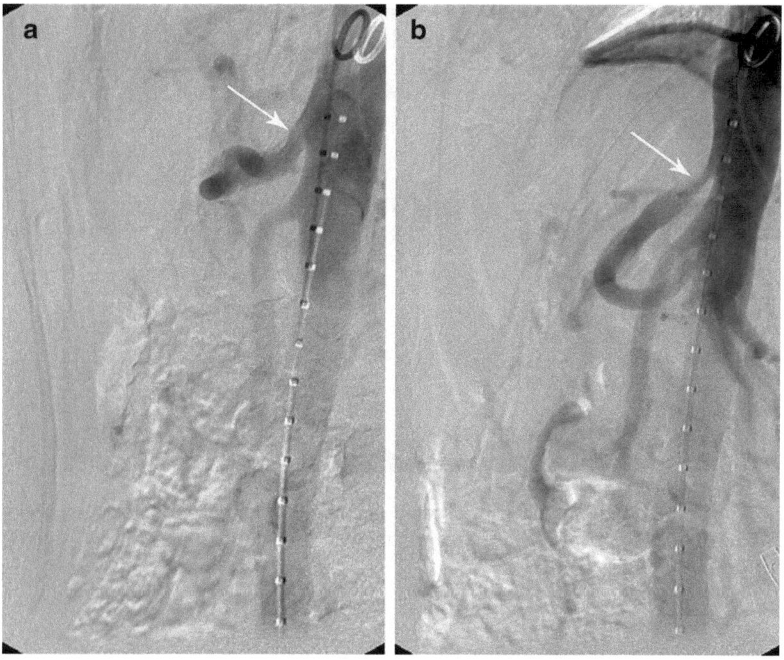

Fig. 27.1 A 50-year-old woman with 15-lb weight loss and upper abdominal pain. (**a**) Lateral aortogram during inspiration demonstrates a widely patent celiac artery origin (arrow). (**b**) Lateral aortogram during expiration demonstrates compression of the celiac artery at the level of the median arcuate ligament (arrow)

etiology of MAL compression may not be clearly imaged with ultrasound. Typically, the Duplex screen is followed by more definitive contrast imaging such as digital, CT or MR angiography.

In the past, conventional angiography with a lateral aortogram and selective celiac and SMA images during full inspiration (Fig. 27.1a) and expiration (Fig. 27.1b) was considered the optimal exam. CT angiography, however, has replaced digital angiography and has the advantage of potentially identifying concomitant abdominal disease and is less invasive (Fig. 27.2). Again, CTA with 2–3-mm-thick axial sections must be performed with inspiration and expiration, with the expectation that the celiac compression will be augmented in the expiratory phase (Fig. 27.3a, b) [13–15]. The CTA may identify a fixed celiac stenosis in both inspiration and expiration, celiac occlusion, abnormal anatomy, mesenteric thrombosis, or atherosclerotic disease which may affect further interventions. It is important to note that incidental identification of celiac artery compression on CT is often unrelated to MALS. For example, in a retrospective review of 744 patients with CT scans, 21 were found to have MALS, but only 3 of the 21 had symptoms [16]. If conventional angiography is performed, the addition of intravascular ultrasound (IVUS) can be done, as an adjunct to contrast imaging [17]. IVUS may identify a more severe stenosis than identified on CTA or lateral angiogram.

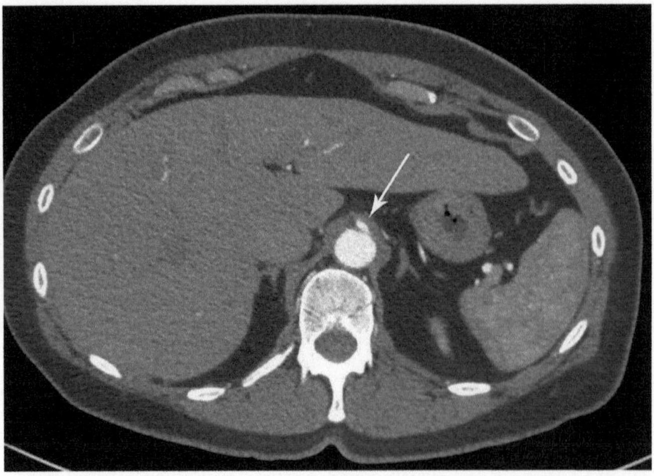

Fig. 27.2 A 38-year-old woman with chronic abdominal pain despite cholecystectomy. Axial images from her CTA identifies a thickened median arcuate ligament (arrow) overlying the celiac artery

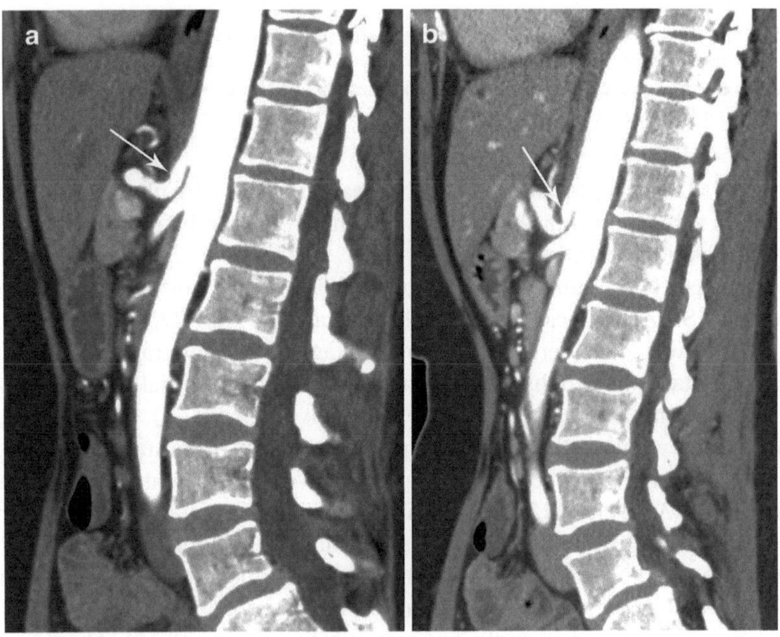

Fig. 27.3 The same 38-year-old woman with sagittal imaging on inspiration and expiration CTA. (**a**) Widely patent celiac artery (arrow) during inspiration. (**b**) High-grade stenosis (arrow) of the celiac artery with expiration

In addition, MALS with significant celiac stenosis has been reported as a cause of pancreaticoduodenal artery aneurysm [18–20]. MRA can be used in a similar manner as CTA for patients with a contrast allergy or in children to avoid radiation. However, expiration phase images are impractical with MRA and may need to be combined with ultrasound imaging to identify dynamic changes in the celiac artery [14]. In addition, MRA may not identify intra-abdominal pathology as well as CT scan.

Injection of Celiac Ganglion and Gastric Tonometry

Because median arcuate compression can be found in both symptomatic and asymptomatic patients, imaging alone may not identify patients who will improve after MAL surgical release. The percutaneous celiac ganglion block has been used for many years to control intractable pain for patients with chronic pancreatitis or intra-abdominal cancers. Although permanent block can be obtained by injecting alcohol, a temporary celiac ganglion injection with local anesthetic performed under CT or fluoroscopic guidance (Fig. 27.4) may help to identify patients who would improve from surgical treatment [21]. Although promising, improvement from ganglion block does not absolutely predict future success from MAL surgical release, and further studies are still necessary.

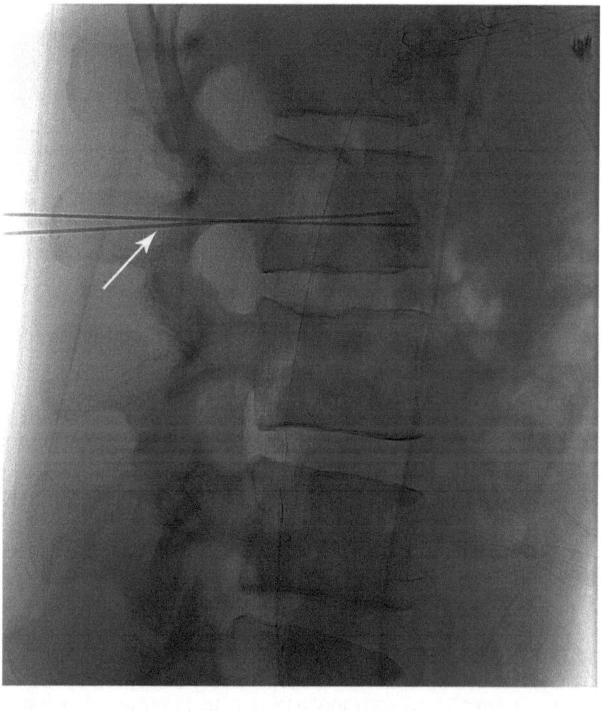

Fig. 27.4 A 25-year-old man with exercise-induced abdominal pain underwent fluoroscopic-guided celiac ganglion temporary block to aid in diagnosis of MALS

Gastric tonometry (See Chap. 6) has also been proposed as a preoperative predictor of success from MAL release. Mensink et al. reported on 43 patients with significant celiac compression of which 30 had ischemia based on gastric exercise tonometry [22]. Of those 30 patients, 29 underwent MAL release and/or revascularization, and 83 % were asymptomatic at 39 months of follow-up. Repeat tonometry in the patients who were asymptomatic was improved in 100 % but only improved in 25 % of patients with persistent symptoms, implicating gastric ischemia an etiology.

Differential Diagnosis

Despite an overlap in symptoms, MALS is distinct from chronic mesenteric ischemia. As opposed to chronic mesenteric ischemia, MALS will not progress to cachexia, bowel gangrene, or death. In addition, MALS typically involves only the celiac artery, although occasionally the ligament can compress the SMA as well. Although initial general symptoms of abdominal pain, postprandial pain, and food fear may lead to the differential diagnosis of both MALS and chronic mesenteric ischemia, careful history and excellent imaging can often easily differentiate between the two diseases.

References

1. Harjola PT. A rare obstruction of the celiac artery. Ann Chir Gynaecol Fenn. 1963;52: 547–50.
2. Dumbar JD, Molnar W, Bemon F, Marable S. Compression of the celiac trunk and abdominal angina. Am J Roentgenol Radium Ther Nucl Med. 1965;45:731–44.
3. Desmond CP, Roberts SK. Exercise-related abdominal pain as a manifestation of the median arcuate ligament syndrome. Scand J Gastroenterol. 2004;39:1310–3.
4. Bech FR. Celiac artery compression syndrome. Surg Clin N Am. 1997;77:409–24.
5. Reilly LM, Ammar AD, Stoney RJ, Ehrenfeld WK. Late results following operative repair for celiac artery compression syndrome. J Vasc Surg. 1985;2:79–91.
6. Brandt LJ, Boely SJ. Celiac axis compression syndrome: a critical review. Dig Dis Sci. 1978;23:633–40.
7. Tribble CG, Harman PK, Mentzer RM. Celiac artery compression syndrome: report of a case and review of the literature. Vasc Surg. 1986;20:120–9.
8. Szilagyi DE, Rian RL, Elliott JP, Smith RF. The celiac artery compression syndrome: Does it exist? Surgery. 1972;72:849–63.
9. Duncan AA. Median arcuate ligament syndrome. Curr Treatment Options in Cardiovasc Med. 2008;10:112–6.
10. Balaban DH, Chen J, Lin Z, et al. Median arcuate ligament syndrome: a possible cause of idiopathic gastroparesis. Am J Gastroenterol. 1997;92:519–23.
11. Richards NG, Neville RF, Sidawy AN, Brody FJ. Celiac artery compression after a gastric bypass. Surg Lapar Endosc Perc Tech Iss. 2014;24(2):e66–9.
12. Sari S, Verim S, Sivrioglu AK. Bozlar U: A rare cause of secondary hypertension: median arcuate ligament compression of the renal artery diagnosed by CT angiography. BMJ Case Rep. 2013 Jun 3;2013. pii: bcr2013009937. doi: 10.1136/bcr-2013-009937.

13. Horton KM, Talamini MA, Fishman EK. Median arcuate ligament syndrome: evaluation with CT angiography. Radiographics. 2005;25:1177–82.
14. Aschenbach R. Compression of the celiac trunk caused by median arcuate ligament in children and adolescent subjects: evaluation with contrast-enhanced MR angiography and comparison with Doppler US evaluation. J Vasc Interv Radiol. 2011;22:556–61.
15. Enterline J. Single injection, inspiratory/expiratory high-pitch dual-source CT angiography for median arcuate ligament syndrome: novel technique for a classic diagnosis. J Cardiovasc Comput Tomogr. 2012;6:357–9.
16. Gümüş H, Gümüş M, Tekbaş G, Önder H, Ekici F, Çetinçakmak M, Bilici A. Clinical and multidetector computed tomography findings of patients with median arcuate ligament syndrome. Clinical Imaging. 2012;36:522–5.
17. Vazquez de Lara F, Higgins C, Hernandez-Vila EA. Median Arcuate Ligament Syndrome Confirmed with the Use of Intravascular Ultrasound. Tex Heart Inst J. 2014;41(1):57–60.
18. Akatsu T, Hayashi S, Yamane T, et al. Emergency embolization of a ruptured pancreaticoduodenal artery aneurysm associated with the median arcuate ligament syndrome. J Gastroenterol Hepatol. 2004;19:482–3.
19. Hildebrand P, Esnaashari H, Franke C, et al. Surgical management of pancreaticoduodenal artery aneurysms in association with celiac trunk occlusion or stenosis. Ann Vasc Surg. 2007; 21:10–5.
20. Armstrong MB, Stadtlander KS, Grove MK. Pancreaticoduodenal artery aneurysm associated with median arcuate ligament syndrome. Ann Vasc Surg. 2014;28:741.e1–5.
21. Lee MJ, Mueller PR, van Sonnenberg E, et al. CT-guided celiac ganglion block with alcohol. AJR Am J Roetgenol. 1993;161:633–6.
22. Mensink PB. Gastric exercise tonometry: the key investigation in patients with suspected celiac artery compression syndrome. J Vasc Surg. 2006;44:277–81.

Chapter 28
Open Surgical Treatment

Audra A. Duncan

Although results of surgical treatment are discussed in Chap. 30, one of the key factors to consider before embarking on open median arcuate ligament (MAL) release is the potential outcomes based on symptoms, patient age, associated comorbidities, and preoperative assessment [1]. Reilly et al. demonstrated that patients with atypical pain patterns, age greater than 60 years old, weight loss less than 20 lbs, and a history of psychiatric disease or alcohol abuse were less likely to improve after MAL release [1]. The patient and surgeon should have a frank discussion regarding the difficulty in predicting postoperative outcomes after MAL release, particularly because of the wide overlap of symptoms of MAL syndrome (MALS) with other gastrointestinal and intra-abdominal pathologies [1].

Open MAL Release

Surgical management, either open or via laparoscopic technique, is nearly always required in order to release the mechanical compression of the fibrous median arcuate band, resect the celiac ganglion, and inspect the celiac artery, often with ultrasound [1–4]. Although endovascular treatment of celiac compression have been reported [5–8], the risk of restenosis or stent compression is high in this generally low-risk, healthy patient group who tolerate open procedures and general anesthesia well.

MAL release is performed through an upper abdominal incision from the xiphoid to several centimeters above the umbilicus. A subcostal incision can be considered depending on the patient's body habitus. A nasogastric tube is placed after

A.A. Duncan, MD (✉)
Division of Vascular and Endovascular Surgery, Department of Surgery,
Mayo Clinic, Rochester, MN, USA
e-mail: duncan.audra@mayo.edu

G.S. Oderich (ed.), *Mesenteric Vascular Disease*,
DOI 10.1007/978-1-4939-1847-8_28

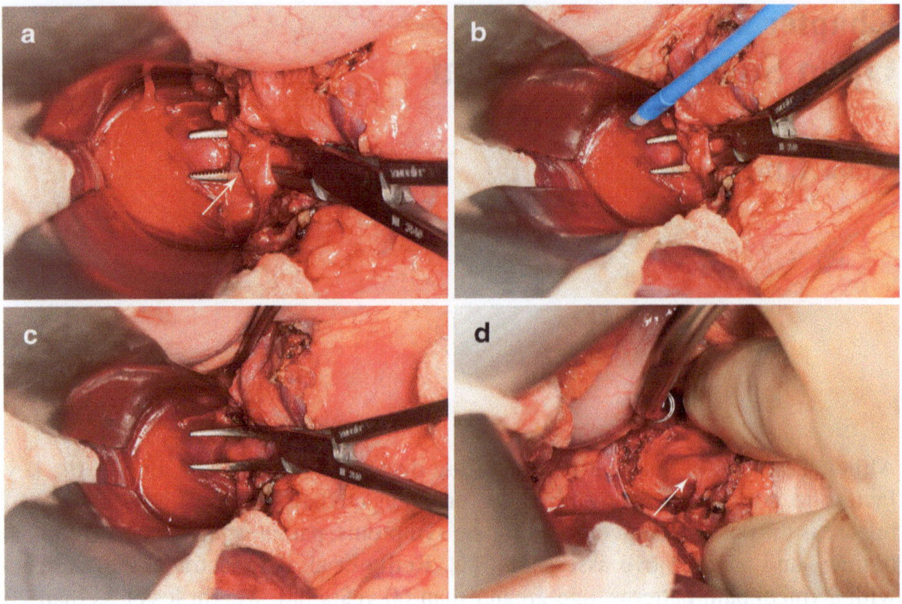

Fig. 28.1 A 45-year-old woman with celiac compression identified on CTA and a 25-lb weight loss with abdominal and back pain. (**a**) The crus of the diaphragm (arrow) is dissected and the ganglion fibers isolated with a right-angle clamp. (**b**) The ganglion fibers are divided with electrocautery. (**c**) The ganglion fibers retract and are excised along with the diaphragmatic fibers. (**d**) The origin of the celiac artery is freed of all surrounding tissue (arrow) and assessed by palpation and ultrasound exam

anesthesia to assure identification of the esophagus during mobilization of the MAL. The diaphragm fibers draped over the aorta are divided proximal to the celiac artery. At this point, the celiac ganglion fibers should be visible and can be divided with cautery or ligated. The celiac artery is then skeletonized of all surrounding nerve and muscle fibers (Fig. 28.1a–d).

Most authors agree that after the celiac artery is inspected and patency assessed, ideally with palpation, Doppler exam, and ultrasound, a decision is made whether celiac artery reconstruction is indicated. Reilly et al recommend celiac reconstruction for all patients with a visible celiac artery deformity, thrill, or pressure gradient [1]. At our institution, all patients undergo intraoperative ultrasound (Fig. 28.2a–c) after open MAL resection, with ~40 % demonstrating residual celiac stenosis despite adequate MAL release [2]. Depending on the length of the stenotic lesion and the proximity to the aorta, either patch angioplasty (bovine pericardium or polyester graft patch) or aortoceliac bypass is recommended. In our early series, patients also had intraluminal dilation but this technique was abandoned due to less favorable success rates. In addition, because of the elongation of the celiac artery in some cases, primary reanastomoses has also been reported.

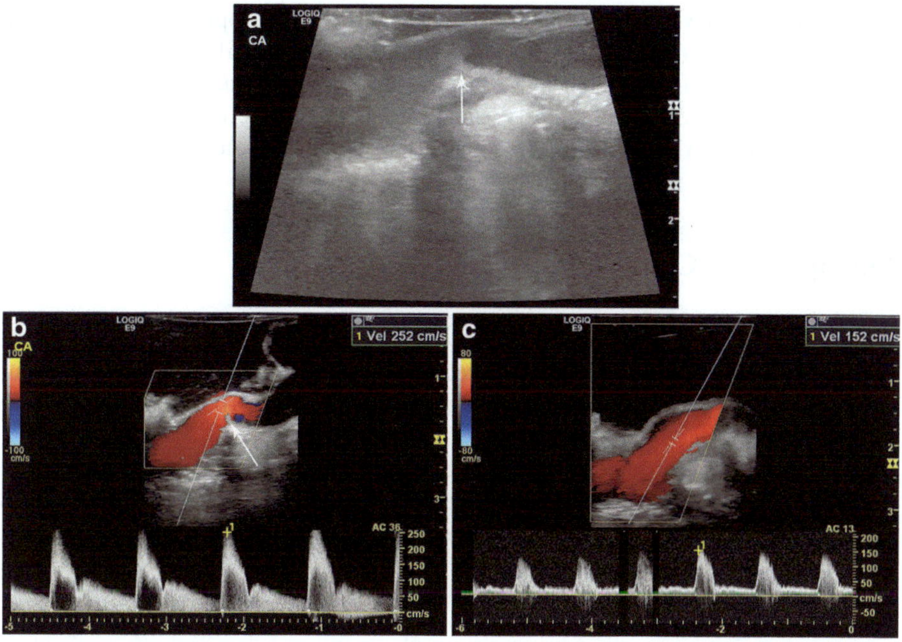

Fig. 28.2 After MAL release in a 37-year-old woman, intraoperative duplex identified a fixed stenosis (arrow) arising from the posterior wall of the celiac artery. (**a**) Gray-scale images identified the stenosis. (**b**) Color flow Doppler confirmed the site of stenosis (arrow) with a peak systolic velocity of 252 cm/s. (**c**) Because of a diminished pulse, the patient underwent a patch angioplasty with bovine pericardium resulting in improvement of the stenosis and improvement of the peak systolic velocity to 152 cm/s

Ganglion Resection

Many authors believe the celiac ganglion resection is the more critical component of the procedure. The ganglion can often be more easily visualized if the percutaneous ganglion injections have been done within 72 h. In our series of five patients with aortoceliac bypass, one had persistent symptoms with a widely patient graft, emphasizing the role of the ganglion in the pain of MALS. In addition, of the 32 patients, 4 had recurrent symptoms, but only 1 of the 4 had recurrent celiac artery stenosis.

Role of Endovascular Treatment

Percutaneous treatment of MALS was first described decades ago to treat recurrent stenosis after open MAL release [5]. However, primary treatment of celiac artery compression either by MAL or an occult malignancy with angioplasty has a high failure rate [6]. Several case reports [6–8] suggest that angioplasty alone, without the preceding removal of the MAL and ganglion fibers, will not be successful. In addition, stents used in a primary fashion are at risk of fracture due to external compression. However, angioplasty can be used to good effect for celiac artery restenosis after MAL release and/or celiac artery bypass or patch angioplasty [5, 9].

Postoperative Care

Patients are permitted to have oral intake the day following surgery if only a MAL release is performed. If celiac artery reconstruction is required, ileus may occur even after a short ischemic time, therefore eating should be delayed until the patient's bowel function returns.

Follow-up imaging can be performed based on clinical exam because celiac artery patency does not always correlate with symptoms. Duplex ultrasound is preferred for follow-up imaging, followed by contrast angiography with or without angioplasty if indicated.

References

1. Reilly LM, Ammar AD, Stoney RJ, Ehrenfeld WK. Late results following operative repair for celiac artery compression syndrome. J Vasc Surg. 1985;2:79–91.
2. Duncan AA. Median arcuate ligament syndrome. Curr Treatment Options in Cardiovasc Med. 2008;10:112–6.
3. Balaban DH, Chen J, Lin Z, et al. Median arcuate ligament syndrome: a possible cause of idiopathic gastroparesis. Am J Gastroenterol. 1997;92:519–23.
4. Desmond CP. Exercise-related abdominal pain as a manifestation of the median arcuate ligament syndrome. Scand J Gastroenterol. 2004;39:1310–3.
5. Saddekni S, Sniderman KW, Hilton S, Sos TA. Percutaneous transluminal angioplasty of nonatherosclerotic lesions. AJR Am J Roentgenol. 1980;135:975–82.
6. Matsumoto AH, Tegtmeyer CJ, Fitzcharles EK, et al. Percutaneous transluminal angioplasty of visceral arterial stenosis: results and long-term clinical follow-up. J Vasc Interv Radiol. 1995;6:165–74.
7. Matsumoto AH, Angle JF, Spinosa DJ, et al. Percutaneous transluminal angioplasty and stenting in the treatment of chronic mesenteric ischemia: results and long-term follow-up. J Am Coll Surg. 2002;194(1 Suppl):S22–31.
8. Cina CS, Safar H. Successful treatment of recurrent celiac axis compression syndrome. A case report. Panminerva Med. 2002;44:69–72.
9. Jimenez JC, Harlander-Locke M, Dutson EP. Open and laparoscopic treatment of median arcuate ligament syndrome. J Vasc Surg. 2012;56:869–73.

Chapter 29
Laparoscopic Transperitoneal Approach

Usah Khrucharoen, Erik P. Dutson, and Juan Carlos Jimenez

The major shift toward less invasive procedures has resulted in general and vascular surgeons with training in minimally invasive surgery becoming more involved in the operative management of median arcuate ligament syndrome (MALS). Pathogenesis of MALS is characterized by extrinsic compression of the celiac artery by dense fibrous tissues of the median arcuate ligament. Balloon angioplasty and stenting as a primary modality in patients with MALS without prior release of the extrinsic compression on the celiac artery has been found to have a high recurrence rate and may result in stent fracture [1]. The traditional surgical therapy for MALS, which has been performed for many years, involves division of the anomalous fibrous diaphragmatic bands overlying the celiac artery, along with the celiac plexus and lymphatic tissues via a midline laparotomy. The laparoscopic median arcuate ligament release technique was successfully performed and reported as early as 2000 by Roayaie et al. [2] and later by Carbonell et al. [3] Excellent clinical outcomes in terms of complete resolution of the symptoms at the 3-month postoperative visit were described with laparoscopic procedures [2]. Laparoscopic median arcuate ligament (MAL) release appears to be efficacious in providing early symptom relief in patients with this syndrome. In a review of comparative outcomes from our institution, only 14 % of patients required additional celiac

U. Khrucharoen, MD
Department of Surgery, David Geffen School of Medicine at UCLA, Los Angeles, CA, USA

E.P. Dutson, MD, FACS
Department of Surgery, Ronald Reagan UCLA Medical Center, Los Angeles, CA, USA
e-mail: EDutson@mednet.ucla.edu

J.C. Jimenez, MD, FACS (✉)
Division of Vascular Surgery, Gonda (Goldschmied) Vascular Center, Ronald Reagan-UCLA Medical Center, Department of Surgery, Division of Vascular Surgery, David Geffen School of Medicine at UCLA, Los Angeles, CA, USA
e-mail: jcjimenez@mednet.ucla.edu

G.S. Oderich (ed.), *Mesenteric Vascular Disease*,
DOI 10.1007/978-1-4939-1847-8_29

revascularization (endovascular or open) compared with the open group [4]. Given its less invasive nature, the laparoscopic MAL release can provide both diagnostic and therapeutic options, especially in younger patients where the question of vascular supply is not entirely clear, and return to work is more rapid. Robotic assistance is one of the most significant recent technological advancements in minimally invasive surgery, which allows surgeons to perform more complex procedures using a minimally invasive approach [5]. With the robotic approach, which we perform in our institution preferentially based on availability, improved visualization related to stereoscopy and precision of movement may represent the optimal treatment modality for MAL release [6]. Purely endovascular treatment of MALS is also a newer option, though not recommended due to concerns about efficacy in the face of external compression as mentioned above. Also, the use of stents in the celiac artery, without previous MAL division, could be complicated by stent compression or fracture [7]. Nevertheless, angioplasty can still be beneficial in cases of recurrent symptoms after surgical decompression of the celiac artery [8]. This chapter covers minimally invasive surgical techniques, including the classic open approach as comparison, for MAL release.

Classic (Open) Approach to MAL Release

According to Tulloch et al., in a retrospective medical record review performed of the patients undergoing laparoscopic and open surgical treatment for MALS from 1999 to 2009 in our institution, five of six patients (83 %) in the open technique group experienced immediate postoperative relief of symptoms. One patient with severe early postoperative abdominal pain was found to have a splenic infarction from intraoperative embolization, and her abdominal pain resolved at 1 month. Three patients (50 %) developed recurrent abdominal pain in the open technique group despite the presence of a patent celiac artery stent on postoperative CT angiography [9].

Surgical Technique

The surgical technique has been recently reported by You et al. [10]. Under general endotracheal anesthesia, a laparotomy incision is performed either as a curvilinear transverse subcostal or a 10-cm long upper midline abdominal incision. The lesser sac and lesser omentum are identified and opened. Downward traction is then applied to the stomach. Dissection is begun along the common hepatic artery and continued in the perivascular plane toward the confluence of the splenic and left gastric arteries to the main trunk of the celiac artery. After skeletonizing the branches of the celiac axis, the arcuate ligament and all of its fibers overlying the celiac axis are divided and dissected. All surrounding ligamentous and ganglionic tissues are sharply dissected and removed down to the aorta and circumferentially mobilized. The abdominal wall is closed in layers.

Laparoscopic Transperitoneal Approach for MALS

As laparoscopic surgery has become more widespread, an increasing number of patients with MALS have been treated with minimally invasive approaches. Roayaie et al. in 2000 described a patient in whom laparoscopy provided a less invasive but equally effective method for decompressing the celiac artery [2]. Several series have demonstrated successful laparoscopic treatment of MALS [4, 9, 11–15]. Our institution has reported two series comparing experience with laparoscopic treatment of MALS to that of the open approach [4, 9]. To our knowledge, this study is the first direct comparison of consecutive patients with MALS treated by open or laparoscopic techniques. Roseborough [7] performed laparoscopic release of the MAL in 15 patients over a 5-year period. In his series, 14 of 15 patients (93 %) subjectively reported significant improvement at a mean follow-up of 44.2 months. One patient remained with severe refractory symptoms. Four patients required open conversion for bleeding. Despite one case of severe pancreatitis, no other complications or deaths were noted. Baccari et al. [12] treated 16 patients with a similar laparoscopic technique over a 7-year period. In this series, two patients required open conversion for bleeding. Fourteen patients were noted to be asymptomatic at postoperative follow-up. Two patients with residual celiac stenosis were symptomatic and completely resolved their abdominal pain after revascularization (aortoceliac bypass and percutaneous transluminal angioplasty/stent). However, patients must be counseled preoperatively that the risk of open conversion is possible with the mean rate of conversion reported in published series nearly 20 % [7, 12].

The minimally invasive approach offers improved visualization of the aorta and celiac trunk to facilitate complete division of the MAL fibers to fully expose the anterior aorta and celiac trunk, which is believed to be the key to success with the operation. Additionally, the patient will incur all of the well-reported benefits of minimally invasive surgery: less bleeding, less pain, decreased need for postoperative pain medications, decreased risk of wound infection, modulated immune response to injury, earlier discharge, faster recovery, and earlier return to work [9]. Despite these benefits, injury to the celiac artery and its major branches, or even the aorta itself, is a serious risk with the minimally invasive approach, and the operative team needs to be prepared for a rapid conversion to the open approach in that circumstance to prevent lethal blood loss. Laparoscopic intraoperative Doppler ultrasound can be used as an adjunct confirmation of adequacy of dissection, as it can objectively assess blood flow in real time [3].

Patient Positioning

To complete the operation safely and efficiently, proper patient positioning and operating room setup are critical. We place the patient in the supine position with legs adducted and arms abducted. The patient's arms are secured with table straps, and obese patients have straps placed on the lower extremities, also for improved security. Pneumatic compression stockings are placed and activated prior to the induction of general anesthesia. These devices counter potentially severe venous stasis resulting from the use of pneumoperitoneum and the reverse Trendelenburg position. Positioning in reverse Trendelenburg provides ideal access to the upper peritoneal space, with a 10°–15° hyperextension of the back to enhance the intra-abdominal working space. A footboard should be routinely used when steep reverse Trendelenburg is employed [16].

Surgical Approaches for Laparoscopic Techniques

Retrogastric Approach (Gastrocolic Ligament Approach)

As described in our study by Tulloch et al., this technique was modified to avoid transection of the muscular body of either the left or right crus and the potential complication of gastroesophageal reflux. To avoid cutting these muscles as a part of the dissection to gain exposure to the MAL, a more inferior approach has been adopted. This consists of dividing the gastrocolic ligament widely inferior to the gastroepiploic artery. This approach would be more suitable for obese patients where the excessive abdominal adiposity creates exposure challenges. Given the laparoscopic approach to the peritoneal space, this allows the dissection to follow a more natural angulation. The overall amount of dissection is decreased via this approach; however, there is some need for an increased level of awareness to protect the celiac branches and the pancreas during the procedure [9].

Operative Technique

After placement of the laparoscopic ports, the peritoneal cavity and the liver surfaces should be inspected for associated pathology. Any suspicious lesion should be biopsied and analyzed by frozen section. A Nathanson liver retractor is inserted via a subxiphoid incision to elevate the left lateral segment of the liver. The greater curvature is elevated with a grasper, and countertraction is placed on the omentum. The initial step in dissection is to divide the gastrocolic ligament widely inferior to the gastroepiploic artery to mobilize the greater curvature of the stomach and gain access to the lesser sac (Fig. 29.1). Division of the gastrocolic ligament is facilitated by the use of the ultrasonic dissector. The stomach is elevated and posterior attachments are divided followed by placing the liver retractor under the posterior gastric wall, elevating the stomach anteriorly and superiorly to expose the superior border of the pancreas.

At this point, approaching the MAL can be performed by three different techniques. The first technique is to follow the right crus of the diaphragm posteriorly to the left crus, which is the most commonly performed approach. The second technique

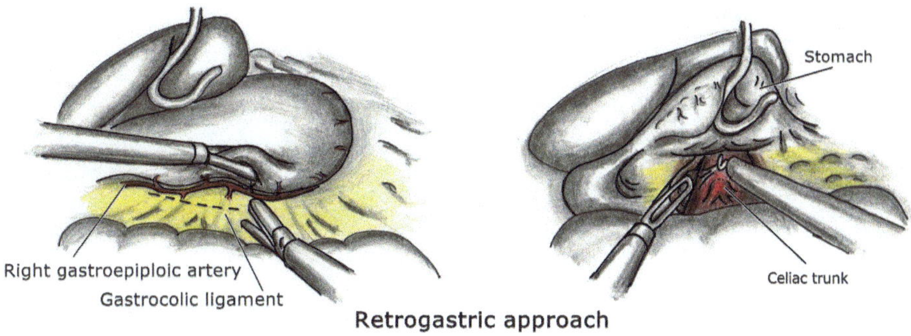

Fig. 29.1 Retrogastric approach

is to start dissection from the left crus posteriorly to the right crus, and the third approach is to follow the branches of the celiac trunk back to the celiac artery until MAL is encountered.

The Right Crus Approach

This technique is the most commonly performed and has been described in several studies [7, 9, 12, 17, 18]. This technique was also the described technique in the pediatric MALS studies by Said et al. and Joyce et al. at the Mayo Clinic, Rochester, MN [17, 18].

Operative Technique

After the stomach is placed on left lateral traction, the right crus of the diaphragm is identified along with the caudate lobe of the liver and the inferior vena cava. The peritoneum over the right crus is opened using the L-hook electrocautery (Fig. 29.2). The esophagus and both the anterior and posterior vagal trunks are carefully identified. The retroesophageal space is then developed. This technique exposes the aorta first and then releases the median arcuate ligament cranially to caudally, directly anterior to the aorta coming onto the celiac artery. The decussation of the right and left crura is dissected to expose the aorta. Dissection proceeds caudally and must remain on the aorta anteriorly without veering off in either direction as there are no named branches until the celiac artery is encountered. The antrum of the stomach and the pancreas will likely need to be retracted caudally. Tight bands and ganglion fibers are lysed using the L-hook electrocautery on a low setting (Fig. 29.3). Because the fibers encountered here are tight and compress the celiac axis from anterior to

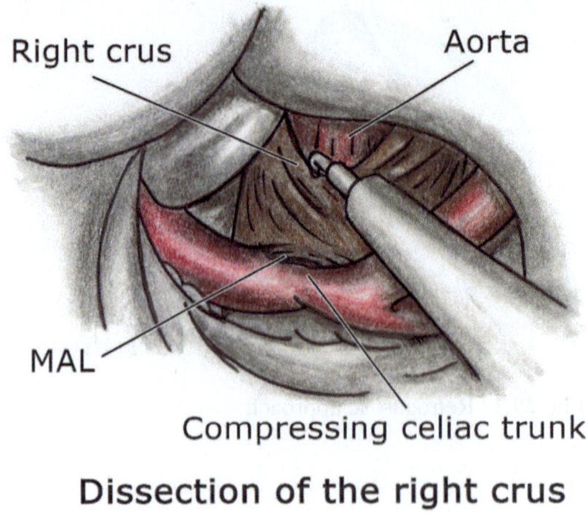

Fig. 29.2 Dissection of the right crus

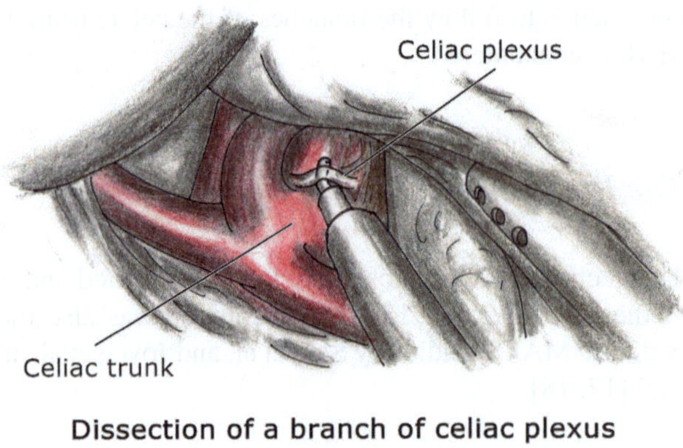

Fig. 29.3 Dissection of a branch of celiac plexus

posterior, these findings make the celiac axis nearly invisible. After one fiber at a time is lysed, the celiac artery will come into view as a bulge on the aorta (Fig. 29.4). Care must be taken not to back-heel (touch with the curved part of the cautery hook) any artery as one is lifting up on the individual fibers. Dissection is continued until the celiac, common hepatic, and left gastric arteries are free with 0.5–1.5 cm in either direction. One can consider re-approximating the crura cephalad to the MAL, though there is no compelling data to suggest that this be performed routinely.

The Left Crus Approach

This approach was described in a retrospective analysis of five consecutive patients who underwent laparoscopic division of the MAL by Nguyen et al. [19].

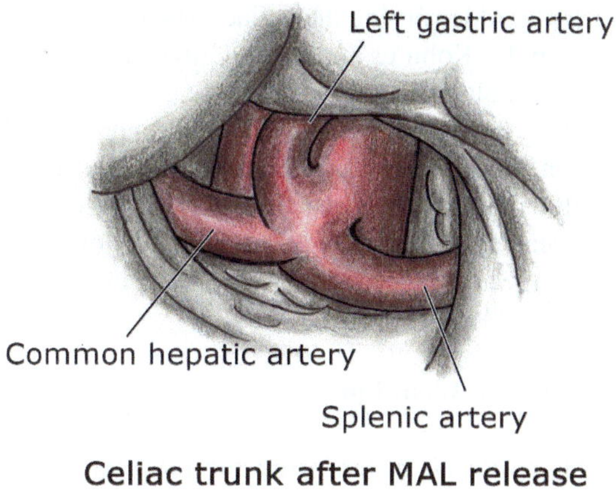

Fig. 29.4 Celiac trunk after MAL release

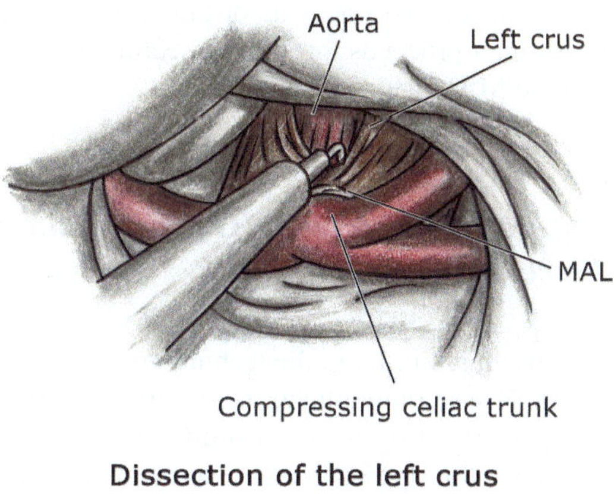

Fig. 29.5 Dissection of the left crus

Operative Technique

After the stomach is retracted superiorly and to the right, a liver retractor is placed under the posterior gastric wall. This technique is started by firstly approached the left crus (Fig. 29.5) and dissecting to the right crus, then to proceed dissecting the preaortic fibrous tissues as described above.

The Vessel Approach

Some surgeons have found this approach to be more beneficial. Roseborough described this technique in his study. In several cases, final exposure of the origin of the celiac artery required retrograde dissection from the more distal celiac artery after first identifying the celiac axis or the hepatic artery distally [7]. A retrospective review by Kohn et al.. of the University of North Carolina, Chapel Hill, described this vascular dissection technique. A total of six patients were identified, two underwent a laparoscopic approach and experienced symptomatic improvement with a mean follow-up at 48.6 months [20]. Vaziri et al. also described this technique, by following the left gastric artery. They reported a case series of three patients with successful outcomes in a short-term follow-up period [13]. This technique was also described in the case reports by Wani et al. [21]

Operative Technique

This approach differs from the preceding description in the following steps: the avascular region of the gastrohepatic omentum (pars flaccida) is opened, and the left gastric artery identified. Using the L-hook electrocautery, dissection follows the left gastric artery and traces its origin up to the celiac trunk until the MAL is encountered, then proceeds through dissecting the preaortic fibrous tissues, celiac plexus, and the MAL as described above.

Antegastric Approach (Gastrohepatic Ligament/Pars Flaccida Approach)

Because it is similar to the technique in gastroesophageal operations such as laparoscopic Nissen fundoplication, this approach for the MAL release has been described and performed by many institutions [14]. A retrospective study by Tulloch et al.. described this approach combined with the right crus technique and demonstrated a technical success rate in the laparoscopic technique group of 80 %. Twenty percent required conversion for bleeding. Operative conversion was required for acute bleeding from the left gastric artery in one patient and the celiac trunk in the other. Both open conversions occurred early in our experience and likely occurred due to subadventitial dissection and excessive thinning of the artery with the ultrasonic dissection. Direct suture repair of the left gastric artery was performed during the first conversion, and patch angioplasty was required to repair the celiac trunk arteriotomy during the second [9].

Operative Technique

The avascular region of the gastrohepatic omentum, also known as the pars flaccida, is identified. A grasper is used on the stomach, retracting it inferiorly and laterally such that tension is placed on the gastrohepatic ligament. An ultrasonic dissector or another cutting/sealing device is used to open the gastrohepatic ligament (Fig. 29.6).

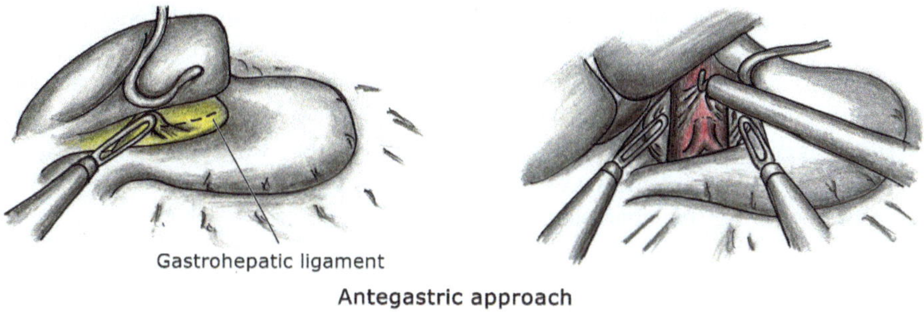

Fig. 29.6 Antegastric approach

The esophagus is dissected circumferentially, exposing the right crus of the diaphragm. The right crus is then isolated inferiorly to the cardia. A Penrose drain or a vascular loop is used to retract the esophagus and/or stomach to gain better exposure of the aortoceliac region. Once the crura of the diaphragm are separated, the abdominal aorta is identified. The preaortic fibrous tissues are divided using the "L"-hook electrocautery as described in the right crus technique. The other two techniques (following left crus and the branches of celiac artery) can also be used. The MAL release is considered complete once the celiac axis is clearly visualized without any residual impinging tissues. This generally results in a visible change in the trunk's position and orientation, albeit sometimes subtle. The trunk has been described as "rising" off the aorta by a small amount.

The Robot-Assisted Technique for MAL Release

Jaik et al. first reported the successful treatment of MALS utilizing a robotic surgical system [6]. Subsequent reports by Antoniou et al. and Meyer et al. also describe the technique of robotic approach for division of the MAL [22, 23]. This technique was also described in a retrospective review performed by Do et al.. from the Ochsner Clinic Foundation, New Orleans, LA. Comparing the outcomes between laparoscopic and robot-assisted treatment of MALS, a total of 16 patients, 8 out of 12 patients (67 %) in the laparoscopic group and 2 out of 4 patients (50 %) in the robot-assisted approach group, reported complete resolution of their abdominal pain in the 20-month follow-up. No intraoperative or perioperative complications nor conversions were reported, though the study size was obviously quite small [24].

In institutions that employ the surgical robotic system, the benefits of robotic surgery may be due to the stereoscopic view of the surgical field, which enhances depth perception, and the improved surgical precision of movement due to the wrist-like articulations of the instruments, enhancing performance in the hard-to-reach areas. This is most obvious if the patient has a somewhat high-riding pancreas, such that the superior border of the pancreas is crowding the area of dissection. The maneuvering around the celiac artery has shown to be improved in terms of the dexterity with the use of the enhanced three-dimensional display inherent to the robotic system when compared to monoscopic laparoscopic systems [10]. However, disadvantages include higher cost and increased operative time and time for equipment setup. Operative time was 168 min in the reported case, in contrast with a mean of 90 min for the laparoscopic technique [12].

Operative Technique

Once a liver retractor is placed exposing the anterior gastric wall, approaching the lesser sac can be performed either with the retrogastric or the antegastric approach.

The robotic system is docked, and meticulous dissection is undertaken in the region of the confluence of the left gastric artery and the hepatic artery. Dissection in this area is carried down until the crura are exposed at the base where the left crus crosses the right crus. In the antegastric approach, the stomach is retracted to the left to gain better exposure. Subsequently, the left gastric artery can be looped with a Penrose drain and also retracted to the left. The right crus dissection is carried out caudally. Upon further dissection, the aorta and celiac artery come into view and the right diaphragmatic crus is seen coursing over the aorta and around the celiac axis. The right crus is then carefully divided. All the fibrous attachments around the aorta and the origin of the celiac artery are meticulously dissected with the L-hook electrocautery along with the celiac nerve plexus and lymphatic tissue. Division of these fibers on the celiac artery is carried out for some distance onto the celiac artery circumferentially until the artery appears to be free of any external compression. Once these maneuvers are completed, the celiac axis will be clearly visualized without any residual kinking and uniform throughout its course.

Essential Equipment

Laparoscope

The Oblique-Viewing (i.e., 30°, 45°) Laparoscope

We generally recommend using this oblique-viewing laparoscope for this procedure because of its flexibility in viewing fixed and deeper structures that may be obscured when using a zero-degree laparoscope. According to the report by Roseborough, performing the operation with the 45° camera in these MAL release procedures had been found to improve the exposure behind the incisura, resulting in conversion of only one of seven patients [7].

The Flexible-Tip Laparoscope

In cases of a high-riding pancreas or difficult exposure, this laparoscope has clear advantages. However, some experience is required to establish its optimal application.

Laparoscopic Trocars

The typical number of 5-mm laparoscopic ports used is four, including a subxiphoid port, an umbilical port, and two lateral ports. An optical 5-mm trocar is used for entering the abdomen midway between the xiphoid and the umbilicus. Additional 5-mm working trocars are placed under videoscopic guidance after first insufflating the abdomen to 15 mmHg with carbon dioxide. A subxiphoid port is used for creating a tract for introducing the Nathanson liver retractor.

Ultrasonic Dissector

The ultrasonic dissector cuts via vibration. The scalpel surface itself cuts through tissue by vibrating in the range of 55–500 Hz. The high-frequency vibration of tissue molecules generates stress and friction in the tissue, which generates heat and causes protein denaturation. Some surgeons prefer this device for dissection of the fibrous tissues around the aorta. However, using this source of energy for dissection of the fibrous tissues around the aorta and its branches, some degree of lateral thermal spread occurs [25–27]. One series described by Baccari et al. showed that 2 patients of the 16 patients were converted to open surgery because of bleeding from the takeoff of the celiac artery from the aorta. This occurred due to a small injury to the proximal part of the thin-walled celiac artery caused by thermal spread from the ultrasonic dissection in one patient and by the coagulating hook in the other patient. Both injuries occurred at the end of the procedure during an attempt to improve the aortoceliac skeletonization by removing the abundant ganglionic tissue encasing the celiac artery. They believe that, during the last steps of the procedure, avoiding high energy and reducing the coagulation setting are advisable [12].

The L-Shaped Hook Monopolar Cautery

The tip of the L-shaped dissector functions as a cutting edge of a knife due to high density. Coagulation, rather than cutting, can be achieved by using the outer side of the "L"-shaped hook. The insulation over the proximal half of the hook prevents unintended cautery burns—so-called stray arcs—to surrounding structures. The common technique for utilizing this device effectively is following a hook-pull-burn sequence by placing sturdy traction on the tissues and then gently sweeping or caressing with the elbow of the wire, creating a more precise and delicate tissue separation [28, 29]. The division of the fibers of the MAL and the surrounding tissues can be better accomplished with the use of a hook cautery [7].

Nathanson Liver Retractor

The liver retractor is used to retract the left lobe of the liver for exposure of the gastroesophageal junction and the gastric cardia. This retractor is placed in a subxiphoid incision, after a subxiphoid port has been removed, then the retractor is introduced transperitoneally by following its distal curve. Once positioned, this device is attached to a self-retaining mechanical arm [30].

Conclusion

Surgical median arcuate ligament release has been the mainstay of treatment for MALS, considering all available options. The surgical techniques for the MAL release include the open technique, the laparoscopic technique, and the robot-assisted approach. The laparoscopic release of MAL is technically feasible and seems to be an appealing modality in centers with experienced laparoscopic surgeons and surgical teams. The retrogastric or antegastric approach facilitates the exposure of the retrogastric surgical field. Approach to deep structures such as the MAL is challenging and can be performed by following either the crura of the diaphragm or the branches of celiac trunk. With the robotic approach, its superior visualization and improved degrees of freedom could represent the optimal treatment modality for MALS in institutions that are properly equipped for robotic surgery. There have been an increasing number of case reports and case series of laparoscopic division of the median arcuate ligament with included technical descriptions of the steps of the procedure [2, 3, 9, 10, 14, 18, 21]. No formal report, however, of the comparison of each technique for the MAL release has been published. The optimal technique for each patient may vary depending on the surgeon's experience, individual patient anatomy, and available equipment and may require switching between approaches during the case for the optimal efficacy and safety. Thus, familiarity with the available approaches prior to embarking on a procedure is well advised.

References

1. Delis KT, Gloviczki P, Altuwaijri M, McKusick MA. Median arcuate ligament syndrome: open celiac artery reconstruction and ligament division after endovascular failure. J Vasc Surg. 2007;46(4):799–802.
2. Roayaie S, Jossart G, Gitlitz D, et al. Laparoscopic release of celiac artery compression syndrome facilitated by laparoscopic ultrasound scanning to confirm restoration of flow. J Vasc Surg. 2000;32:814–7.
3. Carbonell AM, Kercher KW, Heniford BT, et al. Multimedia article. Laparoscopic management of median arcuate ligament syndrome. Surg Endosc. 2005;19:729.
4. Jimenez JC, Harlander-Locke M, Dutson EP. Open and laparoscopic treatment of median arcuate ligament syndrome. J Vasc Surg. 2012;56:869–73.
5. Ballantyne GH. Robotic surgery, telerobotic surgery, telepresence, and telementoring. Review of early clinical results. Surg Endosc. 2002;16:1389–402.
6. Jaik NP, Stawicki SP, Weger NS, Lukaszczyk JJ. Celiac artery compression syndrome: successful utilization of robotic-assisted laparoscopic approach. J Gastrointestin Liver Dis. 2007;16(1):93–6.
7. Roseborough GS. Laparoscopic management of celiac artery compression syndrome. J Vasc Surg. 2009;50:124–33.
8. Cina CS, Safar H. Successful treatment of recurrent celiac axis compression syndrome: a case report. Panminerva Med. 2002;44:69–72.
9. Tulloch AW, Jimenez JC, Lawrence PF, Dutson EP, Moore WS, Rigberg DA, et al. Laparoscopic versus open celiac ganglionectomy in patients with median arcuate ligament syndrome. J Vasc Surg. 2009;50:140–7.
10. You JS, Cooper M, Nishida S, Matsuda E, Murariu D. Treatment of median arcuate ligament syndrome via traditional and robotic techniques. Hawaii J Med Public Health. 2013; 72(8):279–81.
11. El Hayek KM, Titus J, Bui A, Mastracci T, Kroh M. Laparoscopic median arcuate ligament release: are we improving symptoms? J Am Coll Surg. 2013;216:272–9.
12. Baccari P, Civilini E, Dordoni L, Melissano G, Nicoletti R, Chiesa R. Celiac artery compression syndrome managed by laparoscopy. J Vasc Surg. 2009;50(1):134–9.
13. Vaziri K, Hungness ES, Pearson EG, Soper NJ. Laparoscopic treatment of celiac artery compression syndrome: case series and review of current treatment modalities. J Gastrointest Surg. 2009;13(2):293–8.
14. Berard X, Cau J, Déglise S, Trombert D, Saint-Lebes B, Midy D, et al. Laparoscopic surgery for coeliac artery compression syndrome: current management and technical aspects. Eur J Vasc Endovasc Surg. 2012;43(1):38–42.
15. Van Petersen AS, Vriens BH, Huisman AB, Kolkman JJ, Geelkerken RH. Retroperitoneal endoscopic release in the management of celiac artery compression syndrome. J Vasc Surg. 2009;50(1):140–7.
16. William G, Ramesh CR, Giselle H, Sayeed I, Philip RS. Operating room positioning, equipment, and instrumentation for laparoscopic bariatric surgery. In: Philip RS, Bruce DS, Stacy AB, editors. Minimally invasive bariatric surgery. New York: Springer; 2007. p. 87–103.
17. Said SM, Zarroug AE, Gloviczki P, Shields RC. Pediatric median arcuate ligament syndrome: first report of familial pattern and transperitoneal laparoscopic release. J Pediatr Surg. 2010;45:e17–20.
18. Joyce DD, Antiel RM, Oderich G, Gloviczki P, Tung J, Grothe R, Absah I, Zarroug AE. Pediatric median arcuate ligament syndrome: surgical outcomes and quality of life. J Laparoendosc Adv Surg Tech A. 2014;24:104–10.

19. Nguyen T, Neale M, Lane R, Schiavone V, Samra JS, Hugh TJ. Laparoscopic management of the median arcuate ligament syndrome. ANZ J Surg. 2012;82(4):265–8.
20. Kohn GP, Bitar RS, Farber MA, Marston WA, Overby DW, Farrell TM. Treatment options and outcomes for celiac artery compression syndrome. Surg Innov. 2011;18(4):338–43.
21. Wani S, Wakde V, Patel R, Patankar R, Mathur SK. Laparoscopic release of median arcuate ligament. J Minim Access Surg. 2012;8(1):16–8.
22. Antoniou GA, Riga CV, Mayer EK, Cheshire NJ, Bicknell CD. Clinical applications of robotic technology in vascular and endovascular surgery. J Vasc Surg. 2011;53:493–9.
23. Meyer M, Gharagozloo F, Nguyen D, Tempesta B, Strother E, Margolis M. Robotic-assisted treatment of celiac artery compression syndrome: report of a case and review of the literature. Int J Med Robot. 2012;8(4):379–83.
24. Do MV, Smith TA, Bazan HA, Sternbergh 3rd WC, Abbas AE, Richardson WS. Laparoscopic versus robot-assisted surgery for median arcuate ligament syndrome. Surg Endosc. 2013;27(11):4060–6.
25. Družijanić N, Pogorelić Z, Perko Z, Mrklić I, Tomić S. Comparison of lateral thermal damage of the human peritoneum using monopolar diathermy, Harmonic scalpel and LigaSure. Can J Surg. 2012;55(5):317–21.
26. Leigh N, Danial V. Principles of preoperative and operative surgery. In: Townsend Jr CM, Beauchamp RD, Mark Evers B, Mattox KL, editors. Sabiston textbook of surgery: the biological basis of modern surgical practice. 19th ed. Philadelphia: Elsevier Saunders; 2012. p. 236.
27. Awwad JT, Isaacson K. The harmonic scalpel: an intraoperative complication. Obstet Gynecol. 1996;88(4 Pt 2):718–20.
28. Kia H, Johanna M, Klaus J, Bernd K, Thilo S, Lena-Christin C, et al. Ultrasonic scalpel causes greater depth of soft tissue necrosis compared to monopolar electrocautery at standard power level settings in a pig model. BMC Surg. 2012;12:1.
29. Scott-Conner CEH. The SAGES manual: fundamentals of laparoscopy: thoracoscopy, and GI endoscopy. New York: Springer; 2006. p. 92.
30. Bann S, Butler A, Shaul T, Foley R. A technique for insertion of the laparoscopic Nathanson liver retractor. Ann R Coll Surg Engl. 2005;87(6):472–3.

Chapter 30
Results of Open and Laparoscopic Median Arcuate Ligament Release

Juan Carlos Jimenez and Erik P. Dutson

The first case of median arcuate ligament syndrome (MALS) was reported by Harjola in 1963, and Dunbar later described it as a distinct clinical syndrome in his landmark paper in 1965 [1, 2]. This condition is also referred to as celiac artery compression syndrome and Dunbar's syndrome. The median arcuate ligament (MAL) is comprised of a prominent fibrous arch, which traverses the aorta cephalad to the celiac artery origin and bridges the diaphragmatic crura. Preganglionic splanchnic nerves, somatic branches from the phrenic and vagus nerves, parasympathetic preganglionic nerves, and sympathetic postganglionic fibers form the celiac plexus or ganglion, which is immediately adjacent to the MAL.

Median arcuate ligament syndrome and its appropriate treatment continue to raise controversy within the field of vascular surgery. Its existence as a clinical syndrome has been questioned due to the variability of the clinical presentation and a response to treatment that is often difficult to predict. Patients with MALS traditionally present with a variety of chronic abdominal symptoms and radiographic evidence of celiac artery compression or impingement. The pathophysiology of this disorder is poorly understood, and its symptoms have been attributed to both ischemic and neurogenic etiologies. There is conflicting evidence supporting both mechanisms. Many patients with MALS complain of postprandial abdominal pain, thus suggesting a mechanism of disease related to end-organ ischemia. A rich and abundant collateral network in this anatomic region provides evidence against the

J.C. Jimenez, MD, FACS (✉)
Division of Vascular Surgery, Gonda (Goldschmied) Vascular Center, Ronald Reagan-UCLA Medical Center, Department of Surgery, Division of Vascular Surgery, David Geffen School of Medicine at UCLA, Los Angeles, CA, USA
e-mail: jcjimenez@mednet.ucla.edu

E.P. Dutson, MD
Department of Surgery, Ronald Reagan UCLA Medical Center, Los Angeles, CA, USA
e-mail: EDutson@mednet.ucla.edu

G.S. Oderich (ed.), *Mesenteric Vascular Disease*,
DOI 10.1007/978-1-4939-1847-8_30

notion of end-organ ischemia in patients with compression of the celiac artery. Neurogenic compression of the celiac plexus somatic nerves by the MAL may also produce abdominal pain, and therefore, celiac ganglionectomy and removal of somatic visceral nerves associated with ligament release could, in theory, provide pain relief, as does percutaneous celiac plexus block in patients with chronic abdominal pain.

Surgical treatment of MALS consists of division and release of the compressive MAL overlying the celiac artery with or without arterial revascularization. Results in the peer-reviewed literature have demonstrated that symptomatic relief is achieved in a large number of patients with and without reconstruction of the celiac artery [3–5]. Additionally, improvements in laparoscopic and robotic techniques have offered minimally invasive options for treatment of MALS.

Clinical Presentation and Radiographic Evaluation

Patients with MALS present with a variety of abdominal symptoms, which can make diagnosis and optimal patient selection challenging for the vascular surgeon. In a recent published review of the English language literature, we identified 20 retrospective series between 1963 and 2012 reporting outcomes following laparoscopic and open treatment of MALS [6]. Four hundred patients total were identified. In these studies, the most common presenting symptom was abdominal pain ($n=321$; 80 %). Postprandial pain was common; however, it is not present in all patients. Positional and constant pain were also described frequently. Additional signs and symptoms included weight loss ($n=192$; 48 %), abdominal bruit ($n=139$; 35 %), nausea ($n=39$; 9.7 %), and diarrhea ($n=30$; 7.5 %).

Several different radiographic modalities are commonly used to image the MAL and to demonstrate evidence of compression. In our review, abdominal angiography using inspiratory and expiratory views was the most common reported imaging modality used to diagnose MALS (49 %). Ultrasound (33 %) was also frequently used. Computed tomography and magnetic resonance were less commonly used to make the diagnosis. With recent improvements in noninvasive imaging (MR, CT, etc.) at our institution, it is being more routinely used prior to formal angiography. Of note, we routinely use magnetic resonance angiography with expiratory and inspiratory views at our institution during our preoperative assessment of these patients in conjunction with noninvasive duplex imaging.

Several authors have also described the use of gastric exercise tonometry, a measure of gastrointestinal ischemia, for both preoperative and postoperative evaluation in these patients [7]. In a study by Mensink and colleagues reporting outcomes following open MAL release, gastric exercise tomography studies were abnormal in 30 patients [4]. Forty-three patients total were noted to have significant celiac artery compression. After a median follow-up of 39 months, repeated tonometry improved in 100 % of patients who were free of symptoms postoperatively, compared with 25 % in patients with persistent complaints following MAL decompression. Thus, these findings support end-organ ischemia as a key pathophysiologic mechanism in patients with MALS.

Clinical Outcomes: Laparoscopic Division of the Median Arcuate Ligament

The majority of studies reporting outcomes following laparoscopic release of the MAL demonstrate favorable results and symptoms relief following surgical decompression [6]. It should be noted that the current peer-reviewed literature on this topic is largely comprised of small, single-institution series, which may contain significant publication bias toward favorable outcomes. This may magnify the true benefits and downplay the limitations of laparoscopic MAL release.

In our review of the published literature, we identified 121 patients between 1963 and 2012 who underwent laparoscopic MAL division [6]. Immediate postoperative symptomatic improvement was reported in 95 % of patients and only three patients underwent revascularization of the celiac artery (2.4 %). Late recurrence of symptoms (>6 months) was noted in 5.8 % of patients treated. Although the reported incidence of late recurrence in most series is low, a study by Tulloch and colleagues from our institution demonstrated that 50 % ($n=4$) of patients treated with laparoscopic decompression developed early recurrence of symptoms [8]. Three of these patients were noted to have persistent, postoperative celiac artery stenosis and underwent angioplasty and stenting. One patient continued to have postoperative pain despite radiographic evidence of celiac artery patency. Overall in the series, 88 % of patients were no longer taking chronic analgesic medication at a mean follow-up of 14 months.

Subsequent to our published review, other series have been published demonstrating successful outcomes with this technique. In a study by El-Hayek and colleagues, 15 patients underwent laparoscopic MAL release and one patient underwent a robotic-assisted laparoscopic approach (Table 30.1) [9]. The mean age was 34 years and the majority of patients were female (93 %). Ten patients demonstrated a statistically significant decrease in celiac artery velocities following MAL division. Quality of life surveys were returned postoperatively in 86 % of patients and only one patient reported no improvement following laparoscopic MAL release.

Another recent review by Do et al. reported outcomes following laparoscopic MAL release in 16 patients over a 6-year period [10]. Twelve patients were treated with a laparoscopic approach and four patients underwent a robotic-assisted approach. The most common presenting symptom was postprandial abdominal pain. Other symptoms included nausea, vomiting, and weight loss. Five patients had an abdominal bruit on physical examination. The majority of patients laparoscopically treated were women (75 %), and the majority of patients robotically treated were men (75 %). Mean operative times were shorter for the laparoscopic group

Table 30.1 Results of laparoscopic and robotic median arcuate ligament release

Author	Year	Patients	Mean follow-up (months)	Conversion to open	Laparoscopic ligament release	Robotic ligament release	Arterial reconstruc tion	Immediate clinical improvement	No immediate clinical improvement	Recurrence of symptoms
Mak et al.	2013	46	12	0	46	0	0	31	15	0
Joyce et al.	2013	6	13	0	6	0	0	6	6	0
Do et al.	2013	16	22	0	12	4	0	10	6	0
El Hayek et al.	2013	15	15	1	14	1	0	14	1	0
Bernard et al. [16]	2012	11	35	2	11	0	0	10	1	1
Aschenbach et al. [17]	2011	22	NA	0	22	0	0	22	0	NA
Tulloch [18]	2010	12	14	2	12	0	0	12	0	5
Van Petersen et al. [19]	2009	42	20	1	42	0	0	41	1	NA
Baccari et al. [20]	2009	16	28	2	16	0	3	14	2	0
Roseborough [21]	2009	15	44	4	15	0	0	14	1	1
Vaziri et al. [22]	2008	3	6	0	3	0	0	3	0	0
Totals		204	21	12	204	5	3	177	33	7

compared with the robotic-assisted group (101.7 min vs. 145.8 min; $p=0.2$). There was no significant difference in hospital length of stay between the two groups. Eight patients (67 %) in the laparoscopic group and two patients (50 %) in the robotic-assisted group had full symptomatic improvement.

Successful outcomes have also been reported following laparoscopic treatment of MALS in the pediatric population. The peer-reviewed literature is currently limited to two series (excluding case reports) reporting outcomes for MALS in children [11, 12]. In a recent review by Mak and colleagues, 46 pediatric patients (mean age 16.2±0.5 years) underwent laparoscopic release of the MAL [11]. In their series, the condition was more common in females (91 %) than males. Patients were screened with preoperative duplex and subsequent CTA if celiac artery compression was present on noninvasive imaging. Overall, 67 % of patients reported improvement of symptoms following their operation. No intraoperative conversions were required and there were no deaths reported in the series.

In another series by Joyce et al., six patients underwent laparoscopic treatment for MALS over a 3-year period [12]. Similar to Mak's study, the majority of patients were female (83.3 %) with an average age of 15.7±1.5 years. The most common symptoms were postprandial pain (83.3 %) and nausea/vomiting (83.3 %). Other presenting symptoms included epigastric pain (50 %), pain elevated with action (33.3 %), increased bowel activity (16.7 %), and diffuse abdominal pain (16.7 %). Mean operative time and hospital length of stay were 172.5 min and 1.3 days, respectively. Mean peak celiac artery flow (cm/s) was 332.0 preoperatively and decreased to 224.3 postoperatively. A significant improvement from pre- to postsurgical scores was observed in the physical functioning ($p=.03$), mental health ($p=.03$), and self-esteem categories ($p=.03$) of the child assessment. Similarly, there was a significant postsurgical improvement in all categories pertaining to the parent's quality of life ($p=.03$). Improvement was also seen in the parents' perception of their child's physical functioning ($p=.03$), bodily pain/discomfort ($p=.03$), mental health ($p=.03$), and general health perceptions ($p=.03$). No intraoperative or postoperative complications occurred. No patient required celiac artery reconstruction and/or revascularization.

Clinical Outcomes of Open Division of the Median Arcuate Ligament

In our review of the published literature, we identified 279 patients between 1963 and 2012 who underwent open MAL division (Table 30.2) [6]. Arterial reconstruction was performed in 72 patients. Of these patients, 223 (80 %) were reported to have immediate symptomatic improvement and late recurrence of symptoms occurred in 22 patients (9.8 %). The incidence of major postoperative complications noted in our review was 6.5 %. Thrombosed arterial bypass grafts were the most complication (2 %). Other complications included stroke (1.4 %), postoperative

Table 30.2 Results following open release of the median arcuate ligament

Authors	Year	Patients	Mean follow-up (months)	MAL release	Arterial reconstruction	Immediate clinical improvement	No immediate clinical improvement	Recurrence of symptoms
Sultan et al.	2013	11	60	11	3	8	3	0
Tulloch et al.	2010	6	10	6	2	5	1	3
Grotemeyer et al.	2009	18	41	18	7	14	4	0
Mensink	2006	29	39	29	7	24	5	0
Schweizer et al. [23]	2005	8	Range 36–216	8	0	8	0	0
Geelkerken et al.	1990	11	229	11	0	11	0	8
Williams et al. [24]	1985	11	24	11	7	9	2	1
Reilly et al.	1984	51	108	51	35	30	14	14
Rogers et al. [25]	1981	8	60	8	1	6	2	0
Plate et al. [26]	1980	15	Range 18–114	15	0	10	5	NA
Watson et al. [27]	1977	20	27	20	11	18	2	1
Stanley et al. [28]	1971	12	Range 4–42	12	2	9	3	
Marable et al. [29]	1968	30	31	30	0	27	3	NA
Dunbar et al.	1965	13	10	13	0	13	0	NA
Total		290	64	290	75	231	52	27

gastroesophageal reflux disease (1 %), pancreatitis (1 %), hemothorax (0.3 %), and splenic infarction (0.3 %). No procedure-related deaths occurred in any of the papers reviewed for open treatment of MAL.

The landmark study reporting outcomes following open treatment of MAL syndrome was published by Reilly and colleagues in 1985 [13]. This paper is the largest series of patients treated for MAL in the peer-reviewed literature. Fifty-one patients underwent operative treatment for symptomatic celiac artery compression. The majority of patients were female ($n=31$, 76 %). The most common presenting symptom was abdominal pain although atypical pain symptoms were quite diverse in this patient population. These included severe cramping, burning, radiation to the back, and position-related changes. Weight loss occurred in 61 % of the patients and averaged approximately 20 lbs. An epigastric bruit was present in 84 % of patients. The majority of patients in this series (84 %) had undergone prior abdominal operations. Six patients had a documented history of a psychiatric disorder and nine patients had a history of alcohol abuse. Preoperative lateral aortography with inspiratory and expiratory views was performed in all patients prior to operative repair.

Fifty-one patients underwent 55 surgical procedures for division of the MAL in this series. Sixteen patients underwent division of the MAL and celiac ganglionectomy alone. Division of the MAL and the celiac ganglion was performed in conjunction with transceliac arterial dilatation in 17 patients. Celiac artery reconstruction was performed in 18 patients through either resection and primary anastomosis (7 patients) or bypass (11 patients). Saphenous vein and arterial autografts were used as the conduit in the majority of patients ($n=10$).

Forty-four (86 %) patients were available for late follow-up with mean of 9 years. Thirty-three of the patients (77 %) were available for more than 5 years and 20 patients (47 %) were followed for at least 10 years. The authors noted that 68 % of patients were asymptomatic at late follow-up and 32 % had persistent symptoms. Patients who underwent some form of celiac revascularization were more likely to be asymptomatic compared with patients who underwent celiac decompression alone (76 % vs. 53 %, respectively). Late follow-up angiograms in 18 patients demonstrated a widely patent celiac artery in 70 % of asymptomatic patients but a stenosed or occluded celiac artery in 75 % of symptomatic patients. A postprandial pain pattern was associated more often with postoperative symptomatic improvement. Clinical variables associated with worse outcomes were an atypical pain pattern, a history of a psychiatric disorder or alcohol abuse, age greater than 60, and weight loss less than 20 lbs.

A more recent series by Grotemeyer and colleagues demonstrated similar excellent clinical outcomes in a series of 18 patients treated with open MAL division [14]. In this study, 83.3 % of patients were female and the mean age was 46.2 years. All patients were treated with an open surgical technique and 11 underwent a concomitant arterial reconstruction. Mean follow-up was 3.5 years and 15 patients were available for late postoperative evaluation. Eleven of the fifteen patients (73.3 %) were completely free of abdominal symptoms and nine patients gained weight following their operation. Of the 11 patients (55 %) with successful outcomes following surgery, 6 of them had undergone celiac decompression only.

Thus, these outcomes differ slightly from Reilly's series where the majority of patients who were symptom-free underwent some type of arterial reconstruction.

In contrast to the series' mentioned demonstrating good long-term success with open MAL division, Geelkerken and coauthors reported a high rate of recurrence with this technique in their paper published in the *British Journal of Surgery* [15]. In their series, 11 patients underwent open division of the MAL for presumed celiac artery compression syndrome. They noted that three months later, 27 % of patients had recurrent abdominal symptoms. Long-term follow-up (between 15 and 23 years) was available for 8 patients. All eight patients had recurrent symptoms similar to those present prior to their operation. These results are somewhat similar to a series at our institution, which demonstrated late symptomatic recurrence of 50 % following open repair and 42 % following laparoscopic MAL division [8].

Conclusions

The available peer-reviewed evidence demonstrates that division of the MAL in patients with median arcuate ligament syndrome may result in continued symptom relief in the majority of patients. The syndrome appears to have a female predominance and a wide array of presenting clinical symptoms. Arterial reconstruction has been reported to have a positive effect on clinical improvement following open MAL release; however, series reporting outcomes following the laparoscopic approach have demonstrated good results without the need for revascularization. The pathophysiology of this disorder is still not well understood and one of the biggest challenges for the vascular surgeon treating this condition is selecting the optimal patient and predicting successful outcomes. Because the majority of papers are small, single-institution studies, the likelihood that treatment failures and complications are underreported is high. Although there have been no deaths reported following laparoscopic MAL division, open conversion for bleeding from the perivisceral aorta is a potentially morbid and life-threatening complication that needs to be discussed with patients undergoing this procedure.

References

1. Harjola PT. A rare obstruction of the coeliac artery. Report of a case. Ann Chir Gynaecol Fenn. 1963;52:547–50.
2. Dunbar JD, Molnar W, Beman FF, Marable SA. Compression of the celiac trunk and abdominal angina. Am J Roentgenol Radium Ther Nucl Med. 1965;95:731–44.
3. You JS, Cooper M, Nishida S, Matsuda E, Murariu D. Treatment of median arcuate ligament syndrome via traditional and robotic techniques. Hawaii J Med Public Health. 2013;72:279–81.
4. Sultan S, Hynes N, Elsafty N, Tawfick W. Eight years experience in the management of median arcuate ligament syndrome by decompression, celiac ganglion sympathectomy, and selective revascularization. Vasc Endovascular Surg. 2013;47:614–9.

5. Skeik N, Cooper LT, Duncan AA, Jabr F. Median arcuate ligament syndrome: a nonvascular vascular diagnosis. Vasc Endovascular Surg. 2011;45:433–7.
6. Jimenez JC, Harlander-Locke M, Dutson EP. Open and laparoscopic treatment of median arcuate ligament syndrome. J Vasc Surg. 2012;56:869–73.
7. Mensink PB, van Petersen AS, Kolkman JJ, Otte JA, Huisman AB, Geelkerken RH. Gastric exercise tonometry: the key investigation in patients with suspected celiac artery compression syndrome. J Vasc Surg. 2006;44:277–81.
8. Tulloch AW, Jimenez JC, Lawrence PF, Dutson EP, Moore WS, Rigberg DA, et al. Laparoscopic versus open celiac ganglionectomy in patients with median arcuate ligament syndrome. J Vasc Surg. 2009;50:140–7.
9. El Hayek KM, Titus J, Bui A, Mastracci T, Kroh M. Laparoscopic median arcuate ligament release: are we improving symptoms? J Am Coll Surg. 2013;216:272–9.
10. Do MV, Smith TA, Bazan HA, Sternbergh 3rd WC, Abbas AE, Richardson WS. Laparoscopic versus robot-assisted surgery for median arcuate ligament syndrome. Surg Endosc. 2013;27:4060–6.
11. Mak GZ, Speaker C, Anderson K, Stiles-Shields C, Lorenz J, Drossos T, Liu DC, Skelly CL. Median arcuate ligament syndrome in the pediatric population. J Pediatr Surg. 2013;48: 2261–70.
12. Joyce DD, Antiel RM, Oderich G, Gloviczki P, Tung J, Grothe R, Absah I, Zarroug AE. Pediatric median arcuate ligament syndrome: surgical outcomes and quality of life. J Laparoendosc Adv Surg Tech A. 2014;24:104–10.
13. Reilly LM, Ammar AD, Stoney RJ, Ehrenfeld WK. Late results following operative repair for celiac artery compression syndrome. J Vasc Surg. 1985;2:79–91.
14. Grotemeyer D, Duran M, Iskandar F, Blondin D, Nguyen K, Sandmann W. Median arcuate ligament syndrome: vascular surgical therapy and follow up of 18 patients. Langenbecks Arch Surg. 2009;394:1085–92.
15. Geelkerken RH, van Bockel JH, de Roos WK, Hermans J. Coeliac artery compression syndrome: the effect of decompression. Br J Surg. 1990;77:807–9.
16. Berard X, Cau J, Déglise S, Trombert D, Saint-Lebes B, Midy D, Corpataux JM, Ricco JB. Laparoscopic surgery for coeliac artery compression syndrome: current management and technical aspects. Eur J Vasc Endovasc Surg. 2012;43(1):38–42.
17. Aschenbach R, Basche S, Vogl TJ. Compression of the celiac trunk caused by median arcuate ligament in children and adolescent subjects: evaluation with contrast-enhanced MR angiography and comparison with Doppler US evaluation. J Vasc Interv Radiol. 2011;22(4):556–61.
18. Tulloch AW, Jimenez JC, Lawrence PF, Dutson EP, Moore WS, Rigberg DA, Derubertis BG, Quinones-Baldrich WJ. Laparoscopic versus open celiac ganglionectomy in patients with median arcuate ligament syndrome. J Vasc Surg. 2010;52(5):1283–9.
19. van Petersen AS, Vriens BH, Huisman AB, Kolkman JJ, Geelkerken RH. Retroperitoneal endoscopic release in the management of celiac artery compression syndrome. J Vasc Surg. 2009;50(1):140–7.
20. Baccari P, Civilini E, Dordoni L, Melissano G, Nicoletti R, Chiesa R. Celiac artery compression syndrome managed by laparoscopy. J Vasc Surg. 2009;50(1):134–9.
21. Roseborough GS. Laparoscopic management of celiac artery compression syndrome. J Vasc Surg. 2009;50(1):124–33.
22. Vaziri K, Hungness ES, Pearson EG, Soper NJ. Laparoscopic treatment of celiac artery compression syndrome: case series and review of current treatment modalities. J Gastrointest Surg. 2009;13(2):293–8. doi:10.1007/s11605-008-0702-9. Epub 2008 Sep 26. Review.
23. Schweizer P, Berger S, Schweizer M, Schaefer J, Beck O. Arcuate ligament vascular compression syndrome in infants and children. J Pediatr Surg. 2005;40(10):1616–22.
24. Williams S, Gillespie P, Little JM. Celiac axis compression syndrome: factors predicting a favorable outcome. Surgery. 1985;98(5):879–87.
25. Rogers DM, Thompson JE, Garrett WV, Talkington CM, Patman RD. Mesenteric vascular problems. A 26-year experience. Ann Surg. 1982;195(5):554–65.

26. Plate G, Eklöf B, Vang J. The celiac compression syndrome: myth or reality? Acta Chir Scand. 1981;147(3):201–3.
27. Watson WC, Sadikali F. Celiac axis compression: experience with 20 patients and a critical appraisal of the syndrome. Ann Intern Med. 1977;86(3):278–84.
28. Stanley JC, Fry WJ. Median arcuate ligament syndrome. Arch Surg. 1971;103(2):252–8.
29. Marable SA, Kaplan MF, Beman FM, Molnar W. Celiac compression syndrome. Am J Surg. 1968;115(1):97–102.

Part VII
Isolated Mesenteric Artery Dissection

Chapter 31
Clinical Presentation, Etiology, and Diagnostic Considerations of Isolated Visceral Artery Dissections

Ying Huang and Peter Gloviczki

Isolated visceral artery dissection (IVAD) is an uncommon disease with an unpredictable natural history. It is a rare cause of abdominal pain but failure to diagnose it may have disastrous consequences. IVAD includes dissections of the celiac and superior mesenteric arteries (SMA), renal arteries, the inferior mesenteric artery (IMA), and their branches. Although visceral artery dissections can occur with aortic dissections, IVAD has a pathology that is frequently different from that of acute aortic dissection [1–6]. In some of the published literature, the term of "splanchnic artery dissection" was used, which refers to dissection of celiac artery, SMA, or IMA [7–9]. They are four to ten times more common in men than in women and they are more frequently discovered in patients in their fifth to sixth decade of life [2–5, 7, 9–11].

Serious sequelae of IVAD can be rupture and organ ischemia depending on the location and progression of the dissection. Early recognition and appreciation of IVAD are important and will help to initiate an optimal management to prevent life-threatening complications. In this chapter, we will discuss this rare pathology and present the epidemiology, clinical presentation, etiology, and diagnostic considerations of IVAD.

Pathology

In general, dissection starts with a structural weakness in the outer media adjacent to the external elastic media. Once an intimal tear has developed, the intramural hematoma extends longitudinally within the outer media on a course parallel to the

Y. Huang, MD, PhD • P. Gloviczki, MD (✉)
Division of Vascular and Endovascular Surgery, Mayo Clinic, Rochester, MN, USA
e-mail: huang.ying@mayo.edu; gloviczki.peter@mayo.edu

G.S. Oderich (ed.), *Mesenteric Vascular Disease*,
DOI 10.1007/978-1-4939-1847-8_31

blood flow [12]. Secondary ischemia of the media follows the dissection plane and this process disrupts the vasa vasorum of the artery and occasionally induces an aneurysm. The natural course of IVAD is variable and can be limited or it also can progress to thrombosis of the false lumen or to progressive dissection of the vessel, rapid expansion of false lumen with resultant narrowed or obliterated true lumen, or rupture through the adventitia [12–14].

Epidemiology

In a series of 6,666 autopsy cases, the incidence of superior mesenteric artery dissection (SMAD) was 0.06 % [15], a number that is most likely underestimated because of lack of reliable clinical signs and laboratory findings. The incidence of spontaneous renal artery dissection (RAD) was only 0.036–0.049 % of all arterial dissections [16]. Although still rare, reports of IVAD have increased in recent years, largely due to more frequent use of computed tomographic angiography (CTA) [10, 17–22] or magnetic resonance angiography (MRA) [23, 24]. Among the reported dissections of visceral arteries, SMAD has been the most frequent; [5, 7–10, 14, 25–28] dissection of hepatic and splenic artery or IMA is extremely rare, with a number of reported cases of 23 [29, 30], 13 [31], and one [32], respectively, in the English language literature.

Luan et al. reviewed the English language literature and found that 296 patients with isolated SMAD have been reported since Bauerfield et al. first described the disease in 1947; [33] 11 patients (4 %) were diagnosed at autopsy until 1972, there were 35 (12 %) between 1975 and 2001, and 250 (84 %) since 2002 [11].

Clinical Presentation

IVAD shows broad clinical presentations ranging from asymptomatic incidental findings on an abdominal CTA to bowel necrosis or a rupture of a dissecting aneurysm, depending on the location of the dissection, the extent of visceral artery involvement, and the severity of ischemic changes of the abdominal organs. IVAD can be classified as acute and chronic, and if the disease is symptomatic, abdominal pain is the most frequent symptom in most patients.

Superior Mesenteric Artery Dissection (SMAD)

The clinical manifestations of SMAD are diverse. In the acute stage, most patients present with a sudden onset of severe abdominal and/or back pain. The pain is first caused by the dissection itself, which stimulates the mesenteric artery nociceptors.

Table 31.1 Clinical presentations of 296 patients with superior mesenteric artery dissection [11]

Symptom	Number of patients (%)
Abdominal pain	231 (78)
Nausea	27 (9.1)
Vomiting	21 (7.1)
Ileus	11 (3.7)
Bloody stool	10 (3.4)
Diarrhea	8 (2.7)
Emaciation	6 (2.0)
Asymptomatic	47 (16)

Another type of pain, which usually develops somewhat later, is related to intestinal ischemia or a mesenteric hematoma. Other common symptoms are nausea, vomiting, and chronic abdominal pain. Postprandial abdominal pain and bloody stool can be observed if the SMA is stenotic or occluded and in advanced stages when ischemia-induced intestinal mucosal necrosis occurs. Chronic mesenteric ischemia may also present with diarrhea or constipation and weight loss [4, 11, 12, 34–41]. The disease may either regress to an asymptomatic stage or progress to more extensive occlusion of the SMA or a dissecting aneurysm with the risk of bowel ischemia or arterial rupture [34, 35, 42–44].

Luan et al. [11] reviewed 296 patients with SMAD and found that abdominal pain was the most common presentation accounting for 78 % of all symptoms. The cause of the abdominal pain was found to be intestinal ischemia, vasospasm, dissection itself, or an inflammatory response that stimulates the visceral nerve plexus. Other atypical accompanying symptoms are listed in Table 31.1.

On physical examination, patients are usually tender to palpation in the epigastrium or left upper quadrant. Although Froment et al. [45] reported an audible bruit in 17 % of their patients, it was present in only 3.0 % in the review by Luan et al. [11] In a series of 27 patients, recently reported by Kim and associates, periumbilical tenderness was found in 33 % of patients and none had rebound tenderness or peritonitis [41].

Celiac Artery Dissection (CAD)

Approximately one half of the patients with CAD are asymptomatic due to good collateral flow from the SMA [46]. The symptoms are usually nonspecific epigastric pain or postprandial abdominal pain. Sudden onset of epigastric or subcostal pain that resolves spontaneously within 1–5 days is an important sign; it is usually caused by irritation of the celiac nerve plexus or initial contained rupture of the aneurysm [47].

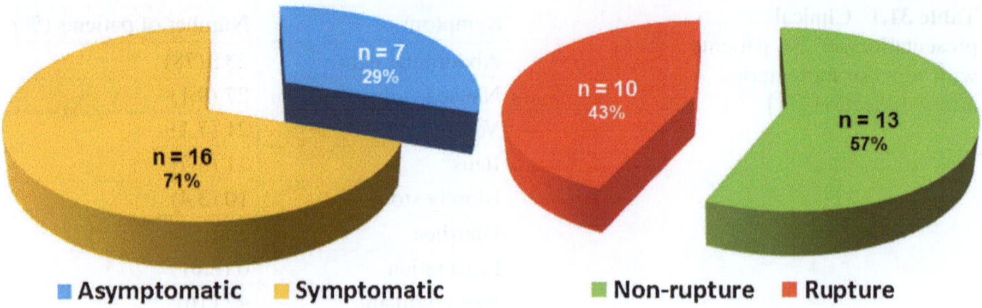

Fig. 31.1 Clinical presentation of 23 reported isolated hepatic artery dissections [29, 30]

In some patients, an abdominal systolic bruit is present [48], although it is a rare finding that may be caused by associated SMA stenosis [47]. The celiac trunk divides into the left gastric artery, the splenic, and the common hepatic arteries (see Chap. 2 on splanchnic artery anatomy), thus all organs downstream of the dissected celiac trunk may suffer from ischemia depending on the involvement and compromised portion of the branch arteries. The clinical picture may include ischemic pancreatitis, gangrenous cholecystitis, ischemic gastropathy, liver ischemia, splenic ischemia with infarctions [49], or a life-threatening hemorrhage due to a rupture of the dissected artery or aneurysm [25, 27, 48, 50–54].

Of the reported 23 cases with hepatic artery dissection (HAD), 71 % have been symptomatic, typically presenting with pain in the epigastrium and right subcostal space (Fig. 31.1). Rupture with abdominal pain and shock occurred in 43 % of cases and rapidly caused death in all cases [29, 30]. Symptoms of splenic artery dissection are usually atypical and may also cause rupture and death of the patient.

The physical examinations and laboratory findings of most patients have been unremarkable except for epigastric tenderness [27, 51, 52]. However, spontaneous CADs must not be overlooked since complications are severe and include extension of the dissection into adjacent vessels, expansion of the false lumen, hemorrhage or organ ischemia, and the development of a celiac or hepatic artery aneurysm. Expansion of a false lumen may lead to rupture or it can result in poor distal perfusion due to compression of the true lumen [8]. Signs of acute liver ischemia are poor prognostic factors and they are associated with death in more than 40 % of the reported cases [47].

Renal Artery Dissections (RAD)

RAD can present either acutely or chronically; the clinical manifestations may vary from sudden onset of severe, persistent, and poorly controlled hypertension to acute flank pain ipsilateral to the site of dissection. Renal ischemia or infarction is a common finding in the acute setting; it occurs in approximately 40 % of the patients [55].

Nonspecific presentations include groin and/or testicular pain, headache, nausea, vomiting, fever, dysuria, hematuria, and blurry vision and these often lead to a delay in diagnosis [55–61]. Chronic RAD is typically encountered during evaluation for renovascular hypertension [56]; either it is asymptomatic or it is a cause of renovascular hypertension [62, 63]. Beroniade and colleagues described three different clinical sequelae of RAD: silent with no apparent ramifications, acute occlusion leading to renal infarction, and chronic dissection leading to renovascular hypertension [16].

Etiology

Compared to aortic dissection which is more common and widely studied, the underlying causes of IVAD are less well known. Possible etiologic factors of IVAD include arteriosclerosis, fibromuscular dysplasia (FMD), inflammatory or infectious disease, cystic medial degeneration (Marfan syndrome), segmental mediolysis arteriopathy, elastic tissue vasculitis, connective tissue disorders (Ehlers-Danlos syndrome) or vasculitis (giant cell arteritis, Takayasu arteritis, and polyarteritis), trauma including iatrogenic injury, hypertension, pregnancy, and a previous surgical history [10, 13, 19, 43, 48, 54, 64–74]. In cases with neither serologic evidence of vasculitis, connective tissue disorders, and inflammatory disorders nor traumatic injury including iatrogenic injury, dissections are classified as "spontaneous."

Superior Mesenteric Artery Dissection (SMAD)

Compared to other IVADs, the etiology of SMAD has been studied the most extensively. SMAD is reported to be most prevalent in Asian ($n = 222$), followed by North American ($n = 36$), European ($n = 29$), and South American ($n = 1$) countries; [11] also, the majority of recent English language publications are from China [24, 39, 40, 74, 75] and South Korea [5, 41, 44]. Given the paucity of reports from the Western countries, this may reflect a possible genetic predisposition to SMAD in the Asian population. Rare causes of SMAD included strangulation due to seat belt injury [65, 76], iatrogenic injury such as contrast passage-induced or aggravated dissection during angiography or stent placement [42, 77–79], dissection after pancreaticoduodenectomy [80], or liver transplantation [81].

With respect to spontaneous isolated SMAD, Solis et al. found that shearing stress was an important mechanism because dissection commonly begins 15–30 mm from the orifice of the SMA, right between the fixed retropancreatic portion of the artery and the more distal mobile portion [65]. On a computer-simulation model, Park et al. [43] observed abnormal mechanical stresses on the anterior wall of convex curvature of the SMA and suggested this might be another possible etiology for dissection. Gender, social habit, and comorbidity may also relate to SMAD [43, 74].

In a series of 51 patients with spontaneous isolated SMAD compared with 38 patients with combined aortic and SMA dissection, Park and colleagues found that spontaneous isolated SMAD was more common in men (90 % vs 71 %, $P=.02$) and occurs less frequently with hypertension (31 % vs 66 %, $P=.001$) [43]. Similar observations were also reported by Li et al. [74]. Spontaneous isolated SMAD was reported to be more frequent in patients with intra-abdominal cancers [43] and in those with a smoking history [74].

Celiac Artery Dissection (CAD) and Hepatic Artery Dissection (HAD)

Spontaneous CAD has typically been associated with hypertension, arteriosclerosis, degeneration of the arterial wall, trauma, pregnancy, and arteriopathy; however, most cases can present without identifiable risk factor [7, 46, 47, 69, 82–84]. Some patients have type IV Ehlers-Danlos syndrome (EDS) [21, 85], also known as the vascular type; it is a rare connective tissue disorder with autosomal dominant transmission (McKusick catalog number 130050) caused by mutations in the COL3A1 gene, resulting in structural alteration of type III collagen [86]. Rare causes of CAD include microtrauma caused by a sudden increase in abdominal pressure, such as weight lifting [47, 84, 87], and rupture of a pancreaticoduodenal arcade aneurysm [88]. Isolated HAD was observed to develop during pregnancy [89] or during selective arteriography done for radioembolization [90].

Renal Artery Dissection (RAD)

RAD is predominantly associated with FMD, especially in chronic cases. Other causes include EDS and atherosclerosis; [2, 55–58, 60] however, many cases present in otherwise healthy individuals [91–94]. Although FMD itself has a female predominance [2], the largest published series of 24 RADs from Mayo Clinic showed a 10:1 male-to-female ratio; [2] this and other publication suggest RAD is a male-predominant disorder [58, 60]. In the first systematic study that included 17 patients, RAD patients were more likely to have history of hypertension, cancer, and connective tissue disorders ($P<.001$), and less likely to have obesity (BMI $\geq$30 kg/m^2), compared with the general population [60]. RAD occurred most frequently in middle-aged men, with a history of hypertension, flank pain, elevated creatinine, and uncontrolled blood pressure at presentation. Associated connective tissue disorders in this study included FMD, EDS, polyarteritis nodosa, gout, or arthritis.

Different types of trauma have also been reported to cause RAD, ranging from blunt trauma to playing football and running marathons [91, 93–96] to iatrogenic trauma due to mal-deployment of endograft during endovascular aneurysm repair (EVAR) [97]. Rare causes included subadventitial angioma of the renal artery [98, 99], cocaine abuse [100], and extracorporeal shock wave lithotripsy [101].

Diagnostic Considerations

Since the clinical presentation is diverse and the disease is rare, early diagnosis of IVAD is rarely established. A thorough history taking and physical examination are essential. Noninvasive imaging studies such as duplex ultrasound (DUS), CTA, MRA, or contrast arteriography are indicated in symptomatic patients suspicious for IVAD. In asymptomatic patients, the diagnosis of IVAD is established only when imaging studies are performed to investigate other abdominal pathologies. Laboratory studies are usually within normal ranges unless ischemic changes of splanchnic organs develop.

Duplex Ultrasound Scanning (DUS)

DUS is a useful tool in the initial assessment of a suspected IVAD or in those patients in whom renal function is compromised. Duplex scanning of the visceral arteries may be helpful in identifying the intimal flap (Figs. 31.2 and 31.3) and the entry or reentry points [11]. DUS is used to assess the flow velocities and resistive index in the renal arteries as well as to evaluate end-organ vascularity. The intestinal wall can also be assessed with a high degree of accuracy by high-resolution

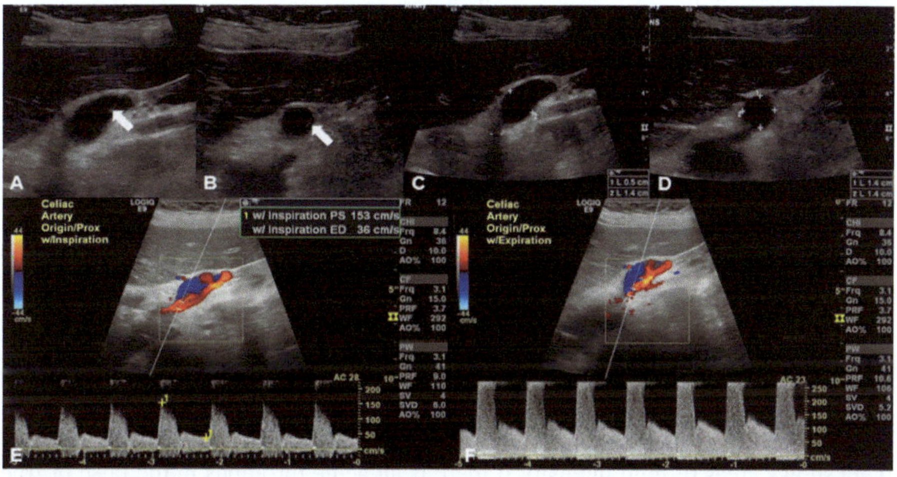

Fig. 31.2 Celiac artery dissection with high-grade stenosis in the proximal celiac artery and distal celiac artery aneurysm. Note changes in flow velocity with inspiration and expiration suggesting median arcuate ligament compression. (**a, b**) *Arrow* indicates intimal flap of the celiac artery dissection. (**c, d**) 1.4 cm celiac artery aneurysm that measured 2.7 cm in length. (**e**) Peak velocity measures 153 cm/s at inspiration. (**f**) Peak velocity measures 401 cm/s at expiration

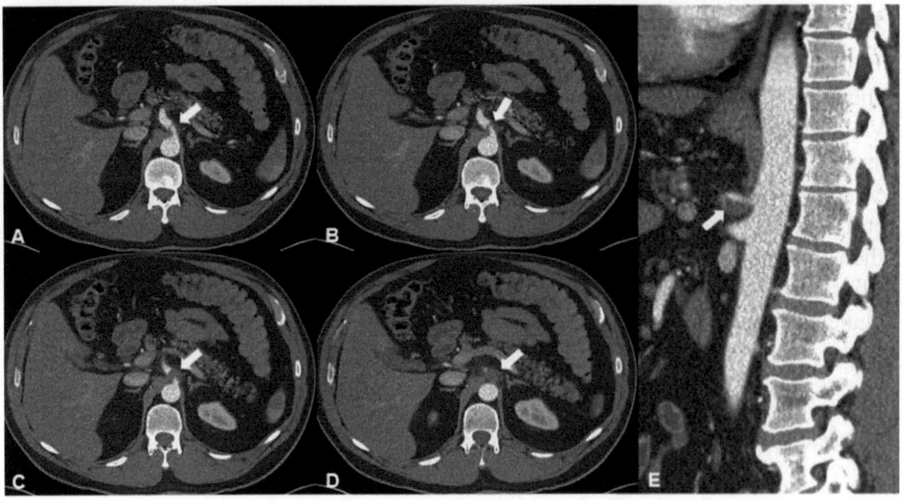

Fig. 31.3 Celiac artery dissection (CAD) extending into the entire splenic artery. (**a**, **b**) *Arrow* indicates intimal flap of the CAD. Within the proximal celiac artery, there is an asymmetric filling defect suggestive of thrombosis. (**c**, **d**) Thrombosed false lumen. (**e**) Thrombosis involving the inferior aspect of the proximal celiac artery with moderate luminal narrowing on sagittal view

transabdominal ultrasound. Transmural hemorrhage, inflammation, and necrotic thickening in the bowel wall can be imaged sonographically [102]. However, this technique is operator-dependent and does not provide the necessary detail to make treatment decisions, considering the anatomy of the affected visceral arteries and their branches, obese patients, patients with considerable bowel gas, and the diagnosis of IVAD may be missed as well. In patients with RAD, preoperative DUS can be performed to evaluate the size of the kidneys, measure the intraparenchymal resistive indexes, and detect renal infarcts which typically appear as wedge-shaped, hypoechoic lesions with absent blood flow on DUS.

Computed Tomographic Angiography (CTA)

When an IVAD is suspected, CTA is the first-line diagnostic modality. CT imaging progressed by leaps and bounds in the past decade, especially with the introduction of interactive multiplanar reconstruction (MPR) /maximum intensity projection (MIP)/3-dimensional (3D) rendering [17, 18, 21, 68]. Plain computed tomography (CT) shows areas of high intensity if there is an acute thrombus in the false or true lumens. Dynamic enhanced CT is helpful to separate the true lumen from the false lumen by an intimal flap [36]. Modern multidetector CT enables imaging with excellent spatial and temporal resolution. In addition to being quick and accurate, it provides the detailed information including intimal flap, anatomy, mural thrombosis, intramural hematoma, true and false lumen, and compromised visceral arteries

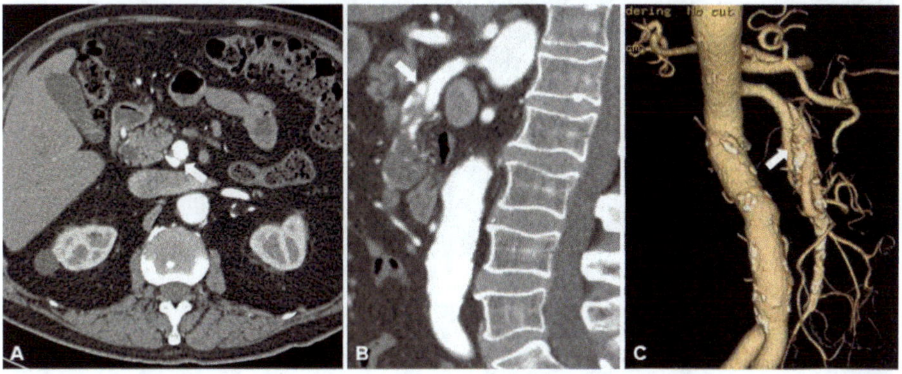

Fig. 31.4 Superior mesenteric artery dissection (SMAD) and aneurysmal dilatation, involving the mid SMA. *Arrow* indicates intimal flap of the SMAD. (**a**) Intimal flap of SMAD on axial view. (**b**) Intimal flap of SMAD on sagittal view; the aneurysm contains significant amount of mural thrombus proximally and completely thrombosed distally. (**c**) Intimal flap of SMAD on 3D reconstruction and moderate amount of peripheral calcification of SMA

with accuracy [21, 39]. An intimal flap separating the proximal portion of the visceral arteries into true and false lumen is a definitive diagnostic finding (Figs. 31.2, 31.3, 31.4, and 31.5); infiltration of the fat surrounding the affected vessel is a well-known secondary sign of acute spontaneous dissection of a visceral artery.

In patients with SMAD, the dissection usually starts within 5–50 mm from the original site [3, 9, 24, 26, 39, 65], where the SMA transitions from an immobile status to a mobile status along the inferior pancreatic margin. At this site, as mentioned before, there is increased shearing force, which may contribute to the intimal tear. The length of SMAD usually varies from 10 to 160 mm [3, 35, 39].

Reviewing CT findings of 34 patients, Jung et al. pointed out that intimal flap, thrombosed false lumen, and aneurysmal dilatation are the most common findings of IVAD [9]. In the symptomatic group, the mean distance from the orifice of the SMA to the intimal flap in 17 SMADs was 19.7 mm (range 6–43 mm); the mean values of the largest diameter and the length of the dissecting artery were 14.7 mm (range 8.4–50 mm) and 85.4 mm (range 33–180 mm), respectively. In four patients with CAD, the mean distance from the orifice to the site of dissection was 10.8 mm (range 9–12 mm). The mean values of the largest diameter and the length of the dissecting artery were 14 mm (range 11–20 mm) and 27.8 mm (range 21–40 mm), respectively. The largest diameter and the length of the dissecting artery in the asymptomatic group were significantly smaller than those of the symptomatic group.

In a recent study of 24 SMADs, an intimal flap which separated the SMA into a true lumen and a false lumen was observed in 83 % of patients; increased SMA diameter occurred in 63 %, 75 % had stenosis of the true lumen, thrombosed false lumen was seen in 63 %, and dissecting aneurysm was present in 30 % [75]. In another study of 27 SMADs, a patent false lumen with both entry and reentry was documented in 19 % of the patients, and partially or completely thrombosed false lumen presented in 81 %; the mean percent of compression of the true lumen occurred in 62 % [41].

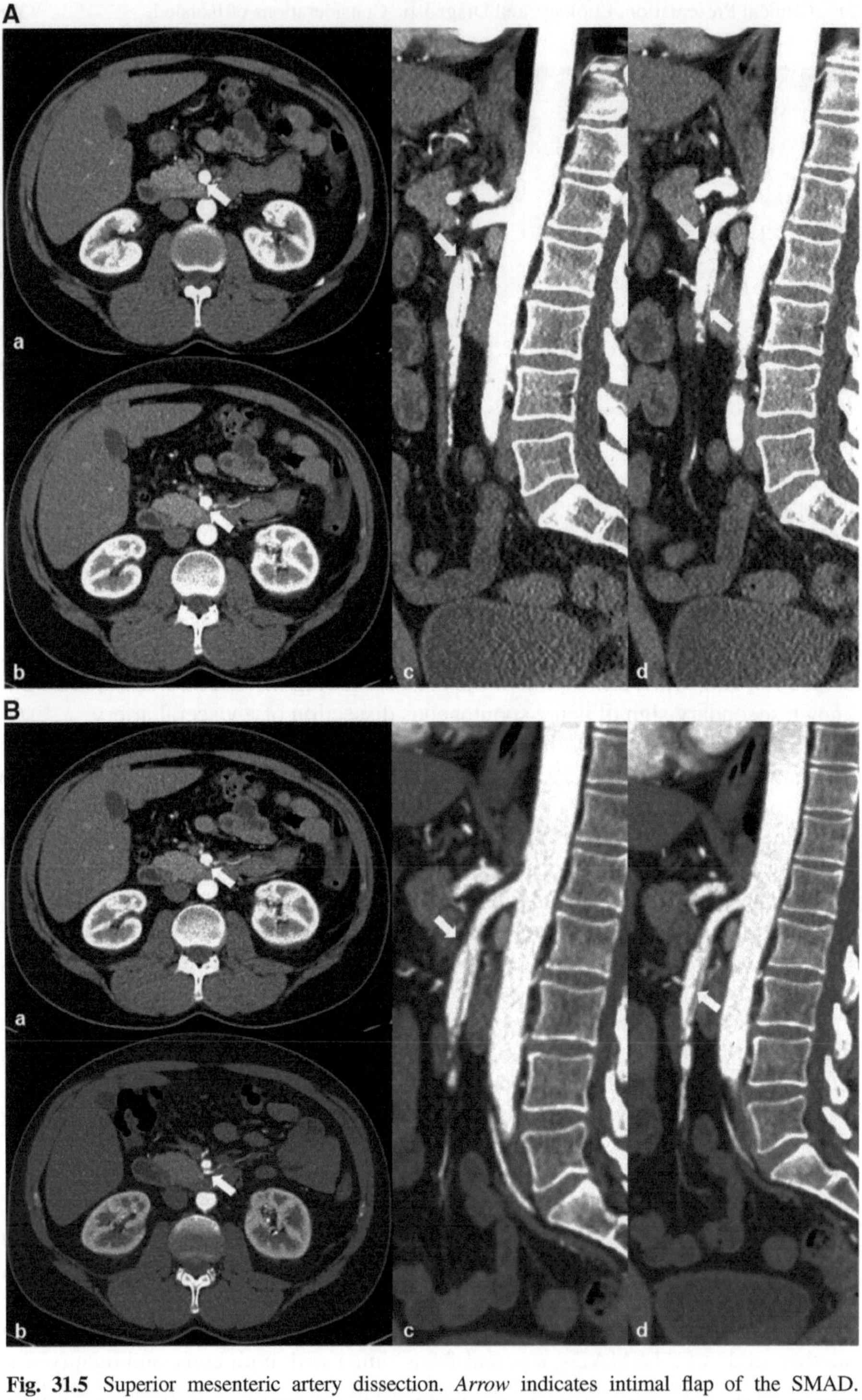

Fig. 31.5 Superior mesenteric artery dissection. *Arrow* indicates intimal flap of the SMAD. (**a**) Dissection begins 4 cm distal to the origin of SMA and extends 5 cm into a jejunal branch. Mild aneurysmal dilatation at the level of the dissection measures 11 mm. (**b**) Follow-up CTA at 4 years, stable SMAD, dilatation with the SMA measuring about 13 mm. *a*, *b* axial view, *c*, *d* sagittal view

Verde et al. reported 24 CADs and 18 SMADs in 38 patients; 30 % of the dissections diagnosed with interactive MPR/MIP/3D rendering were missed on standard imaging planes, and the authors suggested that interactive MPR/MIP/3D rendering can increase diagnostic sensitivity particularly in the setting of pain without any other findings to explain the symptoms [21]. Currently, there is a multitude of classification systems that have been used to distinguish the different types of dissections in the literature and no system is accepted as the gold standard. Based on CT findings, Suzuki et al. [18] classified SMAD into four types: (1) an intimal flap, (2) hematoma of the false lumen or intramural hematoma, (3) an enlarged SMA diameter, and (4) increased attenuation of the fat surrounding the SMA. The authors suggested that the increased attenuation of the fat was an early diagnostic finding.

Sakamoto et al. [19] classified SMAD into four types based on the patency of the false lumen: type I, patent false lumen with both entry and reentry; type II, "cul-de-sac"-shaped false lumen without reentry; type III, thrombosed false lumen with an ulcer-like projection (ULP); and type IV, completely thrombosed false lumen without a ULP. Zerbib et al. [26] described a modified Sakamoto's classification adding the type of "dissecting aneurysm" and the type of "thrombosed SMA." However, the Sakamoto's classification does not take into consideration the patency of the true lumen, which is important to evaluate the mesenteric blood supply and make therapeutic decision.

Cho et al. [3] divided SMAD into two types: (1) double lumen with an intimal flap, with a patent or closed false lumen, and (2) intramural hematoma, which was further subcategorized depending on the presence/absence of SMA stenosis [3]. Dong et al. [24] reported three common findings for SMAD: (1) no identified reentry, (2) patent or partially/completely thrombosed false lumen with larger diameter compared with that of the true lumen, and (3) true lumen compressed by the false lumen.

Most recently, Li et al. [74] proposed a modified morphological classification with subtypes depending on the patency of the true lumen. The following five types were identified: type I, patent false lumen with both entry and reentry; type II, "cul-de-sac"-shaped false lumen without reentry (IIa, patent true lumen; IIb, severe stenosis of the true lumen; IIc, occlusion of the true lumen); type III, thrombosed false lumen with a ULP (IIIa, patent true lumen; IIIb, severe stenosis of the true lumen; IIIc, occlusion of the true lumen); type IV, completely thrombosed false lumen without a ULP (IVa, patent true lumen; IVb, severe stenosis of the true lumen; IVc, occlusion of the true lumen); and type V, dissecting aneurysm. The subtypes of a, b, and c were determined by true lumen residual diameter (TLRD); a dissecting aneurysm of the SMA was defined as an increase in diameter of more than 50 % compared with the normal part of the SMA. According to this classification, of 42 patients studied, 19 % were type I SMAD, 10 % type II, 26 % type III, 38 % type IV, and 7 % type V.

In another classification system, Luan et al. [22] grouped SMAD into four types based on the location of dissection: type A, the dissection was localized at the curved part of the SMA and extended proximally to the SMA ostium; type B, the dissection was limited to the curved part of the SMA; type C, the dissection was localized at the curved part and extended distally, but the ileocolic artery or distal ileal artery was not involved; and type D, the dissection was localized at the curved part and extended distally to the ileocolic artery or distal ileal artery. In their study of 20 patients, the distributions of SMAD in the four types were 25, 30, 10, and 35 %, respectively. Due to the slender nature of the SMA, the imaging examination cannot always detect the entry or reentry site in SMA, and some of the dissections show indefinite distal dissection into the multiple branches. Thus, dissected lesions cannot always be categorized using these classification systems, and the morphological features of the dissection cannot completely predict the outcome and prognosis of the dissection as well.

Magnetic Resonance Angiography (MRA)

MRA is an alternative examination, but it often does not provide the same detail as a CTA. The recognition of the gadolinium-induced nephrogenic system fibrosis substantially limits today the use of contrast-enhanced magnetic resonance imaging (MRI) in patients with a glomerular filtration rate of <60 ml/min. Case report showed that MRI without intravenous contrast media was possible to identify renal infarction by using diffusion-weighted image (DWI) sequence and RAD by using a 3D inflow inversion recovery sequence. This is particularly useful in patients with renal failure [23].

Selective Contrast Arteriography

Before the advent of modern imaging techniques of CTA, the definitive diagnosis of IVAD usually requires selective catheter-based contrast arteriography, which also allows precise determination of the extent of visceral artery involvement, especially of stenotic lesions, evaluation of collateral circulation, and detection of predisposing features [47]. Arterial dissection is characterized by double lumens, string sign, tapered occlusions, occlusions at unusual sites, short segmental narrowings, intimal flaps, irregular stenosis, intraluminal defects, distal pouches, and aneurysms [67]. Currently, mesenteric contrast arteriography is usually not performed for diagnosis unless there are doubts after imaging with CTA or MRA or when it is combined with an endovascular therapy.

Based on angiographic findings, Yun et al. [35] proposed adding total thrombotic occlusion of the SMA to the Sakamoto's classification. Yun et al. also devised an arteriographic classification of three types: type I, patent true and false lumens that show entry and reentry sites; type II, patent true lumen but no reentry flow from the false lumen; type IIa, visible false lumen but no visible reentry site (blind pouch of false lumen); type IIb, no visible false luminal flow (thrombosed false lumen), which usually causes true luminal narrowing; and type III, SMAD with occlusion of SMA. In their study of 32 patients, type I SMAD accounted for

41 %, and it was 50 % for type II (type IIa, 38 %; type IIb, 62 %) and 9 % for type III; the type I lesions were the most common type in asymptomatic patients (70 %), whereas the type II lesions were the most common in symptomatic patients (59 %).

In another series reported by Jia et al. [39], all 17 patients with SMAD were type II (type IIa, 29 %; type IIb, 71 %). However, neither Sakamoto's nor Yun's classification includes the type of "dissecting aneurysm" that is often seen in SMAD patients. Yun et al. also categorized the dissection entry sites into three zones: zone 1, from orifice to 1 cm proximal to the SMA curvature; zone 2, from 1 cm proximal to 1 cm distal to the SMA curvature; and zone 3, from distal to 1 cm distal to the SMA curvature. In their study, 69 % of patients had dissection entry site located in zone 2 [35]. Similar results were also observed by Li et al., with 64 % of entry sites in zone 2 [74].

Although diagnosis of RAD is usually made by CTA or MRA, both imaging studies can miss dissections of smaller branch and end arteries; therefore, renal angiography still remains the gold standard, and it provides information on the extent and nature of the vessel involvement and identifies potential treatment options [61, 92, 99, 103]. In 1970, Hare et al. described the angiographic criteria for diagnosis of RAD, including luminal irregularity associated with aneurysmal dilatation or saccular dissection with segmental stenosis, extension of dissection distal to the first renal artery bifurcation, "cuffing" at branch points, and variable degrees of reversibility documented by subsequent images [104].

Laboratory Studies

Laboratory results can be unremarkable in most of patients with IVAD. With the progression of the disease, laboratory studies related to complications including pancreatitis, intestinal infarction, and liver or renal dysfunction or infarction will be required.

In a review of SMAD, leukocytosis presented in 33 % (27/83) of available patients, and a high level of C-reactive protein (CRP) was noted in 23 % (10/44); results of other laboratory tests are within the normal ranges [11].

Liver function tests including alanine aminotransferase (ALT), aspartate aminotransferase (AST), alkaline phosphatase (ALP), gamma-glutamyl transpeptidase (GGT), prothrombin time (PT), international normalized ratio (INR), albumin, and bilirubin may be helpful in determining if there is hepatic malperfusion and ischemia that might prompt more aggressive management.

If the renal function of the patient needs investigation, evaluation includes serum creatinine (Cr), blood urea nitrogen (BUN), and estimated glomerular filtration rate (eGFR). Laboratory findings associated with acute renal ischemia include leukocytosis, elevated serum lactate dehydrogenase (LDH), microscopic or gross hematuria, proteinuria, and elevated D-dimer. Among the laboratory findings, increased serum creatinine, leukocytosis, and markedly increased level of serum LDH may reflect renal parenchymal cell death [60].

Inflammatory markers, including the erythrocyte sedimentation rate (ESR) and CRP, or specific immunologic or genotype studies according to the etiology of IVAD might be required.

Conclusion

Spontaneous isolated dissection of the visceral arteries is a rare disease. Patients either are asymptomatic or may present with diverse symptoms based on the location of dissection, the extent of visceral artery involvement, and the severity of supplied splanchnic organ ischemia. The diagnosis of symptomatic spontaneous IVAD is based on a high index of suspicion and it can usually be made with DUS and CTA in most patients. The predisposing factors, the type and risk of the lesion, and the natural history of IVAD should be well examined in all patients before therapy is initiated.

References

1. Guthrie W, Maclean H. Dissecting aneurysms of arteries other than the aorta. J Pathol. 1972;108(3):219–35.
2. Edwards BS, Stanson AW, Holley KE, Sheps SG. Isolated renal artery dissection, presentation, evaluation, management, and pathology. Mayo Clin Proc. 1982;57(9):564–71.
3. Cho BS, Lee MS, Lee MK, Choi YJ, Kim CN, Kang YJ, et al. Treatment guidelines for isolated dissection of the superior mesenteric artery based on follow-up CT findings. Eur J Vasc Endovasc Surg. 2011;41(6):780–5.
4. Park YJ, Park KB, Kim DI, Do YS, Kim DK, Kim YW. Natural history of spontaneous isolated superior mesenteric artery dissection derived from follow-up after conservative treatment. J Vasc Surg. 2011;54(6):1727–33.
5. Choi JY, Kwon OJ. Approaches to the management of spontaneous isolated visceral artery dissection. Ann Vasc Surg. 2013;27(6):750–7.
6. Bonardelli S, Battaglia G, Zanotti C, Cervi E, Guadrini C, Giulini SM. Sequential multiple visceral arteries dissections without aortic involvement. Ann Vasc Surg. 2013;27(4):497 e9–13.
7. Takayama T, Miyata T, Shirakawa M, Nagawa H. Isolated spontaneous dissection of the splanchnic arteries. J Vasc Surg. 2008;48(2):329–33.
8. Takach TJ, Madjarov JM, Holleman JH, Robicsek F, Roush TS. Spontaneous splanchnic dissection: application and timing of therapeutic options. J Vasc Surg. 2009;50(3):557–63.
9. Jung SC, Lee W, Park EA, Jae HJ, Chung JW, Park JH. Spontaneous dissection of the splanchnic arteries: CT findings, treatment, and outcome. AJR Am J Roentgenol. 2013;200(1):219–25.
10. D'Ambrosio N, Friedman B, Siegel D, Katz D, Newatia A, Hines J. Spontaneous isolated dissection of the celiac artery: CT findings in adults. AJR Am J Roentgenol. 2007;188(6):W506–11.
11. Luan JY, Li X, Li TR, Zhai GJ, Han JT. Vasodilator and endovascular therapy for isolated superior mesenteric artery dissection. J Vasc Surg. 2013;57(6):1612–20.
12. Subhas G, Gupta A, Nawalany M, Oppat WF. Spontaneous isolated superior mesenteric artery dissection: a case report and literature review with management algorithm. Ann Vasc Surg. 2009;23(6):788–98.

13. Yasuhara H, Shigematsu H, Muto T. Self-limited spontaneous dissection of the main trunk of the superior mesenteric artery. J Vasc Surg. 1998;27(4):776–9.
14. Min SI, Yoon KC, Min SK, Ahn SH, Jae HJ, Chung JW, et al. Current strategy for the treatment of symptomatic spontaneous isolated dissection of superior mesenteric artery. J Vasc Surg. 2011;54(2):461–6.
15. Foord AG, Lewis RD. Primary dissecting aneurysms of peripheral and pulmonary arteries: dissecting hemorrhage of media. Arch Pathol. 1959;68:553–77.
16. Beroniade V, Roy P, Froment D, Pison C. Primary renal artery dissection. Presentation of two cases and brief review of the literature. Am J Nephrol. 1987;7(5):382–9.
17. Furukawa H, Moriyama N. Spontaneous dissection of the superior mesenteric artery diagnosed on multidetector helical CT. J Comput Assist Tomogr. 2002;26(1):143–4.
18. Suzuki S, Furui S, Kohtake H, Sakamoto T, Yamasaki M, Furukawa A, et al. Isolated dissection of the superior mesenteric artery: CT findings in six cases. Abdom Imaging. 2004;29(2):153–7.
19. Sakamoto I, Ogawa Y, Sueyoshi E, Fukui K, Murakami T, Uetani M. Imaging appearances and management of isolated spontaneous dissection of the superior mesenteric artery. Eur J Radiol. 2007;64(1):103–10.
20. Saba L, Sanfilippo R, Atzeni M, Ribuffo D, Montisci R, Mallarini G. Superior mesenteric artery spontaneous and isolated dissection diagnosed by using MDCTA. Eur Rev Med Pharmacol Sci. 2010;14(3):235–8.
21. Verde F, Bleich KB, Oshmyansky A, Black JH, Fishman EK, Johnson PT. Isolated celiac and superior mesenteric artery dissection identified with MDCT: imaging findings and clinical course. J Comput Assist Tomogr. 2012;36(5):539–45.
22. Luan JY, Li X. CT classification and endovascular management of isolated dissection of the superior mesenteric artery with anatomical variations. Eur J Vasc Endovasc Surg. 2014; 47(2):209.
23. Casciani E, Polettini E, Masselli G, Stirati G, Gualdi G. Spontaneous renal artery dissection diagnosed by unenhanced magnetic resonance angiography: case report. Urol Int. 2012; 89(4):486–8.
24. Dong Z, Fu W, Chen B, Guo D, Xu X, Wang Y. Treatment of symptomatic isolated dissection of superior mesenteric artery. J Vasc Surg. 2013;57(2 Suppl):69S–76.
25. Tokue H, Tsushima Y, Endo K. Imaging findings and management of isolated dissection of the visceral arteries. Jpn J Radiol. 2009;27(10):430–7.
26. Zerbib P, Perot C, Lambert M, Seblini M, Pruvot FR, Chambon JP. Management of isolated spontaneous dissection of superior mesenteric artery. Langenbecks Arch Surg. 2010; 395(4):437–43.
27. Oh S, Cho YP, Kim JH, Shin S, Kwon TW, Ko GY. Symptomatic spontaneous celiac artery dissection treated by conservative management: serial imaging findings. Abdom Imaging. 2011;36(1):79–82.
28. Chu SY, Hsu MY, Chen CM, Yeow KM, Hung CF, Su IH, et al. Endovascular repair of spontaneous isolated dissection of the superior mesenteric artery. Clin Radiol. 2012;67(1):32–7.
29. Crowhurst TD, Ho P. Hepatic artery dissection in a 65-year-old woman with acute pancreatitis. Ann Vasc Surg. 2011;25(3):386 e17–21.
30. Pua U. Acute hepatic arterial dissection during transarterial embolotherapy: retrograde infusion in the acute setting is a feasible option. Clin Radiol. 2013;68(4):e222–4.
31. Desinan L, Scott CA, Piai I, Mazzolo GM. Sudden death due to spontaneous rupture in splenic artery atypical dissection with features of vasculitis: case report and review of the literature. Forensic Sci Int. 2010;200(1–3):e1–5.
32. Mei Z, Bao J, Jing Z, Zhao Z. Spontaneous isolated inferior mesenteric artery dissection. Abdom Imaging. 2011;36(5):578–81.
33. Bauersfeld SR. Dissecting aneurysm of the aorta; a presentation of 15 cases and a review of the recent literature. Ann Intern Med. 1947;26(6):873–89.
34. Leung DA, Schneider E, Kubik-Huch R, Marincek B, Pfammatter T. Acute mesenteric ischemia caused by spontaneous isolated dissection of the superior mesenteric artery: treatment by percutaneous stent placement. Eur Radiol. 2000;10(12):1916–9.

35. Yun WS, Kim YW, Park KB, Cho SK, Do YS, Lee KB, et al. Clinical and angiographic follow-up of spontaneous isolated superior mesenteric artery dissection. Eur J Vasc Endovasc Surg. 2009;37(5):572–7.
36. Katsura M, Mototake H, Takara H, Matsushima K. Management of spontaneous isolated dissection of the superior mesenteric artery: Case report and literature review. World J Emerg Surg. 2011;6:16.
37. Carter R, O'Keeffe S, Minion DJ, Sorial EE, Endean ED, Xenos ES. Spontaneous superior mesenteric artery dissection: report of 2 patients and review of management recommendations. Vasc Endovascular Surg. 2011;45(3):295–8.
38. Zhang X, Sun Y, Chen Z, Li X. Therapeutic regimen options for isolated superior mesenteric artery dissection. Vasc Endovascular Surg. 2012;46(3):277–82.
39. Jia ZZ, Zhao JW, Tian F, Li SQ, Wang K, Wang Y, et al. Initial and middle-term results of treatment for symptomatic spontaneous isolated dissection of superior mesenteric artery. Eur J Vasc Endovasc Surg. 2013;45(5):502–8.
40. Pang P, Jiang Z, Huang M, Zhou B, Zhu K, Shan H. Value of endovascular stent placement for symptomatic spontaneous isolated superior mesenteric artery dissection. Eur J Radiol. 2013;82(3):490–6.
41. Kim HK, Jung HK, Cho J, Lee JM, Huh S. Clinical and radiologic course of symptomatic spontaneous isolated dissection of the superior mesenteric artery treated with conservative management. J Vasc Surg. 2014;59(2):465–72.
42. Gobble RM, Brill ER, Rockman CB, Hecht EM, Lamparello PJ, Jacobowitz GR, et al. Endovascular treatment of spontaneous dissections of the superior mesenteric artery. J Vasc Surg. 2009;50(6):1326–32.
43. Park YJ, Park CW, Park KB, Roh YN, Kim DI, Kim YW. Inference from clinical and fluid dynamic studies about underlying cause of spontaneous isolated superior mesenteric artery dissection. J Vasc Surg. 2011;53(1):80–6.
44. Park UJ, Kim HT, Cho WH, Kim YH, Miyata T. Clinical course and angiographic changes of spontaneous isolated superior mesenteric artery dissection after conservative treatment. Surg Today. 2014; doi: 10.1007/s00595-014-0849-9.
45. Froment P, Alerci M, Vandoni RE, Bogen M, Gertsch P, Galeazzi G. Stenting of a spontaneous dissection of the superior mesenteric artery: a new therapeutic approach? Cardiovasc Intervent Radiol. 2004;27(5):529–32.
46. Woolard JD, Ammar AD. Spontaneous dissection of the celiac artery: a case report. J Vasc Surg. 2007;45(6):1256–8.
47. Glehen O, Feugier P, Aleksic Y, Delannoy P, Chevalier JM. Spontaneous dissection of the celiac artery. Ann Vasc Surg. 2001;15(6):687–92.
48. Kang TL, Teich DL, McGillicuddy DC. Isolated, spontaneous superior mesenteric and celiac artery dissection: case report and review of literature. J Emerg Med. 2011;40(2):e21–5.
49. Schaeffer E, Landy C, Masson Y, Nadaud J, Plancade D. Spontaneous celiac trunk dissection complicated by multiple visceral ischaemia: a case report. Ann Fr Anesth Reanim. 2013;32(4):e77–8.
50. Nordanstig J, Gerdes H, Kocys E. Spontaneous isolated dissection of the celiac trunk with rupture of the proximal splenic artery: a case report. Eur J Vasc Endovasc Surg. 2009; 37(2):194–7.
51. Obon-Dent M, Shabaneh B, Dougherty KG, Strickman NE. Spontaneous celiac artery dissection case report and literature review. Tex Heart Inst J. 2012;39(5):703–6.
52. Wang HC, Chen JH, Hsiao CC, Jeng CM, Chen WL. Spontaneous dissection of the celiac artery: a case report and literature review. Am J Emerg Med. 2013;31(6):1000 e3–5.
53. Perini P, Baque J, Chau Y, Sedat J, Batt M. Percutaneous embolization of symptomatic dissecting aneurysms of the celiac artery. Acta Radiol. 2013; doi: 10.1177/0284185113511079.
54. Schrijvers R, Van De Mierop F, De Schepper B, Sprengers D, Dero I, D'Archambeau O, et al. Spontaneous dissection of the celiac trunk: a rare cause of abdominal pain–case report and review of the literature. Acta Gastroenterol Belg. 2013;76(3):335–9.

55. Lacombe M. Isolated spontaneous dissection of the renal artery. J Vasc Surg. 2001; 33(2):385–91.
56. Smith BM, Holcomb 3rd GW, Richie RE, Dean RH. Renal artery dissection. Ann Surg. 1984;200(2):134–46.
57. Alamir A, Middendorf DF, Baker P, Nahman Jr NS, Fontaine AB, Hebert LA. Renal artery dissection causing renal infarction in otherwise healthy men. Am J Kidney Dis. 1997;30(6):851–5.
58. van Rooden CJ, van Baalen JM, van Bockel JH. Spontaneous dissection of renal artery: long-term results of extracorporeal reconstruction and autotransplantation1. J Vasc Surg. 2003; 38(1):116–22.
59. Stawicki SP, Rosenfeld JC, Weger N, Fields EL, Balshi JD. Spontaneous renal artery dissection: three cases and clinical algorithms. J Hum Hypertens. 2006;20(9):710–8.
60. Afshinnia F, Sundaram B, Rao P, Stanley J, Bitzer M. Evaluation of characteristics, associations and clinical course of isolated spontaneous renal artery dissection. Nephrol Dial Transplant. 2013;28(8):2089–98.
61. Garcia-Familiar A, Ortiz-Gutierrez F, De Blas-Bravo M, Sanchez-Abuin J, Rodriguez Saenz de Buruaga V, Egana-Barrenechea JM. Isolated spontaneous renal artery dissection: endovascular management. Ann Vasc Surg. 2014;28(4):1034 e5–8.
62. Ramamoorthy SL, Vasquez JC, Taft PM, McGinn RF, Hye RJ. Nonoperative management of acute spontaneous renal artery dissection. Ann Vasc Surg. 2002;16(2):157–62.
63. Muroya T, Koga S, Maemura K. Chronic renal artery dissection with aneurysm formation treated by stent implantation with coil embolization with detailed intravascular ultrasound evaluation. Catheter Cardiovasc Interv. 2013;81(3):574–7.
64. Vignati PV, Welch JP, Ellison L, Cohen JL. Acute mesenteric ischemia caused by isolated superior mesenteric artery dissection. J Vasc Surg. 1992;16(1):109–12.
65. Solis MM, Ranval TJ, McFarland DR, Eidt JF. Surgical treatment of superior mesenteric artery dissecting aneurysm and simultaneous celiac artery compression. Ann Vasc Surg. 1993;7(5):457–62.
66. Chaillou P, Moussu P, Noel SF, Sagan C, Pistorius MA, Langlard JM, et al. Spontaneous dissection of the celiac artery. Ann Vasc Surg. 1997;11(4):413–5.
67. Matsuo R, Ohta Y, Ohya Y, Kitazono T, Irie H, Shikata T, et al. Isolated dissection of the celiac artery – a case report. Angiology. 2000;51(7):603–7.
68. Sheldon PJ, Esther JB, Sheldon EL, Sparks SR, Brophy DP, Oglevie SB. Spontaneous dissection of the superior mesenteric artery. Cardiovasc Intervent Radiol. 2001;24(5):329–31.
69. Fenoglio L, Allione A, Scalabrino E, Alberto G, Benedetti V, Pomero F, et al. Spontaneous dissection of the celiac artery: a pitfall in the diagnosis of acute abdominal pain. Presentation of two cases. Dig Dis Sci. 2004;49(7–8):1223–7.
70. Batsis JA, Arora AS. Celiac artery dissection: an uncommon cause of abdominal pain and weight loss. Clin Gastroenterol Hepatol. 2005;3(10):xxx.
71. McGuinness B, Kennedy C, Holden A. Spontaneous coeliac artery dissection. Australas Radiol. 2006;50(4):400–1.
72. Tameo MN, Dougherty MJ, Calligaro KD. Spontaneous dissection with rupture of the superior mesenteric artery from segmental arterial mediolysis. J Vasc Surg. 2011;53(4):1107–12.
73. Sugiura T, Imoto K, Uchida K, Yanagi H, Machida D, Okiyama M, et al. Fibromuscular dysplasia associated with simultaneous spontaneous dissection of four peripheral arteries in a 30-year-old man. Ann Vasc Surg. 2011;25(6):838 e9–11.
74. Li DL, He YY, Alkalei AM, Chen XD, Jin W, Li M, et al. Management strategy for spontaneous isolated dissection of the superior mesenteric artery based on morphologic classification. J Vasc Surg. 2014;59(1):165–72.
75. Li N, Lu QS, Zhou J, Bao JM, Zhao ZQ, Jing ZP. Endovascular stent placement for treatment of spontaneous isolated dissection of the superior mesenteric artery. Ann Vasc Surg. 2014;28(2):445–51.
76. Zeebregts CJ, Cohen RA, Geelkerken RH. Posttraumatic dissecting aneurysm of the superior mesenteric artery. Am J Surg. 2004;187(1):98–9.

77. Tajima T, Honda H, Kuroiwa T, Yoshimitsu K, Irie H, Aibe H, et al. Spiral-shaped iatrogenic arterial dissection during superior mesenteric arteriography: a latent risk of diagnostic angiography using the power injector. Comput Med Imaging Graph. 2001;25(5):367–71.
78. Casella IB, Bosch MA, Sousa Jr WO. Isolated spontaneous dissection of the superior mesenteric artery treated by percutaneous stent placement: case report. J Vasc Surg. 2008;47(1):197–200.
79. Yang HJ, Cho YK, Son TJ, Jung YY, Choi SA, Lee SH. Rapidly aggravated dissecting flap by angiography during percutaneous stent placement for acute isolated superior mesenteric artery dissection. Yonsei Med J. 2011;52(5):859–62.
80. Nakai M, Sato H, Sato M, Ikoma A, Sanda H, Nakata K, et al. Endovascular stenting and stent-graft repair of a hemorrhagic superior mesenteric artery pseudoaneurysm and dissection associated with pancreaticoduodenectomy. J Vasc Interv Radiol. 2012;23(10):1381–4.
81. Kokai H, Sato Y, Yamamoto S, Oya H, Kobayashi T, Watanabe T, et al. Isolated dissection of the superior mesenteric artery after living donor liver transplantation: a case report. Transplant Proc. 2012;44(2):588–90.
82. Poylin V, Hile C, Campbell D. Medical management of spontaneous celiac artery dissection: case report and literature review. Vasc Endovascular Surg. 2008;42(1):62–4.
83. Amabile P, Ouaissi M, Cohen S, Piquet P. Conservative treatment of spontaneous and isolated dissection of mesenteric arteries. Ann Vasc Surg. 2009;23(6):738–44.
84. Zhang WW, Killeen JD, Chiriano J, Bianchi C, Teruya TH, Abou-Zamzam AM. Management of symptomatic spontaneous isolated visceral artery dissection: is emergent intervention mandatory? Ann Vasc Surg. 2009;23(1):90–4.
85. Nat A, George T, Mak G, Sharma A, Lebel R. Celiac artery disease and fatal rupture of a hepatic artery aneurysm in the Ehlers-Danlos syndrome. Proc (Bayl Univ Med Cent). 2014;27(2):116–7.
86. Brooke BS, Arnaoutakis G, McDonnell NB, Black 3rd JH. Contemporary management of vascular complications associated with Ehlers-Danlos syndrome. J Vasc Surg. 2010; 51(1):131–8; discussion 138–9.
87. Riles TS, Lin JC. Celiac artery dissection from heavy weight lifting. J Vasc Surg. 2011; 53(6):1714–5.
88. Watanabe A, Kohtake H, Furui S, Takeshita K, Ishikawa Y, Morita S. Celiac artery dissection seen with ruptured pancreaticoduodenal arcade aneurysms in two cases of celiac artery stenosis from compression by median arcuate ligament. J Vasc Surg. 2012;56(4):1114–8.
89. Al Hilli FA. Primary dissecting hepatic artery aneurysm in pregnancy. Cardiovasc Pathol. 2001;10(2):99–101.
90. Brown DB. Hepatic artery dissection in a patient on bevacizumab resulting in pseudoaneurysm formation. Semin Intervent Radiol. 2011;28(2):142–6.
91. Lee SH, Lee HC, Oh SJ, Park MC, Park KJ, Moon YS, et al. Percutaneous intervention of spontaneous renal artery dissection complicated with renal infarction: a case report and literature review. Catheter Cardiovasc Interv. 2003;60(3):335–8.
92. Ullrick SR, Wojtowycz M. Utility of percutaneous treatment in spontaneous renal artery dissection: case report and review of the literature. Semin Intervent Radiol. 2007;24(1):63–7.
93. Iqbal FM, Goparaju M, Yemme S, Lewis BE. Renal artery dissection following marathon running. Angiology. 2009;60(1):122–6.
94. Baroudi S, Bastani B, Balci N, Bieneman BK, Sobti P, Kudva GC. Bilateral renal artery dissection following extreme exertion. Clin Nephrol. 2011;76(4):334–9.
95. Thomas MC, Walker RJ, Packer S. Running repairs: renal artery dissection following extreme exertion. Nephrol Dial Transplant. 1999;14(5):1258–9.
96. Chabrot P, Cassagnes L, Alfidja A, Mballa JC, Nasser S, Guy L, et al. Revascularization of traumatic renal artery dissection by endoluminal stenting: three cases. Acta Radiol. 2010; 51(1):21–6.
97. Lee WH, Jung GS. Renal artery dissection during repositioning of a mal-deployed aortic endograft with suprarenal fixation. Eur J Vasc Endovasc Surg. 2010;40(6):736–8.

98. Acconcia A, Manganelli A. Dissecting aneurysm of renal artery owing to subadventitial angioma. J Urol. 1978;119(2):268–70.
99. Tandon G, Sukhija R. Isolated spontaneous renal artery dissection: a case report and review. Int J Angiol. 2012;21(2):99–102.
100. Edmondson DA, Towne JB, Foley DW, Abu-Hajir M, Kochar MS. Cocaine-induced renal artery dissection and thrombosis leading to renal infarction. WMJ. 2004;103(7):66–9.
101. Orhan O, Kultigin T, Osman K, Yalcin S, Melih A, Niyazi G. An exceedingly rare cause of secondary hypertension: bilateral renal artery dissection possibly secondary to extracorporeal shock-wave lithotripsy (ESWL). Intern Med. 2011;50(21):2633–6.
102. Lo RC, Schermerhorn ML. Mesenteric vascular disease: general considerations. In: Cronenwett JL, Johnston KW, editors. Rutherford's vascular surgery. Eighth ed. Philadelphia: Saunders; 2014. p. 2358–72.
103. Kanofsky JA, Lepor H. Spontaneous renal artery dissection. Rev Urol. 2007;9(3):156–60.
104. Hare WS, Kincaid-Smith P. Dissecting aneurysm of the renal artery. Radiology. 1970;97(2):255–63.

Chapter 32
Open Surgical and Endovascular Revascularizations of Isolated Visceral Artery Dissections

Ying Huang and Peter Gloviczki

Open surgical or endovascular revascularizations for isolated visceral artery dissections (IVADs) are indicated to prevent or treat catastrophic complications, such as arterial rupture or organ ischemia. Spontaneous isolated superior mesenteric artery dissection (SMAD) is the most important IVAD; major complications that require treatment include arterial rupture with bleeding and bowel infarction caused by acute mesenteric ischemia [1–3]. Concerns during the chronic stage are chronic mesenteric ischemia due to decreased blood flow to the gut and progressive dilatation and eventual rupture of the SMA [4].

Interventions for most forms of IVAD serve therefore two purposes: to improve flow and to prevent rupture [5]. In renal artery dissection (RAD), the goal of treatment also includes cure or improvement of renovascular hypertension [6].

Progress in imaging techniques, refinement of open surgical interventions, and development of endovascular interventions significantly improved outcome of IVAD in the past two decades [3, 5, 7–17]. In this chapter, we briefly review the role of conservative management and present techniques and results of open surgical and endovascular therapy.

Conservative Management

Conservative management with regular follow up using different imaging techniques is considered if organ perfusion is not compromised, there is no bleeding, and dissection does not result in aneurysm formation [5, 11, 17–23]. Anticoagulation can be attempted in patients with acute thrombosis of the SMA due to dissection,

Y. Huang, MD, PhD • P. Gloviczki, MD (✉)
Division of Vascular and Endovascular Surgery, Mayo Clinic, Rochester, MN, USA
e-mail: huang.ying@mayo.edu; gloviczki.peter@mayo.edu

G.S. Oderich (ed.), *Mesenteric Vascular Disease*,
DOI 10.1007/978-1-4939-1847-8_32

although regular imaging follow-up is indicated since anticoagulation will fail to control or reverse arterial thrombosis in one of four treated patients [24]. In a group of 24 patients with SMAD who were followed conservatively, progression of the dissection was noted in 29 % on computed tomographic (CT) images, pain recurred in 13 %, and 2 patients died due to bowel infarction [25]. These results suggest that spontaneous isolated SMAD has the potential to progress and may cause fatal complications during medical treatment. Currently, we opt for conservative management in asymptomatic patients and in those with no aneurysm [26, 27]. Detailed medical management is well described in Chap. 33.

Indications for Intervention

Absolute indications for emergency interventions include massive bleeding and hemorrhagic shock due to rupture of the dissected artery or aneurysm or intestinal infarction. Elective open or endovascular interventions are indicated to improve flow through the partially or completely thrombosed artery and to prevent rupture of the aneurysm [5, 11, 16, 23, 25, 28–34]. There is no size threshold for surgery for visceral arterial aneurysm, but in all symptomatic patients and in those with a mesenteric, hepatic, or celiac aneurysm (50 % increase over the diameter of a normal artery) of any size, intervention should be considered; and 2 cm diameter for splenic and renal aneurysms may be a reasonable size to consider intervention [32, 35, 36].

Some authors recommended surgical or endovascular management in SMAD patients with symptoms lasting more than 1 week, aneurysmal dilatations exceeding 2 cm in diameter, severe compression of the true lumen of the SMA >80 %, or SMAD with peritonitis [5, 23, 37, 38].

In cases of hepatic artery dissection (HAD) with long dissections extending to the proper hepatic artery, intervention, usually open surgical bypass, is indicated in patients with inadequate collateral circulation to the liver [39].

In patients with RAD, surgical or endovascular therapy maybe indicated in patients with malignant hypertension or progressive renal failure and in the chronic stage in those with refractory renovascular hypertension [40–45].

Open Surgical Revascularizations

Surgical treatment of the dissected artery includes attempts at repairing the dissected vessel with excision of the intimal flap, with or without thrombectomy. Closure of the artery is usually done with an autologous, bovine pericardial, or prosthetic patch. Excision or ligation of the diseased, dissected or aneurysmal vessel and bypass or interposition graft with saphenous or prosthetic graft are another, more frequently used alternative (Figs. 32.1 and 32.2), while in very rare cases, even small-bowel transplantation can be performed [18, 35, 46].

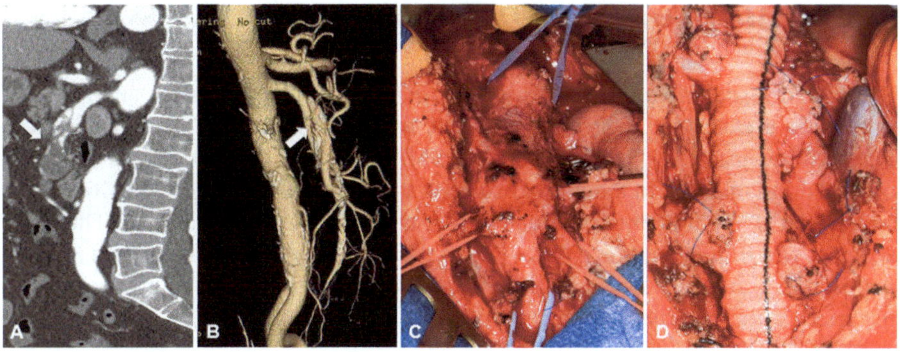

Fig. 32.1 Open surgical repair of thrombosed superior mesenteric artery dissection (SMAD) with aneurysmal dilatation in a 78-year-old male who presented with abdominal pain. (**a**) SMAD on sagittal view of computed tomographic angiography; the aneurysm contains significant amount of mural thrombus proximally and completely thrombosed distally (*arrow*). (**b**) Intimal flap of SMAD (*arrow*) on 3-D reconstruction and moderate amount of peripheral calcification of SMA. (**c**) Intraoperative photograph of the SMAD with the artery and side branches on vessel loops. (**d**) Excision of SMAD, proximal and distal SMA interposition graft using 8 mm Hemashield Dacron graft, and reimplantation of four large jejunal branches

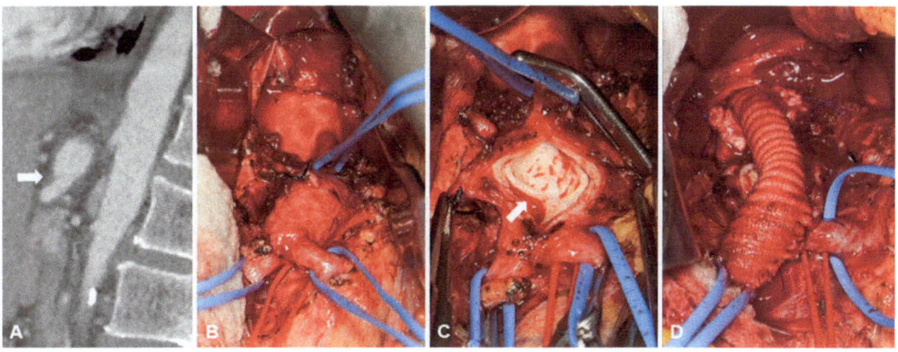

Fig. 32.2 Open surgical repair of celiac artery dissection (CAD) with aneurysmal dilatation in a 61-year-old male with progressive epigastric pain. (**a**) CAD on sagittal view of computed tomographic angiography; thrombosed proximal celiac artery with distal aneurysm with dissection (*arrow*). (**b**) Intraoperative photograph of the CAD with branches on vessel loops. (**c**) The CAD was opened. Note dissection flap in the artery (*arrow*). (**d**) Repair with aorto-distal celiac artery 8 mm Hemashield Dacron interposition graft with extension of the distal anastomosis onto the common hepatic artery

Many of the revascularization procedures are similar to those used for acute or chronic mesenteric ischemia or for atherosclerotic or true aneurysms of the visceral vessels. For detailed techniques of these procedures, the readers should consult Chaps. 11, 16, and 17, regarding open mesenteric revascularization.

Superior Mesenteric Artery Dissection (SMAD)

Surgical revascularization procedures have been performed using antegrade or retrograde aorto-SMA or a retrograde iliac artery-SMA bypass or an SMA-SMA interposition graft; bypass between the SMA and right gastroepiploic artery or transposition of SMA to the more distal aorta was also reported [12, 38, 46–49].

Dong et al. reported the technique of surgical fenestration of the SMA. The target segment was transected, the intimal flap of the proximal stump was excised, and the flap in the distal artery was reattached to the wall with sutures. The two stumps of the artery were then reanastomosed in an end-to-end fashion [38].

Celiac Artery Dissection (CAD) and Hepatic Artery Dissection (HAD)

The surgical procedure can be performed via an upper midline or chevron incision. The aneurysm is approached through the gastrohepatic ligament, the lesser sac is entered and the crus of the diaphragm divided if the aorta needs to be dissected, and a bypass is performed between the supraceliac aorta and the celiac trunk using Dacron or, in a patient with an infected field, with a vein graft [50, 51].

In patients with HAD, saphenous vein graft is usually preferred because of the small size of the hepatic artery distal to the dissection [52]. Rarely, the inferior mesenteric vein can be used for autologous bypass [39].

Renal Artery Dissection (RAD)

Open repair of RAD is a technically demanding procedure. Standard aortorenal bypass with vein or Dacron or autologous internal iliac artery is indicated in patients when the dissection only involves the main renal artery or a short segment of its primary branches [40, 53].

Extra-anatomic reconstruction (splenorenal or hepatorenal bypass) can also be performed. Ex vivo reconstruction in these patients is frequently required to salvage the ischemic kidney, treat hypertension, or prevent rupture of the artery. This technique is used in patients when vascular lesions are located more distally and extend into the secondary or tertiary branches of the renal artery [6, 40, 53]. Once exteriorized for the repair, the kidney is perfused with chilled Collins' solution and packed with ice [6, 40]. In some patients, extracorporeal repair and autotransplantation of the kidney into the pelvis were reported [40, 53, 54].

Reported clinical success of open surgical revascularization has ranged from 71 to 91 % [40, 55]. Complications may include loss of the kidney (8–27 %), acute thrombosis of the renal artery (6–12 %), and late restenosis (15 %) [6, 40, 53, 56–58].

Endovascular Revascularization

Nowadays, with improved interventional technologies and rapid development of endovascular materials, catheters, and stents, minimal invasive percutaneous endovascular treatment has become an attractive alternative to surgical revascularization for IVAD. Endovascular therapies include catheter-directed thrombolytic therapy, coil embolization, and placement of bare metal or covered stents. The specific application of endovascular treatment should be tailored to the needs of the patient, according to clinical presentation and the location and extent of dissection [14, 16, 27, 33, 59, 60].

Catheter-Directed Thrombolytic Therapy

Catheter-directed thrombolytic therapy of acutely thrombosed and dissected visceral arteries has been reported, with mixed results. Secondary procedures, including stenting [61] and laparotomy [2, 62], are frequently needed. Most success with catheter-directed thrombolysis (CDT) was achieved in patients with renal artery thrombosis due to dissection [42–44, 56]. In cases of RAD with acute renal artery thrombosis, CDT using urokinase [42, 43] and tissue plasminogen activator (rt-PA) [44], or combined with aspiration thrombectomy under antithrombotic protection with glycoprotein IIb/IIIa inhibitor [56], has been used successfully before stent placement in hemodynamically stable patients and achieved good early results.

Embolization

Sufficient collateral flow is essential to avoid organ infarction if we use embolization for IVAD to occlude visceral arteries. Successful embolizations of renal and celiac artery dissections have been reported [63]. Takeda et al. [60] reported on treatment of CAD with coils. Platinum-fiber coils (Cook Medical) and detachable Amplatzer Vascular Plugs (AVPs) I, II, and/or IV (AGA Medical, Golden Valley, MN, USA) were embolization materials used. Perini et al. recommend that the diameter of the AVPs is approximately 30–50 % larger than that of the treated artery [45].

Li et al. suggested coil embolization to occlude the false lumen and stent placement to improve flow through the true lumen in patients with type V SMAD [25]. However, the need for coil embolization in such patients has been questioned since placement of self-expandable stent will reduce the aneurysm size with gradual resolution of the false lumen and the increase in diameter of the true lumen [34, 38, 64, 65].

Stenting Visceral Arteries

At present, there are no evidence-based data that support the choice of the best type of stent for each specific IVAD. For principles of visceral artery stenting and the use of balloon or self-expandable stents, or covered or bare metal or nitinol stents, the readers should consult Chaps. 13, 14, and 18. Precise positioning and good flexibility are requirements for the stent used in the treatment of IVAD. Careful planning includes selection of the length of the stent that can be deployed at the location, the size of entry and reentry sites, measurement of the length of the broad-based pseudoaneurysm, and the severity of arterial stenosis [16] (Fig. 32.3).

Because of the radial strength, conformability, and sufficient length, self-expandable stents are recommended in the management of IVAD. Numerous stents such as WALLSTENT (Boston Scientific, Natick, MA), Zilver or Zilver 635® stent (Cook Medical, Bloomington, IN), SMART or PRECISE stent (Cordis, Miami Lakes, FL), Palmaz Blue stent (Cordis, Bridgewater, NJ), Xpert (Abbott Vascular, Abbott Park, IL), Astron Pulsar (Biotronik AG, Switzerland) have been used with diameters of up to 8 mm and overall lengths of up to 100 mm. Stents with a diameter 10 % greater than the diameter of the proximal artery are usually chosen [5, 16, 25, 31, 35, 58, 60, 66–68]. Sinus-SuperFlex nitinol stent (OptiMed, Ettlingen, Germany) was used with success by one group for RAD [56]. For short dissection, a balloon-expandable stent can be considered [33, 60]. However, the balloon-expandable stent is stiffer and the resulting axial force is greater so it should be avoided in the curved, second segment of SMA. Although covered stent was reported to treat a ruptured SMAD [26], a potential disadvantage is that it obliterates side branches of the treated artery. Covered stent, however, was also used with success to treat SMAD [69, 70].

Occasionally, laparotomy can be combined with transmesenteric endovascular approach and retrograde mesenteric stenting (hybrid treatment) [15, 49]. Intravascular ultrasound (IVUS) may be helpful to identify the true and false lumen, image the flap, and even establish the site of the tear in the artery.

The double-coaxial technique (mother-and-child technique) might be helpful to facilitate the delivery of stent to a complex lesion [71]. In patient with large discrepancy in diameters between proximal and distal arteries, two stents of different calibers with an overlap of 1.5 cm were suggested [14]. Chu et al. pointed out that in long dissection, coverage of a short segment at the entry tear by the stent graft or even bare stent can yield good result with gradual resolution of the mural hematoma on follow-up CTA images [16].

Currently, endovascular treatment with stenting is increasingly used in patients with RAD [43, 44, 56]. The risk of acute occlusion after stent placement, however, must be weighed in each case. Considering the lesion needs to be completely covered, long stents are frequently needed; however, long stents are more thrombogenic than short stents. Thus, stent thrombosis is also a concern. When the dissection extends into the renal hilum, the risk of renal infarct and further extension of the dissection with placement of a stent is high [56].

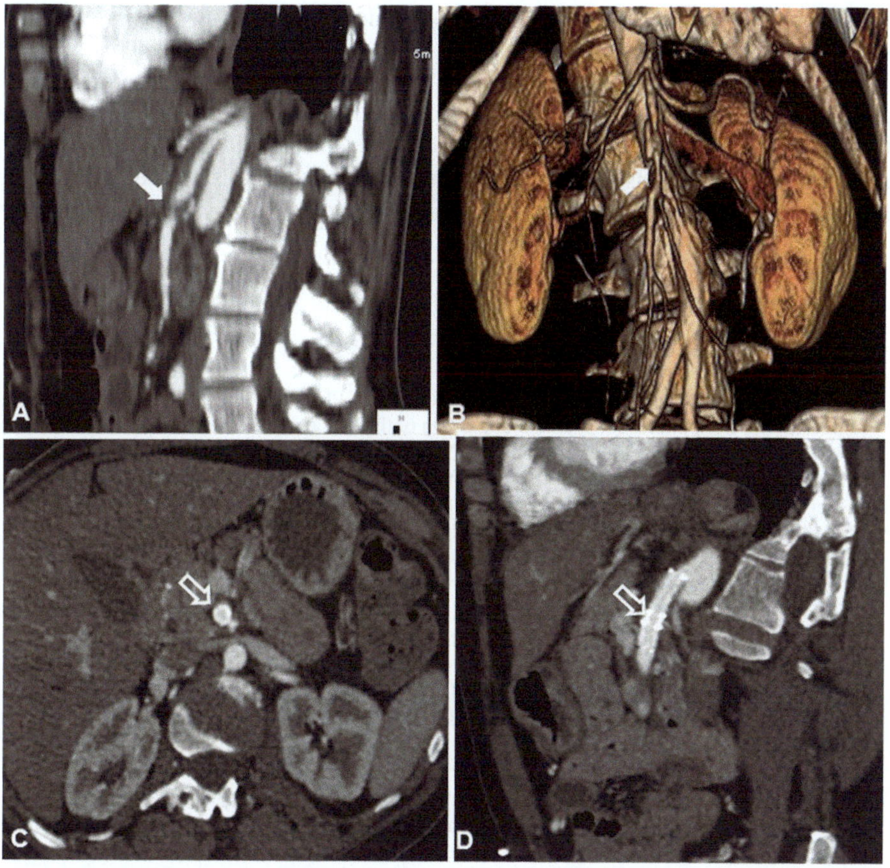

Fig. 32.3 Endovascular repair of partially thrombosed superior mesenteric artery dissection (SMAD) with self-expandable stents. (**a**) SMAD on sagittal view of computed tomographic angiography; the aneurysm contains significant amount of mural thrombus in mid SMA (*arrow*) with patent artery distally. (**b**) Intimal flap of SMAD (*arrow*) on 3-D reconstruction. (**c**) Axial view of computed tomographic angiography after stent placement in the SMA showed well-stented SMA (*hollow arrow*), and there was no evidence of intramural thrombosis. (**d**) On sagittal view of computed tomographic angiography, the involved SMA segment was fully covered by two stents (*hollow arrow*), and there was no evidence of intramural thrombosis, SMA stenosis, or compression (Courtesy of Timur P. Sarac, MD, Cleveland Clinic, Cleveland, OH)

Conclusions

Treatment options for IVAD are largely dependent on the clinical presentation, acute or chronic symptoms, the location and extent of the dissection, and the size of the aneurysm. For asymptomatic patients and some mildly symptomatic patients with no or small aneurysm, conservative treatment with or without anticoagulation or antiplatelet medication is recommended; however, close follow-up with imaging studies using duplex ultrasound scanning or CTA is required to detect any progression of the dissection. Open or endovascular revascularization is indicated in patients who fail to conservative therapy or in those who present acutely with organ ischemia or infarcts, arterial occlusion without collateral circulation, or rupture. Because of the less invasive nature, endovascular procedure is considered first in all patients, although open surgery is still frequently needed to attempt to save the organ or the life of the patient if catastrophic complications occur.

References

1. Leung DA, Schneider E, Kubik-Huch R, Marincek B, Pfammatter T. Acute mesenteric ischemia caused by spontaneous isolated dissection of the superior mesenteric artery: treatment by percutaneous stent placement. Eur Radiol. 2000;10(12):1916–9.
2. Javerliat I, Becquemin JP, D'Audiffret A. Spontaneous isolated dissection of the superior mesenteric artery. Eur J Vasc Endovasc Surg. 2003;25(2):180–4.
3. Suzuki S, Furui S, Kohtake H, Sakamoto T, Yamasaki M, Furukawa A, et al. Isolated dissection of the superior mesenteric artery: CT findings in six cases. Abdom Imaging. 2004;29(2):153–7.
4. Sakamoto I, Ogawa Y, Sueyoshi E, Fukui K, Murakami T, Uetani M. Imaging appearances and management of isolated spontaneous dissection of the superior mesenteric artery. Eur J Radiol. 2007;64(1):103–10.
5. Min SI, Yoon KC, Min SK, Ahn SH, Jae HJ, Chung JW, et al. Current strategy for the treatment of symptomatic spontaneous isolated dissection of superior mesenteric artery. J Vasc Surg. 2011;54(2):461–6.
6. Muller BT, Reiher L, Pfeiffer T, Muller W, Hort W, Voiculescu A, et al. Surgical treatment of renal artery dissection in 25 patients: indications and results. J Vasc Surg. 2003;37(4):761–8.
7. Bauersfeld SR. Dissecting aneurysm of the aorta; a presentation of 15 cases and a review of the recent literature. Ann Intern Med. 1947;26(6):873–89.
8. Sheldon PJ, Esther JB, Sheldon EL, Sparks SR, Brophy DP, Oglevie SB. Spontaneous dissection of the superior mesenteric artery. Cardiovasc Intervent Radiol. 2001;24(5):329–31.
9. Furukawa H, Moriyama N. Spontaneous dissection of the superior mesenteric artery diagnosed on multidetector helical CT. J Comput Assist Tomogr. 2002;26(1):143–4.
10. Hirai S, Hamanaka Y, Mitsui N, Isaka M, Kobayashi T. Spontaneous and isolated dissection of the main trunk of the superior mesenteric artery. Ann Thorac Cardiovasc Surg. 2002;8(4):236–40.
11. Zhang WW, Killeen JD, Chiriano J, Bianchi C, Teruya TH, Abou-Zamzam AM. Management of symptomatic spontaneous isolated visceral artery dissection: is emergent intervention mandatory? Ann Vasc Surg. 2009;23(1):90–4.
12. Katsura M, Mototake H, Takara H, Matsushima K. Management of spontaneous isolated dissection of the superior mesenteric artery: case report and literature review. World J Emerg Surg. 2011;6:16.
13. van Uden DJ, Verhulst F, Robers-Brouwer H, Reijnen MM. Images in vascular medicine. Endovascular intervention for a spontaneous isolated superior mesenteric artery dissection. Vasc Med. 2011;16(1):79–80.
14. Lim EH, Jung SW, Lee SH, Kwon BS, Park JY, Koo JS, et al. Endovascular management for isolated spontaneous dissection of the superior mesenteric artery: report of two cases and literature review. J Vasc Interv Radiol. 2011;22(8):1206–11.
15. Nomura Y, Yamaguchi M, Kitagawa A, Okada T, Okita Y, Sugimoto K. Hybrid management of ruptured isolated superior mesenteric artery dissecting aneurysm. J Vasc Surg. 2011;54(6):1808–11.

16. Chu SY, Hsu MY, Chen CM, Yeow KM, Hung CF, Su IH, et al. Endovascular repair of spontaneous isolated dissection of the superior mesenteric artery. Clin Radiol. 2012; 67(1):32–7.
17. Jibiki M, Inoue Y, Kudo T. Conservative treatment for isolated superior mesenteric artery dissection. Surg Today. 2013;43(3):260–3.
18. Cho BS, Lee MS, Lee MK, Choi YJ, Kim CN, Kang YJ, et al. Treatment guidelines for isolated dissection of the superior mesenteric artery based on follow-up CT findings. Eur J Vasc Endovasc Surg. 2011;41(6):780–5.
19. Park YJ, Park KB, Kim DI, Do YS, Kim DK, Kim YW. Natural history of spontaneous isolated superior mesenteric artery dissection derived from follow-up after conservative treatment. J Vasc Surg. 2011;54(6):1727–33.
20. Choi JY, Kwon OJ. Approaches to the management of spontaneous isolated visceral artery dissection. Ann Vasc Surg. 2013;27(6):750–7.
21. Peng K, Gao Y, Chu E, Shen B, Gao D, Luo J. CT angiography features of the involved arterial branches of the spontaneous isolated superior mesenteric artery dissection. Zhonghua Wei Chang Wai Ke Za Zhi. 2014;17(3):264–7.
22. Park UJ, Kim HT, Cho WH, Kim YH, Miyata T. Clinical course and angiographic changes of spontaneous isolated superior mesenteric artery dissection after conservative treatment. Surg Today. 2014; doi:10.1007/s00595-014-0849-9.
23. Kim HK, Jung HK, Cho J, Lee JM, Huh S. Clinical and radiologic course of symptomatic spontaneous isolated dissection of the superior mesenteric artery treated with conservative management. J Vasc Surg. 2014;59(2):465–72.
24. Luan JY, Li X. Computed tomography imaging features and classification of isolated dissection of the superior mesenteric artery. Eur J Vasc Endovasc Surg. 2013;46(2):232–5.
25. Li DL, He YY, Alkalei AM, Chen XD, Jin W, Li M, et al. Management strategy for spontaneous isolated dissection of the superior mesenteric artery based on morphologic classification. J Vasc Surg. 2014;59(1):165–72.
26. Amabile P, Ouaissi M, Cohen S, Piquet P. Conservative treatment of spontaneous and isolated dissection of mesenteric arteries. Ann Vasc Surg. 2009;23(6):738–44.
27. Kang UR, Kim YH, Lee YH. Endovascular stent graft for treatment of complicated spontaneous dissection of celiac artery: report of two cases. Korean J Radiol. 2013;14(3):460–4.
28. Glehen O, Feugier P, Aleksic Y, Delannoy P, Chevalier JM. Spontaneous dissection of the celiac artery. Ann Vasc Surg. 2001;15(6):687–92.
29. Cho YP, Ko GY, Kim HK, Moon KM, Kwon TW. Conservative management of symptomatic spontaneous isolated dissection of the superior mesenteric artery. Br J Surg. 2009;96(7): 720–3.
30. Mousa AY, Coyle BW, Affuso J, Haser PB, Vogel TR, Graham AM. Nonoperative management of isolated celiac and superior mesenteric artery dissection: case report and review of the literature. Vascular. 2009;17(6):359–64.
31. Baldi S, Zander T, Rabellino M, Maynar M. Endovascular management of a spontaneous dissecting aneurysm of the superior mesenteric artery: case report and discussion of treatment options. Ann Vasc Surg. 2009;23(4):535 e1–4.
32. Subhas G, Gupta A, Nawalany M, Oppat WF. Spontaneous isolated superior mesenteric artery dissection: a case report and literature review with management algorithm. Ann Vasc Surg. 2009;23(6):788–98.
33. Zhang T, Zhang X, Jiang J, Zhou B. Endovascular treatment of isolated spontaneous celiac artery dissection. Vascular. 2012;20(2):118–20.
34. Jia ZZ, Zhao JW, Tian F, Li SQ, Wang K, Wang Y, et al. Initial and middle-term results of treatment for symptomatic spontaneous isolated dissection of superior mesenteric artery. Eur J Vasc Endovasc Surg. 2013;45(5):502–8.
35. Morris JT, Guerriero J, Sage JG, Mansour MA. Three isolated superior mesenteric artery dissections: update of previous case reports, diagnostics, and treatment options. J Vasc Surg. 2008;47(3):649–53.

36. Gobble RM, Brill ER, Rockman CB, Hecht EM, Lamparello PJ, Jacobowitz GR, et al. Endovascular treatment of spontaneous dissections of the superior mesenteric artery. J Vasc Surg. 2009;50(6):1326–32.
37. Zerbib P, Perot C, Lambert M, Seblini M, Pruvot FR, Chambon JP. Management of isolated spontaneous dissection of superior mesenteric artery. Langenbecks Arch Surg. 2010;395(4): 437–43.
38. Dong Z, Fu W, Chen B, Guo D, Xu X, Wang Y. Treatment of symptomatic isolated dissection of superior mesenteric artery. J Vasc Surg. 2013;57(2 Suppl):69S–76.
39. Higashiyama H, Ishii M, Fujimoto K, Oka Y, Uehara T, Kumada K, et al. Dissecting aneurysm of the hepatic artery caused by an isolated spontaneous celiac trunk dissection. Ann Vasc Surg. 2014;28(5):1316.e7–13.
40. Lacombe M. Isolated spontaneous dissection of the renal artery. J Vasc Surg. 2001;33(2): 385–91.
41. Misrai V, Peyromaure M, Poiree S, Marteau V, Laurian C. Spontaneous dissection of branch renal artery – is conservative management safe and effective? J Urol. 2006;176(5):2125–9.
42. Lupattelli T, Basile A, Iozzelli A, Quarenghi M, Nano G, Casana R, et al. Thrombolytic therapy followed by stenting for renal artery dissection secondary to blunt trauma. Emerg Radiol. 2005;11(3):164–6.
43. Jeon YS, Cho SG, Hong KC. Renal infarction caused by spontaneous renal artery dissection: treatment with catheter-directed thrombolysis and stenting. Cardiovasc Intervent Radiol. 2009;32(2):333–6.
44. Abdel-Kerim A, Cassagnes L, Alfidja A, Gageanu C, Favrolt G, Dumousset E, et al. Management of isolated non-traumatic renal artery dissection: report of four cases. Acta Radiol. 2012;53(4):401–5.
45. Perini P, Baque J, Chau Y, Sedat J, Batt M. Percutaneous embolization of symptomatic dissecting aneurysms of the celiac artery. Acta Radiol. 2013; doi:10.1177/0284185113511079.
46. Picquet J, Abilez O, Penard J, Jousset Y, Rousselet MC, Enon B. Superficial femoral artery transposition repair for isolated superior mesenteric artery dissection. J Vasc Surg. 2005;42(4): 788–91.
47. Tsuji Y, Hino Y, Sugimoto K, Matsuda H, Okita Y. Surgical intervention for isolated dissecting aneurysm of the superior mesenteric artery – a case report. Vasc Endovascular Surg. 2004; 38(5):469–72.
48. Kochi K, Orihashi K, Murakami Y, Sueda T. Revascularization using arterial conduits for abdominal angina due to isolated and spontaneous dissection of the superior mesenteric artery. Ann Vasc Surg. 2005;19(3):418–20.
49. Luan JY, Li X, Li TR, Zhai GJ, Han JT. Vasodilator and endovascular therapy for isolated superior mesenteric artery dissection. J Vasc Surg. 2013;57(6):1612–20.
50. Untereiner X, Kretz B, Camin-Kretz A, Tibuleac A, Gu WM, Faller B, et al. Dissecting aneurysm of the celiac trunk: a case report. Ann Vasc Surg. 2014;28(4):1037.e1–4.
51. Jung SC, Lee W, Park EA, Jae HJ, Chung JW, Park JH. Spontaneous dissection of the splanchnic arteries: CT findings, treatment, and outcome. AJR Am J Roentgenol. 2013;200(1): 219–25.
52. Crowhurst TD, Ho P. Hepatic artery dissection in a 65-year-old woman with acute pancreatitis. Ann Vasc Surg. 2011;25(3):386 e17–21.
53. van Rooden CJ, van Baalen JM, van Bockel JH. Spontaneous dissection of renal artery: long-term results of extracorporeal reconstruction and autotransplantation1. J Vasc Surg. 2003; 38(1):116–22.
54. Slavis SA, Hodge EE, Novick AC, Maatman T. Surgical treatment for isolated dissection of the renal artery. J Urol. 1990;144(2 Pt 1):233–7.
55. Reilly LM, Cunningham CG, Maggisano R, Ehrenfeld WK, Stoney RJ. The role of arterial reconstruction in spontaneous renal artery dissection. J Vasc Surg. 1991;14(4):468–77; discussion 77–9.
56. Pellerin O, Garcon P, Beyssen B, Raynaud A, Rossignol P, Jacquot C, et al. Spontaneous renal artery dissection: long-term outcomes after endovascular stent placement. J Vasc Interv Radiol. 2009;20(8):1024–30.

57. Tandon G, Sukhija R. Isolated spontaneous renal artery dissection: a case report and review. Int J Angiol. 2012;21(2):99–102.
58. Garcia-Familiar A, Ortiz-Gutierrez F, De Blas-Bravo M, Sanchez-Abuin J, Rodriguez Saenz de Buruaga V, Egana-Barrenechea JM. Isolated spontaneous renal artery dissection: endovascular management. Ann Vasc Surg. 2014;28(4):1034 e5–8.
59. Takeda H, Matsunaga N, Sakamoto I, Obata S, Nakamura S, Hayashi K. Spontaneous dissection of the celiac and hepatic arteries treated by transcatheter embolization. AJR Am J Roentgenol. 1995;165(5):1288–9.
60. Takach TJ, Madjarov JM, Holleman JH, Robicsek F, Roush TS. Spontaneous splanchnic dissection: application and timing of therapeutic options. J Vasc Surg. 2009;50(3):557–63.
61. Yoon YW, Choi D, Cho SY, Lee DY. Successful treatment of isolated spontaneous superior mesenteric artery dissection with stent placement. Cardiovasc Intervent Radiol. 2003;26(5): 475–8.
62. Hwang CK, Wang JY, Chaikof EL. Spontaneous dissection of the superior mesenteric artery. Ann Vasc Surg. 2010;24(2):254 e1–5.
63. Mudrick D, Arepally A, Geschwind JF, Ronsivalle JA, Lund GB, Scheel P. Spontaneous renal artery dissection: treatment with coil embolization. J Vasc Interv Radiol. 2003;14(4):497–500.
64. Li N, Lu QS, Zhou J, Bao JM, Zhao ZQ, Jing ZP. Endovascular stent placement for treatment of spontaneous isolated dissection of the superior mesenteric artery. Ann Vasc Surg. 2014; 28(2):445–51.
65. Jia Z, Zhao J, Jiang G. Regarding "Management strategy for spontaneous isolated dissection of the superior mesenteric artery based on morphologic classification". J Vasc Surg. 2014; 59(3):876–7.
66. Yang HJ, Cho YK, Son TJ, Jung YY, Choi SA, Lee SH. Rapidly aggravated dissecting flap by angiography during percutaneous stent placement for acute isolated superior mesenteric artery dissection. Yonsei Med J. 2011;52(5):859–62.
67. Obon-Dent M, Shabaneh B, Dougherty KG, Strickman NE. Spontaneous celiac artery dissection case report and literature review. Tex Heart Inst J. 2012;39(5):703–6.
68. Pang P, Jiang Z, Huang M, Zhou B, Zhu K, Shan H. Value of endovascular stent placement for symptomatic spontaneous isolated superior mesenteric artery dissection. Eur J Radiol. 2013;82(3):490–6.
69. Tsai HY, Yang TL, Wann SR, Yen MY, Chang HT. Successful angiographic stent-graft treatment for spontaneously dissecting broad-base pseudoaneurysm of the superior mesenteric artery. J Chin Med Assoc. 2005;68(8):397–400.
70. Nakai M, Sato H, Sato M, Ikoma A, Sanda H, Nakata K, et al. Endovascular stenting and stent-graft repair of a hemorrhagic superior mesenteric artery pseudoaneurysm and dissection associated with pancreaticoduodenectomy. J Vasc Interv Radiol. 2012;23(10):1381–4.
71. Muroya T, Koga S, Maemura K. Chronic renal artery dissection with aneurysm formation treated by stent implantation with coil embolization with detailed intravascular ultrasound evaluation. Catheter Cardiovasc Interv. 2013;81(3):574–7.

Chapter 33
Results of Medical, Interventional, and Surgical Treatment

John H. Landau and Adam H. Power

The phenomenon of spontaneous isolated visceral artery dissection (SIVAD) is a rare entity that can involve the celiac artery, SMA, IMA, or their branch vessels. It was first described in 1947 by Bauersfeld [1], and published literature since that time has shown 296 reported cases of spontaneous isolated SMA dissection (SISMAD) [2], 72 cases of spontaneous isolated celiac artery dissection (SICAD) [3], and one case of spontaneous isolated IMA dissection (SIIMAD) [4]. While the early case reports of SIVAD showed this to be a diagnosis made at the time of autopsy which uniformly resulted in death, advances in diagnostic imaging technology and techniques for surgical and endovascular intervention have led to more favorable results in recent years. To date, no randomized controlled trials have been performed to evaluate the outcomes of medical management, endovascular repair, and open surgical repair of SIVAD due to its rarity. While no consensus has been reached on the optimal modality of treatment, favorable outcomes have been described using each of these three approaches.

Role of Medical Management and Results

Medical management of SIVAD may include bowel rest, analgesia, IV rehydration, parenteral nutrition, blood pressure control, anticoagulation, and antiplatelet therapy. These treatment strategies are employed to provide symptom relief and prevent an

J.H. Landau, MD • A.H. Power, MD, MPhil (✉)
Department of Vascular Surgery, London Health Sciences Centre,
Victoria Hospital, Western University, London, ON N6A 5 W9, Canada
e-mail: John.Landau@londonhospitals.ca; Adam.Power@lhsc.on.ca

G.S. Oderich (ed.), *Mesenteric Vascular Disease*,
DOI 10.1007/978-1-4939-1847-8_33

existing dissection from progressing, which can result in expansion of the false lumen and true lumen narrowing, aneurysmal degeneration, end-organ malperfusion and necrosis, or vessel rupture.

Several authors have tried to define the optimal patient population in which to utilize conservative medical management alone [2, 3, 5, 6]. In general, patients who are asymptomatic and have SIVAD discovered incidentally on imaging should undergo initial conservative medical management. In patients who present with symptoms of abdominal pain, nausea, vomiting, or diarrhea but show no evidence of intestinal necrosis or impending vessel rupture, it is reasonable to begin with medical therapy, but these patients require close follow-up. Patients with new-onset, unremitting, or recurring symptoms secondary to their dissection, or those with progression of their dissection on follow-up imaging concerning for vessel narrowing or impending rupture, require further endovascular or surgical management (Fig. 33.1). Follow-up clinical evaluation and imaging beginning 1 week to 3 months after discharge and repeated at 6 months, 1 year, and annually are recommended given the absence of good long-term data to describe the natural history of this disease process.

In patients who are suitable candidates for medical management, the role of anticoagulation and antiplatelet therapy is unclear. The rationale for these therapies is the prevention of thrombosis and distal microemboli. While this strategy has traditionally been advocated in the medical management of SIVAD [3, 7],

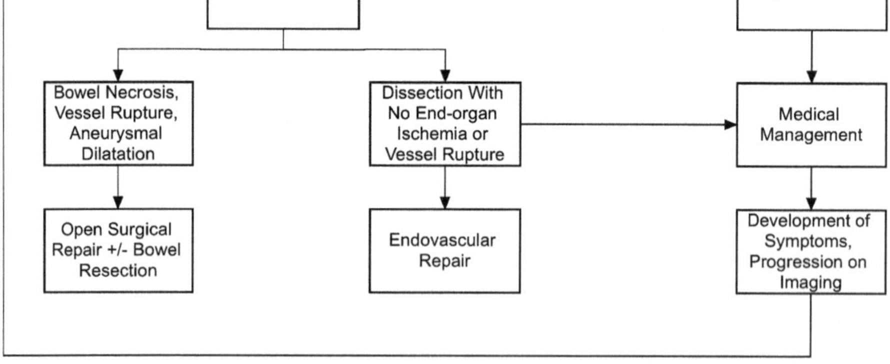

Fig. 33.1 Proposed treatment algorithm for patients presenting with SIVAD

recent studies have failed to demonstrate significant benefit. In the largest case series of patients with SISMAD treated medically to date, Park et al. [8] analyzed 46 patients treated with medical management. Twelve patients received some combination of anticoagulation or antiplatelet therapy in their cohort, while 38 received neither. There was no difference observed in the clinical course of these two groups over a median follow-up period of 28 months, suggesting that anticoagulation and antiplatelet agents may not be necessary in the medical management of SIVAD. Furthermore, Takayama et al. [9] describe a cohort of 18 patients with dissections in the celiac, SM, common hepatic, and splenic arteries who were managed with medical management alone without anticoagulation or antiplatelet therapy, and all showed good outcomes over a mean follow-up time of 20.9 months. Moreover, a literature review of 291 cases of SISMAD performed by Luan et al. [2] evaluated 209 patients treated with medical management and failed to show any significant difference in outcomes between those treated with and without anticoagulation. In the absence of level I evidence, it can be said that patients have been successfully treated both with and without anticoagulation and antiplatelet therapy.

Results of conservative management in the treatment of SIVAD have been favorable. The majority of asymptomatic patients, as well as a significant number of symptomatic patients without evidence of vessel rupture or bowel necrosis, have been treated exclusively with medical management without the need for further intervention. A review of the literature in patients with SISMAD has shown that out of 291 reported cases, 209 (72 %) were treated with medical management alone [2]. Of these 209 patients, 156 (75 %) were managed successfully and 53 (25 %) required further treatment. In those patients that were managed unsuccessfully with medical treatment, 13 (6 %) died and were diagnosed at autopsy after no formal targeted visceral vessel management, 6 (3 %) required further hospitalization and medical management, 21 required endovascular intervention (10 %), 10 required open surgical intervention (5 %), 2 required bowel resection (1 %), and 1 patient received a hybrid repair with transmesenteric stenting of the SMA (Table 33.1). Compared to patients receiving endovascular or surgical intervention in SISMAD, patients receiving medical management have been shown to be younger on average and have less compression of their true lumen on initial imaging. Additionally, patients treated with medical management alone required shorter hospital stay [14]. Medical therapy is the most common approach to SICAD as well as having been used in 45–63 % of cases [3].

Follow-up data shows that SIVAD may often be a self-limiting event with very few long-term complications. Patients who present during the acute stage of their dissection with symptoms of abdominal pain, nausea, vomiting, and diarrhea are often symptomatic from the arterial dissection itself rather than from complications of the dissection (Fig. 33.2). With medical management, most patients see gradual resolution of their symptoms and follow-up imaging shows radiographic resolution with stable or improved dissection, partial or complete false lumen thrombosis, and an increase in true lumen diameter [3, 5–9].

Table 33.1 Reported cases of medical, endovascular, and open surgical treatment of SIVAD

Vessel	# of cases	Medical	Endovascular	Open surgery	Secondary interventions	Complications
Celiac	72	47	6	19	None	None
SMA	291	209	40	42	Open surgery – 10	1 patient thrombosed open surgical repair on follow-up but remained asymptomatic
					Bowel resection – 2	1 patient thrombosed stent on follow-up but was asymptomatic
					Endovascular – 22	1 patient had progressive aneurysmal dilatation after stenting and received a second stent
					Hybrid – 1	
IMA	1	0	0	1	0	None

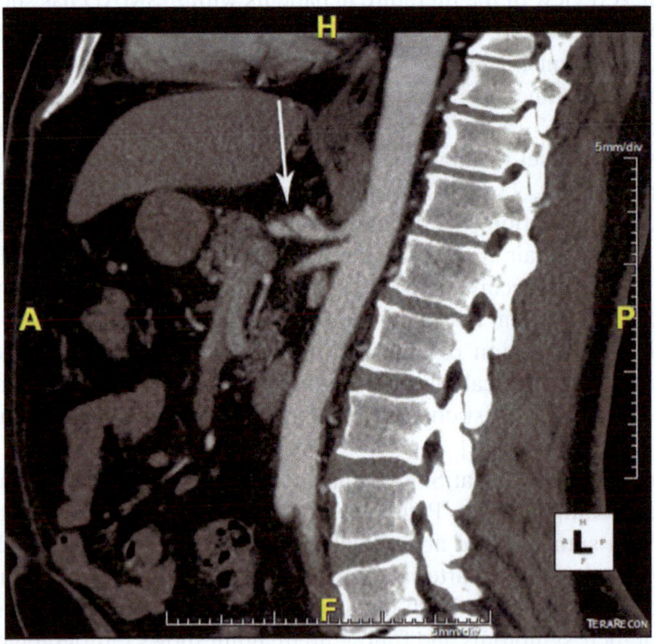

Fig. 33.2 Spontaneous dissection of the celiac artery treated successfully with conservative medical management

Results of Open Surgical Repair

Open surgical repair of SIVAD was first described in a report of isolated SMA dissection by Sisteron and Vieville in 1975 [10]. Since that time, open surgical repair has been described in 19 cases of SICAD and 43 cases of SISMAD. While these open surgical approaches were originally considered the mainstay of treatment for any SIVAD, more recently, endovascular approaches and conservative medical management have become more common. Currently, the suggested indications for open surgical repair in SIVAD include suspected end-organ necrosis requiring exploratory laparotomy, vessel rupture, and thrombosis or significant narrowing of the true lumen. Additionally, surgery can be considered in patients managed expectantly with persistent or recurring abdominal pain, progressive aneurysmal dilatation of the affected vessel segment, and false lumen expansion causing progressive narrowing of the true lumen.

Of the 19 cases of open surgery in SICAD reported, approaches have included bypass to the hepatic artery with prosthetic or autogenous vein graft in 14 patients, resection of the celiac artery with direct anastomosis of the hepatic artery to the celiac ostium in 3 patients, and ligation of the celiac artery without revascularization in 2 patients [3]. Eighteen of these procedures were performed during the initial phase of diagnosis, and only one after failure of conservative medical management, defined as worsening pain and propagation of the dissection [11]. No perioperative deaths have been reported in this patient population. Additionally, limited short-term follow-up ranging from 6 to 36 months shows these reconstructions to be durable, with all patients being asymptomatic on follow-up and evidence of stable repairs on imaging.

Out of 43 cases of open surgery in SISMAD, approaches have included aorto-mesenteric bypass in 9 patients, resection of SMA dissection with interposition graft in 6 patients, SMA to right gastroepiploic artery bypass in 3 patients, SMA to right common iliac artery bypass in 2 patients, transposition of the SMA to the aorta in 2 patients, SMA ligation in 1 patient, and a combination of intimectomy, thrombectomy, and endoaneurysmorrhaphy with or without patch angioplasty in 13 patients. The operative details for the remaining seven patients were not described [2]. Thirty-three cases were done at primary presentation, while the remaining ten cases were secondary interventions after failed conservative medical management. Two of the cases required bowel resection at the time of reconstruction due to bowel ischemia and necrosis. There have been no reported cases of patients needing surgical re-intervention after open surgery or endovascular treatment. Surgery has been generally performed on an emergent, acute, or subacute basis after the diagnosis of SISMAD, though in some cases patients required intervention up to 2 years after the first presentation of symptoms [12]. After successful surgical treatment, patients have all done well with relief of their symptoms and evidence of patent repairs at up to 5 years. Patients who have been treated with open surgical repair have been shown to be older and require a longer stay in hospital than those receiving endovascular interventions or medical treatment alone [13]. Only one case of failure after surgical intervention has been described. The patient in question received a saphenous vein graft bypass between the SMA and right common iliac artery as a primary intervention. During follow-up, the bypass thrombosed due to competitive flow in the native SMA but the patient continued to be asymptomatic at 5 years.

The single known reported case of SIIMAD was treated with open surgical repair [4]. The patient initially presented with abdominal pain and was found to have dissection of the IMA on CT scan. Conservative medical management was utilized initially but the patient complained of progressive abdominal pain and developed peritonitis on exam with an elevated white blood cell count and fever. Open thrombectomy, intimectomy, and patch angioplasty of the IMA were performed. On follow-up, the patient was asymptomatic with evidence of a patent repair on CT.

Surgical management of SIVAD has shown to be a durable intervention with excellent results up to 5 years with a smaller incidence of reported treatment failures than conservative medical management. However, its use has declined in recent years due to the emergence of endovascular techniques. Despite endovascular advances, open surgery still plays a role in the appropriate patient population, particularly in those that require exploratory laparotomy for bowel ischemia.

Results of Endovascular Repair

Endovascular intervention for SIVAD was first described by Leung et al. [14] with the use of a self-expanding bare metal stent in a symptomatic patient with SISMAD. Since that time, there have been a number of different endovascular approaches to SIVAD described in the literature and it has become an increasingly common intervention. While the role of endovascular intervention has yet to be strictly defined, it has been used increasingly in symptomatic patients without evidence of arterial rupture or end-organ ischemia and/or necrosis and in patients who fail a trial of conservative medical management [2, 3, 5, 6, 14–16].

A series of six cases of SICAD treated with endovascular intervention reported the use of coil embolization of the celiac artery and its associated branches in two patients, hybrid repair involving coil embolization of the celiac artery dissection and open hepatic artery bypass in one patient, and stenting of the celiac artery with a covered stent in three patients. These patients had a wide spectrum of presentations ranging from asymptomatic to abdominal pain with shock and intraperitoneal hematoma. Patients were embolized with coils alone or coils and Amplatzer occluder plugs (St. Jude Medical, Plymouth, MN) depending on the extent of their dissection and involvement of branches. None of the patients with embolization received antiplatelet or anticoagulation therapy on discharge, and all of the patients had resolution of symptoms with persistent occlusion of the celiac artery on follow-up imaging up to 18 months. Patients with celiac artery stenting all had self-expanding covered stents placed. Lifelong antiplatelet therapy was used in one of these cases, but no mention was made of antiplatelet therapy in the other two. Follow-up at up to one year showed these patients to be asymptomatic with patent stents and false lumen thrombosis. It should be noted that all six of these patients had confirmed patency on imaging of their SMA with adequate collateralization to the celiac artery before intervention. The presence of stenosis, occlusion, or concomitant dissection in the SMA should serve as a contraindication to embolization, as absence of collateral flow through the gastroduodenal artery from the SMA may devascularize the pancreas, liver, and spleen. Even in the context of celiac stenting, a compromised SMA could lead to catastrophic visceral ischemia in the setting of stent occlusion.

Endovascular intervention in SISMAD has included a broader range of treatment options all aimed at sealing off the false lumen and maintaining true lumen patency. A series of 53 patients with endovascular treatment reported its use as the primary treatment modality in 40 patients and as a secondary intervention after conservative medical management failed in the other 13 [2]. Treatment strategies have included self-expanding bare metal or covered stents, balloon-expandable bare metal or covered stents, balloon angioplasty, coil embolization of SMA branch vessels, and catheter-directed infusion of a vasodilator.

Stenting of the SMA is by far the most common endovascular treatment for SISMAD. Self-expanding stents have been used most often due to their flexibility and the fragility of the dissected visceral artery, but balloon-expandable stents have also been used successfully. Both brachial and femoral approaches have been described with no difference in technical success rates. In a review of 51 cases of endovascular stent placement in SISMAD, 38 patients received stents as a primary intervention and 13 underwent stenting after failure of conservative medical management [2]. Stenting has shown to be a durable repair on short-term follow-up, with only two failures reported in these 51 cases. One patient demonstrated stent occlusion 17 months after placement, though the patient remained asymptomatic [14], and a second patient had progressive aneurysmal dilatation of the false lumen at 4 months which was treated successfully with placement of a second stent. Coil embolization of the false lumen as an adjunct to endovascular stenting has also been described separately in a patient receiving intervention after failure of conservative medical management [13]. The remaining 49 patients above did well and were asymptomatic with false lumen thrombosis and patent stents on imaging during follow-up as long as 38 months. Endovascular stenting in SISMAD was used almost exclusively in patients who were symptomatic or as a secondary intervention in asymptomatic patients who failed conservative medical treatment. Compared to patients receiving initial conservative medical management, patients receiving initial endovascular stenting for SISMAD were more likely to have a higher degree of true lumen compression [13, 15]. Additionally, patients receiving stenting for SISMAD have been shown to have shorter fasting times than those treated with conservative medical management, and shorter hospital stays than open surgical repair [5, 17]. Patients have received a variety of antiplatelet therapies after stent placement including aspirin and/or clopidogrel ranging from 6 months to lifelong treatment.

Recently, a study by Luan et al. [2] demonstrated the use of catheter-directed infusion of papaverine into the true lumen in SISMAD both as a primary intervention and as an adjunct to stenting. The proposed benefit of this treatment is that local infusion of a vasodilator such as papaverine can relieve vasospasm in the distal branches of the SMA which often occurs after dissection. Thus, there is an increase in blood flow to the intestines and therefore a decrease in the possibility of bowel necrosis in the acute phase of a dissection. In this cohort, 11 symptomatic SISMAD patients were treated initially with local papaverine infusion, and 7 of these patients required further intervention in the form of endovascular stenting of the SMA because of persistent abdominal pain after 24 h. During a mean follow-up of 14.9 months, patients receiving papaverine treatment either as primary intervention or as an adjunct to stenting were asymptomatic with a patent SMA seen on imaging.

Balloon angioplasty, coil embolization, and catheter-directed thrombolysis are not regularly used in treatment of SISMAD, and only one instance of each treatment modality has been described in the literature [18]. Iwase et al. [19] describe a patient with SISMAD seen on both CT and intravascular ultrasound that was treated with balloon angioplasty and post-procedure anticoagulation with resolution of symptoms and no complications on follow-up. Sakamoto et al. [20] report a case of a patient presenting with abdominal pain and anemia who was found to have dissection in the SMA extending into the middle colic artery with an associated ruptured pseudoaneurysm. This was treated with coil embolization and the patient recovered well postoperatively. Finally, Li et al. [13] describe a case of catheter-directed thrombolysis in a patient with SISMAD and complete thrombosis of the SMA. On follow-up, the patient was asymptomatic with no progression of the dissection seen on CT imaging.

Endovascular treatment in SIVAD has been shown to be a viable treatment option. While the literature has shown excellent results in the short term, more long-term data must be obtained to evaluate its safety and efficacy as little to no information exists on the rate of long-term stent occlusion or dissection recurrence. Additionally, the true indications for endovascular intervention remain unclear and it is difficult to ascertain if some patients would have done just as well with conservative medical management alone.

References

1. Bauersfeld SR. Dissecting aneurysm of the aorta: a presentation of 15 cases and a review of the recent literature. Ann Intern Med. 1947;26(6):873–89.
2. Luan JY, Li X, Li TR, Zhai GJ, Han JT. Vasodilator and endovascular therapy for isolated superior mesenteric artery dissection. J Vasc Surg. 2013;57(6):1612–20.
3. Neychev V, Krol E, Dietzek A. Unusual presentation and treatment of spontaneous celiac artery dissection. J Vasc Surg. 2013;58(2):491–5.
4. Mei Z, Bao J, Jing Z, Zhao Z. Spontaneous isolated inferior mesenteric artery dissection. Abdom Imaging. 2011;36(5):578–81.
5. Jia ZZ, Zhao JW, Tian F, Li SQ, Wang K, Wang Y, Jiang LQ, Jiang GM. Initial and middle-term results of treatment for symptomatic spontaneous isolated dissection of superior mesenteric artery. Eur J Vasc Endovasc. 2013;45(5):502–8.

6. Kim HK, Jung HK, Cho J, Lee JM, Huh S. Clinical and radiologic course of symptomatic spontaneous isolated dissection of the superior mesenteric artery treated with conservative management. J Vasc Surg. 2014;59(2):465–72.
7. Cho YP, Ko GY, Kim HK, Moon KM, Kwon TW. Conservative management of symptomatic spontaneous isolated dissection of the superior mesenteric artery. Br J Surg. 2009;96(7):720–3. (Cons mgmt. w/ anticoagulation).
8. Park YJ, Park KB, Kim DI, Do YS, Kim DK, Kim YW. Natural history of spontaneous isolated superior mesenteric artery dissection derived from follow-up after conservative treatment. J Vasc Surg. 2011;54(6):1727–33.
9. Takayama T, Miyata T, Shirakawa M, Nagawa H. Isolated spontaneous dissection of the splanchnic arteries. J Vasc Surg. 2008;48(2):329–33.
10. Sisteron A, Vieville C. Aneurysmes des arteres a destine digestive: observations personnelles. In: Courbier R, editor. Chirurgie des arteriopathies digestives. Paris: Expansion Scientifique Francaise; 1975. p. 197–202.
11. Takach TJ, Madjarov JM, Holleman JH, Robicsek F, Roush TS. Spontaneous splanchnic dissection: application and timing of therapeutic options. J Vasc Surg. 2009;50(3):557–63.
12. Tsuji Y, Hino Y, Sugimoto K, Matsuda H, Okita Y. Surgical intervention for isolated dissecting aneurysm of the superior mesenteric artery–a case report. Vasc Endovascular Surg. 2004; 38(5):469–72.
13. Li DL, He YY, Alkalei AM, Chen XD, Jin W, Li M, Zhang HK. Management strategy for spontaneous isolated dissection of the superior mesenteric artery based on morphologic classification. J Vasc Surg. 2014;59(1):165–72.
14. Leung DA, Schneider E, Kubik-Huch R, Marincek B, Pfammatter T. Acute mesenteric ischemia caused by spontaneous isolated dissection of the superior mesenteric artery: treatment by percutaneous stent placement. Eur Radiol. 2000;10(12):1916–9.
15. Gobble RM, Brill ER, Rockman CB, Hecht EM, Lamparello PJ, Jacobowitz GR, Maldonado TS. Endovascular treatment of spontaneous dissections of the superior mesenteric artery. J Vasc Surg. 2009;50(6):1326–32.
16. Dong Z, Fu W, Chen B, Guo D, Xu X, Wang Y. Treatment of symptomatic isolated dissection of superior mesenteric artery. J Vasc Surg. 2013;57(2):69S–76.
17. Min SI, Yoon KC, Min SK, Ahn SH, Jae HJ, Chung JW, Ha J, Kim SJ. Current strategy for the treatment of symptomatic spontaneous isolated dissection of superior mesenteric artery. J Vasc Surg. 2011;54(2):461–6.
18. Yun WS, Kim YW, Park KB, Cho SK, Do YS, Lee KB, Kim DI, Kim DK. Clinical and angiographic follow-up of spontaneous isolated superior mesenteric artery dissection. Eur J Vasc Endovasc Surg. 2009;37(5):572–7.
19. Iwase K, Sando K, Ito T, Mikata S, Mizushima T, Kainuma S, Sumitsuji S. Isolated dissecting aneurysm of the superior mesenteric artery: intravascular ultrasound (IVUS) images. Hepatogastroenterology. 2007;54(76):1161–3. (balloon angioplasty).
20. Sakamoto I, Ogawa Y, Sueyoshi E, Fukui K, Murakami T, Uetani M. Imaging appearances and management of isolated spontaneous dissection of the superior mesenteric artery. Eur J Radiol. 2007;64(1):103–10.

Part VIII
Mesenteric Aneurysms

Chapter 34
Clinical Presentation, Etiology, Diagnostic Considerations, Treatment, and Results

Ying Huang, Leonardo Reis de Souza, Gustavo S. Oderich, and William M. Stone

Visceral artery aneurysms (VAAs), also named splanchnic artery aneurysms, are defined as those affecting the celiac artery, superior mesenteric artery (SMA), inferior mesenteric artery (IMA), and their branches, with dilation or enlargement of the artery to more than 1.5 times of its normal diameter. VAAs are a rare entity, with an incidence in the general adult population ranging from 0.1 to 2 % up to 10 % in the elderly population based on autopsy review. Regardless of the etiology, the natural history of most VAAs appears to be one of progressive enlargement leading to eventual rupture. The mortality associated with ruptured VAA ranges from 10 to 90 % [1–5]. With the development of modern imaging technologies and increased utilization of imaging studies, such as duplex ultrasound (DUS), computed tomography angiography (CTA), and magnetic resonance angiography (MRA), a growing number of VAAs before their rupture have been detected. The majority of VAAs are splenic artery aneurysms (SAAs), accounting for 60 %, followed by hepatic artery aneurysms (HAAs, 20 %), superior mesenteric artery aneurysms (SMAAs, 5.5 %),

Y. Huang, MD, PhD
Division of Vascular and Endovascular Surgery, Mayo Clinic, Rochester, MN, USA
e-mail: Huang.Ying@mayo.edu

L.R. de Souza, MD
Division of Vascular and Endovascular Surgery, Mayo Clinic, Rochester, MN, USA

Masters Degree Program from the Department of Surgery, Universidade Federal do Rio Grande do Sul, Porto Alegre, Brazil
e-mail: reissouza@gmail.com

G.S. Oderich, MD, FACS (✉)
Division of Vascular Surgery, Mayo Clinic, Rochester, MN, USA

Gonda Vascular Center, Mayo Clinic, Rochester, MN, USA
e-mail: oderich.gustavo@mayo.edu

W.M. Stone, MD
Department of Surgery, Mayo Clinic, Scottsdale, AZ, USA
e-mail: stone.william@mayo.edu

G.S. Oderich (ed.), *Mesenteric Vascular Disease*,
DOI 10.1007/978-1-4939-1847-8_34

celiac artery aneurysms (CAAs, 4 %), gastric artery aneurysms (GAAs, 4 %), jejunal, ileal, and colic artery aneurysms (3 %), pancreaticoduodenal artery aneurysms (PDAAs, 2 %), gastroduodenal artery aneurysms (GDAAs, 1.5 %), and inferior mesenteric artery aneurysms (IMAAs, < 1 %). Among all VAAs, HAAs have the highest rate of rupture [6].

Clinical presentations of VAAs varied from incidentally diagnosed asymptomatic aneurysms to catastrophic rupture. Presentation varies largely and is dependent upon the location, size, and etiology of the aneurysm. By far most VAAs are incidental findings noted on cross-sectional imaging studies performed for unrelated symptoms. Taken into consideration the risk of rupture and the resultant high mortality, timely diagnosis and optimal treatment are essential to prevent life-threatening complications. Current management strategies include conservative treatment with imaging surveillance in selected cases and open surgical and endovascular therapies for patients at increased risk of rupture. However, since natural history of this rare disease is poorly understood, there is no consensus regarding treatment guidelines of VAAs. In this chapter, we will have a comprehensive review of VAAs in terms of clinical presentation, etiology, diagnostic considerations, and treatment in order to propose acceptable treatment guidelines for this unusual disorder. Renal artery aneurysms (RAAs) are not discussed in this topic.

Clinical Presentation

Majority of VAAs are asymptomatic, especially SAAs. For symptomatic patients, the most frequent symptom is abdominal pain; clinical manifestations varied according to the etiology, size, and location of the aneurysm. Acute abdominal pain and hemodynamic collapse or hemorrhagic shock are frequently encountered in cases of rupture. Mycotic aneurysms usually present with fever and abdominal pain.

Splenic Artery Aneurysms (SAAs)

Symptomatic SAAs can cause abdominal pain in the epigastrium or in the left upper quadrant, but other possible symptoms are anorexia, nausea, and vomiting. On rare occasions, patient may present with "double rupture" phenomenon that occurs after initial tamponade of splenic artery hemorrhage into the lesser sac, which can prolong free rupture into the retroperitoneum by as long as 4 days [6]. Splenic arteriovenous fistulae caused by rupture are characterized by the symptoms and signs of portal hypertension such as splenomegaly, barometric portal hypertension, esophageal varicosis, gastrointestinal bleeding, ascites, and diarrhea. The most frequent sign is machinery-type bruit over the left flank [7]. Pseudoaneurysms of the splenic artery may also rupture into adjacent structures, including the gastrointestinal tract, pancreatic duct, and splenic vein, and can even form pancreatic pseudocysts [6].

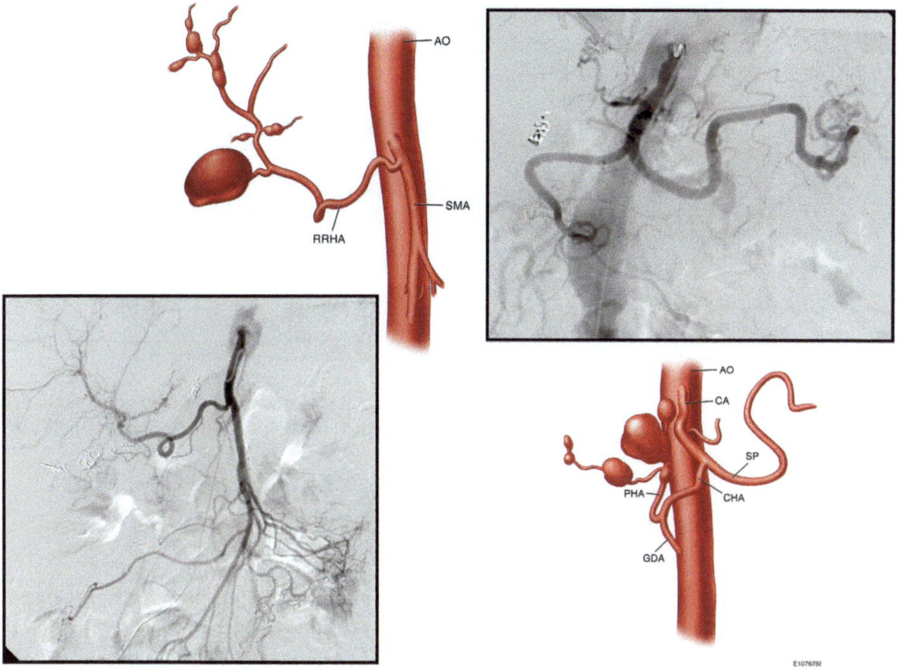

Fig. 34.1 Multiple intrahepatic aneurysms in a patient with polyarteritis nodosa treated by coil embolization and corticosteroid therapy

Hepatic Artery Aneurysms (HAAs)

If an HAA is intrahepatic and has a conspicuous dimension, it can present with Quincke's triad of right upper quadrant pain, jaundice, and hemobilia (Fig. 34.1). Abdominal discomfort and back pain are vague symptoms that may be caused by rapidly expanding aneurysms. Rupture can be seen with equal frequency into the peritoneal cavity or hepatobiliary tract. HAA with erosion into the stomach is a rare but serious cause of upper and lower gastrointestinal bleeding. Patients with hepatic artery pseudoaneurysms developed after liver transplantation usually present with intra-abdominal or gastrointestinal bleeding within 2 months after transplantation. In many cases, there is evidence of intra-abdominal infection, and bile-containing drainage often precedes the rupture of these pseudoaneurysms. [6]

Superior Mesenteric Artery Aneurysms (SMAAs)

Non-ruptured SMAAs are more likely to cause symptoms compared with other VAAs; in addition to abdominal pain, patients may present with nausea, vomiting, gastrointestinal bleeding, or weight loss (Fig. 34.2). The high mortality rate is due to a free rupture into the peritoneal cavity with accompanying intestinal ischemia [6].

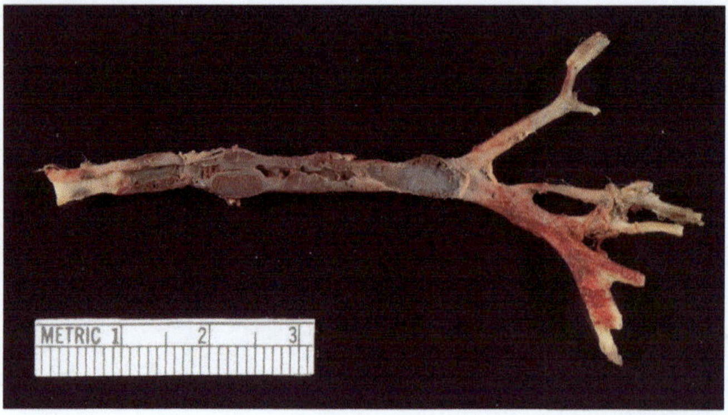

Fig. 34.2 Autopsy specimen with multiple small superior mesenteric artery branch aneurysms in a patient with indeterminate connective tissue disorder who died of ruptured visceral artery aneurysm

Celiac Artery Aneurysms (CAAs)

Most CAAs are symptomatic, presenting with vague abdominal pain. Patients experiencing biliary obstruction may also present with gastrointestinal bleeding and jaundice. The "double rupture" phenomenon seen in SAAs is reported in nearly 25 % of ruptured CAAs [6].

Gastric Artery Aneurysms (GAAs) and Gastroepiploic Artery Aneurysms (GEAAs)

More than 90 % of reported GEAAs are ruptured on initial presentation, resulting in hemorrhage into the peritoneum. They usually present with mild epigastric pain, hemoperitoneum, and hemorrhagic shock requiring some form of intervention [6].

Pancreaticoduodenal Artery Aneurysms (PDAAs) and Gastroduodenal Artery Aneurysms (GDAAs)

Symptoms arising from PDAAs and GDAAs are most often vague and include epigastric abdominal pain that may radiate to the back (Fig. 34.3). Other symptoms may include gastrointestinal bleeding, hypotension, emesis, diarrhea, and jaundice. Of 74 GDAAs reported between 1956 and 2011, a gastrointestinal hemorrhage secondary to rupture of the aneurysm was the most common clinical presentation (52 %), followed by abdominal pain (46 %); only 7.5 % of the patients were asymptomatic. Rupture of a PDAA can cause potentially fatal bleeding into the retroperitoneal space, abdominal cavity, or gastrointestinal tract [6, 8].

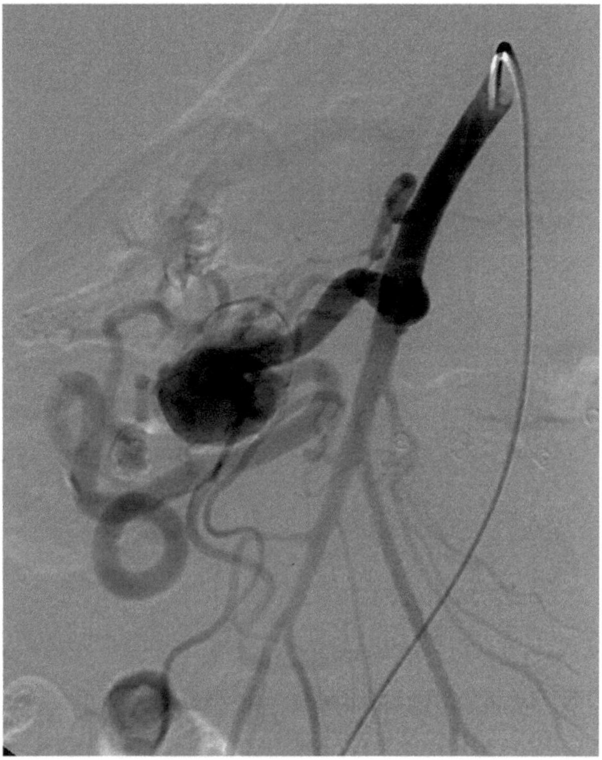

Fig. 34.3 Large gastroduodenal branch artery aneurysm

Inferior Mesenteric, Jejunal, Ileal, and Colic Artery Aneurysms

Although abdominal pain and hypovolemic shock are seen in approximately 85 % of the cases [6, 9], around 50 % of inferior mesenteric artery aneurysms (IMAAs) are asymptomatic. On reviewing 54 IMAAs, 21 were associated with SMA (Fig. 34.4) and CA occlusion [10]. For middle colic artery aneurysms, patients usually present with abdominal pain, vomiting, and a sudden unexpected drop in hemoglobin [11].

Epidemiology and Etiology

The etiology of VAAs differs for true aneurysms versus pseudoaneurysms. Causes of true VAAs include atherosclerosis, medial degeneration, collagen vascular diseases, and fibromuscular dysplasia (FMD). Other factors such as multiparity, portal hypertension, and posttransplant status have been associated specifically with VAA formation. Of 927 liver transplant recipients, 21 developed VAAs (2.3 %); the majority involved hepatic and splenic arteries [12]. Rare medical conditions, such as von Recklinghausen's disease, type VI Ehlers-Danlos syndrome (EDS), and

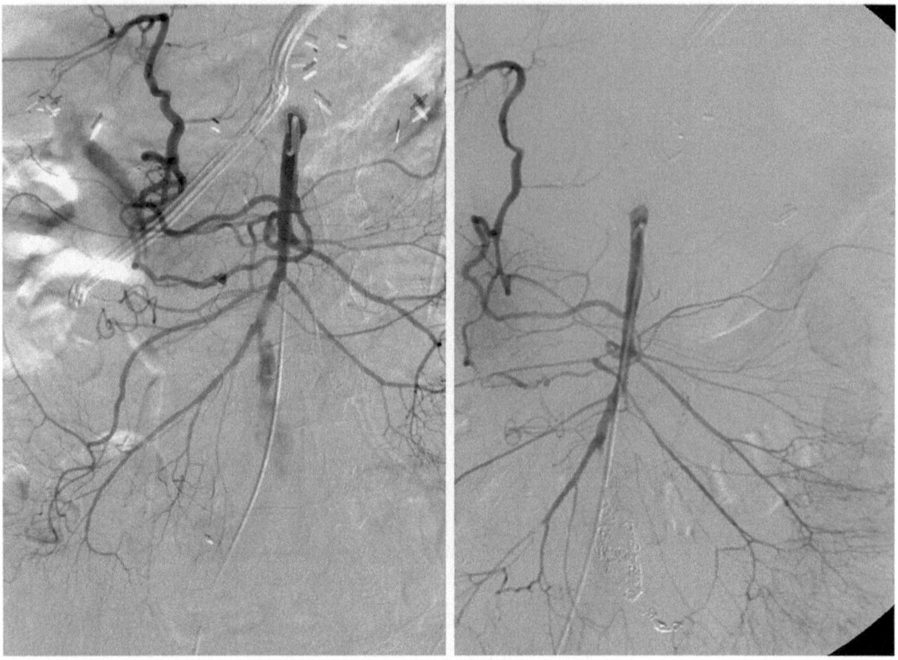

Fig. 34.4 SMA branch aneurysm treated by coil embolization

polyarteritis nodosa (PAN), have been implicated in the development of VAAs. Reported case series have demonstrated the association of multiple VAAs with systemic arteritis, endocarditis with septic emboli, connective tissue disorders, and even excessive acetaminophen use [6].

Visceral pseudoaneurysms, defined as a tear in the vessel wall with resultant peri-artery hematoma, seem to be less frequent than true aneurysms and can be caused by trauma, iatrogenic interventions (from surgical, laparoscopic, or interventional treatments), inflammatory conditions (pancreatitis), or infectious disease (mycotic aneurysm) [13].

Splenic Artery Aneurysms (SAAs)

The incidence of SAAs in the general population based on autopsy studies and angiography series has been estimated between 0.01 % and 0.78 %, and 10 % in an elderly population autopsy series.

Most SAAs are related to atherosclerosis, arterial fibrodysplasia, and arteritis; most patients are young. Associated risk factors include female gender, with a ratio of 4:1 over male, multiparity, and portal hypertension. The association between SAA and portal hypertension has been documented, especially in patients undergoing orthotopic liver transplantation. Eleven evaluated patients with known portal hypertension or cirrhosis showed a likely SAA incidence ranging from 10 % to 20 %, 114 with one study reporting an incidence as high as 50 % [6].

Pseudoaneurysm formation associated with pancreatitis has been attributed to digestion of the splenic artery by pancreatic enzymes. Splenic artery pseudoaneurysm formation associated with chronic pancreatitis represents the leading cause of hemosuccus pancreatitis and is a challenging clinical scenario [6].

Hepatic Artery Aneurysms (HAAs)

The incidence of HAAs is estimated to be less than 0.4 % in the general population, and with increasing use of hepatobiliary instrumentation and manipulation, the incidence appears to increase. Hepatic artery pseudoaneurysm formation after liver transplantation is estimated to be 1–2 %. The male-to-female ratio is 3:2, and the age of presentation is closer to a mean of 60 years old if trauma etiologies are excluded [6].

Most HAAs are atherosclerotic, accounting for approximately 30 % of cases. Arterial dysplasia, trauma, PAN, and biliary diseases have also been implicated in the formation of HAA [6]. Rare cause is post vascular endothelial growth factor (VEGF) receptor tyrosine-kinase inhibitor (RTKI) therapy in a female patient with I^{131}-refractory, differentiated, metastatic thyroid cancer [14]. In a Mayo Clinic series of 36 true HAAs, the most commonly associated comorbidity was hypertension, which occurred in 72 % of patients [15].

Superior Mesenteric Artery Aneurysms (SMAAs)

SMAAs appear to affect men and women equally, with most patients presenting at ages older than 50 years. Incidence based on autopsy studies is reportedly 1 in 12,000 to 1 in 19,000 [6].

The most common etiology of SMAAs continues to be infection; mycotic etiologies account for 60 % of all SMAAs. Other conditions related to true SMAA formation include atherosclerosis, connective tissue disease, pancreatitis, and trauma in the development of SMA pseudoaneurysms. [6]

Celiac Artery Aneurysms (CAAs)

Prevalence of CAAs based on autopsy review is about 1 in 8000. The majority of CAAs are found in men (66 %) and are discovered in patients at an average age of 56 years. Historically, the primary cause of CAAs was infection, while in contemporary clinical experience, atherosclerosis and congenital or developmental medial defects are main etiologies of CAAs [6].

Gastric Artery Aneurysms (GAAs) and Gastroepiploic Artery Aneurysms (GEAAs)

The etiology of GAAs and GEAAs has been attributed to atherosclerosis in 30 % of cases, trauma in 25 %, and infection in 15 %. Comorbid conditions include peptic ulcer disease, vasculitis, and pancreatitis. There is a reported male predominance, with initial presentation in the sixth or seventh decade of life. The majority of these aneurysms are located along the left or right gastric artery.

Pancreaticoduodenal Artery Aneurysms (PDAAs) and Gastroduodenal Artery Aneurysms (GDAAs)

Both are male predominant diseases with a ratio of 4:1 over female and present in the sixth decade of life. Factors associated with the formation of PDAAs include atherosclerosis, local infection, trauma, pancreatitis, FMD, congenital anomalies, and compression of the celiac axis by the median arcuate ligament (MAL) [8, 16]. Of 131 PDAAs reported between 1895 and 2014, 62 % were associated with occlusion or stenosis of the celiac axis, with 16 % attributed to compression by a MAL [17].

Atherosclerosis and pancreatitis are the two most common risk factors for GDAAs. The pancreaticoduodenal artery is the main collateral pathway between the celiac axis and the SAM. Increased blood flow in the pancreaticoduodenal artery, as compensation for occlusion or stenosis of the SMA or celiac axis, may cause a GDAA. [3, 18] In a review of the English literature over a 25-year period from 1970 to 1995, pancreatitis was found to be the most common associated condition with GDAAs accounting for 47 % of all cases followed by ethanol abuse (25 %), peptic ulcer disease (17 %), and cholecystectomy (3 %) [3]. As for pseudoaneurysms, inflammation with the most common cause being pancreatitis [19].

Inferior Mesenteric, Jejunal, Ileal, and Colic Artery Aneurysms

Connective tissue disorders that may contribute to the etiology of these aneurysms include Marfan's syndrome, EDS, FMD, hereditary hemorrhagic telangiectasia, Osler-Weber-Rendu disease, and Kawasaki's disease. Other described etiologies may include alpha one antitrypsin deficiency, infections (specifically tuberculosis), trauma, or iatrogenic injury during previous procedures [11]. A large series from the Mayo Clinic reported eight patients with these mesenteric branch aneurysms, noting that most of the patients had a significant smoking history and used alcohol [20].

Among 54 IMAAs reported between 1861 and 2012, atherosclerosis is the most common cause, accounting for 41 %. Other reported causes are mycotic, polyarteritis nodosa, Takayasu's disease, iatrogenic, aortitis, segmental mediolytic arteritis, tuberculous, Behcet's disease, and neurofibromatosis [10].

The common causes of middle colic artery aneurysm are atherosclerosis, angiodysplasia, arteritis, and infection. Among these, segmental arterial mediolysis (SAM) is the most common. [9] The etiologies of jejunal and ileal artery aneurysms remain poorly defined.

Rupture Risk

Rupture rate of VAAs largely depends on aneurysm location, shape, size, and etiology. Aneurysm rupture in the setting of circulatory collapse is a devastating clinical scenario, with perioperative mortality rates reported from 20 to 70 % [6]. The risk of rupture seems higher for pseudoaneurysms than for true aneurysms, and ruptures are more frequent in the hepatic artery (80 %), pancreatic arteries (75 %), and SMA (38 %).

Splenic Artery Aneurysms (SAAs)

SAAs have a relatively low rupture rate of less than 2 % in cases not associated with pregnancy. Although rare, the mortality for ruptures in nonpregnant patients is approximately 25–36 % [1, 3]. This rate nearly doubles in pregnant patients (65–75 %), with fetal mortality of 95 %, [21] and patients with portal hypertension (>50 %) [22]. Colonoscopy was the procedure reported most frequently associated with rupture. Common medications associated with rupture included anticoagulants, thrombolytics, and recombinant granulocyte-colony stimulating factor. Portal hypertension is an additional significant risk factor, associated with nearly 20 % of all SAA ruptures [6].

Other Splanchnic Aneurysms

Among all VAAs, HAAs have the highest rate of rupture, with reported rate varied from 60 to 80 %; mortality rates associated with rupture are high, ranging from 20 to 70 %. Rupture rates are 38–50 % for SMAAs with an associated mortality rate of 30–90 %. Rupture rates range from 10 to 20 % for CAAs, with a mortality of 50 %. It is 68 % for PDAAs, 56 % for GDAAs, and 90 % for GEAAs. The gastrointestinal or biliary tract is the site of rupture in 65 % of cases, whereas rupture into the retroperitoneal space occurs in 35 % of cases. In one series, 75 % of PDAAs presented as ruptured, with 50 % mortality. The mortality rate with rupture of a GDAA is about 40 %, with the highest mortality rate comes from rupture into the duodenum approaching 21 %. Less frequently, patients with GDAA can present with retroperitoneal or intraperitoneal bleeds with a 19 % mortality rate [6, 18].

Diagnostic Considerations

A thorough history including predisposing factors and past surgical intervention and physical examinations is essential for diagnosis. A pulsatile abdominal mass with or without a bruit on auscultation can be the sole warning sign and should initiate prompt diagnostic workup to preclude the worst outcome. Noninvasive imaging studies such as duplex ultrasound (DUS), CTA or MRA, or contrast arteriography are indicated in symptomatic patients suspicious for VAA. In asymptomatic patients the diagnosis of VAA is established only when imaging studies are performed to investigate other abdominal pathologies. It should be kept in mind that investigations that involve exposure of the fetus to radiations should be avoided or kept to a minimum.

Duplex Ultrasound (DUS)

DUS is a useful tool in the initial assessment of a suspected VAA, especially in pregnant patients to evaluate size of the aneurysm, mural thrombosis, as well as arteries proximal and distal to the aneurysm. It is very useful during long-term follow-up of small aneurysms treated conservatively. In the diagnostic evaluation of unstable patients, the use of a CT scan, MRI, or angiography has a limited role primarily because of their time-consuming nature, and the use of bedside ultrasound to detect intra-abdominal free fluid aids in the diagnosis of the less common causes of antepartum hemorrhage caused by rupture of a VAA [23]. However, this technique is operator dependent, and the detection of VAA might be missed in obese patients and those patients with visceral branch aneurysms or with considerable bowel gas.

Computed Tomography Angiography (CTA)

CTA has the advantage of being noninvasive and localizing the aneurysm with its relations to surrounding structures, size measurements, and evaluation of collateral flow and identifying areas of bleeding masking an aneurysm and is necessary for procedure planning (Fig. 34.5). Usually, the diagnosis of a VAA can be made with cross-sectional imaging, especially in visceral branch aneurysms. In patients with pancreatitis, CT scan can reveal a homogeneously enhancing structure within or adjacent to a pseudocyst which is highly suggestive of an associated pseudoaneurysm.

Magnetic Resonance Angiography (MRA)

MRA is an alternative examination, but it often does not provide the same detail as a CTA. In patients with renal failure, MRA is usually required for operative planning.

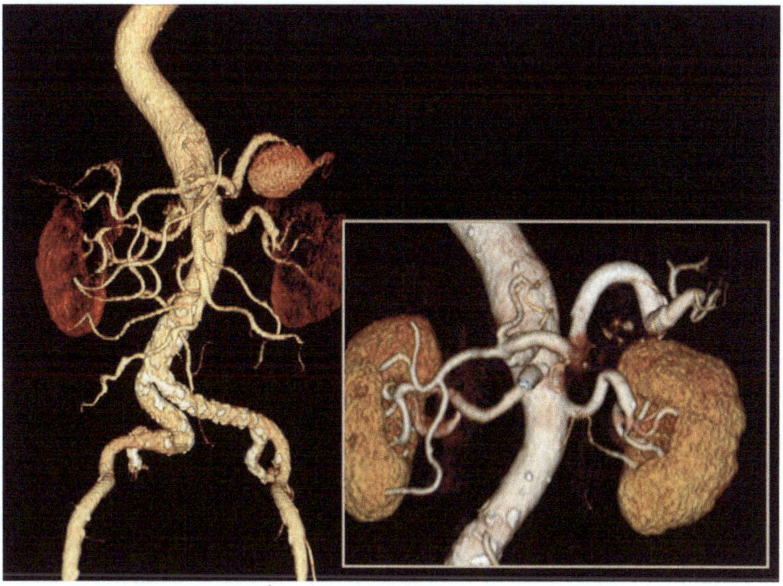

Fig. 34.5 Computed tomography angiography prior and after treatment of splenic artery aneurysm by stent graft

Selective Arteriography

Nowadays, catheter-based contrast angiography is seldom served as a diagnostic modality (Fig. 34.3). Instead, it is more frequently used in combination with percutaneous endovascular therapy of the VAA or diagnosis of visceral branch aneurysms, which are difficult to define the related anatomy with noninvasive imaging studies. Selective mesenteric angiography is a prerequisite to delineate the anatomy upon proceeding with endovascular treatment, which includes location of the aneurysm, inflow and outflow, collaterals, and tortuosity of the involved arteries. However, VAAs may not be visualized when mural thrombus or considerable thrombus present within the aneurysm.

Laboratory Studies

Laboratory results can be unremarkable in most of patients with VAA. Considering the variety of etiologies, standard white blood cell count, serum inflammatory markers, erythrocyte sedimentation rate and C-reactive protein, antibody and hepatitis panels, tuberculin skin testing, arteriography, and biopsy may be informative in diagnosing the etiology.

Treatment Modalities

The purpose of treatment of VAA is to exclude the aneurysmal sac from the systemic circulation while ideally preserving distal blood flow, while in case of rupture, the aim is immediate resuscitation and cessation of bleeding. Due to lack of natural history and prospective studies, there is no consensus regarding treatment guidelines for VAAs. Current treatment modalities include conservative treatment and open surgical or endovascular therapies. The choice of the therapeutic option is made on individual basis and depends on the symptom, the location of the aneurysm, and general condition of the patient and the risk of organ ischemia.

Observation

Observation is reserved for small aneurysms with relatively low risk of rupture. However, close imaging surveillance is required for early detection of rapid expansion in certain type of VAAs. In the report from the Mayo Clinic, of 168 patients with SAAs who underwent observation for a mean period of 75 months, only 10 % of the half patients monitored with serial imaging were noted to have aneurysm growth averaging 0.06/cm/year. No rupture or other complications related to the SAAs occurred, and only 3 of the original 168 patients (1.8 %) required intervention due to aneurysm growth [24]. The Cleveland Clinic reported similar results after reviewing 66 SAAs with observation; the average growth rate was 0.2/mm/year over 3.1 follow-up years. There were no ruptures or other complications attributed to the aneurysms in the observed group [25].

Indications for Interventions

Indications for interventions for VAAs are considered to be asymptomatic VAAs > 20 mm in size, rapidly increasing in size during surveillance ≥ 0.5 cm/year, symptomatic and ruptured VAAs, and pseudoaneurysms. Pancreaticoduodenal aneurysms are prone to rupture and should be treated at any size diameter. Ruptured VAAs should be treated emergently. In addition, because of the high risk of rupture, regardless of size, mycotic aneurysms, female patients of childbearing age or pregnant, or orthotopic liver transplant recipients are indicated for intervention for SAA; SMAA, CAA, multiple or non-atherosclerotic HAAs, and other branch aneurysms require intervention [5, 15]. Of all the mesenteric branch artery aneurysms, colic aneurysms are the most likely to rupture; therefore, they should be considered for intervention at an early stage [20].

Open approaches are reserved for cases with tortuous, angulated, or short vessels which are not amenable to the endovascular approach, those who require preservation of end-organ perfusion [11], mycotic aneurysms [26], or those who fail to endovascular intervention. Endovascular treatment is preferred for anatomically suitable patient with a hostile abdomen or abdominal sepsis, pancreatic inflammation, and high surgical risk.

Open Surgical Techniques

Treatment of VAAs with open surgery has been established as a safe and durable standard. Currently open repair is primarily researched for aneurysms involving branch vessels or bifurcation of critical vessels that cannot be incorporated with stent grafts or sacrificed with coil embolization or liquid agents. This is often the case of mid SMA trunk aneurysms or distal hepatic artery aneurysms. An open surgical approach allows for direct visualization of end organs and concomitant disease processes and is useful for determining the need for arterial reconstruction if intestinal viability is compromised. Open techniques include aneurysmectomy, aneurysmal ligation with or without bypass, and end-organ resection. The choice of technique depended on anatomic localization and the need for downstream revascularization which is largely dependent on the adequacy of collaterals. Some authors suggested to revascularize both the celiac artery and SMA whenever feasible. Intraoperative duplex ultrasound scanning during visceral revascularizations can help to optimize technical success and outcome [27]. Expeditious ligation of both the proximal and distal branches is generally performed without the need for reconstruction in the case of frank rupture and hemodynamic collapse and often during elective cases if adequate collateralization to end organs is present. Any small bowel ischemia may require resection. Minimally invasive surgical approach includes laparoscopic clipping as well as robotic assisted interventions [6].

Endovascular Techniques

Endovascular therapy has become the primary treatment modality whenever possible. The advent of minimally invasive endovascular therapy has provided an alternative to surgery in anatomically suitable patient in whom VAA needs to be treated, with the early benefits of reduced hospital stay and faster recovery. The most commonly used endovascular methods are coiling to induce thrombosis and stenting to exclude the aneurysm; access via the right femoral or left brachial artery is preferred. The use of endovascular approaches continues to expand with modern techniques and the development of endovascular materials. Endovascular management of ruptured VAAs has also been reported as a feasible option but should only be used in selective stable cases. However, some anatomical conditions may constrain these techniques, such as vessel tortuosity, aneurysm of the artery supplying an organ that has multiple arterial sources, main branch originating from the aneurysm, etc. Potential complications including visceral ischemia caused by sacrifice of the

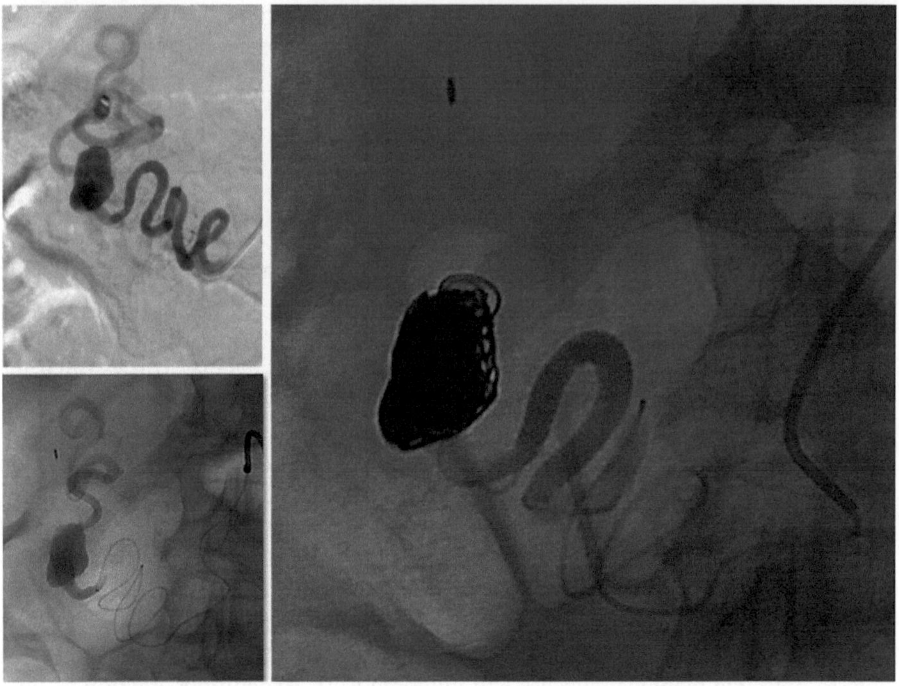

Fig. 34.6 Treatment of gastroduodenal branch aneurysm by coil embolization

involved visceral artery, coil migration with resultant embolization of non-treated artery, end-organ thrombosis, vessel recanalization, persistence of the aneurysm, stent thrombosis, or restenosis should be taken into consideration. Prolonged imaging follow-up is also required for these patients since long-term durability after endovascular treatment is not well understood.

Transcatheter Embolization

Reported embolic materials include nitinol coils (Fig. 34.6), cyanoacrylate glue, thrombin, and even ethyl alcohol. The rate of glue polymerization can be altered for precision targeting using ethiodized oil dilution. A 5 F, 6 F, or 7 F long sheath is crucial to accommodate catheter to a target vessel; a 3 F microcatheter is useful for interventions in the distal aspect of an arterial bed for selective deployment of embolization material. Both true and pseudoaneurysms of the splanchnic circulation can be managed with embolization. Endovascular exclusion to ablate both inflow and outflow can be achieved by placement of coils first distally to the sac and then proximally to the sac. For aneurysms supplied by terminal branches, the sac can be directly injected or coiled [6]. Coil embolization is a well-known technique for the treatment of saccular aneurysms, but it can become challenging in wide neck; therefore, self-expandable stent or covered stent-assisted coil embolization

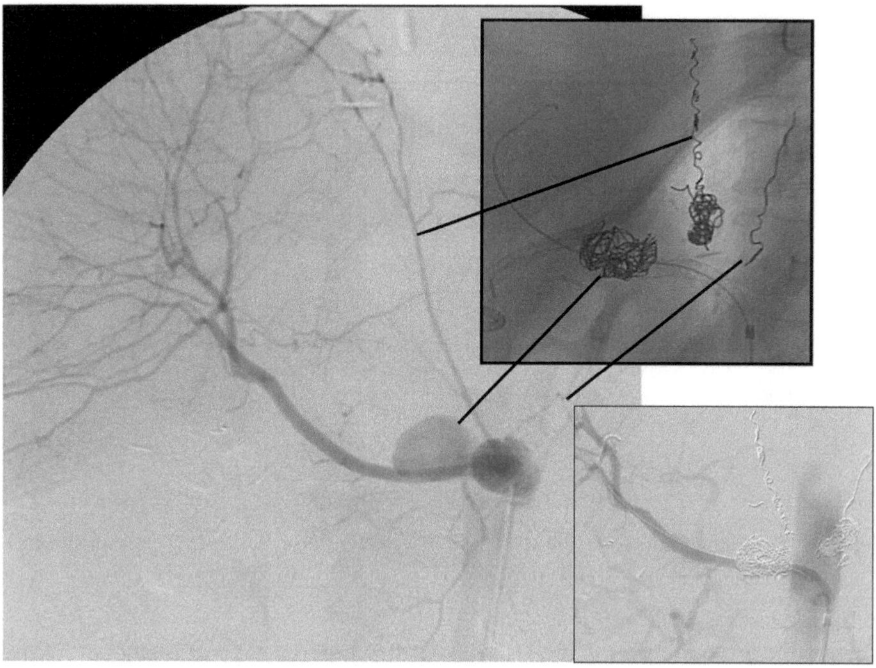

Fig. 34.7 Treatment of proximal hepatic artery aneurysm by covered stent with coil embolization of side branches

techniques were used in the treatment of such aneurysms such as SAA [28] and CAA [29] to allow selective embolization of the aneurysm sac and blood supply to the distal artery and avoid migration of the coils which may lead to distal embolization. Also, proximal embolization alone should not be performed because the aneurysm may recruit a robust vascular supply in a retrograde manner. Clipping, coiling, and thrombin injection may also be achieved laparoscopically or robotically in appropriately selected patients [11].

Covered Stents and Stent Grafts

Requirements for stent grafting are the presence of suitable sealing zones (Fig. 34.7) proximally and distally to the aneurysm, the absence of a critical vessel takeoff from the aneurysm sac to be excluded, and an arterial access that permits safe navigation of the stent graft deployment system to the target location.

Flow-Diverting Stents

Flow-diverting stents (FDSs) are designed to slow and laminate blood flow inside an aneurysm (Fig. 34.8) allowing an organized thrombus to form while maintaining flow in the main artery and branch vessels. They reduce the flow velocity, by up to 90 %.

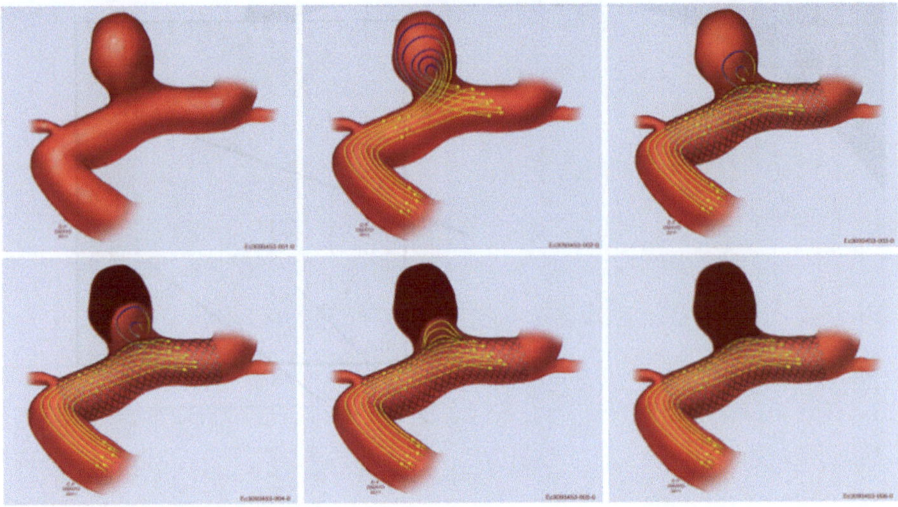

Fig. 34.8 Diagram of flow diversion stents with progressive thrombosis of saccular aneurysm

The results are quite promising with a significant percentage of aneurysm thrombosis and shrinkage during follow-up and without any branch vessel occlusion [30–32]. In a review article, Sfyroeras et al. reported 26 VAAs treated by FDSs; Cardiatis multilayer stents (Cardiatis, Isnes, Belgium) were used in all patients except two: one SAA was treated using the Pipeline embolization device (ev3, Plymouth, MN) and the other SMAA with the SILK arterial reconstruction device (Balt Extrusion, Montmorency, France). Three patients with Cardiatis multilayer stent developed early in-stent thrombosis in SMA, splenic, and hepatic artery, respectively, possibly due to the poor runoff and patients' noncompliance with dual-antiplatelet therapy [30].

Specific Issues

Splenic Artery Aneurysms

Aneurysms located in the proximal or middle third of the splenic artery may be treated by open or endovascular techniques. Endovascular treatment is preferable and can be done with preservation of the flow using small profile stent grafts. To overcome tortuosity, use of brachial approach and coaxial system is recommended (Figs. 34.9, 34.10, and 34.11). Alternatively if this is not possible, open repair with simple excision and with proximal and distal ligation of the artery and splenic preservation may be considered. For aneurysms located in the distal third, resection with splenectomy is most often performed. In symptomatic cases, splenectomy or

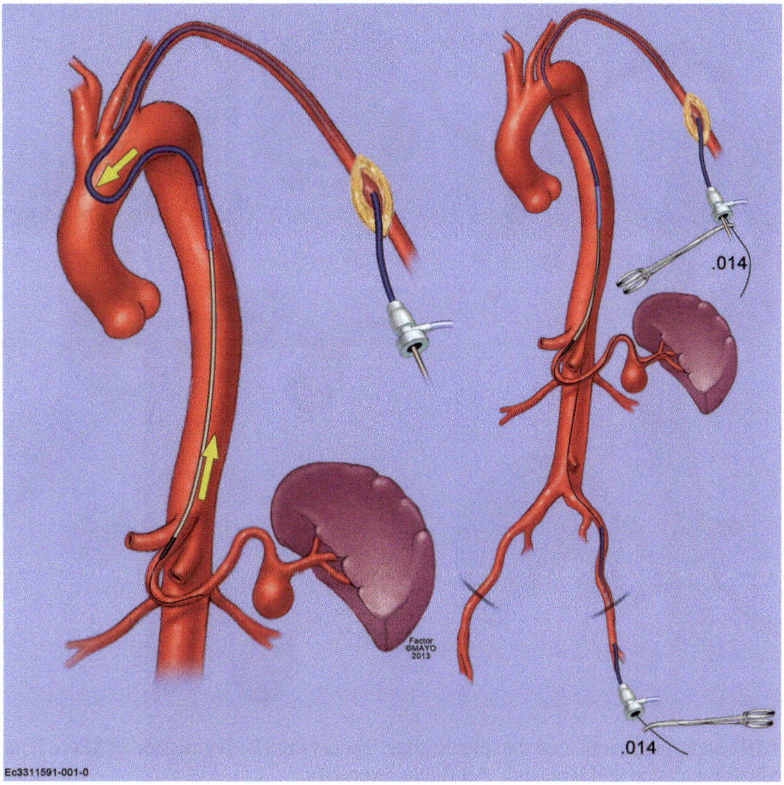

Fig. 34.9 Coaxial system for difficult cases from brachial approach (By permission of Mayo Foundation for Medical Education and Research. All rights reserved)

splenopancreatectomy is usually performed with ligation of the splenic artery through caesarian section laparotomy [21]. To visualize the splenic artery, dissection proceeds with mobilization of the splenocolic ligament. The splenic flexure is then mobilized away from the retroperitoneum and abdominal wall. The aneurysm sac can be identified with palpation or intraoperative ultrasound. Currently, these procedures can be performed with open or laparoscopic intervention, as well as robotic surgical repair [6].

Endovascular therapy has emerged as an effective option in the management of SAAs. Treatment usually includes coil embolization, a combination with other techniques. For SAA arising from the splenomesenteric trunk, the feared complication is dislodgment or misplacement of coils into the SMA with consequent bowel ischemia. In addition, the rapid flow of blood in the SMA (500–600 mL/min) may prevent thrombosis of the aneurysms if coil embolization alone is attempted. A suitable neck allows for direct embolization of the aneurysm and reduces the risk of distal migration [33].

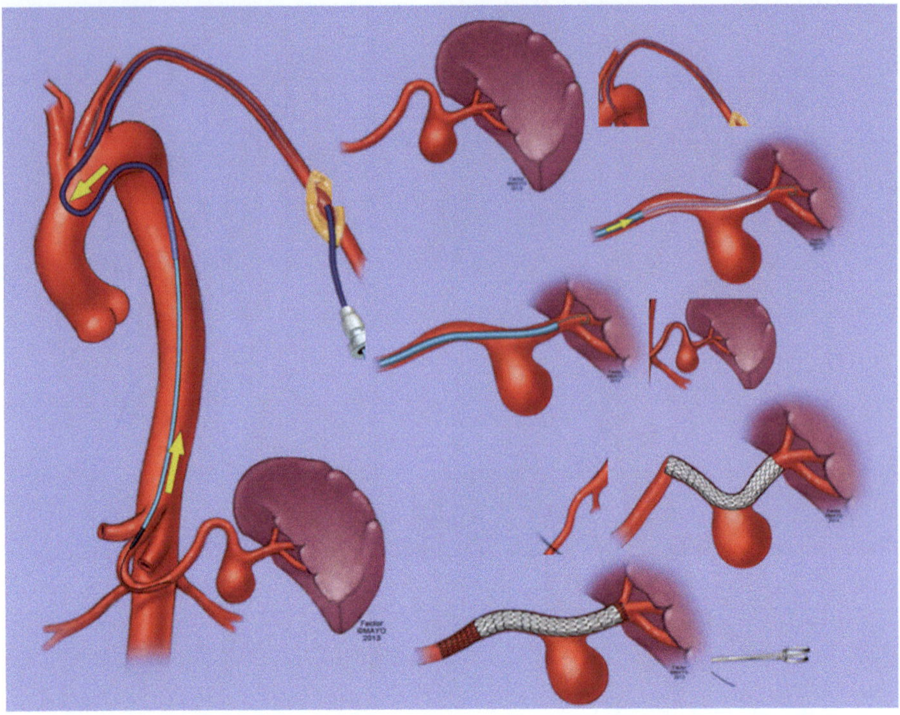

Fig. 34.10 Stent-graft technique for splenic artery aneurysms (By permission of Mayo Foundation for Medical Education and Research. All rights reserved)

Hepatic Artery Aneurysms

Open surgical repair of HAAs depends largely on the anatomic location of the lesion, adequate collateral flow, condition of the liver, and overall medical status of the patient. HAAs are accessible through a right subcostal incision. Techniques include excision, ligation with or without bypass using autologous vein or graft, and, if needed, hepatic resection. Common HAAs can generally be treated with simple ligation or endovascular ablation because the gastroduodenal artery (GDA) provides sufficient collateral flow in most patients. HAAs distal to the GDA can be treated by arterial reconstruction or other methods to restore blood flow to the end organ if the revascularization is straightforward. Aneurysms located within the parenchyma may be treated with resection, ligation, or embolization. If the hepatic artery is ligated, an increase in oxygen content of the portal vein blood through splanchnic arteriovenous shunting occurs. Therefore, hepatic artery ligation should never be performed in the presence of cirrhosis or any other condition where the liver function is compromised. If the proper or right hepatic artery is ligated, the gall bladder is at risk for necrosis, and cholecystectomy should be performed simultaneously [6].

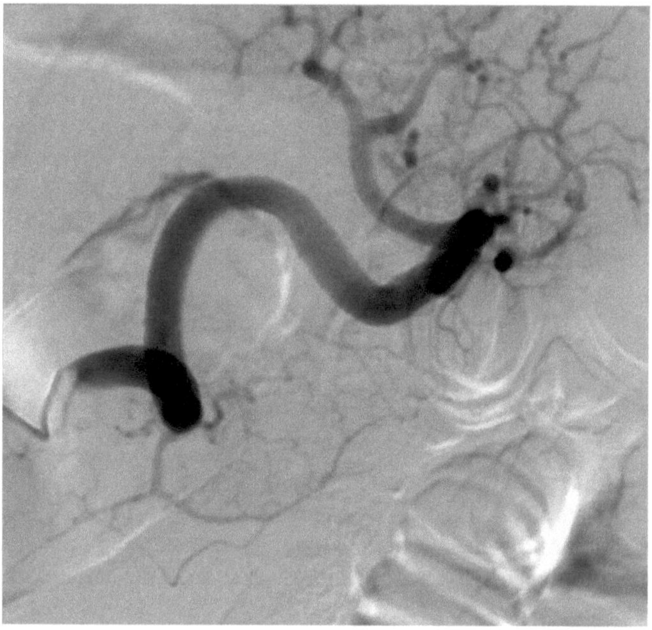

Fig. 34.11 Completion angiography of splenic artery stent graft

Embolization is suitable for lesions located within the hepatic parenchyma. However, patients undergoing embolization should be watched carefully for hepatic parenchymal necrosis, which may require operative intervention or drainage. Custom-made aortic endograft with a single fenestration for the hepatic artery, together with a visceral covered stent, was reported to treat a patient with hepatic artery pseudoaneurysm after liver transplantation [34].

Superior Mesenteric Artery Aneurysms

SMAAs can be treated surgically with aneurysmectomy, arterial reconstruction, and, rarely, simple ligation. It is important to take into account that SMAAs have a predilection for mycotic or inflammatory etiology, in such cases, polytetrafluoroethylene (PTFE) or Dacron grafts should not be used. Ligation of SMA proximal and distal to the aneurysm with reliance on collateral flow through the celiac trunk and inferior mesenteric artery (IMA) is feasible; however, careful intraoperative assessment of intestinal viability is mandatory and may be accomplished by clinical evaluation, fluorescein dye, or Doppler flow study. Open exposure of SMA and surrounding tissue or organ has been described in Chapters 11 and 32. Coil embolization and stent graft placement have been reported in the treatment of SMAA.

Celiac Artery Aneurysms

Open surgery with simple ligation of the celiac trunk, aneurysmectomy, aneurysmorrhaphy, reimplantation of the celiac trunk, and autogenous or prosthetic bypass grafting represents a valid treatment option, especially in elective cases. The need for arterial reconstruction depends largely on aneurysm location and the adequacy of collaterals. In the emergency setting of rupture, simple ligation with postprocedural observation for ischemia can be also applied. Endovascular surgery includes embolization of the celiac trunk or stent grafting.

Pancreaticoduodenal and Gastroduodenal Artery Aneurysms

Suggestions for the management of both aneurysms include surgical ligation, endovascular embolization, and stent graft placement. With respect to open surgery, in addition to ligation of the aneurysm, a partial pancreatectomy or pancreaticoduodenectomy may need to be performed. Revascularization of the celiac axis is indicated in these cases to correct the underlying etiology. Vascular reconstruction is not essential after resection of a GDAA unless there is celiac artery occlusion, as ligation of the GDA may cause gangrene of the gallbladder and stomach, splenic necrosis, or other disastrous consequences. In cases with celiac compression by an MAL, some authors have suggested a resection of the ligament after definitive aneurysm treatment; however, the necessity of surgical decompression of the celiac axis in such patients is controversial [6, 17, 18].

Coil embolization techniques are generally preferred for these aneurysms, and limited case reports have reported promising success rates [6]. Because these aneurysms are often associated with celiac axis occlusion, it is important to determine presence of adequate collaterals prior to embolization. Ruptured aneurysms can be effectively treated by immediate embolization, which has a lower mortality rate than surgical treatment [8].

Gastric and Gastroepiploic Artery Aneurysms

Open surgical repair includes aneurysmectomy and exclusion with or without arterial revascularization. For nonemergent aneurysms, using a laparoscopic approach has also been reported with success. Emergent or ruptured cases are usually managed with open laparotomy; however, with the advent of endovascular techniques, it becomes the first treatment of choice if vessel anatomy allows. Coil embolization is an accepted form of treatment of these aneurysms. When performing embolization in saccular aneurysms of the GDAs, isolation of the aneurysm neck may be sufficient, but if the aneurysm has a short neck, both proximal and distal embolization should be performed. [6]

Inferior Mesenteric, Jejunal, Ileal, and Colic Artery Aneurysms

Open surgical treatment includes ligation of the aneurysm, with arterial reconstruction to maintain blood flow on the basis of the status of the intestinal circulation. Naito et al. [35] first reported a successful endovascular treatment for middle colic artery aneurysm, and there have been some reports of successful endovascular treatment [36].

Results

Open Surgical Treatment

According to literature, open surgical repair of VAAs provides good early results with early mortality < 2.0 % [37–39] and durable late outcomes. Pulli et al. [37] reported 59 VAA repairs in 55 patients, which included 30 SAA repairs. Approximately 70 % of VAAs were repaired with open revascularization. Early mortality was 1.8 %, one early death occurred due to acute pancreatitis; early major complication rate was 3.6 %, one retroperitoneal hematoma and one acute pancreatitis developed after operation; all three events occurred in patients with SAA, resulting in an early mortality of 3.3 % and early morbidity of 6.6 % with SAA repair. Mean follow-up was 82 months, 10-year survival rate was 80 %, and aneurysm-related, complication-free survival rate was 75 %. Of 74 patients who underwent open repair, Marone et al. [38] reported an early mortality of 1.3 %; the only one death was due to acute mesenteric ischemia secondary to acute thrombosis of a 6 mm ePTFE graft for an SMAA repair. Early morbidity was 9.4 % (7/74). At a mean follow-up of 42 months, survival rates were 100 % at 1 year and 85 % at 5 years. To be noticed, both studies included RAAs.

Ghariani and colleagues [39] reported 60 patients who underwent open surgical repair for 78 VAAs; 30 were treated without arterial revascularization (CAA, 3; HAA, 2; SAA, 19; SMAA, 1; GDAA, 3; PDAA, 2), 48 required revascularization (CAA, 20; HAA, 18; SMAA, 10). Of 45 bypass grafts, 30 (67 %) were prosthetic grafts, 9 (20 %) were autologous venous grafts, and 6 (13 %) were arterial grafts. In-hospital mortality was 1.7 %, the only one death occurred after gastrointestinal bleeding from gastric metastases of a kidney cancer. Pulmonary and gastrointestinal complications were the two most common postoperative complications, accounting for 18 % ($n = 11$). Among the gastrointestinal complications, acute pancreatitis ($n = 4$) and colonic ischemia ($n = 3$) were the most frequent. At a mean follow-up of 42 months, survival rates were 98 % at 1 year and 97 % at 5 years, and thereafter primary patency rates at the same time points were 98 and 95 %, respectively.

In a randomized controlled trial, 14 open SAA repairs were compared with 15 laparoscopic repairs; direct anastomosis was performed on 3 patients in each group. Open surgical conversion occurred in 13 % of laparoscopic patients. Laparoscopic repair

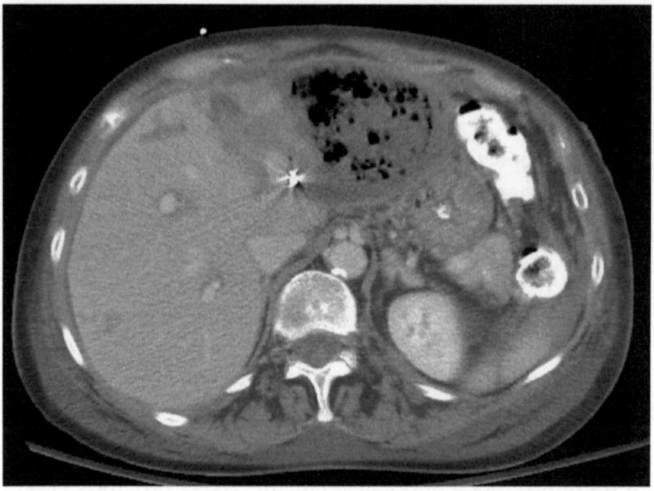

Fig. 34.12 Liver abscess after coil embolization for ruptured intrahepatic aneurysm

was associated with shorter procedures, lower morbidity, quicker resumption of oral diet, earlier drain removal, and shorter hospital stay. During a mean follow-up of 50 months, two of the three patients underwent laparoscopic anastomosis developed late thromboses. The study confirmed the clinical benefits of ablative procedures under laparoscopy, but long-term patency for laparoscopic anastomoses was poor [40].

Endovascular Therapy

Complications following endovascular therapy include distal thromboembolic event, nontarget vessel embolization, coil migration, end-organ infarction, neck recanalization, [41] and stent thrombosis. Splenic atrophy or infarct has been reported in 20–40 % of cases following endovascular treatment of distal or hilar splenic artery aneurysms. [5] Long-term outcomes after endovascular treatment are not well defined. Liver infarct with abscess formation can also occur with embolization (Fig. 34.12).

Tulsyan et al. [42] reviewed endovascular treatment of 20 VAAs and 28 visceral artery pseudoaneurysms. Coil embolization was used in 96 % of patients; N-butyl-2-cyanoacrylate was used in 19 %. Technical success was 98 %. Thirty-day mortality was 8.3 %, all four deaths occurred after urgent or emergent treatment, and causes of death were unrelated to aneurysm except one patient died from recurrent gastrointestinal bleeding after embolization of a GDAA. Postembolization syndrome developed in three patients (6 %) after splenic artery embolization. Among 77 % of patients with follow-up CT imaging at a mean of 16 months, 97 % achieved complete exclusion of the aneurysm.

In a large retrospective case series from the Mayo Clinic, Fankhauser and colleagues [43] reported 185 visceral aneurysms (true aneurysm, 36 %; pseudoaneurysm, 64 %) treated by endovascular therapy. Coil embolization alone was used alone in 75 % of patients and in combination with other techniques in 11 %. Technical success was 98 %. Thirty-day mortality was 6.2 % and aneurysm-related mortality was 3.4 %; 30-day reintervention rate was 3 %. During follow-up of 1.4 years, two patients (1.1 %) reported aneurysm-related complications, including one bile duct ischemia related to GDAA coiling that required hepaticojejunostomy, and another sepsis following splenic infarction managed by emergent splenectomy [43].

Yasumoto et al. followed 46 VAAs treated with coil packing, mean follow-up was 37 months, and compaction and recanalization occurred in two (4 %) and 12 aneurysms (26 %), respectively. The authors suggested that insufficient embolization with low packing density and large aneurysms might contribute to coil compaction and recanalization [44]. Koganemaru et al. studied 23 patients with VAAs (SAA, 15; HAA, 2; GDAA, 2; CAA, 2; PDAA, 1; GEAA, 1) who underwent coil embolization at a mean follow-up of 18 months. MRA demonstrated complete aneurysmal occlusion in 22 patients (96 %); neck recanalization was found in one of the eight patients (13 %) using a neck preservation technique, at 9 and 20 months after embolization; complete hemodynamic status after embolization was determined in 21 patients (91 %); asymptomatic localized splenic infarction was confirmed in one patient (4 %) [41].

With respect to covered stent in the treatment of VAAs, Künzle et al. [45] reported 13 cases with CTA follow-up at a mean of 28 months. Jo-Graft and Graftmaster (Abbott, Rangendingen, Germany), Viabahn (W. L. Gore and Associates, Flagstaff, Arizona), and Fluency (Bard, Tempe, Arizona) covered stents were used. Noticeably, eight pseudoaneurysms and four RAAs were included in this study. Early mortality was 11 %; there was one VAA-related death from hemorrhagic shock and sepsis after successful endovascular repair of HAA. The two late stent thromboses occurred in one patient with SAA and another with RAA.

Balderi et al. reported five VAAs treated using Cardiatis multilayer stent; stent occlusion was observed in one patient with HAA at 6 months and another with SAA at 24 months [31]. However, no major consequences developed because of the developed collaterals.

Open vs Endovascular therapy

A retrospective single institution study over nearly 15 years, between 1991 and 2005, was performed at Mount Sinai in New York. Fifty-nine patients with 61 aneurysms involving branches of the superior mesenteric and celiac arteries were identified of which 24 underwent the traditional open treatment and 35 had an endovascular approach. The authors reported an 89 % success rate with the endovascular technique with the use of coil embolization or covered stent. [46] A group from Milan,

Italy, treated 94 patients with VAA/VAPA between 1988 and 2010, 74 with open surgery and the remaining 20 with endovascular technique. Early mortality was 1.3 % after open surgery and 0 % after endovascular intervention; early morbidities were similar, around 10 % for both groups [38]. In two European centers (France, UK), 32 patients were treated between 1995 and 2010, 17 VAAs in 16 patients with open repair, 15 VAAs in 15 patients with endovascular repair. There was no significant difference between open repair and endovascular patients in terms of 30-day mortality (6.3 % vs 0 %) and complication rate (25 % vs 6.7 %). The only one death occurred after emergent endovascular repair of a ruptured infected SAA. The mean length of stay was significantly higher after open repair (17 vs 4 days, $P<.001$). During more than 1 year follow-up, there is no late aneurysm-related death. Not including the seven RAAs in this study, two patients with open repair had reintervention due to lengthy graft or anastomosis stenosis; one SAA patient with endovascular treatment underwent reintervention at 2 years because of a reperfusion of the aneurysmal sac [47].

Conclusions

VAAs are a rare entity; however, aneurysm rupture, which is the catastrophic complication, may lead to a mortality rate up to 90 % according to the location of the aneurysm. Timely diagnosis of VAA is the most important, and individualized treatment is tailored based on the symptoms and signs, size, location, anatomy, and etiology of the aneurysm, as well as patient's surgical risk. Currently, there is no consensus regarding treatment guidelines. Asymptomatic patients with VAA < 2.0 cm in diameter can be observed with close imaging follow-up which includes DUS, CTA, or MRA. In general, interventions are indicated in symptomatic or ruptured VAAs, pseudoaneurysms, asymptomatic patients with aneurysm > 2.0 cm, and aneurysm with rapid increase in size ≥ 0.5 cm/year. Besides, due to the high risk of rupture, regardless of size or symptom, interventions are also recommended in female patient of childbearing age or pregnant and orthotopic liver transplant recipient who harbors an SAA, and patient with visceral branch aneurysms. Surgical repair includes excision of the VAA with or without revascularization or organ resection; endovascular therapy includes embolization and placement of covered stents. Regardless of the procedure performed, revascularization must be considered when there is inadequate or no collateral flow to maintain end-organ perfusion. Long-term results of open repair of VAAs are durable; endovascular treatment, as a promising alternative to open surgery especially in anatomically suitable and high risk patients, provides good short-term results; however, its long-term results are not yet well known. Follow-up data from randomized controlled trials and prospective studies are required to justify the treatment strategy for VAAs.

References

1. Stanley JC, Wakefield TW, Graham LM, Whitehouse Jr WM, Zelenock GB, Lindenauer SM. Clinical importance and management of splanchnic artery aneurysms. J Vasc Surg. 1986;3(5):836–40.
2. Carr SC, Pearce WH, Vogelzang RL, McCarthy WJ, Nemcek Jr AA, Yao JS. Current management of visceral artery aneurysms. Surgery. 1996;120(4):627–33; discussion 33–4.
3. Shanley CJ, Shah NL, Messina LM. Common splanchnic artery aneurysms: splenic, hepatic, and celiac. Ann Vasc Surg. 1996;10(3):315–22.
4. Messina LM, Shanley CJ. Visceral artery aneurysms. Surg Clin North Am. 1997;77(2): 425–42.
5. Cordova AC, Sumpio BE. Visceral artery aneurysms and pseudoaneurysms – should they all be managed by endovascular techniques? Ann Vasc Dis. 2013;6(4):687–93.
6. Lakin RO, Kashyap VS. Splanchnic Artery Aneurysms. In: Cronenwett JL, Johnston KW, editors. Rutherford's vascular surgery. 8th ed. Philadelphia: Saunders; 2014. p. 2220–35.
7. Barbaros U, Ozemir IA, Aksakal N, Tukenmez M, Kilic B, Agcaoglu O, et al. Laparoscopic surgery of the splenic artery and vein aneurysm with spontaneous arteriovenous fistula. Surg Laparosc Endosc Percutan Tech. 2013;23(3):e127–30.
8. Takase A, Akuzawa N, Hatori T, Imai K, Kitahara Y, Aoki J, et al. Two patients with ruptured posterior inferior pancreaticoduodenal artery aneurysms associated with compression of the celiac axis by the median arcuate ligament. Ann Vasc Dis. 2014;7(1):87–92.
9. Sarcina A, Bellosta R, Magnaldi S, Luzzani L. Aneurysm of the middle colic artery–case report and literature review. Eur J Vasc Endovasc Surg. 2000;20(2):198–200.
10. Edogawa S, Shibuya T, Kurose K, Sasaki K, Tomita H. Inferior mesenteric artery aneurysm: case report and literature review. Ann Vasc Dis. 2013;6(1):98–101.
11. Moskowitz R, Rundback J. Middle colic artery branch aneurysm presenting as spontaneous hemoperitoneum. Ann Vasc Surg. 2014;28(7):1797.e15-7. doi:10.1016/j.avsg.2014.05.001.
12. Cron DC, Coleman DM, Sheetz KH, Englesbe MJ, Waits SA. Aneurysms in abdominal organ transplant recipients. J Vasc Surg. 2014;59(3):594–8.
13. Lagana D, Carrafiello G, Mangini M, Dionigi G, Caronno R, Castelli P, et al. Multimodal approach to endovascular treatment of visceral artery aneurysms and pseudoaneurysms. Eur J Radiol. 2006;59(1):104–11.
14. Wiegering A, Ritter CO, Allolio B, Buck AK, Germer CT, Lorenz U. Early development of a celiac trunk aneurysm during anti-vascular endothelial growth factor receptor therapy. Surgery. 2014;155(4):729–30.
15. Abbas MA, Fowl RJ, Stone WM, Panneton JM, Oldenburg WA, Bower TC, et al. Hepatic artery aneurysm: factors that predict complications. J Vasc Surg. 2003;38(1):41–5.
16. Sgroi MD, Kabutey NK, Krishnam M, Fujitani RM. Pancreaticoduodenal artery aneurysms secondary to median arcuate ligament syndrome may not need celiac artery revascularization or ligament release. Ann Vasc Surg. 2014. doi:10.1016/j.avsg.2014.05.020. [Ahead of print]
17. Armstrong MB, Stadtlander KS, Grove MK. Pancreaticoduodenal artery aneurysm associated with median arcuate ligament syndrome. Ann Vasc Surg. 2014;28(3):741 e1–5 e1.
18. Habib N, Hassan S, Abdou R, Torbey E, Alkaied H, Maniatis T, et al. Gastroduodenal artery aneurysm, diagnosis, clinical presentation and management: a concise review. Ann Surg Innov Res. 2013;7(1):4.
19. Bergert H, Hinterseher I, Kersting S, Leonhardt J, Bloomenthal A, Saeger HD. Management and outcome of hemorrhage due to arterial pseudoaneurysms in pancreatitis. Surgery. 2005;137(3):323–8.
20. Tessier DJ, Abbas MA, Fowl RJ, Stone WM, Bower TC, McKusick MA, et al. Management of rare mesenteric arterial branch aneurysms. Ann Vasc Surg. 2002;16(5):586–90.
21. Sadat U, Dar O, Walsh S, Varty K. Splenic artery aneurysms in pregnancy – a systematic review. Int J Surg. 2008;6(3):261–5.

22. Lee PC, Rhee RY, Gordon RY, Fung JJ, Webster MW. Management of splenic artery aneurysms: the significance of portal and essential hypertension. J Am Coll Surg. 1999;189(5): 483–90.
23. Jackson HT, Diaconu SC, Maluso PJ, Abell B, Lee J. Ruptured splenic artery aneurysms and the use of an adapted fast protocol in reproductive age women with hemodynamic collapse: case series. Case Rep Emerg Med. 2014;2014:454923.
24. Abbas MA, Stone WM, Fowl RJ, Gloviczki P, Oldenburg WA, Pairolero PC, et al. Splenic artery aneurysms: two decades experience at Mayo clinic. Ann Vasc Surg. 2002;16(4):442–9.
25. Lakin RO, Bena JF, Sarac TP, Shah S, Krajewski LP, Srivastava SD, et al. The contemporary management of splenic artery aneurysms. J Vasc Surg. 2011;53(4):958–64; discussion 65.
26. Ruddy JM, Dodson TF, Duwayri Y. Open repair of superior mesenteric artery mycotic aneurysm in an adolescent girl. Ann Vasc Surg. 2014;28(4):1032 e21–4 e21.
27. Oderich GS, Panneton JM, Macedo TA, Noel AA, Bower TC, Lee RA, et al. Intraoperative duplex ultrasound of visceral revascularizations: optimizing technical success and outcome. J Vasc Surg. 2003;38(4):684–91.
28. Stella N, Palombo G, Taddeo C, Rizzo L, Taurino M. Stent-assisted coil embolization of a complex wide-neck splenic artery aneurysm. Ann Vasc Surg. 2013;27(8):1187 e5–8 e5.
29. Plaza-Martinez A, Genoves-Gasco B, Cester-Ves D, Gomez-Palones FJ. Endograft-assisted coil embolization of a celiac trunk aneurysm. Ann Vasc Surg. 2014;28(1):263 e1–5 e1.
30. Sfyroeras GS, Dalainas I, Giannakopoulos TG, Antonopoulos K, Kakisis JD, Liapis CD. Flow-diverting stents for the treatment of arterial aneurysms. J Vasc Surg. 2012;56(3):839–46.
31. Balderi A, Antonietti A, Pedrazzini F, Sortino D, Vinay C, Grosso M. Treatment of visceral aneurysm using multilayer stent: two-year follow-up results in five consecutive patients. Cardiovasc Intervent Radiol. 2013;36(5):1256–61.
32. Sfyroeras GS, Liapis CD. Endovascular management of visceral artery aneurysms with flow-diverting stents. Ann Vasc Surg. 2014;28(4):1080.
33. Wong SS, Lindsay TF, Roche-Nagle G. Anomalous splenic artery aneurysm. Vascular. 2013; 21(2):105–8.
34. Verzini F, Biello A, Marucchini A, Parente B, Parlani G, Cao P. Total endovascular solution for complex visceral aneurysms. J Vasc Surg. 2013;58(5):1412–6.
35. Naito A, Toyota N, Ito K. Embolization of a ruptured middle colic artery aneurysm. Cardiovasc Intervent Radiol. 1995;18(1):56–8.
36. Ham EM, Cho BS, Ye JB, Mun YS, Choi YJ, Kwon OS. The endovascular treatment of a ruptured aneurysm of the middle colic artery combined with an isolated dissection of superior mesenteric artery: report of a case. Vasc Endovascular Surg. 2014;48(4):352–5.
37. Pulli R, Dorigo W, Troisi N, Pratesi G, Innocenti AA, Pratesi C. Surgical treatment of visceral artery aneurysms: A 25-year experience. J Vasc Surg. 2008;48(2):334–42.
38. Marone EM, Mascia D, Kahlberg A, Brioschi C, Tshomba Y, Chiesa R. Is open repair still the gold standard in visceral artery aneurysm management? Ann Vasc Surg. 2011;25(7):936–46.
39. Ghariani MZ, Georg Y, Ramirez C, Lebied E, Gaudric J, Chiche L, et al. Long-term results of surgical treatment of aneurysms of digestive arteries. Ann Vasc Surg. 2013;27(7):954–8.
40. Tiberio GA, Bonardelli S, Gheza F, Arru L, Cervi E, Giulini SM. Prospective randomized comparison of open versus laparoscopic management of splenic artery aneurysms: a 10-year study. Surg Endosc. 2012 Jun 30. [Ahead of print].
41. Koganemaru M, Abe T, Nonoshita M, Iwamoto R, Kusumoto M, Kuhara A, et al. Follow-up of true visceral artery aneurysm after coil embolization by three-dimensional contrast-enhanced MR angiography. Diagn Interv Radiol. 2014;20(2):129–35.
42. Tulsyan N, Kashyap VS, Greenberg RK, Sarac TP, Clair DG, Pierce G, et al. The endovascular management of visceral artery aneurysms and pseudoaneurysms. J Vasc Surg. 2007;45(2): 276–83; discussion 83.
43. Fankhauser GT, Stone WM, Naidu SG, Oderich GS, Ricotta JJ, Bjarnason H, et al. The minimally invasive management of visceral artery aneurysms and pseudoaneurysms. J Vasc Surg. 2011;53(4):966–70.

44. Yasumoto T, Osuga K, Yamamoto H, Ono Y, Masada M, Mikami K, et al. Long-term outcomes of coil packing for visceral aneurysms: correlation between packing density and incidence of coil compaction or recanalization. J Vasc Interv Radiol. 2013;24(12):1798–807.
45. Kunzle S, Glenck M, Puippe G, Schadde E, Mayer D, Pfammatter T. Stent-graft repairs of visceral and renal artery aneurysms are effective and result in long-term patency. J Vasc Interv Radiol. 2013;24(7):989–96.
46. Sachdev U, Baril DT, Ellozy SH, Lookstein RA, Silverberg D, Jacobs TS, et al. Management of aneurysms involving branches of the celiac and superior mesenteric arteries: a comparison of surgical and endovascular therapy. J Vasc Surg. 2006;44(4):718–24.
47. Cochennec F, Riga CV, Allaire E, Cheshire NJ, Hamady M, Jenkins MP, et al. Contemporary management of splanchnic and renal artery aneurysms: results of endovascular compared with open surgery from two European vascular centers. Eur J Vasc Endovasc Surg. 2011;42(3):340–6.

Index

G.S. Oderich (ed.), *Mesenteric Vascular Disease*,
DOI 10.1007/978-1-4939-1847-8

N

T

U

V

MIX
Papier aus verantwortungsvollen Quellen
Paper from responsible sources
FSC® C105338

If you have any concerns about our products,
you can contact us on
ProductSafety@springernature.com

In case Publisher is established outside the EU,
the EU authorized representative is:
Springer Nature Customer Service Center GmbH
Europaplatz 3, 69115 Heidelberg, Germany

Printed by Libri Plureos GmbH
in Hamburg, Germany